Radiation Oncology: Research and Practice

Radiation Oncology: Research and Practice

Edited by Andra Quinn

hayle
medical

New York

Hayle Medical,
750 Third Avenue, 9th Floor,
New York, NY 10017, USA

Visit us on the World Wide Web at:
www.haylemedical.com

ISBN: 978-1-63241-700-8

Cataloging-in-Publication Data

Radiation oncology : research and practice / edited by Andra Quinn.
    p. cm.
Includes bibliographical references and index.
ISBN 978-1-63241-700-8
1. Cancer--Radiotherapy. 2. Cancer--Treatment. 3. Tumors--Radiotherapy.
4. Radiation--Methods. 5. Oncology. I. Quinn, Andra.
RC271.R3 R33 2019
615.842--dc23

Table of Contents

Preface

Radiation therapy or radiotherapy is a cancer therapy using ionizing radiation that is aimed at killing or controlling malignant cells of a tumor. It may be curative if the cancer is localized to one part of the body. It can also be used as a part of adjuvant therapy in order to prevent tumor recurrences after surgery, along with other systemic therapies such as chemotherapy, hormone therapy and immunotherapy. Ionizing radiation acts against the cancer by damaging the DNA of cancerous tissue therefore resulting in cellular death. The primary types of radiation therapy are external beam radiation therapy, intraoperative radiotherapy, brachytherapy, contact X-ray brachytherapy, etc. Radiotherapy may be used as a palliative treatment or as a therapeutic treatment. The topics covered in this extensive book deal with the core aspects of radiation oncology. From theories to research to practical applications, case studies related to all contemporary topics of relevance to this field have been included in this book. Scientists and students actively engaged in radiation oncology will find this book full of crucial and unexplored concepts.

This book is a comprehensive compilation of works of different researchers from varied parts of the world. It includes valuable experiences of the researchers with the sole objective of providing the readers (learners) with a proper knowledge of the concerned field. This book will be beneficial in evoking inspiration and enhancing the knowledge of the interested readers.

In the end, I would like to extend my heartiest thanks to the authors who worked with great determination on their chapters. I also appreciate the publisher's support in the course of the book. I would also like to deeply acknowledge my family who stood by me as a source of inspiration during the project.

Editor

Light and shadows of a new technique: is photon total-skin irradiation using helical IMRT feasible, less complex and as toxic as the electrons one?

Michela Buglione[1*] ⓘ, Luigi Spiazzi[2], Mauro Urpis[1], Liliana Baushi[1], Rossella Avitabile[2], Nadia Pasinetti[1], Paolo Borghetti[1], Luca Triggiani[1], Sara Pedretti[1], Federica Saiani[2], Alfredo Fiume[2], Diana Greco[1], Stefano Ciccarelli[1], Alessia Polonini[2], Renzo Moretti[2] and Stefano Maria Magrini[1]

Abstract

Background: Radiotherapy is one of the standard treatments for cutaneous lymphoma and Total Skin Electrons Beam Irradiation (TSEBI) is generally used to treat diffuse cutaneous lymphoma and some cases of localized disease. Helical IMRT (HI) allows to treat complex target with optimal dose distribution and organ at risk sparing, so helical tomotherapy has been proposed as alternative technique to TSEBI but only one preliminary report has been published.

Methods: Three patients treated (from May 2013 to December 2014) with Helical IMRT, with a total dose between 24 and 30 Gy, were retrospectively evaluated. Data about dosimetric features, response and acute toxicity were registered and analyzed.

Planned target coverage was compared with daily in vivo measures and dose calculation based on volumetric images used for set up evaluation as well.

Results: The patients had a mean measured surface fraction dose ranging from 1.54 Gy up to 2.0 Gy. A planned target dose ranging from 85 to 120% of prescription doses was obtained. All doses to *Organs At Risk* were within the required constraints. Particular attention was posed on "whole bone marrow" planned V_{10Gy}, V_{12Gy} and V_{20Gy} values, ranging respectively between 23 and 43%, 20.1 and 38% and 9.8 and 24%. A comparison with the *theoretical* homologous values obtained with TSEBI has shown much lower values with TSEBI.

Even if treatment was given in sequence to the skin of the upper and lower hemi-body, all the patients had anaemia, requiring blood transfusions, leukopenia and thrombocytopenia.

Conclusion: Based on our limited results TSEBI should still be considered the standard method to treat total skin because of its pattern of acute and late toxicities and the dose distribution. In this particular case the better target coverage obtained with HI can be paid in terms of worse toxicity. Helical IMRT can instead be considered optimal in treating large, convex, cutaneous areas where it is difficult to use multiple electrons fields in relation with the clinical results and the limited and reversible toxicities.

Keywords: Total skin irradiation, Total skin electrons beam irradiation - TSEBI, Photons, Radiotherapy, Bone marrow, Primary cutaneous lymphoma (PCL), Toxicity

* Correspondence: michela.buglione@unibs.it
[1]Radiation Oncology Department, University and Spedali Civili Hospital – Brescia, P.le Spedali Civili 1 –, 25123 Brescia, Italy
Full list of author information is available at the end of the article

Background

Primary cutaneous lymphomas (PCL) are a group of heterogeneous diseases with a typical skin involvement and generally without systemic signs or symptoms, besides that the final stages of Mycosis Fungoides (MF) and Sèzary Syndrome (SS). MF/SS can be classified, according to TNMB classification, into four clinical stages depending on extension of skin involvement (in percentage of body surface), lymph node metastases, visceral involvement or presence of Sèzary cells in blood [1]. Age, type and disease extension, visceral metastases, increased LDH at diagnosis are recognized as prognostic factors [1–3].

Radiotherapy (RT) for PCL has been used in different clinical settings. In patients with solitary nodules of MF, or localized skin B/T disease, RT is the treatment of choice. The treatment of advanced-stage MF-SS is more complex and the final objective is to maintain clinical remission or stabilization of disease, improving quality of life.

Many studies report the efficacy of RT in patients featuring a set of localized lesions (up to three or four lesions covering less than 5% of the body). Routinely, these lesions are treated with a 6–9 MeV single direct electron beam, using a bolus to increase the dose to the cutaneous surface up to 95%. The standard prescribed dose varies from 30.6–36.0 Gy at 1.8–2.0 Gy per fraction. Recurrence rate is about 30% while 92% of patients obtain complete response [4–7].

Low dose large electron fields to treat the entire skin (Total Skin Electron Beam Irradiation, TSEBI) are used for advanced MF allowing a generalized and superficial treatment. [8, 9]. With the already known different standard techniques [10–13], however, it is extremely difficult to obtain a uniform dose distribution, considering the irregular shape of the human body surface [14].

Modern RT techniques have a goal not only to improve cancer cure rate, but also to reduce the treatment related adverse effects. Modern RT techniques have a proven capability to create highly conformal dose distributions, allowing the physicians to escalate the dose within the target volume and to spare adjacent organs at risk (OAR). The clinical use of Tomotherapy® induced radiation oncologists to use this technique to treat cutaneous circumferential localized lesions [15] and to think to use it to perform total skin irradiation. A preliminary report about the use of HI for total skin photon beam cutaneous irradiation has been already published [16]. We report a retrospective analysis on clinical/dosimetric data of three patients with diffuse cutaneous lymphoma treated with HI.

Methods

From May 2013 to December 2014 three patients were treated with total skin photon radiotherapy. The first (#1) had MF (stage IVA1; T4N0M0); the second (#2) had diffuse cutaneous and systemic localizations of cutaneous T cell lymphoma; the third (#3) had a diagnosis of Granulomatous MF (stage II) (Table 1). After receiving adequate information about the technique and the possible acute and late effect of the treatment, all the patients accepted it and signed the informed consent.

Immobilization and target definition

To obtain the better immobilization of the patient and treatment reproducibility, also in prevision of IGRT evaluations, set-up was obtained using vacuum-lock system and 5 points head & neck and abdominal thermoplastic masks. Gross tumor volume (GTV) included regions with evident disease (plaques). The *CTV-skin* included

Table 1 Patient's features, RT prescriptions and response

	Patient #1 (female)	Patient #2 (male)	Patient #3 (male)
Diagnosis	MF (stage IVA1; T4N0M0) with erythrodermic disease,	Diffuse cutaneous and systemic localizations of cutaneous T cell lymphoma,	Granulomatous MF (stage II) slack skin
Previous treatments	Chemotherapy and UVB-PUVA, but never treated with radiotherapy	Different types of cutaneous therapies (PUVA), chemotherapy and localized RT, and finally proposed for palliative total-skin irradiation	Previously untreated
Prescribed dose (Median target dose)	27.0Gy/1.8Gy/fr (upper body) 26.0Gy/2.0Gy/fr (lower body) (22.05Gy/1.47Gy/fr Gy for the scalp and eyelids) 23 days split in between the two	28.8Gy/1.8Gy/fr (upper body) 28.8Gy/1.8Gy/fr (lower body) 15 days split in between the two	30.4 Gy/1.9 Gy/fr (upper body) 30.0 Gy/2 Gy/fr (lower body) 8 days split in between the two
Compensative electrons boost on "under-dosed" regions	One field electron boost (upper back) after the end of the photon treatment.	4 electron field boosts (right arm, left arm, inguinal, right foot dorsum). During the split between the first and the second part of the photon treatment	9 electron field boosts (right and left forearm, right and left arm, right back, left back, internal right thigh). During the split between the first and the second part of the photon treatment
Response to RT and duration	Short complete remission (6 months)	Short complete remission (6 months)	Complete remission (4 years)

the entire body surface with a thickness of 5 mm. GTV plus 5 mm was included in CTV. PTV was defined as CTV plus 5 mm geometrical external margin and 7 mm internal margin. (Fig. 1). PTV was divided in PTV_eval (the intersection of PTV and the patient body contour) and OPTV, (PTV portion outside body contour).

Optic nerves, lens, eyes, lacrimal glands, cochlea, mandibles, parotids, thyroid, great vessels and heart, lungs, humeral heads, femoral heads, liver, stomach, intestinal cavity, spleen, kidneys, bladder, breast, rectum and uterus (for #1), testicles, penis and corpora cavernosa (for #2 and #3) were defined as OAR. Bone marrow was defined as the tissue within cortical bone of sternum, ribs, cranial, pelvic and long bones [17, 18].

The defined IGRT protocol included two daily MVCT, one at the beginning and one at the end of the volume in order to better evaluate the patient's set-up along the all volume [25]. The median differences between the two MVCT revealed movements, were applied for the treatment.

To compare bone marrow dose resulting from the use of different techniques (electrons versus photons), and even if with the limits of the absence of a TPS calculating the real electrons dose distribution, a theoretical planned DVH was retrospectively obtained considering the percentage depth dose (PDD) applied to patients treated with electrons (30.0 Gy; 86% at 7 mm). With the same intent, a bone marrow volume included in the superficial body layer was created. It was obtained with an automatic symmetrical contraction of the contoured external body volume of different extent (2 to 28 mm). Considering a dose prescription for TSEBI (28.8 Gy in 16 fraction), estimated DVH points were calculated, combining bone marrow volume included in the superficial layers and the measured dose curve in the conditions of the TSEBI setup. (Fig. 2).

Clinical dose prescription

The prescribed doses were different for the three patients (Table 1) but always within the therapeutic range. Considering the 160 cm maximal target length in Tomotherapy® and to allow partial bone marrow recovery, the treatment was always delivered in two consecutive sessions of 13–16 fractions each. Upper body and lower body were treated

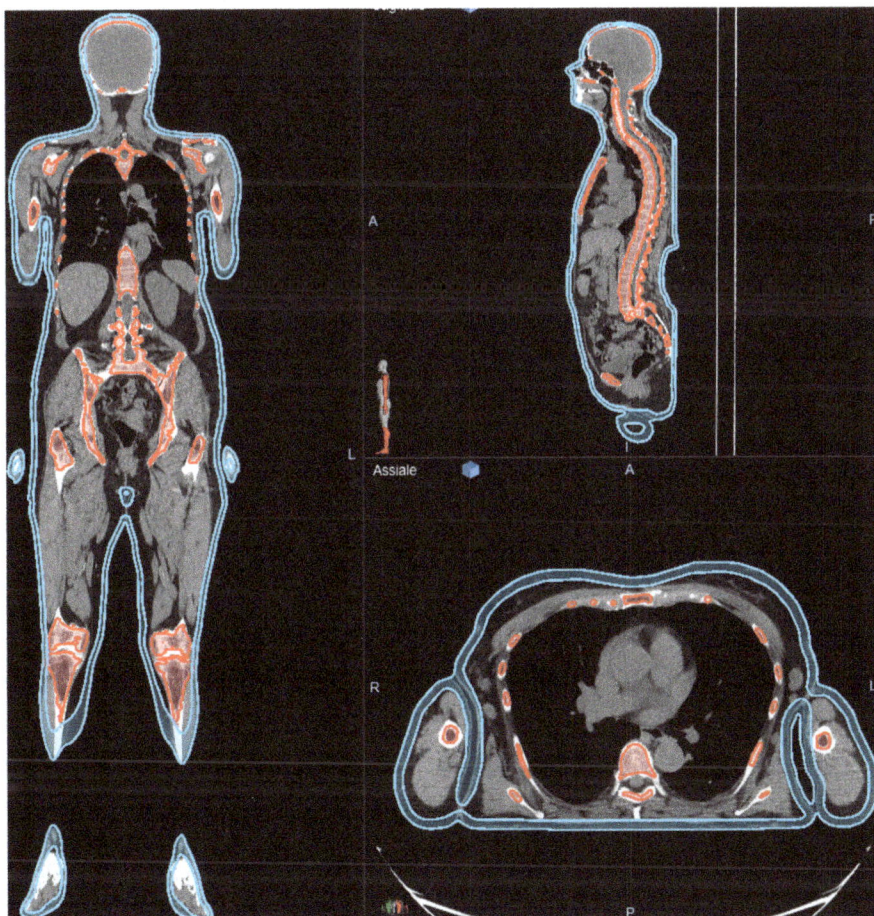

Fig. 1 Target and bone marrow contouring

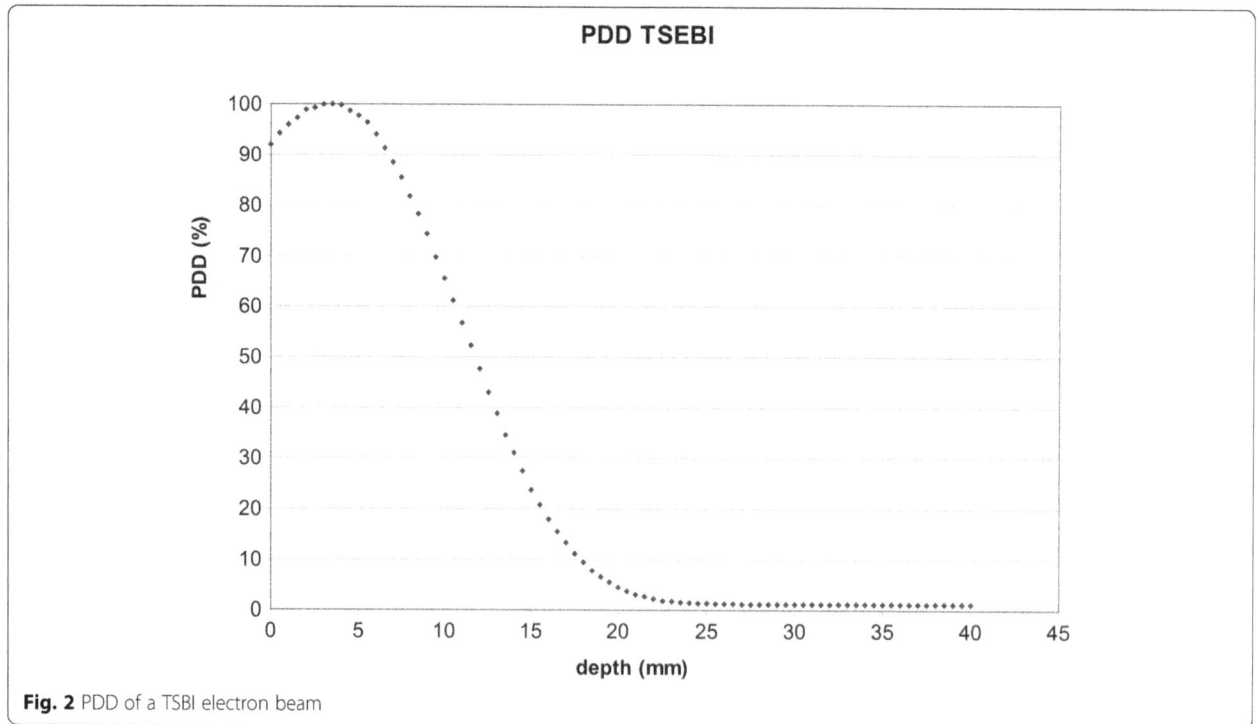

Fig. 2 PDD of a TSBI electron beam

posing the junction in a stable section of the body depending on each patient anatomy and set-up. The treatments were delivered 5 days a week for all the patients and all the sessions. All the patients had electron boosts to compensate under dosages (Table 1) or to treat macroscopic disease. In order to avoid over/under dosage in the treatments junctions, both the upper and the lower regions had two steps gradient regions, 5 cm each.

Physical features of the treatment

The treatments were delivered with Helical IMRT (Tomotherapy®) with MVCT for set-up verification. All the plans were calculated with a 5 cm collimator. To reach a more homogeneous dose distribution, both PTV_eval and OPTV were divided in multiple sub-volumes during the optimization process. The OPTVs were included separately in the optimization to have a planned photon fluency that could expand beyond the planning CT body and treat efficiently the patients' skin.

To reach adequate lungs and lens DVH values, the respective PRV were blocked during the optimization process. Other inner ad hoc volumes, obtained as a contraction of 2 cm of the body contours, were created and completely blocked in the optimization process to avoid internal organ irradiation. Eye Lens with 6 mm margin were, as well, completely blocked. All plans were elaborated with Helical Irradiation and computed with calculation grid fine. [19]. The plans characteristics of the different patients are reported in Table 2.

All plans underwent three different kinds of Quality Assurance (QA) procedures: a) multiple standard pretreatment dosimetric QA with measurements of the dose delivered to two phantoms (A1SL Exradin -Standard Imaging ionization chamber- in a cheese phantom; PTW Octavius chambers array for planar doses); b) daily delivered dose calculations based on MVCTs, co-registered with the planning CT (DODA, Dose of the day); c) in vivo *dosimetry* performed with Gafchromic films (EBT3®).

The Gaf-chromic films were positioned on the patients' skin, in points considered at higher risk for dose distribution alterations. Lower and upper posterior aspect of torso, lateral aspect of the right and left arm, forehead, cheek, nape, scapula, sternum, right and left thigh, right and left hand dorsum, right and left foot dorsum, abdomen, pubic region, skin over fibula and medial/lateral aspect of right and left tibia were considered.

The exact positions of Gaf dosimeters were recorded to estimate, from daily dose distribution, the expected doses to match the result with. The films were handled according to AAPM TG-55 report [20].

Response assessment

Patients were evaluated weekly during the treatment, one time 1 month after the end of the treatment and then every 3 months. Complete response was defined as complete disappearance of cutaneous lesions. Disease recurrence was defined in a multidisciplinary team (radiation oncologist, dermatologist and hematologist).

Light and shadows of a new technique: is photon total-skin irradiation using helical IMRT...

5

Table 2 Tomotherapy® plan characteristics

Pat	Treatment session	Plan	Duration (min)	N. rotations	N. fractions	Number of PTV sub-volumes used in optimization	Number of region at risk used in optimization
#1	Upper Hemibody	#1 U1	22.6	45.3	3	56	33
		#1 U2	22.6	43.7	12	56	25
	Lower Hemibody	#1 L1	23.6	19	10	14	14
		#1 L2	23.6	19	3	14	14
#2	Upper Hemibody	#2 U1	27.1	56	8	59	27
		#2 U2	28.9	56	8	68	28
	Lower Hemibody	#2 L1	40.0	50.1	3	45	35
		#2 L2	40.0	50.1	13	46	34
#3	Upper Hemibody	#3 U1	27.2	52.7	3	61	45
		#3 U2	27.2	52.7	13	74	56
	Lower Hemibody	#3 L1	29.4	83.9	15	71	42

Toxicity evaluation

Acute toxicity was defined as cutaneous and haematological damage appearing during the treatment and within 3 months after the end of radiotherapy. Adverse events occurring more than 3 months after the end of radiotherapy were defined as late toxicity. All the toxic events were defined with the CTCAE.4 scale. The possible relationship between clinical toxicity and dosimetric parameters was evaluated. The follow up was continued for all the patients (every 3 months) after the end of the treatment to evaluate late toxicity and outcomes.

Statistical analysis

Results were compared with the z-test when a sample of data was compared with a reference value. t-Student test was used for paired data when two samples of data were compared. The differences were considered statistically significant if $p < 0,01$ to account for the high number of tests performed.

Results
Target dose

Deviation of planning median dose from the prescribed one were within 3% and therefore considered acceptable.

The planned doses per fraction to the target were compared with the DODA calculated for each fraction. Dose-volume points did not result significantly different, but in the few cases where the average DODAs were significantly higher than the provisional ones (eg. for patient #2 average D2% of the "lower volume" 2.1 Gy (SD 0.05 Gy) vs 2.1 Gy; average D95% 1.1 Gy (SD 0.06 Gy) vs 0.9 Gy; average D2% of the "upper volume" 2.3 Gy (SD 0.03 Gy) vs 2.2 Gy). Differences between the in vivo measures and DODA mean values for the different regions of the three patients were statistically different only in selected sites (upper back, right hand and foot

dorsum for patient #1; the back and forearms for patient #2; the back, shoulders, harms and forearms for patient #3). Table 3 reports the target DVH outcomes for the patients obtained by means of Tomotherapy treatment planning. Cumulative plans are considered for each patient's session. The results are calculated for the PTV_eval contours. The data show that the best target coverage was obtained in patient #3.

Organs at risk dose

Doses to the different OARs were within the safe limits. Higher mean doses were evident in superficial organs as lacrimal glands in pat #3 (16.7 Gy) parotids in all patients (range 18.1–20.9 Gy), thyroid (range 7.5–17.5 Gy), testicles respectively 27.0 Gy and 18.7 Gy for pat #2 and #3. The doses of all defined OAR are reported in Table 4.

Some structures had a large mean dose variation between the three patients. Lacrimal glands, parotids and thyroid mean variation was due to patient

Table 3 Target dose volume points

Treatment session	Target DVH points (Gy)			
	DVH point	Patient #1	Patient #2	Patient #3
Upper hemi body: #1: 27/1.8 Gy #2: 28.8/1.8 Gy #3: 28.8/1.8 Gy	D (10 ml)	30.8	34.1	35.7
	D (2%)	30.0	33.1	34.9
	D (50%)	*26.4*	*28.5*	*30.9*
	D (90%)	22.4	22.2	23.8
	D (95%)	19.4	19.7	19.8
Lower hemi body: #1: 26/2 Gy #2: 28.8/1.8 Gy #3: 27.0/1.8 Gy	D(10 ml)	29.6	33.6	35.3
	D (2%)	28.9	33.0	34.5
	D (50%)	*25.7*	*28.5*	*30.9*
	D (90%)	23.1	19.7[a]	28.5
	D (95%)	21.7	14.2[a]	27.5

[a]electron field boost performed in the under dosage regions

Table 4 Previsional OAR's mean doses and *DODA average mean doses CL's (99,7% 3 σ)*

Organs	Plans total mean dose (Gy)			DODAs mean doses CL – 3σ(Gy)		
	Pat #1	Pat #2	Pat #3	Pat #1	Pat #2	Pat #3
Bowel (abdominal cavity)	1.1	10.9	3.9	0.89–0.93	8.7–9.0	4.6–4.8
Brain	4.5	3.2	4.6	4.3–4.5	3.1–3.6	4.5–4.6
Cord	3.1	6.7	6.1	3.2–3.6	6.69–6.73	6.1–6.9
Oesophagus	3.6	8.1	5.9	3.6–3.7	7.9–8.0	5.7–5.8
Heart	3.3	4.6	5.4	3.26–3.30	4.55–4.59	5.4–5.5
Lacrimal glands	3.1	3.3	16.7	3.9–4.6	3.7–3.8	13.3–13.6
Lens	1.9	2.2	5.9	2.1–2.7	2.2–2.4	6.2–6.5
Liver	2.4	4.3	4.3	2.3–2.4	4.2–4.3	4.4–4.5
Lungs	2.3	3.5	3.1	2.17–2.20	3.36–3.38	3.30–3.32
Parotids	20.9	19.5	18.1	19.5–20.3	16.7–18.2	18.5–18.7
Thyroid	17.5	14.4	7.5	14.1–14.7	14.5–14.7	6.9–7.0
Oral cavity	5.5	2.7	2.5	5.2–5.5	2.69–2.72	2.36–2.42
Spleen	2.7	4.6	9.9	2.5–2.6	4.3–4.6	9.4–9.6
Kidneys	3.1	3.8	3.3	3.0–3.2	3.56–3.58	3.34–3.39
Stomach	2.4	2.1	2.1	1.6–1.6	1.96–1.98	2.07–2.11
Bladder	11.0	2.6	1.4	9.1–9.4	2.30–2.34	1.31–1.31
Rectum	15.9	4.8	1.6	13.6–13.8	4.6–4.8	1.44–1.46
Uterus	13.8	/	/	10.8–11.3	/	/
Testicles	/	27.0	18.7	/	27.2–28.8	19.9–20.2
Penis and corpora cavernosa	/	24.0	9.9	/	22.3–22.4	7.5–8.0

anatomy, while bladder, rectum and bowel cavity mean doses where affected both by patient anatomy and by the choice of upper and lower plans overlapping regions.

The differences between the DODA to the single organs and the planned ones were not statistically significant. The mean doses to the internal OARs are all < 1.0 Gy per fraction; the confidence limit of organs DODAs mean doses are shown in Table 4. Organs generally received lower doses than the planned ones.

Bone marrow dose

The median and mean whole bone marrow cumulative doses for the entire treatment (upper plus lower plan) were 4.0 Gy and 8.5 Gy for patient #1; 4.5 Gy and 10.1 Gy for patient #2 and 6.5 Gy and 12.0 Gy for patient #3. These average cumulative doses were given in two consecutive sessions. Therefore, while the fraction of the bone marrow included in the upper part of the body is receiving a dose, the lower part of the body (and the corresponding bone marrow fraction) is not; the reverse is also true.

Whole bone marrow planned V_{10Gy}, V_{12Gy} and V_{20Gy} values were 23%, 20% and 10% for patient #1; 37%, 34.1% and 23% for patient #2, 43%, 39% and 24% for patients #3. (Figs 3, 4, 5).

With TSEBI, the provisional values of bone marrow V_{10Gy}, V_{12Gy} and V_{20Gy} were lower than those obtained with photons. In particular they were respectively 17%, 14.5%, 9.6% for patient #1; 14.5%, 13.7% and 9.4% for patient #2, 6.6%, 5.1% and 2.8% for patients #3. Median bone marrow dose for TSEBI would have been 0.4 Gy, 0.35 Gy and 0.35 Gy respectively for patient #1, #2 and #3; the average bone marrow dose would have been 3.6 Gy, 3.3 Gy and 1.3 Gy, respectively. (Fig. 6).

Acute toxicity

Non-haematological toxicity

All patients had transient G2–3 skin toxicity with erythema and epitheliolysis, especially in sites with non-homogeneous dose distribution (axillary, inguinal regions and fingers). All patients experimented alopecia, nails alterations and oral mucositis (G2–3). All patients had plantar feet pain during 2 months after the end of treatment. All the symptoms were controlled with specific supportive care.

Haematological toxicity

All patients experienced anaemia requiring blood support and neutropenia requiring growth factors. Thrombocytopenia was evident in two patients

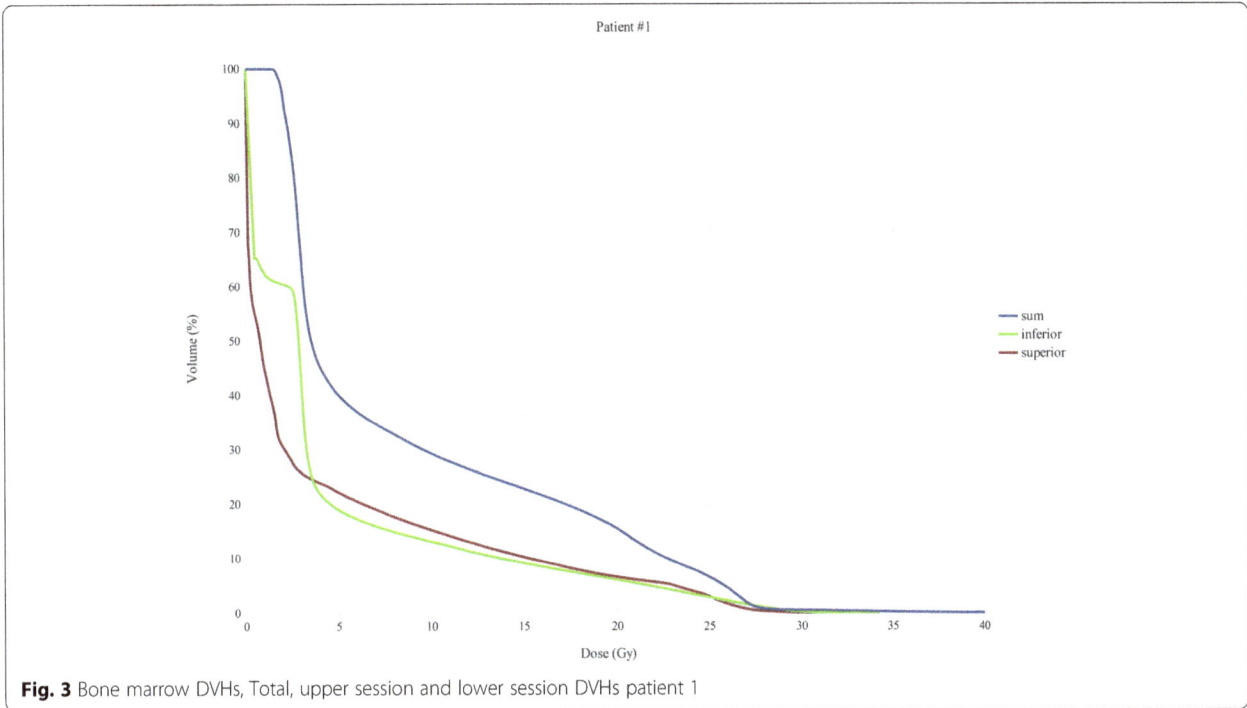

Fig. 3 Bone marrow DVHs, Total, upper session and lower session DVHs patient 1

and recovered within 6 months after RT. Haematological toxicity has been worse, including prolonged thrombocytopenia, in Patient #3. *Patient #1* had G2 anaemia twice, during the lower body and upper body treatment; G3 thrombocytopenia and G2 neutropenia. The haematological toxicity increased during the treatment in parallel with the increase of RT dose to the bone marrow. All the acute toxicities recovered within 2 months after the end of the treatment. *Patient #2* had G1 anaemia, G3 neutropenia and G1 thrombocytopenia at the end of both sessions, treated with blood transfusions and growth factors. Anemia, neutropenia and thrombocytopenia were respectively G2, G1 and G3 for *Patient #3* at the end of the

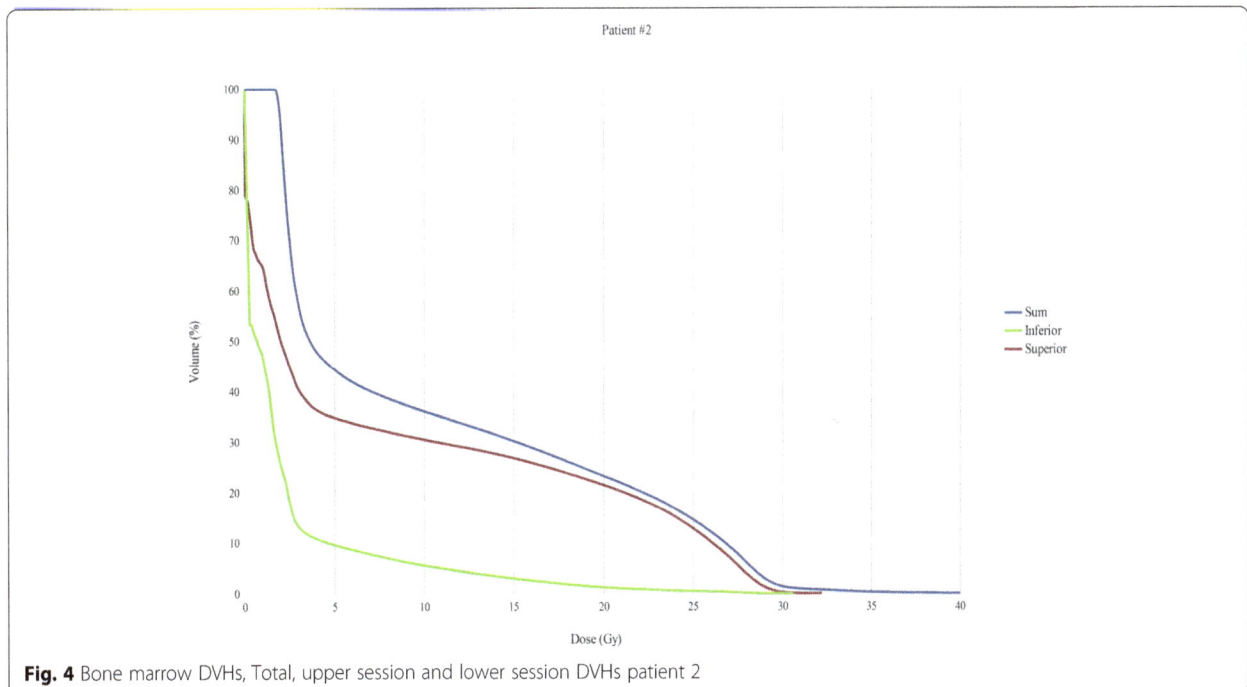

Fig. 4 Bone marrow DVHs, Total, upper session and lower session DVHs patient 2

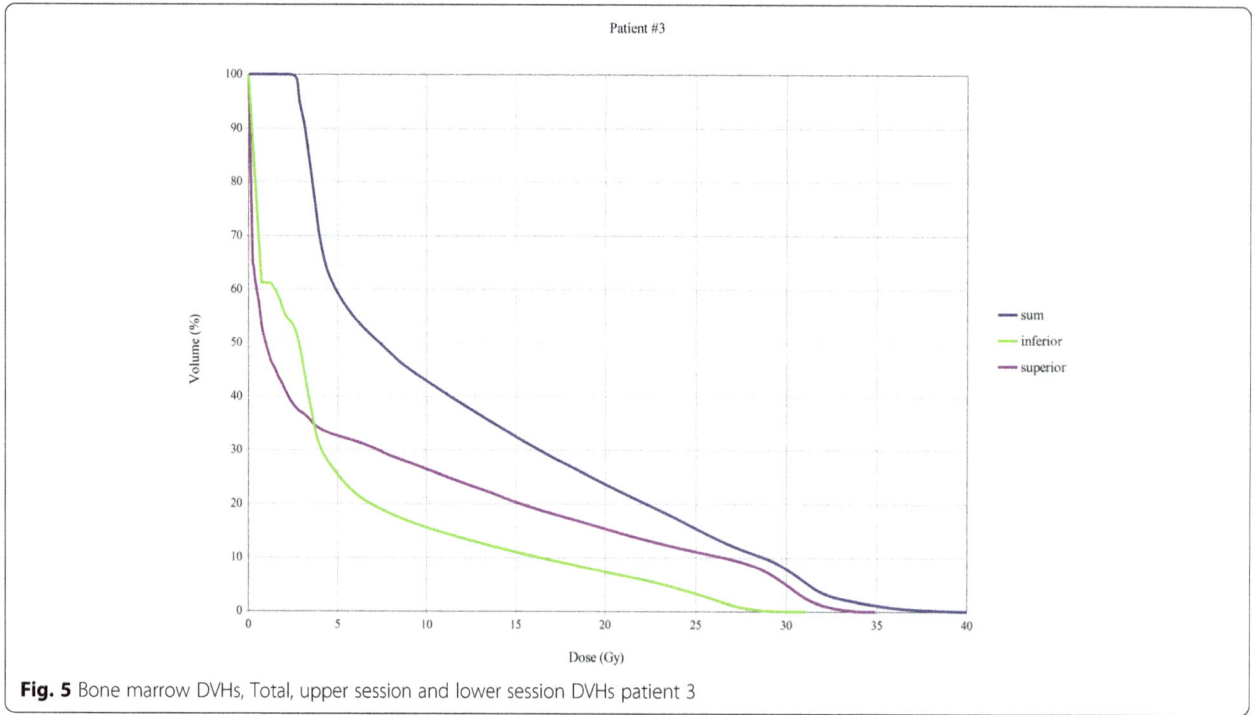

Fig. 5 Bone marrow DVHs, Total, upper session and lower session DVHs patient 3

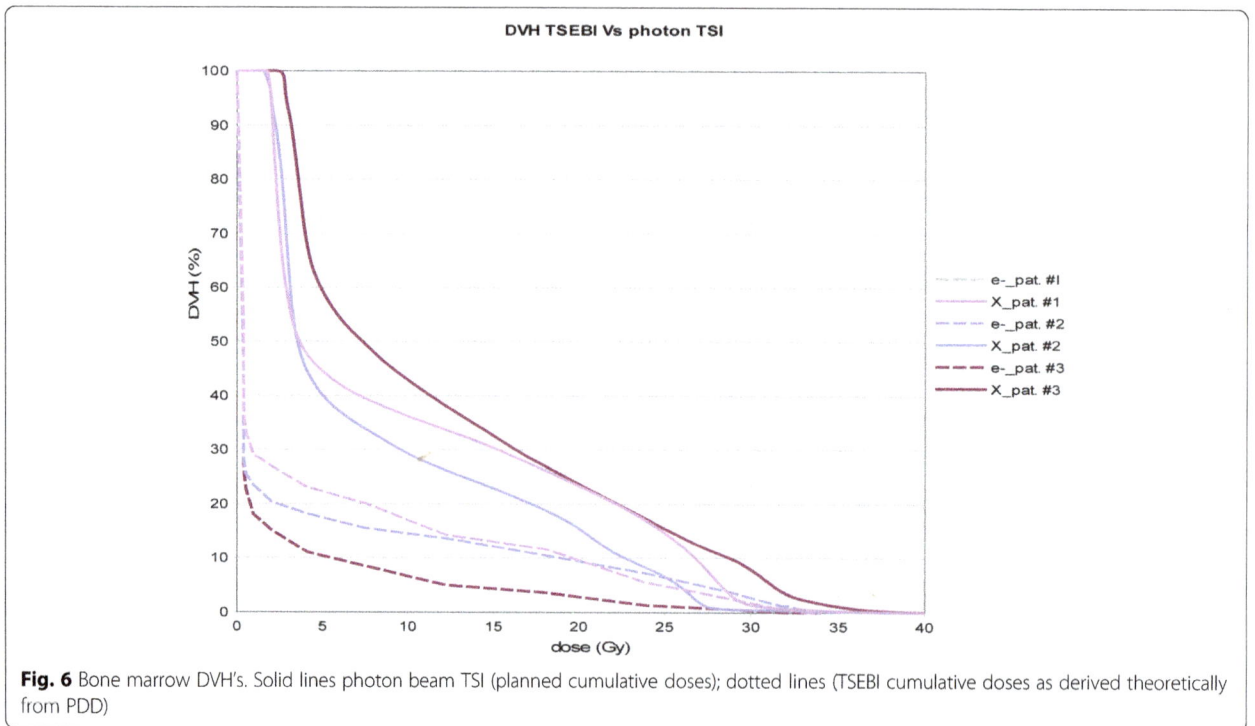

Fig. 6 Bone marrow DVH's. Solid lines photon beam TSI (planned cumulative doses); dotted lines (TSEBI cumulative doses as derived theoretically from PDD)

Light and shadows of a new technique: is photon total-skin irradiation using helical IMRT...

9

treatment. All the acute toxicities but thrombocytopenia (70,000/ULt 3 years after the end of RT) recovered within 2 months after the end of the treatment.

Response

The immediate disease response was good in all the patients. In one patient, treated with radical intent, the response was durable. (Table 1).

Discussion

Large electrons fields perpendicular to the body of the patient, who is standing and rotated in 6 differently angled positions, are used to treat the entire skin, when indicated, according to the most used technique, the Stanford one [21]. The physical distribution of electrons [22] requires the use of fields perpendicular to the surface of the target and do not allow to treat concave or convex volumes with a homogeneous dose. With Total Skin Electron Beam Irradiation (TSEBI) a 2.0 Gy/fraction to the whole skin is delivered in 2 days (three body positions a day), and the patient is treated 5 days a week. No hematological toxicity is generally reported for TSEBI [23]. Nevertheless, this treatment is not considered *simple*, mostly for its duration and the need of adequate patient compliance. Additional complexity is due to difficulties in dosimetry and to the required equipment.

In recent years the use of sophisticated technologies allowed to treat targets close to OAR's, and irregular volumes. There are some experiences suggesting the use of IMRT and Helical IMRT with IGRT to treat irregularly shaped body parts, like cutaneous circumferential targets on legs, arms, scalp or face [15, 24]. Image guided IMRT (also helical) is increasingly used to treat other complex targets, such as bone marrow in its entirety and the entire cranio-spinal volume [25–28].

The experience here reported revealed different critical issues using Tomotherapy® to treat a total skin volume. The problems are mostly related to treatment set-up, dosimetry, planning and verification, dose distribution to organs at risk, acute and late toxicity.

Treatment set up

Patient's compliance has to be adequate due to set up complexity (vac-lock, double thermoplastic mask, long daily treatment duration). Set-up and repositioning relevance has been emphasized also in other similarly demanding helical IMRT experiences, as total bone marrow-irradiation [29]. Not all the patients are able to reproduce and maintain the defined position, especially during the advanced phases of the treatment, when skin toxicity is more pronounced. This observation has been made also in the single, already published experience of total skin irradiation with helical IMRT, where the differences between the planning and the treatment position

were about 3 mm, as measured during daily controls before and after each fraction [16]. Difficulties in the treatment set-up could be responsible of the statistically significant differences reported in the present paper between the planned, DODAs and gaf-measured doses during the treatment.

Target coverage and homogeneity

The surface dose, reported in the unique already published experience of TSI with helical IMRT, is 84 cGy on the lesion (range 73.6 to 89.4 cGy) [16]. Our patients had a mean measured surface dose/fraction ranging between 1.54 Gy and 2 Gy. In general, we obtained a planned target dose ranging from 85 to 120% of prescription doses. Nonetheless, it was possible to identify hot and cold regions and to manage them; for this reason, re-planning was an important part of the process. This is clearly an advantage over the standard TSEBI technique approach, where it is not possible to correct for the inhomogeneous dose distribution [21].

OAR dose distribution

The median doses to internal OARs, in the other published report, were 29.3 Gy and 24.7 Gy for the parotid and thyroid gland, respectively; 8.0 Gy for the brain; 5.2 and 6.8 Gy for liver and spleen; 3.8, 2.5 and 2.1 Gy for spinal cord, brain stem and lens, respectively. The authors report also median doses to lungs (4.5/4.7 Gy), heart (3.3 Gy) and kidneys (3.9/4.3 Gy) [16]. In our series, we reported mean organ doses and all the doses received by the OARs were largely within the accepted dose constraints and in line with those reported in the previous experience. As expected, doses to superficial organs were higher than those to the deeper ones, due to the photon characteristic depth curve.

Bone marrow dose

Haematopoietic bone marrow is very radiation sensitive and it can be considered the most important OAR for this treatment because, particularly in districts as cranial bones, ribs and sternum, it is very close to the target (< 1 cm). Up to 30–40% of total bone marrow could be within the first 3 cm of the outer body layer. Bone marrow total dose was carefully analyzsed, also in relation with haematological toxicity and it was demonstrated a correlation with bone marrow RT dose.

In patients treated with radio-chemotherapy for cervical cancer, with a median pelvic RT dose of 45.0 Gy (range, 36.0–50.4) and a median *point A* dose (in patients undergoing intracavitary implants using low-dose-rate brachytherapy) of 85.0 Gy (range, 75.0–87.0), pelvic bone marrow V_{10Gy} values of > 90% are related to higher rates of hematologic G3-G4 toxicities and delays in chemotherapy administration [29]. Similarly, Albuquerque et al.

reports, in patients who received 45.0 Gy with concurrent weekly cisplatin for cervical cancer, a significant increase of Grade 2–3 hematologic toxicity when ≥80% of whole pelvic bone received 20.0 Gy [30, 31]. The RT total body dose used to induce aplasia, conditioning bone marrow transplantation, is 12.0 Gy with a twice a day fractionation regimen (2.0 Gy/fraction) [31, 32].

Chen-Hsi Hsieh et al. identified the bone of the spine (cervical, thoracic, lumbar and sacrum) as *haematopoietic bone marrow*. Right and left iliac crest, right and left femurs, right and left pelvic bone, ribs and cranial theca, were not included in the bone marrow volume. The median doses reported in their experience ranged between 4 Gy (lumbar spine and sacrum) to 9 Gy (iliac crests), to > 12 Gy (femurs and pelvic bones). All these parameters can be used as a reference to evaluate bone marrow dosimetric results for the present series also considering that bone marrow was outlined in its entirety. The planned mean doses were 8.5 Gy for the first patient and, respectively, 10.1 and 12.0 Gy for patients #2 and #3. The average DODAs were slightly but significantly higher for the *first lower plan* and for the *second upper plan*, for the first patient and slightly lower for both the upper plans for the third patient. However, the skin of the upper and the lower hemi-body have been treated sequentially, with an interval up to about 3 weeks between the two treatment sessions. Thus, only about half of the bone marrow was directly exposed in each of the two sessions. It could therefore be considered that while part of the marrow is accumulating damage, the other is not (or not to the same extent) or is recovering.

The bone marrow mean and median doses are slightly higher for patient #3, probably in relation with treatment planning optimization. This could be the reason for protracted thrombocytopenia of patient #3, along with the shorter interval between the first and the second session of the treatment (Table 1). In fact, the total mean dose of 12.0 Gy was delivered during the entire treatment (31 fractions) with a mean dose per fraction of 0.4 Gy.

The average bone marrow doses given with photon TSI, even if are much lower than those used as a conditioning regimen in bone marrow transplantation, are sufficient to induce bone marrow toxicity. In fact, this is what happened with low dose TBI used in different trials to obtain bone marrow disease control in follicular lymphomas. [33, 34] The bone marrow dose volume points for a hypothetical TSEBI treatment, with the same dose regimen, would have been significantly lower for all patients. Since this is the main cause of hematological toxicity, it can be considered as a limiting factor for the use of this technique to treat total skin. In fact, one out of only three patients had late thrombocytopenia.

Toxicity

As far as toxicity is concerned, doses to the internal organs (abdominal cavity, kidney, spleen and eyes) are lower than those defined as "constraints" but they are higher than those given using electrons that is less than 0.3 Gy on average to organs located at a depth of more than 3 cm. (Fig. 4).

Although a direct comparison between the toxicity related to HT and TSEBI is not possible, due to the very small number of HT treated cases, data from the literature (6) and from our experience with TSEBI point to a substantial similarity of the skin/nails damage and of the other non-hematologic toxicities induced by the two techniques. Superficial organs as lacrimal glands, thyroid, and lenses receive similar or lower doses than those given with TSEBI, and the resulting toxicity does not seem to be substantially different.

However, TSEBI hematologic toxicity is scarce, whereas all our patients had different degrees (G2–3) of hematologic toxicity (even if patient #1 marrow doses were close to those expected with TSEBI).

Conclusions

Based on previous published experiences of the use of Helical IMRT to treat large and complex superficial volumes, this is the second report on total skin treatments with photons performed with this technique.

As expected, dose homogeneity has been better than with TSEBI and a durable remission has been obtained in the unique patients treated with radical intent.

Even if a relative increase in bone marrow toxicity was expected, its extent was unexpected, considering also the split course nature of the treatment.

Therefore, according to our results, TSEBI should still be considered the standard method to treat total skin because of its pattern of acute and late toxicities and further use of helical IMRT for this treatment discouraged: the better target coverage obtained with HI is not clearly related to better clinical response and can possibly induce worse toxicity.

On the other hand, considering the data published, the clinical results and the limited and reversible toxicities in treating volumes smaller than total skin, Helical IMRT can be considered optimal in treating large, convex, cutaneous areas where it is difficult to use multiple electrons fields.

Abbreviations

CR: Complete response; CTV: Clinical target volume; DODA: Dose of the Day. Calculation of daily delivered dose based on the verification MVCT; DVH: Dose volume histogram; Dy%: Dose at least received from y% of volume (y is a number between 0 and 100); GTV: Gross tumor volume; HI: Helical IMRT; IGRT: Image guided radiation therapy; IMRT: Intensity modulated Radiation Therapy; MF: Micosis Fungoides; MVCT: Megavoltage computed tomography; OAR: Organs at risk; OPTV: Outside the body surface PTV; PCL: Primary cutaneous lymphomas; PD: Progressive disease; PR: Partial response; PRV: Planning organ at Risk Volume; PTV: Planning target volume; QA: Quality Assurance; RT: Radiotherapy; SS: Sèzary Syndrome; TSEBI: Total skin electron beams irradiation; V_{xGy}: Percentage of volume receiving at least X Gy (X is a number)

Authors' contributions

MB: treated the patients, collected and analysed the data; wrote and revised the paper. LS: performed the treatment planning, collected and analysed the data; wrote and revised the paper. MU: treated the patients and collected the data. LB: treated the patients and collected the data. RA: performed the treatment planning. NP: treated the patients. PB: treated the patients. LT: treated patients and collected the data. SP: treated the patients. FS: performed the treatment planning. AF: performed the treatment planning. DG: treated the patients. SC: treated the patients. AP: helped in the treatment planning. SMM: revised the paper. All authors read and approved the final manuscript.

Competing interests

The authors declare that they have no competing interests.

Author details

[1]Radiation Oncology Department, University and Spedali Civili Hospital – Brescia, P.le Spedali Civili 1 –, 25123 Brescia, Italy. [2]Medical Physics, Spedali Civili Hospital – Brescia, P.le Spedali Civili 1 –, 25123 Brescia, Italy.

References

1. Olsen E, Vonderheid E, Pimpinelli N, et al. Revisions to the staging and classification of mycosis fungoides and Sezary syndrome: a proposal of the International Society for Cutaneous Lymphomas (ISCL) and the cutaneous lymphoma task force of the European Organization of Research and Treatment of Cancer (EORTC). Blood. 2007;110:1713–22.
2. Arulogun SO, Prince HM, Ng J, et al. Long-term outcomes of patients with advanced-stage cutaneous T-cell lymphoma and large cell transformation. Blood. 2008;112:3082–7.
3. Yen A, McMichael A, Kilkenny M, et al. Mycosis fungoides: an Australian experience. Australas J Dermatol. 1997;38(Suppl. 1):S86–90.
4. Hoppe R. Mycosis Fungoides: radiation terapy. Dermatol Ther. 2003;16:347–54.
5. Cotter GW, Baglan RJ, Wasserman TH, et al. Palliative radiation treatment of cutaneous mycosis Fungoides a dose response. Int J Radiat Oncol Biol Phys. 1983;9:1477–80.
6. Elsayad K, Kriz J, Moustakis C, Scobioala S, Reinartz G, Haverkamp U, Willich N, Weishaupt C, Stadler R, Sunderkötter C, Eich HT. Total skin Electron beam for primary cutaneous T-cell Lymphoma. Int J Radiat Oncol Biol Phys. 2015; 93(5):1077–86. https://doi.org/10.1016/j.ijrobp.2015.08.041.
7. Pedretti S, Urpis M, Leali C, Borghetti P, Baushi L, Sala R, Tucci A, Greco D, Pasinetti N, Triggiani L, Rossi G, Calzavara-Pinton P, Magrini SM, Buglione M. Primary cutaneous non-Hodgkin lymphoma: results of a retrospective analysis in the light of the recent ILROG guidelines. Tumori. 2017; https://doi.org/10.5301/tj.5000606.
8. Goujon E, Truc G, Pétrella T, Maingon P, Jeudy G, Collet E, Galliot C, Dalac-Rat S. Total skin electron beam for early-stage mycosis fungoides: immediate results and long term follow-up in 68 patients. Ann Dermatol Venereol. 2009;136(3): 249–55. https://doi.org/10.1016/j.annder.2008.11.017.
9. Gettler SL. Fung MA efficacy of treatments for mycosis fungoides and Sezary syndrome: nationwide survey responses. Dermatol Online J. 2005;11(3):6.
10. Karzmack C. 1987. Total skin electron therapy: technique and dosimetry. Report no. 23.
11. Piotrowski T, Malicki J. The rotary dual technique for total skin irradiation in the treatment of mycosis fungoides - a description of applied method. Rep Pract Oncol Radiother. 2006;11:29–37.
12. Hensley F, Major G, Edel C, Hauswald H, Bischof M. Technical and dosimetric aspects of the total skin electron beam technique implemented at Heidelberg University Hospital. Rep Pract Oncol Radiother. 2014;19:135–43.
13. Podgorsak EB, Pla C, Pla M, et al. Physical aspects of a rotational total skin electron irradiation. Med Phys. 1983;10:159–68.
14. Gamble LM, Farrell TJ, Jones GW, Hayward JE. Two-dimensional mapping of underdosed areas using radiochromic film for patients undergoing total skin electron beam radiotherapy. Int J Radiat Oncol Biol Phys. 2005; 62(3):920–4.
15. Mazzeo E, Rubino L, Buglione M, Antognoni P, Magrini SM, Bertoni F, Parmiggiani M, Barbieri P, Bertoni F. The current management of mycosis Fungoides and Sèzary syndrome and the role of radiotherapy: principles and indications. Rep Pract Oncol Radiother. 2013;19(2):77–91. Review
16. Hsieh CH, Shueng PW, Lin SC, Tien HJ, Shiau AC, Chou YH, Wu MH, Wang JY, Chen CK, Chen YJ. Helical irradiation of the total skin whit dose painting to replace total skin electron beam therapy for therapy-refactory cutaneous CD4+ T-cell lymphoma. Biomed Res Int; 2013. https://doi.org/10.1155/2013/717589.
17. Morrison SJ, Scadden DT. The bone marrow niche for haematopoietic stem cells. Nature. 2014;505(7483):327–34. https://doi.org/10.1038/nature12984.
18. Clarke B. Normal Bone Anatomy and Physiology. Clin J Am Soc Nephrol. 2008;3(Suppl 3):S131–9. https://doi.org/10.2215/CJN.04151206.
19. Piotrowski T, Czajka E, Bak B, Kazmierska J, Skorska M, Ryczkowski A, Adamczyk M, Jodda A. Tomotherapy: implications on daily workload and scheduling patients based on three years' institutional experience. Technol Cancer Res Treat. 2014;13:233–42.
20. Niromand-rad A, Blackwell CR, Coursey BM, Gall KP, Galvin JM, MacLaughlin WL, Meigooni AS, Ravinder N, Rodgers JE, Soares CG. Radiochromic film dosimetry: recommendations of AAPM radiation therapy committee task group 55. Med Phys. 1998;25(11):2093–115.
21. Hoppe RT, Fuks Z, Bagshaw MA. The rationale for curative radiotherapy in mycosis fungoides. Int J Radiat Oncol Biol Phys. 1977;2:843–51.
22. Gahbauer R, Landberg T, Chavaudra J, Dobbs J, Gupta N, Hanks G, Horiot J-C, Johansson K-A, Möller T, et al. Physical characteristics of electron beams. Journal of the ICRU. 2004;4:1. https://doi.org/10.1093/jicru/ndh009. Oxford University Press
23. Jones GW, Kacinski BM, Wilson LD, et al. Total skin electron irradiation in the management of mycosis fungoides: consensus of the European organization fo the research and treatment of Cancer (EORTC) cutaneous lymphoma project group. J Am Acad Dermatolo. 2002;47:364–70.
24. Ostheimer C, Janich M, Hübsch P, Gerlach R, Vordermark D. The treatment of extensive scalp lesions using coplanar and non-coplanar photon IMRT: a single institution experience. Radiat Oncol. 2014;9:82.
25. Corvò R, Zeverino M, Vagge S, Agostinelli S, Barra S, et al. Helical tomotherapy targeting total bone marrow after total body irradiation for patients with relapsed acute leukemia undergoing an allogeneic stem cell transplant. Radiother Oncol. 2011;98:382–6.
26. Han C, Schultheisss TE, Wong JYC. VMAT in total marrow irradiation Dosimetric study of volumetric modulated arc therapy fields for total marrow irradiation. Radiother Oncol. 2012;102:315–20.
27. Wong JYC, Rosental J, Liu A, Schuktheiss T, et al. Image guided Total marrow irradiation using helical Tomotherapy in patients with multiple myeloma and acute leukemia undergoing hematopoietic cell transplantation. Int J Radiat Oncol Biol Phys. 2009;73(1):273–9.
28. Takahashi Y, Stefano Vagge MD, Agostinelli S, Han E, Matulewicz L, et al. Multi-institutional Feasibility Study of a Fast Patient Localization Method in Total Marrow Irradiation With Helical Tomotherapy: A Global Health Initiative by the International Consortium of Total Marrow Irradiation. Int J Radiat Oncol Biol Phys. 2015;91(1):30–8.
29. Mell LK, Kochanski JD, Roeske JC, Haslam JJ, et al. Dosimetric predictors of acute hematologic toxicity in cervical cancer patients treated with concurrent cisplatin and intensity-modulated pelvic radiotherapy. Int J Radiat Oncol Biol Phys. 2006;66:1356–65.

30. Albuquerque K, Giangreco D, Morrison C, Siddiqui M, et al. Radiation-related predictors of hematologic toxicity after concurrent chemoradiation for cervical cancer and implications for bone marrow-sparing pelvic IMRT. Int J Radiat Oncol Biol Phys. 2011;79:1043–7.

31. Aristei C, Santucci A, Corvo R, Gardani G, et al. In haematopoietic SCT for acute leukemia TBI impacts on relapse but not survival: results of a multicentre observational study. Bone Marrow Transplantation. 2013;48:908–14.

32. Hank B, O'Reilly R, Cunningham I, Kernan N, Yaholom J, Brochstein J, et al. Total body irradiation for bone marrow transplantation: the Memorial Sloan-Kettering Cancer Center experience. Radiother Oncol. 1990; 18(Suppl 1):68–81.

33. Richaud PM, Soubeyran P, Eghbali H, et al. Place of low-dose total body irradiation in the treatment of localized follicular non-Hodgkin's lymphoma: results of a pilot study. Int J Radiat Oncol Biol Phys. 1998;40(2):387–90.

34. Meerwaldt JH, Carde P, Burgers JM, et al. Low-dose total body irradiation versus combination chemotherapy for lymphomas with follicular growth pattern. Int J Radiat Oncol Biol Phys. 1991;21(5):1167–72.

Stereotactic body radiotherapy based treatment for hepatocellular carcinoma with extensive portal vein tumor thrombosis

Yongjie Shui[1], Wei Yu[1,4], Xiaoqiu Ren[1,4], Yinglu Guo[1,4], Jing Xu[1,4], Tao Ma[2], Bicheng Zhang[1], Jianjun Wu[3], Qinghai Li[3], Qiongge Hu[1], Li Shen[1], Xueli Bai[2], Tingbo Liang[2] and Qichun Wei[1,4]*

Abstract

Background: There is currently no worldwide consensus for the management of hepatocellular carcinoma (HCC) with portal vein tumor thrombus (PVTT). We evaluated the efficacy of stereotactic body radiotherapy (SBRT) as the initial treatment for HCC with extensive PVTT based on a relatively large number of patients.

Methods: In our multidisciplinary approach for patients with hepatobiliary tumors, SBRT is recommended for unresectable HCC with PVTT or those with contraindication for transarterial chemoembolization (TACE). The aim is to shrink the tumor thrombus and preserve adequate portal venous flow, thus facilitating subsequent treatments such as TACE and tumor resection. In the present study, 70 continuous cases of HCC patients with extensive PVTT initially treated with SBRT were studied. The median follow-up period was 9.5 months (range, 1.0–21.0 months). The dynamic changes of tumor thrombosis with time after SBRT were also analyzed.

Results: The median survival time for the whole group was 10.0 months (95% CI, 7.7–12.3 months), with a 6- and 12-month overall survival (OS) rate of 67.3%, and 40.0% respectively. Patients who received combined SBRT and TACE showed significantly longer OS than those without indication for TACE after SBRT (12.0 ± 1.6 vs. 3.0 ± 1.0 months). Patients with good response to radiation usually had better survival. SBRT was well tolerated in our patient series.

Conclusions: In conclusion, SBRT used as the initial treatment for HCC patients with extensive PVTT originally unsuitable for resection or TACE can achieve adequate thrombus shrinkage and portal vein flow restoration in the majority of cases. It could thus offer the patients an opportunity to undergo further treatment such as resection or TACE procedure. Such therapeutic strategy may result in survival advantage, especially for those who do receive combined modality with SBRT.

Keywords: Hepatocellular carcinoma, Portal vein tumor thrombosis, Stereotactic body radiotherapy, Transarterial chemoembolization

* Correspondence: Qichun_Wei@zju.edu.cn
This work has been accepted for a "ePoster presentation" at the 13th IHPBA
World Congress taking place in Geneva, Switzerland, 4-7 September 2018
(presentation code "EP01B-015")
[1]Department of Radiation Oncology, The Second Affiliated Hospital, Zhejiang
University School of Medicine, Jiefang Road 88, Hangzhou 310009, People's
Republic of China
[4]Ministry of Education Key Laboratory of Cancer Prevention and Intervention,
Zhejiang University Cancer Institute, Hangzhou 310009, People's Republic of
China
Full list of author information is available at the end of the article

Background

Hepatocellular carcinoma (HCC) is the sixth most prevalent cancer worldwide [1]. In China, HCC is the fourth most commonly diagnosed cancer and the third leading cause of cancer death [2]. Macrovascular invasion (MVI) is common in HCC; in such case, tumor cells invade the portal veins, hepatic veins, or the inferior vena cava in the liver [3, 4]. Portal vein tumor thrombus (PVTT) is the most common form of MVI in HCC, with an incidence ranging from 44 to 62.2% [5]. About 10% to 60% of HCC patients have PVTT at the time of diagnosis [6, 7]. Although the survival rate of patients with HCC has been improved recently, the prognosis for those with PVTT remains poor, as their median survival is only 2–4 months via supportive care [8]. Overall, PVTT plays a major role in predicting the therapeutic outcome and clinical staging of HCC [9, 10].

There is currently no widely-accepted consensus for the management of HCC with PVTT. According to some guidelines in Europe and America, HCC with PVTT is regarded as Stage C per Barcelona Clinic Liver Cancer (BCLC) Staging system, and sorafenib alone is recommended as the treatment of choice [11]. In Southeast Asian countries, modalities including surgery, radiotherapy, transarterial chemoembolization (TACE), and/or sorafenib are involved in the multidisciplinary treatment of HCC with PVTT [12, 13]. Surgical treatment is recommended for suitable HCC patients with type I/II PVTT [14–16]. However, the management of HCC with extensive portal vein involvement remains complicated and controversial. Patients with PVTT extended to the main portal vein or the contralateral branch had no survival benefit after surgical treatment [17]. TACE has been contraindicated in the treatment of HCC patients with PVTT involving the main trunk and/or first branch of the portal vein due to potential risk of liver infarction and hepatic failure resulting from ischemia [6, 18]. Several recent reports have shown that selected patients with PVTT may benefit from more aggressive treatment modalities [6, 19] such as a combination of radiotherapy and TACE. So far, few studies have investigated the efficacy of stereotactic body radiotherapy (SBRT) for the treatment of PVTT [20–22].

SBRT has emerged as a new technology which delivers large dose of radiation to a target in a few fractions. By taking advantage of the technologic advancements in precise radiation dose delivery, respiratory motion management, and daily image guidance, SBRT enables accurate targeting of multiple high-dose radiation beams to treat a tumor volume, typically over 1 to 5 fractions. Characterized by rendering a higher biologically effective dose (BED) than conventionally fractionated radiotherapy, minimal invasiveness and decreased morbidity, SBRT can be finished in a week. Such relatively short treatment course may post less interference with other therapeutic measures which may also benefit the patient sequentially in time.

In our multidisciplinary management for patients with hepatobiliary tumors, SBRT is recommended for patients with unresectable HCC with PVTT and those with contraindication for TACE. The aim is to shrink the tumor thrombus and preserve adequate portal venous flow, thus facilitating subsequent treatments such as TACE or tumor resection. In the present report, 70 continuous HCC with extensive PVTT initially treated with SBRT were analyzed. The therapeutic response, survival, safety, and treatment strategy were discussed.

Methods

Patient population and radiation treatment

This retrospective study was performed with the approval of our local ethics committee. From December 2015 to June 2017, 70 continuous HCC patients with PVTT received SBRT at the Second Affiliated Hospital, Zhejiang University School of Medicine. The diagnosis of HCC was based on the American Association for the Study of Liver Disease (AASLD) guideline [23]. Portal vein invasion was identified by the presence of a low-attenuation intraluminal filling defect adjacent to the primary tumor as discerned from contrast-enhanced computed tomography (CT). Cheng's classification of PVTT was applied in this study, and comprised of four levels based on the extent of tumor thrombus in the portal vein (Fig. 1): type I_0, tumor thrombus found only under microscopy; type I, tumor thrombus involving segmental or sectoral branches of the portal vein or above; type II, tumor thrombus involving the right/left portal vein; type III, tumor thrombus involving the main portal vein; and type IV, tumor thrombus involving the superior mesenteric vein [24]. Basic criteria for SBRT: (1) tumor thrombus involving the main trunk and/or first branches of the portal vein, unsuitable for surgery or TACE; (2) an Eastern Cooperative Oncology Group (ECOG) performance status (PS) of 0–2; (3) no refractory ascites; (4) Child–Pugh class A and B, or class C with good performance status; (5) no previous radiotherapy to the liver; and (6) more than 700 cc of uninvolved liver. A preliminary estimate of the uninvolved liver volume was made using 3D imaging software (IQQA-Liver, EDDA Technology Inc., Princeton, NJ, USA), whereas its exact volume was verified from the subsequent SBRT planning dosimetry (Eclipse software, Varian® Medical Systems, Palo Alto, CA).

All patients were immobilized in a stereotactic body frame (Karity, Guangzhou, China) with customized vacuum cushion and abdominal compression for control of respiratory motion. Oral contrast agent (50 ml of 3%

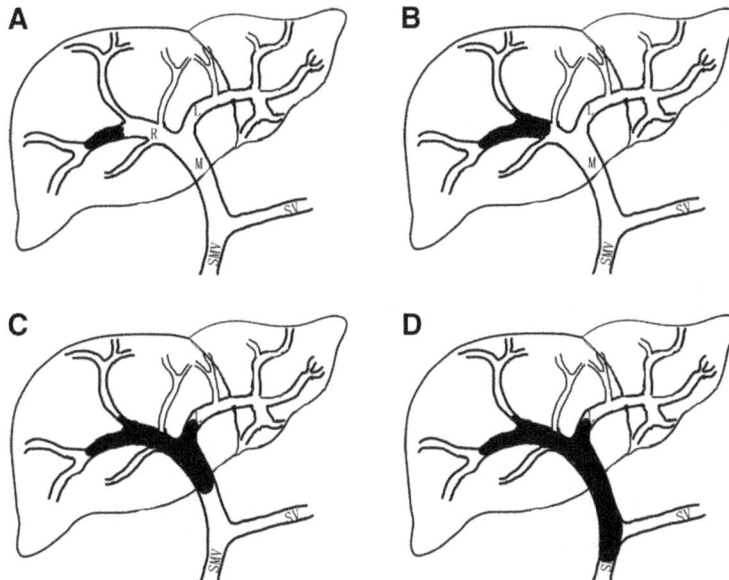

Fig. 1 Cheng's classification of hepatocellular carcinoma with portal vein tumor thrombus. **a** type I, tumor thrombus involving segmental or sectoral branches of the portal vein or above; **b** type II, tumor thrombus involving the right/left portal vein; **c** type III, tumor thrombus involving the main portal vein; **d** type IV, tumor thrombus involving the superior mesenteric vein

Ioversol) was administered before CT simulation. Four-dimensional contrast-enhanced computed tomography (4DCT) simulation (Light Speed RT, GE) was performed at 2.5-mm slice thickness. For breathing movement amplitude too small to be detected during 4DCT scanning, scans were taken at end-expiration phase, end-inspiration phase, and during quiet free-breathing under abdominal compression. The CT scan during free breathing was then used for treatment planning. The gross tumor volume (GTV) represented the tumor thrombosis visualized on the contrast enhanced CT, and magnetic resonance (MR) images. If the primary hepatic lesion was small (less than 5 cm) and adjacent to the PVTT, both portal vein tumor thrombus and the primary lesion were contoured as the GTV. Internal target volume (ITV) was defined as the volumetric sum of GTVs in the multiple phases. The planning target volume (PTV) included ITV with 3–5 mm margins, to account for daily set-up variations. PTV was adjusted manually to minimize overlapping the gastrointestinal tract when indicated. The mean volume of PTV was 390.8 ± 37.6 cm^3, varying widely from a minimum of 63.0 cm^3 to a maximum of 1452.9 cm^3. Plans were devised such that the prescription dose was prescribed at the isodose line encompassing > 95% of the PTV. The preferred maximum dose within the PTV was between 110 and 130% of the prescribed dose. The median prescription dose to PTV was 40 Gy (range, 25–50) in five fractions administered over a week. Organs at risk (OARs) included liver, kidneys, stomach, duodenum, small intestine, colon and spinal cord. Dose-volume planning objectives for the OARs were defined as follows

(Table 1): normal liver, mean dose ≤15 Gy; bilateral kidney, mean dose ≤12 Gy; and spinal cord, maximal dose<27 Gy. The maximal dose to 1 cc (D1cc) was limited to 31 Gy for the gastrointestinal tract including stomach, duodenum, small intestine and colon. Normal liver volume was defined as the total liver volume minus the PTV. Target and OAR contouring were performed using Varian Dosimetrist and Oncologist software (Eclipse software, Varian® Medical Systems, Palo Alto, CA). Treatment was delivered with a Varian® Trilogy™ linear accelerator (Varian® Medical Systems, Palo Alto, CA) using X-ray beams of 6–10 MV energy. Daily image guidance was performed by means of kilovoltage cone-beam CT, with

Table 1 Dose-volume constraints to organs at risk

Organs at risk	Constraints (5 Fractions)
Liver	mean dose ≤15 Gy, >700 cc
Kidney	mean dose ≤12 Gy V18 < 33%
Spinal cord	maximal dose < 27 Gy
Stomach	V31 < 1 cc V20 < 3 cc
Duodenum	V31 < 1 cc V20 < 3 cc
Small intestine	V31 < 1 cc V20 < 3 cc
Colon	V31 < 1 cc V20 < 10 cc

Abbreviations: Vxx = the volume or percentage of organ receiving more than the xx Gy

patients' 3D positioning verified prior to each radiation treatment session.

Evaluation

Patients were assessed weekly for toxicities in the first month after SBRT, monthly for the following two months, and once every three months thereafter. Treatment-associated acute and late toxicities were scored according to the Common Terminology Criteria for Adverse Events (CTCAE; version 3.0). Tumor response was assessed using the modified Response Evaluation Criteria in Solid Tumors (mRECIST) criteria [25]. The response of PVTT to SBRT was evaluated by dynamic contrast enhanced CT and/or MRI at 1, 3, and then every 3 months after SBRT. Biochemical response was assessed in patients with elevated alpha-fetoprotein (AFP) level before radiotherapy and defined as either a ≥ 50% reduction or normalization of the AFP level within one month after SBRT.

Follow-up and statistical analysis

The cutoff date for the last follow-up was February 28, 2018, for the censored data analysis. The median follow-up period was 9.5 months (range: 1.0–21.0). The overall survival (OS) was calculated from the start of SBRT to the date of either death or the last follow-up visit. The Kaplan-Meier method was used to analyze the OS, with log-rank test used to examine group differences. Cox regression model was used for multivariate analysis. All statistical analyses were performed using SPSS software package (version 20.0; SPSS Inc., Chicago). A p-value of <0.05 was considered statistically significant.

Results

A total of 70 HCC patients with PVTT were irradiated and included in this analysis. Table 2 shows the patients' characteristics, classification of PVTT and radiotherapy scheme. The median age at diagnosis of PVTT was 53.8 years (range: 25–75). The median time from primary HCC diagnosis to SBRT treatment was 7 months (range: 0–85). The median time interval between diagnosis of PVTT and SBRT treatment was 1.2 months (range 0–12). Tumor thrombosis involving the first order portal vein branches without main portal vein involvement (TypeII) was found in 42 patients (60%). Twenty- seven patients (38.6%) had tumor thrombosis invading the main trunk (Type III), one patient (1.4%) had tumor thrombosis invaded the superior mesenteric vein, portal vein main trunk and both first branches (Type IV).

Twenty patients (28.6%) received SBRT alone. Another 46 (65.7%) patients received TACE (1–5 cycles, median 2.4 cycles) after SBRT; among them, 3 underwent further radioactive seeds implantation, and one received

Table 2 Patient characteristics

Characteristics	n (%)
Age, y	
≥ 50	48 (68.6)
< 50	22 (31.4)
Gender	
Male	59 (84.3)
Female	11 (15.7)
Therapeutic modalities	
SBRT alone	20 (28.6)
SBRT+TACE	46 (65.7)
SBRT+Surgery	4 (5.7)
Dose, Gy	
≤ 35.0	29 (41.4)
≥ 40.0	41 (58.6)
Types of PVTT	
II	42 (60.0)
III	27 (38.6)
IV	1 (1.4)
HBsAg	
Negative	12 (17.1)
Positive	58 (82.9)
Child-Pugh classification	
A	45 (64.3)
B	24 (34.3)
C	1 (1.4)
PS (ECOG)	
0	56 (80.0)
1	14 (20.0)
Origination of PVTT	
Right branch	49 (70.0)
Left branch	21 (30.0)
AFP, ng/L	
≤ 20	13 (18.6)
21 ~ 399	17 (24.3)
≥ 400	40 (57.1)
PLT, 10^9/L	
≥ 100	39 (55.7)
< 100	31 (44.3)
HGB, g/L	
≥ 120	42 (60.0)
< 120	28 (40.0)
TBIL, μmol/L	
≥ 20	34 (48.6)
< 20	36 (51.4)
Albumin, g/L	

Table 2 Patient characteristics (Continued)

Characteristics	n (%)
≥ 35	41 (58.6)
< 35	29 (41.4)
ALT, U/L	
≥ 50	25 (35.7)
< 50	45 (64.3)
AST, U/L	
≥ 50	48 (68.6)
< 50	22 (31.4)

Abbreviations: SBRT Stereotactic body radiotherapy, Types types of tumor thrombi, HBsAg Hepatitis B surface antigen, PS Performance status, ECOG Eastern Cooperative Oncology Group, AFP Alpha–fetoprotein, PLT Platelet, HGB Hemoglobin, TBIL Total bilirubin, ALT Alanine aminotransferase, AST Aspartate aminotransferase

radiofrequency ablation (RFA) after TACE. The final 4 (5.7%) patients underwent surgery, including 3 with respective liver lobectomy at 3, 8 and 10 weeks after SBRT, and one patient underwent liver transplantation 4 weeks after SBRT.

PVTT response

Fifty-three cases had contrast-enhanced CT/MRI around 4 weeks after SBRT, partial response (PR), stable disease (SD), and progression disease (PD) were observed in 41 (77.4%), 8 (15.1%), and 4 (7.5%), respectively. While none had achieved complete response (CR) by this time point, there were 5 patients (9.4%) reached near CR with minimal residual disease less than 10% of original enhanced size. Local control (LC) (inclusive of partial and stable response) was thus achieved in 92.5% of the treated lesions.

At 3 months after SBRT, 62 patients were assessed for PVTT therapeutic responses. CR, PR, and SD were observed in 6 (9.7%), 43 (69.4%), and 4 (6.4%) of the patients, respectively. LC (inclusive of CR, PR and SD) was achieved in 85.5% of the treated lesions. The rest 9 patients (14.5%) had PD, including 3 cases having developed PD at the first follow-up.

Six months after SBRT, assessments of PVTT therapeutic response were done in 31 patients, CR, PR, SD, and PD were observed in 10 (32.2%), 16 (51.6%), 2 (6.4%), and 3 (9.8%) (including 1 case evaluated as PD beforehand) patients, respectively. Sixteen patients had follow-up imaging around 9 months after SBRT, and the respective CR and PR rate were 56.25% (9 patients) and 43.75% (7), with the corresponding figures at 12 months being 66.7% (10) and 33.3% (5).

Of the 57 patients with elevated AFP levels before SBRT, 29 patients (54.7%) exhibited ≥50% reduction in the AFP levels within one month after SBRT, with 6 cases (11.3%) had AFP in the normal range.

Overall survival

With median follow-up period of 9.5 months, 25 patients (35.7%) were still alive at the time of the current analysis. The median survival time for the whole group was 10.0 months (95% CI, 7.7–12.3), with 6- and 12-month OS rates of 67.3%, and 40.0%, respectively (Fig. 2a).

Median survival times were 12.0 ± 1.6 and 3 ± 1.0 months for those receiving TACE after SBRT and SBRT alone, respectively. Patients who received combined treatments of SBRT and TACE showed significantly longer OS than those unable to undergo TACE after SBRT ($p < 0.001$; Fig. 2b). The 6- and 12-month OS rates were 82.8%, and 49.7% for patients receiving SBRT plus TACE, and 30.0%, and 10.0% for those receiving SBRT alone. Four patients underwent tumor resection after SBRT, with 1 patient died at the fourth month while the other 3 were alive at their respective follow-up time of 13, 15 and 15 months.

The median survival time for patients with PR, SD and PD of the PVTT at 3 months after completion of SBRT was 13.0, 8.0 and 4.0 months respectively. The median survival for the 6 patients with CR was deficiency because only 2 patients died at seventh and eleventh month. The other 4 patients remained alive, with 1 patient assessed at 15-month and 3 at 16-month follow-up points after SBRT. The median survival times for patients with LC (inclusive of CR, PR and SD) of the PVTT were better than those with PD after SBRT (13.0 vs. 4.0 months, $p < 0.001$) (Fig. 2c).

Interestingly, patients with PVTT at the left branch location seemed to have longer median OS than those with thrombosis in the right branch of portal vein (13.0 vs. 8.0 months, $P = 0.079$) (Fig. 2d, Table 3).

Toxicity

Patients tolerated the SBRT generally well, since a very mild pattern of acute toxicity was observed. No treatment-related deaths or serious adverse events were seen within 3 months after SBRT. Acute radiation side effects were mild, including nausea, vomiting, anorexia, and abdominal pain in some cases. Grade-3 leukopenia and thrombocytopenia were seen in 5 (7.1%) and 4 (5.7%) patients, respectively. Grade-3 liver enzyme and bilirubin elevation were found in 3 (4.3%) and 8 (8.6%) cases, while grade-3 albumin decrease was seen in 11 (15.7%). No grade-4 hematologic toxicity, liver enzyme, bilirubin and albumin level change was seen. No radiation induced liver disease was encountered in the entire patient group. Later toxicities such as gastrointestinal stenosis, bleeding, perforation and ulcer were not observed during the follow-up periods.

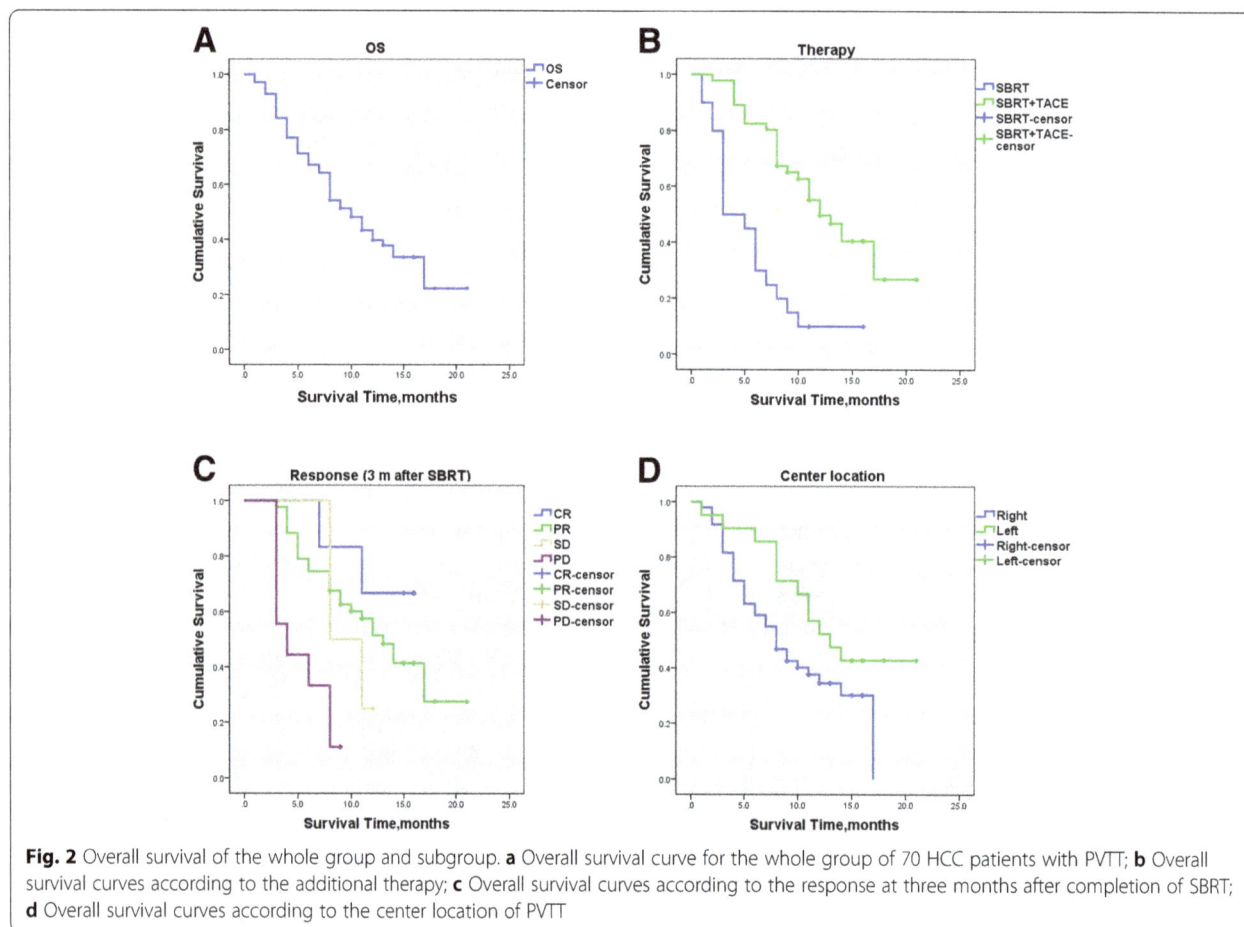

Fig. 2 Overall survival of the whole group and subgroup. **a** Overall survival curve for the whole group of 70 HCC patients with PVTT; **b** Overall survival curves according to the additional therapy; **c** Overall survival curves according to the response at three months after completion of SBRT; **d** Overall survival curves according to the center location of PVTT

Only one patient (1.4%) showed progression of Child-Pugh class from A to C within 3 months after SBRT, while progression from class B to C was observed in 2 cases. All these 3 patients were deteriorated due to intrahepatic tumor progression. Downgrading of Child-Pugh class from B to A was observed in 3 cases.

Discussion

In the present study, SBRT was used as the first therapy for the management of HCC patients with extensive PVTT. These patients were originally unsuitable for surgery or had contraindication for TACE. SBRT induced prominent response in the PVTT. The objective response rate at 1, 3, 6 months were 77.4%, 79.1% and 83.8%, respectively. Within 1 month after SBRT, 5 cases reached near CR, i.e., minimal residual disease less than 10% of initial lesion. Remarkably, the CR rate increased with time, from 9.7% at 3 months to 32.2% at 6 months after SBRT. For the 16 patients with imaging reassessment at 9 months after treatment, more than half achieved CR. Progression after SBRT was found in about 17.1% of the cases, with most PD occuring within the first 3 months. In our series, 4 patients had PD of the

PVTT within 1 month, 6 between 1 and 3 months, and only 2 patients at 6 months. To the best of our knowledge, this appears to be the first report describing the dynamic changes of tumor thrombosis after SBRT.

Around 70% of our PVTT cases shrank to a degree of PR in the first few weeks. Most achieved restoration of portal vein flow, which relieved the associated symptoms and made it feasible for patients to endure further interventional therapies. The strategy seems practical to shrink the thrombosis and restore the portal flow by SBRT, thus enable the patients to have the opportunity to receive subsequent treatments, such as tumor resection or TACE procedure.

The median survival time from the start of SBRT for this patient series was 10.0 months, with the respective 6- and 12-month OS rates of 67.3% and 40.0%. Published results concerning SBRT in the treatment of PVTT are scarce, and median survival time has been reported to vary from 8 to 13 months, with 1-year OS rate from 43.2 to 50.3% [22, 26, 27]. In a prospective study of phase I and II trials reported by Bujold et al. [28], 56 HCC patients with tumor thrombosis showed a 1-year OS rate of 44% after SBRT, with which our result seems

Table 3 Analysis of prognostic factors for survival

	N	Median survival (month; 95% CI)	p values
Gender			0.13
Male	59	11.0 (7.6–14.4)	
Female	11	8.0 (1.5–14.5)	
Age, y			0.033
<50	22	17.0 (17.0–17.0)	
≥ 50	48	8.0 (6.3–9.7)	
AFP, ng/L			0.438
≤ 20	14	8.0 (2.9–13.1)	
21–399	18	14.0 (11.9–16.1)	
≥ 400	38	8.0 (5.6–10.4)	
Additional treatment after RT			0.00
SBRT alone	20	3.0 (1.1–4.9)	
SBRT+TACE	46	12.0 (8.9–15.1)	
Radiation Dose			0.376
≤ 27.5Gy	4	3.0 (0–8.9)	
30–35Gy	25	8.0 (6.8–9.2)	
≥ 40Gy	41	11.0 (7.7–14.3)	
Origination of PVTT			0.079
Right branch	49	8.0 (5.8–10.2)	
Left branch	21	13.0 (8.5–17.5)	
Type of tumor thrombosis			0.107
Type II	42	8.0 (5.5–10.5)	
Type III	27	14.0 (8.6–19.4)	
Response (3 m after SBRT)			0.000
CR	6	*	
PR	43	13.0 (10.0–16.0)	
SD	4	**	
PD	9	4.0 (1.1–6.9)	

Abbreviations: *SBRT* Stereotactic body radiotherapy, *AFP* Alpha-fetoprotein, *RT* Radiotherapy, *CR* Complete response, *PR* Partial response, *SD* Stable disease, *PD* Progressive disease. * The medium survival for patients with CR was not reported because only two patients died in 7th and 11th month. The other four patients were alive, 1 patient with 15 months follow-up, 3 patients with 16 months follow-up after SBRT. ** In the four patients with SD, 3 patients died in the 8th, 8th and 11th month, the other patient was alive with 12 months follow-up

comparable. With a median survival time of 12 months, our patients who got the chance to receive TACE after SBRT had longer survival time that is comparable to the results of the previous reports [27]. It is remarkable that patients in the present study were originally considered to harbor unresectable tumor or had contraindication for TACE. This subgroup of patients was expected to have lower OS rate. In view of such adverse baseline characteristics, the therapeutic outcome with median OS of 10 months seems satisfactory.

For the 5 patients who achieved near CR within the first few weeks, all were alive at the last follow-up times

of 20, 17, 17, 16, and 10 months respectively. Those had CR at 3 months after SBRT also showed longer OS. Patients with good PVTT response to SBRT usually have better survival. As for the radiation dose, patients receiving 40 Gy or more seems to have longer OS (Table 3). Hence, We suggest higher radiation dose (≥40Gy in 5 fractions) for the SBRT treatment of PVTT, with the aim of achieving adequate therapeutic response and better survival.

The natural history of HCC patients with PVTT dictates only 2.4–4 months of survival duration [8]. Although Sorafenib provided a significant survival benefit in randomized phase III trials, the gain was modest (2–3 months) [29, 30]. Radiotherapy may improve survival chance for such patients. Yeh et al. reported a large series of HCC with PVTT treated by conventional three-dimensional conformal radiotherapy (3D-CRT), but the median survival time was only 7.0 months [31]. Matsuo et al. compared the efficacy of SBRT with 3D-CRT in the management of PVTT and better therapeutic results for the former was observed, with 1-year OS rates of 49.3% in SBRT group vs. 29.3% in 3D-CRT group. Taking all the results into consideration, SBRT seems to be of therapeutic benefit for HCC patients with PVTT, especially for those who had contraindication for TACE or surgery.

SBRT was well tolerated in our patient series. Only mild radiation acute side effects were observed in some of cases. No treatment-related deaths or serious adverse events were encountered. Furthermore, no radiation induced liver disease was observed, even in those receiving TACE after SBRT. Those who experienced deterioration of liver function were mainly due to intrahepatic tumor progression. The low toxicity of SBRT in the management of PVTT was in line with the results of other SBRT studies [26, 27].

There are several limitations of the present study that should be addressed. First, only contrast enhanced CT and/or MRI were used for the assessment of PVTT response, at 1, 3, and then every 3 months after SBRT. If liver vessel Doppler scan had been utilized in this study, the portal vein blood flow changes after SBRT might have been detected with higher frequency. Since Doppler exams could be repeated in shorter intervals, more information could have been collected in this respect. Second, the study was retrospective, with widely varied therapeutic modalities after SBRT for this group of patients, including TACE, surgical resection, and one liver transplantation. In addition, some patients received different number of TACE sessions. These could represent sources of bias for the observed data, and one should be cautious in the interpretation of the clinical outcomes. A well designed prospective study is warranted to validate the results.

Conclusions

SBRT can be used as the first-line therapy for HCC patients with extensive PVTT originally considered unsuitable for surgical resection or TACE. The dynamic change of tumor thrombosis in time after SBRT has been described. Thrombus shrinkage and portal vein flow restoration can be achieved in the majority of cases. Thereafter, SBRT may enable patients to pursue consolidative local treatments, such as surgery and TACE procedure. Such therapeutic strategy may result in improved survival benefit, especially for those who do receive further therapies after SBRT.

Abbreviations

3D-CRT: Three-dimensional conformal radiotherapy; AFP: Alpha-fetoprotein; CTCAE: Common Terminology Criteria for Adverse Events; D1cc: Maximal dose to 1 cc; HCC: Hepatocellular carcinoma; LC: Local control; mRECIST: Modified Response Evaluation Criteria in Solid Tumors; OARs: Organs at risk; OS: Overall survival; PD: Progressive disease; PR: Partial response; PVTT: Portal vein tumor thrombus; SBRT: Stereotactic body radiotherapy; SD: Stable disease; TACE: Transarterial chemoembolization

Acknowledgements
The authors would like to thank Professor Steve P. Lee from Department of Radiation Oncology, UCLA for editorial assistance.

Funding
This study was supported by the National Natural Science Foundation of China (Grant No. 81572952).

Authors' contributions

YJS participated in the design of the study and wrote the manuscript; WY and JX carried out the clinical data analysis and participated in writing of the manuscript; XQR, YLG, and BCZ interpreted the clinical data; TM and JJW contribute with the clinical data of TACE; QHL and QGH read and interpreted the CT and MRI image. LS, XLB and TBL contribute with the clinical data of surgery and radiotherapy; QCW conceived the study and wrote the manuscript. All authors read and approved the final manuscript.

Competing interests

The authors declare that they have no competing interests.

Author details
[1]Department of Radiation Oncology, The Second Affiliated Hospital, Zhejiang University School of Medicine, Jiefang Road 88, Hangzhou 310009, People's Republic of China. [2]Department of Hepatobiliary and Pancreatic Surgery, Zhejiang Provincial Key Laboratory of Pancreatic Disease, The Second Affiliated Hospital, Zhejiang University School of Medicine, Hangzhou 310009, People's Republic of China. [3]Department of Radiology, The Second Affiliated Hospital, Zhejiang University School of Medicine, Hangzhou 310009, People's Republic of China. [4]Ministry of Education Key Laboratory of Cancer Prevention and Intervention, Zhejiang University Cancer Institute, Hangzhou 310009, People's Republic of China.

References
1. Siegel RL, Miller KD, Jemal A. Cancer Statistics, 2017. CA Cancer J Clin. 2017; 67(1):7–30.
2. Chen W, Zheng R, Baade PD, et al. Cancer statistics in China, 2015. CA Cancer J Clin. 2016;66(2):115–32.
3. Roayaie S, Blume IN, Thung SN, et al. A system of classifying microvascular invasion to predict outcome after resection in patients with hepatocellular carcinoma. Gastroenterology. 2009;137(3):850–5.
4. Yuan BH, Yuan WP, Li RH, et al. Propensity score-based comparison of hepatic resection and transarterial chemoembolization for patients with advanced hepatocellular carcinoma. Tumour Biol. 2016;37(2):2435–41.
5. Zhang ZM, Lai EC, Zhang C, et al. The strategies for treating primary hepatocellular carcinoma with portal vein tumor thrombus. Int J Surg. 2015; 20:8–16.
6. Chan SL, Chong CC, Chan AW, Poon DM, Chok KS. Management of hepatocellular carcinoma with portal vein tumor thrombosis: Review and update at 2016. World J Gastroenterol. 2016;22(32):7289–300.
7. Zhong JH, Peng NF, You XM, et al. Tumor stage and primary treatment of hepatocellular carcinoma at a large tertiary hospital in China: A real-world study. Oncotarget. 2017;8(11):18296–302.
8. Schöniger-Hekele M, Müller C, Kutilek M, Oesterreicher C, Ferenci P, Gangl A. Hepatocellular carcinoma in Central Europe: prognostic features and survival. Gut. 2001;48(1):103–9.
9. Li SH, Wei W, Guo RP, et al. Long-term outcomes after curative resection for patients with macroscopically solitary hepatocellular carcinoma without macrovascular invasion and an analysis of prognostic factors. Med Oncol. 2013;30(4):696.
10. Li SH, Guo ZX, Xiao CZ, et al. Risk factors for early and late intrahepatic recurrence in patients with single hepatocellular carcinoma without macrovascular invasion after curative resection. Asian Pac J Cancer Prev. 2013;14(8):4759–63.
11. Bruix J, Sherman M. Management of hepatocellular carcinoma: an update. Hepatology. 2011;53(3):1020–2.
12. Cheng S, Yang J, Shen F, et al. Multidisciplinary management of hepatocellular carcinoma with portal vein tumor thrombus - Eastern Hepatobiliary Surgical Hospital consensus statement. Oncotarget. 2016;7(26): 40816–29.
13. Kokudo T, Hasegawa K, Matsuyama Y, et al. Survival benefit of liver resection for hepatocellular carcinoma associated with portal vein invasion. J Hepatol. 2016;65(5):938–43.
14. Chen XP, Qiu FZ, Wu ZD, et al. Effects of location and extension of portal vein tumor thrombus on long-term outcomes of surgical treatment for hepatocellular carcinoma. Ann Surg Oncol. 2006;13(7):940–6.
15. Peng ZW, Guo RP, Zhang YJ, Lin XJ, Chen MS, Lau WY. Hepatic resection versus transcatheter arterial chemoembolization for the treatment of hepatocellular carcinoma with portal vein tumor thrombus. Cancer. 2012; 118(19):4725–36.
16. Chok KS, Cheung TT, Chan SC, Poon RT, Fan ST, Lo CM. Surgical outcomes in hepatocellular carcinoma patients with portal vein tumor thrombosis. World J Surg. 2014;38(2):490–6.
17. Katagiri S, Yamamoto M. Multidisciplinary treatments for hepatocellular carcinoma with major portal vein tumor thrombus. Surg Today. 2014;44(2): 219–26.
18. Omata M, Lesmana LA, Tateishi R, et al. Asian Pacific Association for the Study of the Liver consensus recommendations on hepatocellular carcinoma. Hepatol Int. 2010;4(2):439–74.
19. Kudo M, Matsui O, Izumi N, et al. JSH consensus-based clinical practice guidelines for the management of hepatocellular carcinoma: 2014 update by the liver cancer study group of Japan. Liver Cancer. 2014;3(3–4):458–68.
20. Yu JI, Park HC. Radiotherapy as valid modality for hepatocellular carcinoma with portal vein tumor thrombosis. World J Gastroenterol. 2016;22(30):6851–63.
21. Matsuo Y, Yoshida K, Nishimura H, et al. Efficacy of stereotactic body radiotherapy for hepatocellular carcinoma with portal vein tumor thrombosis/inferior vena cava tumor thrombosis: evaluation by comparison

Stereotactic body radiotherapy based treatment for hepatocellular carcinoma with extensive portal...

21

with conventional three-dimensional conformal radiotherapy. J Radiat Res. 2016;57(5):512–23.

22. Xi M, Zhang L, Zhao L, et al. Effectiveness of stereotactic body radiotherapy for hepatocellular carcinoma with portal vein and/or inferior vena cava tumor thrombosis. PLoS One. 2013;8(5):e63864.

23. Bruix J, Sherman M. Management of hepatocellular carcinoma. Hepatology. 2005;42(5):1208–36.

24. Shuqun C, Mengchao W, Han C, et al. Tumor thrombus types influence the prognosis of hepatocellular carcinoma with the tumor thrombi in the portal vein. Hepatogastroenterology. 2007;54(74):499–502.

25. Lencioni R, Llovet JM. Modified RECIST (mRECIST) assessment for hepatocellular carcinoma. Semin Liver Dis. 2010;30(1):52–60.

26. Lee SU, Park JW, Kim TH, et al. Effectiveness and safety of proton beam therapy for advanced hepatocellular carcinoma with portal vein tumor thrombosis. Strahlenther Onkol. 2014;190(9):806–14.

27. Kang J, Nie Q, Du R, et al. Stereotactic body radiotherapy combined with transarterial chemoembolization for hepatocellular carcinoma with portal vein tumor thrombosis. Mol Clin Oncol. 2014;2(1):43–50.

28. Bujold A, Massey CA, Kim JJ, et al. Sequential phase I and II trials of stereotactic body radiotherapy for locally advanced hepatocellular carcinoma. J Clin Oncol. 2013;31(13):1631–9.

29. Llovet JM, Ricci S, Mazzaferro V, et al. Sorafenib in advanced hepatocellular carcinoma. N Engl J Med. 2008;359(4):378–90.

30. Cheng AL, Kang YK, Chen Z, et al. Efficacy and safety of sorafenib in patients in the Asia-Pacific region with advanced hepatocellular carcinoma: a phase III randomised, double-blind, placebo-controlled trial. Lancet Oncol. 2009;10(1):25–34.

31. Yeh SA, Chen YS, Perng DS. The role of radiotherapy in the treatment of hepatocellular carcinoma with portal vein tumor thrombus. J Radiat Res. 2015;56(2):325–31.

3

Development of a PMMA phantom as a practical alternative for quality control of gamma knife® dosimetry

Jae Pil Chung[1], Young Min Seong[1], Tae Yeon Kim[2], Yona Choi[2], Tae Hoon Kim[3], Hyun Joon Choi[4], Chul Hee Min[4], Hamza Benmakhlouf[5], Kook Jin Chun[2*] and Hyun-Tai Chung[6*]

Abstract

Background: To measure the absorbed dose rate to water and penumbra of a Gamma Knife® (GK) using a polymethyl metacrylate (PMMA) phantom.

Methods: A multi-purpose PMMA phantom was developed to measure the absorbed dose rate to water and the dose distribution of a GK. The phantom consists of a hemispherical outer phantom, one exchangeable cylindrical chamber-hosting inner phantom, and two film-hosting inner phantoms. The radius of the phantom was determined considering the electron density of the PMMA such that it corresponds to 8 g/cm^2 water depth, which is the reference depth of the absorbed dose measurement of GK. The absorbed dose rate to water was measured with a PTW TN31010 chamber, and the dose distributions were measured with radiochromic films at the calibration center of a patient positioning system of a GK Perfexion. A spherical water-filled phantom with the same water equivalent depth was constructed as a reference phantom. The dose rate to water and dose distributions at the center of a circular field delimited by a 16-mm collimator were measured with the PMMA phantom at six GK Perfexion sites.

Results: The radius of the PMMA phantom was determined to be 6.93 cm, corresponding to equivalent water depth of 8 g/cm^2. The absorbed dose rate to water was measured with the PMMA phantom, the spherical water-filled phantom and a commercial solid water phantom. The measured dose rate with the PMMA phantom was 1.2% and 1.8% higher than those measured with the spherical water-filled phantom and the solid water phantom, respectively. These differences can be explained by the scattered photon contribution of PMMA off incoming ^{60}Co gamma-rays to the dose rate. The average full width half maximum and penumbra values measured with the PMMA phantom showed reasonable agreement with two calculated values, one at the center of the PMMA phantom (LGP6.93) and other at the center of a water sphere with a radius of 8 cm (LGP8.0) given by Leksell Gamma Plan using the TMR10 algorithm.

Conclusions: A PMMA phantom constructed in this study to measure the absorbed dose rates to water and dose distributions of a GK represents an acceptable and practical alternative for GK dosimetry considering its cost-effectiveness and ease of handling.

Keywords: Gamma knife, PMMA phantom, Quality control, Absorbed dose rate to water, Dose distribution, Penumbra, Scattered photon contribution

* Correspondence: chunkj@korea.ac.kr; htchung@snu.ac.kr
[2]Department of Accelerator Science, Korea University Sejong Campus, 2511 Sejong-ro, Sejong 30019, Korea
[6]Department of Neurosurgery, Seoul National University College of Medicine, 101 Daehak-ro Jongno-gu, Seoul 03080, Korea
Full list of author information is available at the end of the article

Background

The absorbed dose to water and dose distribution penumbra are essential parameters that need to be accurately determined in radiation therapy because their values are directly applied to build treatment plans. For the measurement of the absorbed dose to water, two protocols are generally used in radiotherapy: TG-51, published by the American Association of Physicists in Medicine (AAPM) in 1999, and TRS-398, published by the International Atomic Energy Agency (IAEA) in 2004 [1, 2]. Both protocols require calibration of the ionization chamber in a water-filled parallelepiped phantom for ^{60}Co beam and dosimetric measurement using the calibrated chamber in the user beam with a same or similar phantom. Other conditions required for this measurement, such as the source to surface distance (SSD), field size (FS), reference depth, etc., are well described in the protocols.

However, when we attempted to apply these protocols to the Gamma Knife® (GK; Elekta AB, Stockholm, Sweden), we confronted problems in applying the conditions of the protocols. First, the conditions specified for the calibration are no longer valid in a GK. In the GK, approximately 200 gamma-ray beams are focused into the patient positioning system (PPS) calibration center instead of being irradiated along a certain direction. Therefore, it is not possible to define a specific SSD, FS, or other parameters of the standard protocols, and unique conditions must be established. Second, no water phantom has been used in the absorbed dose to water measurement of the GK [3]. This dose is usually measured with phantoms made of two types of plastics, acrylonitrile butadiene styrene (ABS) and solid water (Gamex Model 457, SUN NUCLEAR Co., Melbourne, FL, USA). Although the different radiological characteristics between the plastic phantom and the water phantom must be carefully taken into account, they are neglected in most instances. In order to overcome this factor, the authors developed a spherical water-filled phantom with an equivalent water depth (EWD) of 8 g/cm^2 and showed that there could be approximately a 2% difference in dose rates measured by the spherical water-filled phantom and two ABS phantoms [4]. Although it is expected that the spherical water-filled phantom provides a more accurate value of the absorbed dose rate to water, there are practical obstacles for using this kind of phantom in ordinary clinical settings due to difficulties in management and risk of damage at the center of the GK during measurement. The solid water phantom (Leksell Gamma Knife Dosimetry Phantom, Elekta, Stockholm, Sweden) represents an alternative because it should have a response to radiation equivalent to water. However, because of its high price, this option is not likely to be generally accepted. Recently, IAEA published a technical reports series no.483 (IAEA TRS-483) [5] and provided a code of practice for dose determination of non-standard fields. IAEA TRS-483 recommended to use plastic phantoms and presented the output correction factors for several combinations of ion chambers and two phantoms from the GK manufacturer. Though it can be accepted as a standard in the clinical sites, it did not provide correction factors for other phantom materials and there are still debates on the exact values of the correction factors such as the study from Mirzakhanian et al. [6].

In this study, we developed a polymethyl metacrylate (PMMA) phantom for GK dosimetry that will be of great use for general GK dosimetry. A calibration factor to convert the measured value to the absorbed dose rate to water was determined by comparing the dose rates of a GK Perfexion measured with the PMMA phantom to those obtained with the spherical water-filled phantom. This factor was also verified by two independent Monte Carlo simulations. For quality assurance of the absolute dose rate measurement and relative dose distribution with the same phantom, two types of inner phantoms were manufactured to accommodate an ionization chamber and radiochromic films.

Methods

Construction of the PMMA phantom

A multi-purpose PMMA phantom for measurement of the absorbed dose to water and dose distributions of a GK was constructed. The phantom material was chosen to be PMMA, which was recommended by IAEA as a water substitute and is commonly used in radiation dosimetry. Considering the geometrical distribution of the ^{60}Co sources in a GK, the phantom was designed to be cylindrically symmetric, and the radius was intended to be 8.00 g/cm^2 of equivalent water depth, which was suggested by IAEA/AAPM [5] as the reference depth for measurement of the absorbed dose rate to water in GK dosimetry. The physical radius of the phantom was determined via an electron density comparison between the PMMA and water [7]. The electron density of the PMMA was calculated as follows:

$$\rho_{\text{PMMA}}^{\text{el}} = \rho_{\text{PMMA}}^{\text{mass}} \times \left[\sum_i f_i \left(\frac{z}{A} \right)_i \right], \qquad (1)$$

where $\rho_{\text{PMMA}}^{\text{mass}}$ is the bulk density of PMMA, f_i is the fraction by weight of the atom i, and $\left(\frac{z}{A} \right)_i$ is the atomic number weight ratio. The radius of the phantom was then obtained from the following equation:

$$r_{PMMA} = r_{EWD} \frac{\rho^{el}_{H_2O}}{\rho^{el}_{PMMA}}, \qquad (2)$$

where r_{PMMA} is the physical radius of the PMMA phantom, r_{EWD} is the equivalent water depth, $\rho^{el}_{H_2O}$ is the electron density of water, and ρ^{el}_{PMMA} is the electron density of PMMA.

The phantom consisted of an outer phantom and exchangeable inner phantoms, as well as one chamber-hosting inner phantom and two film-hosting inner phantoms. One of the film-hosting inner phantoms was designed to set the film in the xy-plane (axial plane) of the Leksell stereotactic coordinate system, and the other was in the xz-plane (sagittal plane). The detailed structure of phantom was drawn using AutoCAD 2D and 3D tools (version 2014, Autodesk Inc.) and the PMMA was machined to a tolerance of 0.002 cm. To minimize deformation of the PMMA due to heat generated by machining, soluble cutting oil was applied continuously during the process. Schematic diagrams of the PMMA phantom and photographs of the outer and inner phantoms are presented in Fig. 1. The radius of the hemispherical portion of the outer phantom was 6.93 cm. The outer phantom was firmly attached to the Leksell G-frame (Elekta AB, Stockholm, Sweden) as shown in Fig. 1c. Each inner phantom was tightly fitted into the outer

phantom with the smallest possible air gap to allow the entire phantom to be approximated as homogeneous. There was a directional guide on each phantom to maintain the relative orientation.

Measurement of absorbed dose to water

For the measurement of the absorbed dose rate to water, a PTW TN31010 ionization chamber and a Keithley 6517B electrometer (Keithley Instruments Inc., Cleveland, OH, USA) were used to measure the dose rate of the 16-mm collimator from a Gamma Knife Perfexion. The PTW TN31010, with a nominal sensitive volume of 0.125 cm^3 and inner radius of 0.275 cm, is recommended for the measurement of dose rate in the GK by the manufacturer. Calibration of the ionization chamber in terms of the absorbed dose to water was carried out at the dosimetry laboratory of the Korea Research Institute of Standards and Science (KRISS), which is a national standard institute in Korea associated with the International Bureau of Weights and Measures (BIPM). A Mensor Model 2105 precision barometer (MENSOR Corp., San Marcos, USA) was used for pressure measurement, and an ASL F250 precision thermometer (Automatic Systems Laboratories, Croydon, UK) was used for temperature measurement. The barometer and thermometer were calibrated annually at the Center for Thermometry and the Center for Mass and Related Quantities, KRISS. Temperature and pressure were measured simultaneously with the ionization

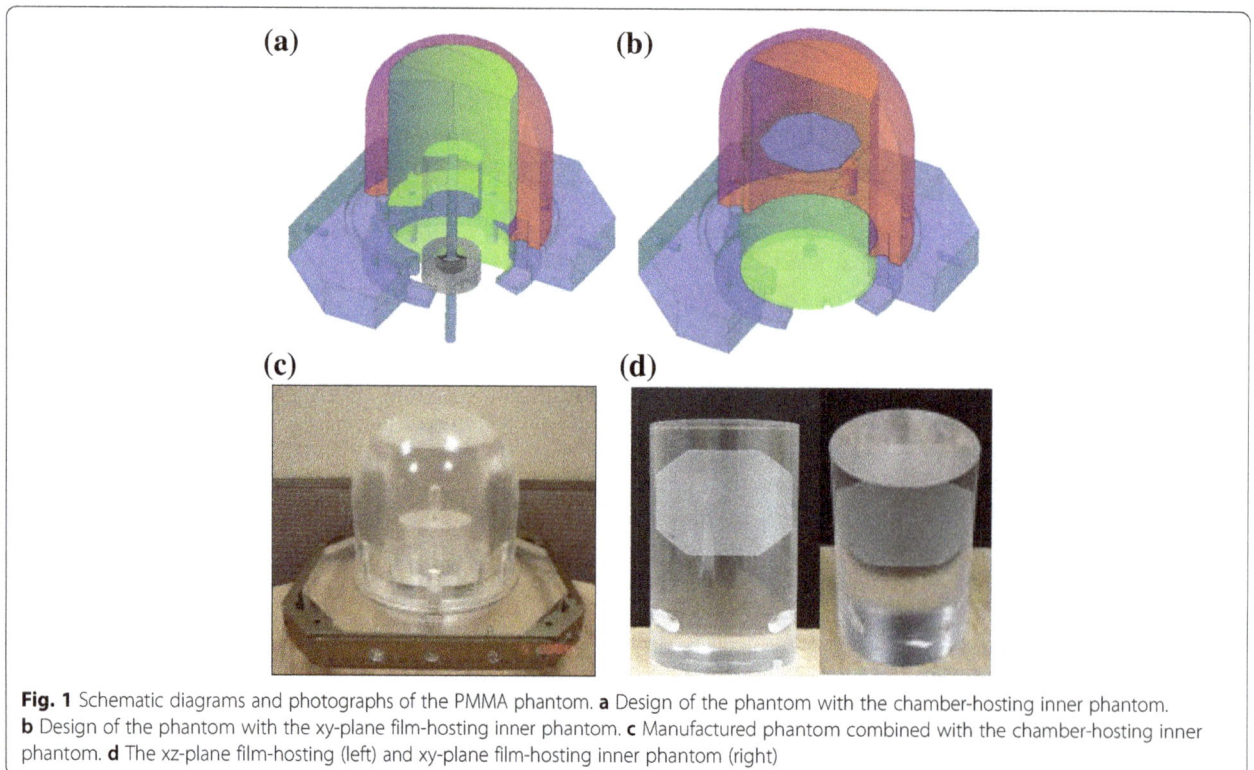

Fig. 1 Schematic diagrams and photographs of the PMMA phantom. **a** Design of the phantom with the chamber-hosting inner phantom. **b** Design of the phantom with the xy-plane film-hosting inner phantom. **c** Manufactured phantom combined with the chamber-hosting inner phantom. **d** The xz-plane film-hosting (left) and xy-plane film-hosting inner phantom (right)

current. The absorbed dose rate to water of the 16-mm collimator of a GK Perfexion™ (Elekta AB, Stockholm, Sweden) was measured with the PTW TN31010 chamber inserted into the chamber-hosting inner phantom (Fig. 2a). To estimate the contribution by the scattered photon in the phantom material, the dose rate at the center of a spherical water-filled phantom was also measured (as shown in Fig. 2b) and used as a reference value. The structure and material of the spherical water-filled phantom were described in detail in a previous report [4]. For the comparison, the commercial solid water phantom (Elekta, Sweden) was also used for measurement of the dose rate (Fig. 2c).

Monte Carlo simulation of the scattering contribution

Seco and Evans [7] reported that the electron-density scaling method considering only Compton scattering can predict primary photon fluences in commonly used plastic materials to within a 0.5% difference from those in water by Monte Carlo simulations with a 1-MeV photon pencil beam with a diameter of 0.1 mm. The remaining discrepancies can be attributed to other scattered photon contributions, and their effects cannot be generally predicted because they depend on various factors such as the phantom geometry, beam shape, and beam energy. In the present study, the effect of the scattered photons in the PMMA phantom was measured by comparing the dose rates measured in the PMMA phantom and the water-filled phantom. To verify the measured value, Monte Carlo simulations were performed with a simplified geometry. The absorbed doses to a water sphere with a diameter of 5.5 mm located at the center of a spherical water phantom with a radius of 8.0 cm and a spherical PMMA phantom with a radius of 6.93 cm were simulated. The diameter of 5.5 mm was chosen to be the same as the diameter of the active volume of the PTW 31010 ionization chamber. The standard chemical composition of PMMA $(C_5O_2H_8)_n$ and a mass density of 1.1847 g/cm^3 were used in the simulation. The geometry of a GK Perfexion was obtained from the vendor. Three independent Monte Carlo simulations were performed. In a simulation with Geant 4 version 10.02 [8], five runs with 1.92×10^{10} histories were executed for each phantom, and their averaged values were compared. The PENELOPE low-energy electromagnetic model of Geant4 was used, and the range cut value was 0.1 mm for all kinds of particles. When the dose distributions generated by this simulation were compared with those from Leksell Gamma Plan (LGP) version 11.0 [9], the pixels with absorbed doses larger than or equal to 20% of the maximum dose showed global gamma index pass rates of 99.4% and 99.5% under 1 mm/3% criteria in the axial and sagittal planes, respectively. In another simulation with Geant 4 version 10.02 [8], which was performed by a separate team with independent code generation, a phase space file for the 16-mm

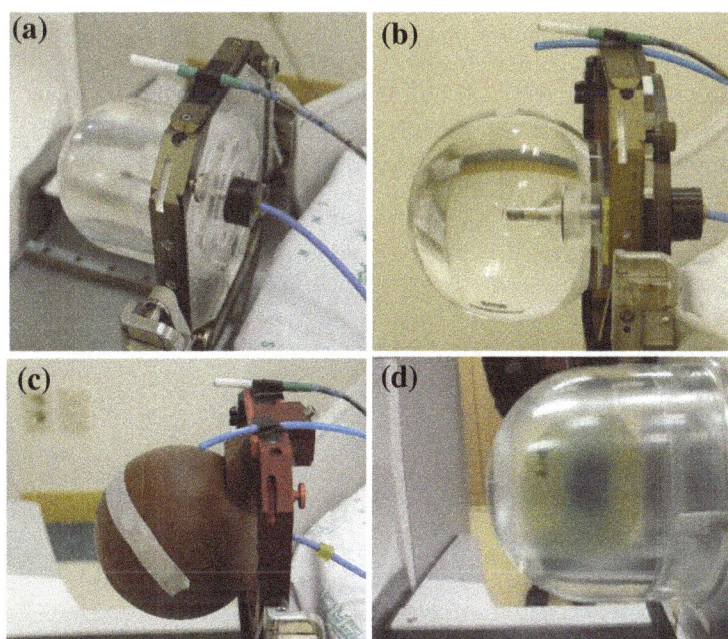

Fig. 2 Pictures of the experimental setup for measurement of the absorbed dose to water with different phantoms. a The PMMA phantom with a PTW 31010 ionization chamber was mounted to the Leksell Gamma Knife Perfexion for dose rate measurement. b The spherical water-filled phantom with a PTW 31010 ionization chamber. c A solid water phantom with a PTW 31010 ionization chamber. d The PMMA phantom with the xz-plane film-hosting inner phantom. The film shows the dose distribution of the 16-mm collimator in the xz-plane

collimator along a single direction was built by generating 1.08×10^{10} photons from the ^{60}Co source. The generated phase space file had 3.33×10^8 particles. Using the phase space file, six simulation runs with 6.66×10^8 histories were performed for each phantom and the averaged values were compared. The physics model of Geant 4 and the range cut value were the same as in the simulation described above. In the third simulation, the user-code penEasy Imaging v. 2010-09-02 [10, 11], which is based on the MC-system, PENetration and Energy Loss of Positrons and Electrons (PENELOPE) 2008 [12], was used. A phase space file (provided by Elekta Instrument AB) describing a 16-mm Perfexion beam was used as the input source. The absorbed dose to a water sphere with a 2.75-mm radius placed in an 8.0-cm spherical water phantom and 6.93-cm PMMA phantom was calculated. The transport parameters used in these MC calculations can be found in Benmakhlouf et al. [13].

Measurement of the beam profile

The beam profiles using the 16-mm collimator of six GK Perfexion™ units were measured using GafChromic™ MD-V3 films (International Specialty Products, Wayne, NJ, USA). Full width half maximum (FWHM) values and the physical penumbra, which is defined as the distance from the dose level of 80% to the dose level of 20%, were measured [14]. The films were cut into 6×6-cm^2 octagonal pieces to be fitted into the film-hosting inner phantom. The films were calibrated by irradiating 5, 10, 15, 20, 25, 30, 35, 40, 45, 50, 55, and 60 Gy at the maximum using the 16-mm collimator. The analysis of the irradiated films followed standard procedures of radiochromic film dosimetry [14]. The films were scanned using an EPSON Expression 10000XL scanner with a transparency unit (Seiko-Epson Co, Nagano, Japan). The scanned images were analyzed with ImageJ and homemade LabVIEW software. More detailed film handling procedures are described in a previous report [15]. In brief, the films were scanned with 300 DPI resolution and the red channel values were converted to optical densities. Absorbed doses were obtained by fitting the calibration data points with a third-order polynomial using the commercial software package, Origin 2015 (OriginLab Corp, Northhampton, MA, USA). One-dimensional dose distributions along the x-axis (right to left), y-axis (posterior to anterior), and z-axis (head to feet) were analyzed and compared with LGP.

Results

Construction of the PMMA phantom

The atomic compositions of the PMMA were analyzed using the element analysis (EA) technique at the Korea Research Institute of Chemical Technology. The bulk density was obtained by measuring the weights of three

0.9981 ± 0.0002 cm^3 cubic pieces ten times each. The bulk density of the PMMA was 1.185 ± 0.001 g/cm^3. The atomic compositions of the PMMA and the calculated electron density are shown in Table 1. The unknown material was assumed to be evenly distributed and to have an atomic number weight ratio of 0.5. Its contribution to the resultant electron density was negligible because the actual radius of the phantom was not affected by their existence. The radius of the PMMA phantom was determined to be 6.93 cm for a corresponding equivalent water depth of 8.00 g/cm^2. The alignment of the center of the active volume of the PTW TN31010 ionization chamber to the PPS calibration center was investigated by computed tomography (CT) images taken using a GE Light Speed Ultra CT (GE Healthcare Korea, Seoul, Korea) (Fig. 3a). The measured coordinate values of the effective point of the PTW 31010 ionization chamber deviated by 0.2 mm along the x-axis only. The deviations of the film-holding inner phantoms were less than or equal to 0.1 mm along a direction perpendicular to the dose distribution measuring plane (Fig. 3b, c).

Measurement of absorbed dose rate to water

The measured absorbed dose rate to water with the 16-mm collimator was 1.666 ± 0.015 Gy/min for the PMMA phantom, 1.647 ± 0.015 Gy/min for the water-filled phantom, and 1.637 ± 0.015 Gy/min for the solid water phantom. The dose rate measured with the PMMA phantom was 1.2% higher than that measured with the spherical water-filled phantom and 1.8% higher than that measured with the solid water phantom.

The experimental factor to convert a measured dose rate in the PMMA phantom to the dose rate in the water-filled phantom was 0.989 ± 0.013. The first Geant4 simulation using no phase space file provided a conversion factor of 0.9883 ± 0.0004, and the second Geant4 simulation using a phase space file showed a conversion factor of 0.9893 ± 0.0006. The PENELOPE-simulated conversion factor was 0.986 ± 0.002. The differences between the simulated conversion factors and the experimental values were 0.1%, 0.0% and 0.3%, respectively.

Table 1 Chemical composition and electron density of the PMMA used as the phantom material

Component	fi	Z/A	$\rho_{e,PMMA}$	$\rho_{e,PMMA}/\rho_{e,water}$
H	0.081	0.992162	0.639	1.155
C	0.595	0.499542		
O	0.317	0.500031		
unknown	0.007	0.500		

Legend: f_i is the fraction by weight of the atom i, Z/A is the atomic number weight mass ratio, $\rho_{e,PMMA}$ is the electron density of PMMA and $\rho_{e,PMMA}/\rho_{e,water}$ is the ratio of the electron densities of PMMA and water

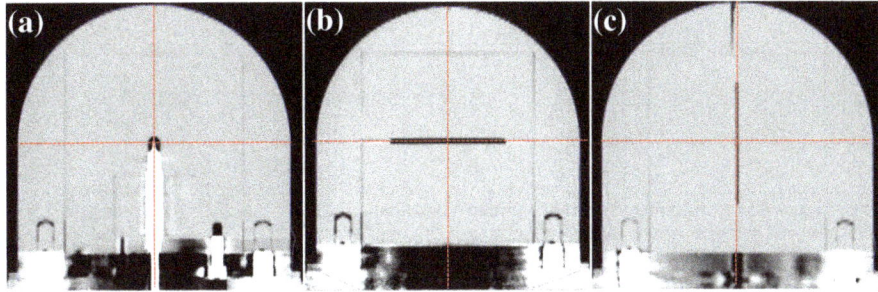

Fig. 3 Reconstructed coronal computed tomography images of the PMMA phantom with different inner phantoms. In each figure, the crossing point of the dashed lines is the PPS calibration center of a GK. **a** The effective point of the PTW TN31010 ionization chamber is 0.2 mm off in the x-direction (right-left). **b** The xy-plane film position is well matched with the xy-plane. **c** The xz-plane film position is well matched with the xz-plane

Measurement of the beam profile

The optical densities from the dose calibration films were fitted with a third-order polynomial to convert the optical density to the absorbed dose, and the adjusted R^2 value of the fitting curve was 0.9997. Typical one-dimensional beam shapes taken at the center of the PMMA are given in Fig. 4. The calculated beam shapes given by LGP using the TMR10 algorithm are given together [9]. The average values of the FWHM and penumbra measured using the PMMA phantom at six GK Perfexion sites are shown in Table 2.

For comparison, measured values using the solid water phantom at a single GK Perfexion site are also given. Two calculated results, one at the center of the PMMA phantom (LGP 6.93) and the other at the center of a water sphere with a radius of 8.0 cm (LGP 8.0), were obtained in the dose distributions given by LGP using the TMR10 algorithm. The TMR10 algorithm took into account only the geometry of the phantoms and neglected inhomogeneous electron densities between materials.

Discussion

Measurement of the absorbed dose rate to water

The difference between the absorbed dose rate to water measured with the PMMA phantom and those with the water-filled spherical phantom and the solid water phantom can be explained by the radius of the PMMA phantom having been determined based on elemental analysis of the PMMA, bulk density measurement and electron density calculation. However, the scattered effect of the PMMA body off the incoming ^{60}Co beam could cause additional contribution to the measurement of dose rate at the center of the PMMA phantom, whereas the photon beam scattered from the thin (5 mm) spherical PMMA shell of the water-filled phantom was attenuated mostly by the water before it arrived to the chamber at the center of the water-filled phantom. Therefore, the 1.2% difference seemed to be mainly due to the scattered photon contribution. Another possible reason for this difference may be the geometrical effect between the PMMA phantom and the water-filled phantom, although the hemispherical geometry of the PMMA phantom was nearly identical to the spherical shape of the water-filled phantom as long as the effective area of the GK is concerned, and its contribution to the dose rate should be negligible.

The comparison of the measured dose rate between the solid water phantom and the spherical water-filled phantom showed a difference of 0.6%, and this could also be due to the scattered photon contribution of the

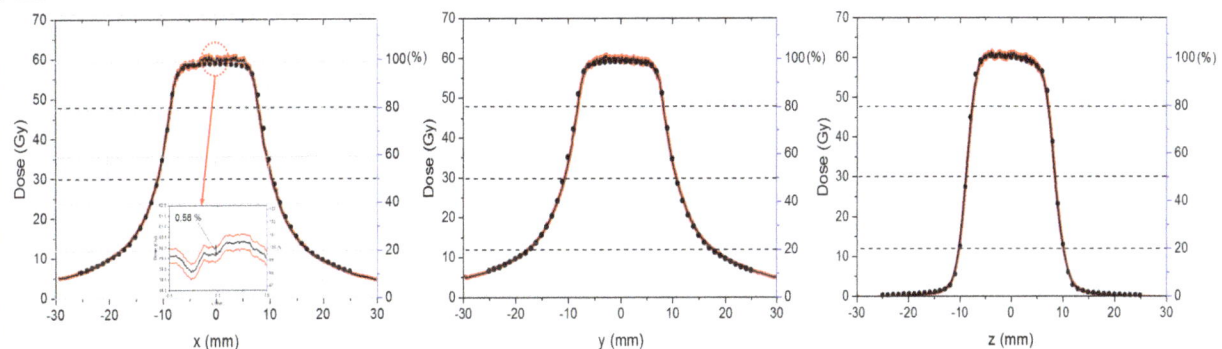

Fig. 4 One-dimensional dose distributions using the 16-mm collimator of a Gamma Knife Perfexion. The solid lines indicate measured distributions in the PMMA phantom, and the solid circles indicate results calculated by the GK treatment planning program at the center of a sphere with an 8.0-cm radius. The measured data are expressed a band and its half width is one standard deviation of each point

Table 2 FWHM and penumbra values measured in the PMMA phantom and the solid water phantom (SW) and calculated by LGP

Axis	FWHM (mm)				Penumbra (mm)			
	PMMA	LGP6.93[a]	SW	LGP8.0[b]	PMMA	LGP6.93[a]	SW	LGP8.0[b]
x	21.83 ± 0.25	21.68	21.57 ± 0.27	21.75	9.58 ± 0.22	9.04	8.76 ± 0.19	9.03
y	22.10 ± 0.32	21.68	21.56 ± 0.27	21.75	9.86 ± 0.18	9.04	8.96 ± 0.23	9.03
z	17.46 ± 0.11	17.39	17.41 ± 0.17	17.44	2.72 ± 0.10	3.09	2.65 ± 0.14	2.55

Legend: [a]Calculated by Leksell Gamma Plan at the center of the PMMA phantom (LGP6.93)
[b]Calculated by Leksell Gamma Plan and at the center of a sphere with a radius of 8.0 cm (LGP8.0)

solid water material to the dose rate. These results are consistent with the recently reported round-robin dose rate measurement in which the dose rate measured with a PTW 31010 ionization chamber in a hemispherical liquid water phantom was 0.4% larger than the dose rate measured in the Elekta solid water phantom under the TG-51 protocol [16].

Measurement of the beam profile

The FWHM values measured in the PMMA phantom were closer to the calculated values at the center of the 8.0-cm sphere than the values measured in the solid water phantom. However, all the FWHM values were within a range with variations less than 0.4 mm. Penumbras showed larger variations from the calculated values. In general, the PMMA showed wider penumbra than those from LGP8.0, while the values from the solid water phantom were narrower. This difference was due to the wider width of the 20% dose line in the PMMA phantom, which can be explained by the greater scattering contribution in the PMMA phantom compared to that in phantoms composed of other materials.

Uncertainty analysis

A detailed uncertainty budget based on the relative standard uncertainties for the measurements of the absorbed dose rate to water and the beam profile are tabulated in Tables 3 and 4. The contributing uncertainty components were classified as either statistical (type A) or systematic (type B) uncertainties, and their

values are listed [17]. The main features of the uncertainty components are described as follows.

The uncertainty for the calibration factor of the chamber may be provided in the calibration certificate. The uncertainty for the displacement of the ionization chamber can be measured by moving the reference phantom in 0.1-cm steps. Although the change in the dose rate in the x- and y-axes was less than 0.03%, the change along the z-axis was 0.15%. The uncertainty of the alignment of the PMMA phantom with the PPS calibration center of the GK was determined by the difference of the coordinates between the phantom center at (99.8, 100, 100) and the PPS calibration center at (100, 100, 100).

The uncertainty of calibration curve fitting represents the overall uncertainty introduced during the fitting procedure performed to obtain the calibration curve.

Using the PMMA phantom proposed in this study for GK dosimetry may be a good choice because it provides a solution to the problem for how the dose rate should be measured in a water phantom. However, the other conditions required by the standard protocols, such as a single directional beam, source to surface distance of 100 cm, and measurement depth of 5 g/cm^2, cannot be achieved yet. To do so would require an additional factor to correct these differences by applying a dose correction factor measured in a standard library at a clinical site. Or, the generalized beam quality correction factor suggested by Alfonso et al. [18] could be obtained by Monte Carlo simulations considering the conditions of field size, geometry, phantom material, and beam quality. However, there are no published reports on this

Table 3 The uncertainty components for measurement of the absorbed dose rate to water

Uncertainty component	Type A (%)	Type B (%)
Calibration factor of the ionization chamber, $N^c_{D_w,Q_0}$		0.50
Ionization current measurement	0.01	0.02
Temperature and pressure measurement		0.056
Scattered photon contribution	0.01	1.28
Displacement of the ionization chamber	0.01	0.15
Alignment of the PMMA phantom with the PPS calibration center		0.20
Long-term stability of the ionization chamber		0.12
Standard relative combined uncertainty	1.40	

Legend: A PTW TN31010 ionization chamber was used for measurements of the FWHM and penumbra at the patient positioning system (PPS) calibration center

Table 4 The uncertainty components for measurements of the FWHM and penumbra

Uncertainty component	Type A (%)	Type B (%)
Optical density measurement	0.10	0.02
Intensity resolution		0.002
Uniformity of the radiochromic film		0.50
Temperature and relative humidity measurements		0.056
Alignment of the PMMA phantom with the PPS calibration center		0.20
Positioning of the radiochromic film inside the phantom		0.16
Calibration curve fitting		1.33
Measurements of FWHM and penumbra	0.02	0.01
Standard relative combined uncertainty	1.45	

Legend: GafChromic™ MD-V3 films were used for the measurement of absorbed dose rate to water at the patient positioning system (PPS) calibration center

generalized correction factor for the GK, except for a technical report and a study on relative output correction factors for different size collimators [13, 19].

Conclusions

A PMMA phantom was constructed for the measurement of the absorbed dose rates to water and the dose distribution of a GK. The phantom was characterized with the composition of the hemispherical outer phantom fixed firmly to the Leksell Gamma frame and the exchangeable inner phantoms. The radius of the PMMA phantom corresponding to an equivalent water depth of 8 g/cm^2 was determined from the electron density calculation, but a factor of 0.989 was necessary to convert the measured value to a dose rate absorbed to water. The FWHM and penumbra values measured using the phantom showed reasonable agreement to the calculated values, although more sophisticated handling of the scattered photon contribution seemed to be necessary to explain the wider penumbra in the measured beam shapes. The PMMA phantom in this study represents an acceptable and practical alternative for GK dosimetry considering its cost-effectiveness and ease of handling. For reference, the cost of manufacturing the phantom including the PMMA price and phantom design was forty thousand dollars, which is economical compared with that of purchasing a commercial phantom. The phantom is ready to be commercialized upon request.

Abbreviations

(AAPM): American Association of Physicists in Medicine (AAPM); ABS: Acrylonitrile butadiene styrene; BIPM: International Bureau of Weights and Measures; CT: Computed tomography; EWD: Equivalent water depth; FS: Field size; FWHM: Full width half maximum; GK: Gamma knife; IAEA: International Atomic Energy Agency; KRISS: Korea Research Institute of Standards and Science; PMMA: Polymethyl metacrylate; PPS: Patient positioning system; SSD: Source to surface distance

Acknowledgements

This work was supported by the research project 'Development of absolute measurement technology of absorbed dose to water for radiotherapy radiation using micron-size water calorimeter' with contract number 2015M2A2A4A02044791 granted by the Ministry of Science and ICT (MSIT). This study was also supported by the research project 'Standardization of accurate measurement technology for determining absorbed dose to water of Gamma Knife radiosurgery facility' with grant number 10069168 by the Korea Agency for Technology and Standards.

Funding

This study was supported by the Ministry of Science and ICT (contract number: 2015M2A2A4A02044791) and by the Korea Agency for Technology and Standards (grant number: 10069168).

Authors' contributions

Concept and design: JP, HT, and KJ. Treatment planning: HT and GK. Experiment: JP, HT, KJ, YM, and YN. Data analysis: JP, HT, KJ, HJ, and TH. Simulation: HT, TY, CH, and HB. Manuscript preparation: JP, HT, and KJ. All authors read and approved the final manuscript.

Competing interests

The authors declare that they have no competing interests.

Author details

[1]Center for Ionizing Radiation, Division of Metrology for Quality of Life, Korea Research Institute of Standards and Science, 267 Gajeong-ro, Yuseong-gu, Daejon 34311, Korea. [2]Department of Accelerator Science, Korea University Sejong Campus, 2511 Sejong-ro, Sejong 30019, Korea. [3]Department of Nuclear Engineering, Hanyang University College of Engineering, Seoul 04763, Korea. [4]Department of Radiation Convergence Engineering, Yonsei University, 1 Yeonsedae-gil, Heungeop-myeon, Wonju 26493, Korea. [5]Department of Medical Radiation Physics and Nuclear Medicine, Karolinska University Hospital, SE-17176 Stockholm, Sweden. [6]Department of Neurosurgery, Seoul National University College of Medicine, 101 Daehak-ro Jongno-gu, Seoul 03080, Korea.

References

1. Almond PR, Biggs PJ, Coursey BM, et al. AAPM's TG-51 protocol for clinical reference dosimetry of high-energy photon and electron beams. Med Phys. 1999;26:1847–970.
2. Andreo P, Burns DT, Hohfeld K, et al. Absorbed dose determination in external beam radiotherapy: an international code of practice for dosimetry based on standards of absorbed dose to water. Technical report series no. 398 (V.11b). Vienna: IAEA; 2004.
3. Maitz AH, Wu A, Lunsford LD, et al. Quality assurance for gamma knife stereotactic radiosurgery. Int J Radiat Oncol Biol Phys. 1995;32:1465–71.
4. Chung HT, Park Y, Hyun S, al e. Determination of the absorbed dose to water for the 18-mm helmet of a gamma knife. Int J Radiat Oncol Biol Phys. 2011;79:1580–7.
5. Andreo P, Burns DT, Hohfeld K, et al. Dosimetry of small static fields used in external beam radiotherapy: an international code of practice for reference and relative dose determination. Technical report series no. 483. Vienna: IAEA; 2017.
6. Mirzakhanian L, Benmarkhlouf H, Tessier F, et al. Determination of $k_{Qmsr, Qo}$ factors for ion chambers used in the calibration of Leksell gamma knife Perfextion model using EGSnrc and PENELOPE Monte Carlo codes. Med Phys. 2018;45:1748–57.

7. Seco J, Evans PM. Assessing the effect of electron density in photon dose calculations. Med Phys. 2006;33:540–52.

8. Allison J, Amako K, Apostolakis J, et al. Recent developments in GEANT4. Nucl Instrum Methods Phys Res A. 2016;835:186–225. https://geant4.web.cern.ch/publications

9. Xu AY, Bhatnagar J, Bednarz G, et al. Dose difference between the three dose calculation algorithms in Leksell gamma plan. J Appl Clin Med Phys. 2014;15:89–99.

10. Badal-Soler A. Development of advanced geometric models and acceleration technique for Monte Carlo simulation in Medical Physics. Ph.D. Thesis. Barcelona: Universitat Politècnica de Catalunya; 2008.

11. Sempau J, Badal A, Brualla L. A PENELOPE-based system for the automated Monte Carlo simulation of clinacs and voxelized geometries application to far-from-axis fields. Med Phys. 2011;38:5887–95.

12. Salvat F, Fernandez JM, Sempau J. PENELOPE-2008, A code system for Monte Carlo simulation of electron and photon transport. Issy-les-Moulineaux: OECD Nuclear Energy Agency; 2009.

13. Benmakhlouf H, Johansson J, Paddick I, et al. Monte Carlo calculated and experimentally determined output correction factors for small field detectors in Leksell gamma knife Perfexion beams. Phys Med Biol. 2015;60:3959–73.

14. Niroomand-Rad A, Blackwell CR, Coursey BM, et al. Radiochromic film dosimetry: recommendations of AAPM radiation therapy committee task group 55. American Association of Physicists in Medicine. Med Phys. 1998; 25(11):2093–115.

15. Chung JP, Oh SW, Seong YM, et al. An effective calibration technique for radiochromic films using a single-shot dose distribution in gamma knife. Physica Medica. 2016;32:368–78.

16. Drzymala RE, Alvarez PE, Bednarz G, et al. A round-robin gamma stereotactic radiosurgery dosimetry inter-institution comparison of calibration protocols. Med Phys. 2015;42:6745–56.

17. EAL Task Force. Public Reference, Expression of the uncertainty of measurement in calibration, European co-operation for accreditation, EA-4/02; 1999.

18. Alfonso R, Andreo P, Capote R, et al. A new formalism for reference dosimetry of small and nonstandard fields. Med Phys. 2008;35:5179–86.

19. Johansson J and Gorka B. Application of a new formalism for absolute dosimetry of the Leksell Gamma Knife. Stockholm: Elekta Instrument AB; 2012. SE-10393, Reference No. SSM 2010/2201 and project No. 4017003–06.

4

Comparing simultaneous integrated boost vs sequential boost in anal cancer patients: results of a retrospective observational study

Pierfrancesco Franco[1]* ⓘ, Berardino De Bari[2], Francesca Arcadipane[1], Alexis Lepinoy[3], Manuela Ceccarelli[4], Gabriella Furfaro[1], Massimiliano Mistrangelo[5], Paola Cassoni[6], Martina Valgiusti[7], Alessandro Passardi[7], Andrea Casadei Gardini[7], Elisabetta Trino[1], Stefania Martini[1], Giuseppe Carlo Iorio[1], Andrea Evangelista[4], Umberto Ricardi[1] and Gilles Créhange[8]

Abstract

Background: To evaluate clinical outcomes of simultaneous integrated boost (SIB) - intensity modulated radiotherapy (RT) in patients with non metastatic anal cancer compared to those of a set of patients treated with 3-dimensional conformal RT and sequential boost (SeqB).

Methods: A retrospective cohort of 190 anal cancer patients treated at 3 academic centers with concurrent chemo-RT employing either SIB or SeqB was analysed. The SIB-group consisted of 87 patients, treated with 2 cycles of Mitomycin (MMC) and 5-Fluorouracil (5FU) using SIB-IMRT delivering 42-45Gy/28–30 fractions to the elective pelvic lymph nodes and 50.4-54Gy/28-30fractions to the primary tumor and involved nodes, based on pre-treatment staging. The SeqB group comprised 103 patients, treated with MMC associated to either 5FU or Capecitabine concurrent to RT with 36 Gy/20 fractions to a single volume including gross tumor, clinical nodes and elective nodal volumes and a SeqB to primary tumor and involved nodes of 23.4 Gy/13 fractions. We compared colostomy-free survival (CFS), overall survival (OS) and the cumulative incidence of colostomy for each radiation modality. Cox proportional-hazards model addressed factors influencing OS and CFS.

Results: Median follow up was 34 (range 9–102) and 31 months (range 2–101) in the SIB and SeqB groups. The 1- and 2-year cumulative incidences of colostomy were 8.2% (95%CI:3.6–15.2) and 15.0% (95%CI:8.1–23.9) in the SIB group and 13.9% (95%CI: 7.8–21.8) and 18.1% (95%CI:10.8–27.0) in the SeqB group. Two-year CFS and OS were 78.1% (95%CI:67.0–85.8) and 87.5% (95%CI:77.3–93.3) in the SIB group and 73.5% (95%CI:62.6–81.7) and 85.4% (95%CI: 75.5–91.6) in the SeqB, respectively. A Cox proportional hazards regression model highlighted an adjusted hazard ratio (AdjHR) of 1.18 (95%CI: 0.67–2.09;$p = 0.560$), although AdjHR for the first 24 months was 0.95 (95%CI: 0.49–1.84; $p = 0.877$) for the SIB approach.

Conclusions: SIB-based RT provides similar clinical outcomes compared to SeqB-based in the treatment of patients affected with non metastatic anal cancer.

Keywords: Anal cancer radiotherapy, Concomitant radio-chemotherapy, Simultaneous integrated boost, Sequential boost, Overall treatment time

* Correspondence: pierfrancesco.franco@unito.it
[1]Department of Oncology, Radiation Oncology, University of Turin, Via Genova 3, 10126 Turin, Italy
Full list of author information is available at the end of the article

Background

Concurrent chemo-radiation (RT-CHT) is presently considered as a standard therapeutic option in patients affected with squamous cell carcinoma of the anal canal [1, 2]. The association of pelvic radiotherapy (RT) to concomitant 5-fluorouralcil (5-FU) and mitomycin C provides high rates of complete responders (around 90%) and consistent results in terms of disease-free survival (DFS), up to 70–75% for early disease (T1-T2 tumors) and 60–65% for more advanced stages (T3-T4 or node positive tumors) at 3 years [2–4]. When RT is delivered with conventional techniques, the toxicity profile can be important, as observed in the 5-FU/MMC arm of the RTOG 9811 trial, with grade 3–4 events as high as 48% for skin and 61% for hematologic toxicity [5]. As a result, treatment breaks can be necessary with a prolongation of overall treatment time (OTT) and consequent detrimental effects on clinical outcomes [6]. Intensity-modulated radiotherapy was shown to reduce the rates of ≥ G3 acute gastrointestinal and skin toxicity and that of ≥ G2 hematologic events [7, 8]. Moreover, oncological results in terms of both local control (LC) colostomy-free (CFS) and overall survival (OS) seems promising with this treatment strategy [9, 10]. In anal cancer patients, macroscopic primary and nodal disease and elective volumes are treated to different total nominal doses [11]. In the sequential boost approach (SeqB), this can be achieved through the progressive boosting of selected target regions harboring the macroscopic disease [12]. Target volumes are progressively shrinking and boost dose is added on top of the previous sequence [13]. In the simultaneous integrated boost (SIB) strategy, a differential dose per fraction is delivered to selected sub-regions during the same treatment session, heading to different total nominal doses given to target volumes in the same number of fractions [1]. Consequently, SIB provides a reduction in OTT compared to the sequential boost approach, with a potential beneficial effect on clinical outcomes in the context of a highly repopulating tumor such as anal cancer [14]. To evaluate the potential impact of different treatment strategies on clinical outcomes, we compared data of 2 cohorts of anal cancer patients treated either with SeqB or SIB approaches, in terms of CFS as primary endpoint, after adjusting for known prognostic factors, and in terms of OS and cumulative incidence of colostomy as secondary endpoints.

Methods

In this multi-centre retrospective observational study, we compared clinical outcomes of patients affected with anal cancer. Consecutive patients treated between 2007 and 2015 at the Radiation Oncology Departments of 3 academic Institutions were enrolled, namely a) University of Turin, Italy, b) University Hospital 'Jean Minjoz',

Besançon, France and c) Centre 'Georges François Leclerc', Dijon, France. Clinical data were retrieved from local clinical databases by 2 different operators (FA and AL) and merged together on a common database used for the present analysis. The frame of the final dataset was agreed by the 2 centres. Briefly, all patients enrolled had a histologically confirmed diagnosis of anal squamous cell carcinoma (both anal canal and margin). Tumor stage was defined according to the indications of the American Joint Committee on Cancer (2002 version) and patients with clinical stage T1-T4, N0-N3, M0 were included. Patients having clinical T1 N0 tumors of the anal margin were excluded, because they were submitted to local excision. Pre-treatment clinical evaluation included complete medical history, physical examination and complete laboratory testing. Staging included a chest, abdomen and pelvis computed tomography scan (CT), a magnetic resonance imaging (MRI) of the pelvic region and positron-emission tomography (PET). A subset of patients within the SIB group, treated in center a), also received inguinal sentinel lymphnode biopsy (SLNB) for inguinal nodal staging. Patients in the SeqB, treated in centres b) and c), did not receive any SLNB procedure because of a different staging policy. Patients were followed-up according to local clinical practice and vital status was clinically updated in 2016. Written informed consent for treatment was obtained for all patients. The Ethical Review Board of each Institutional Hospital approved the present study.

Radiotherapy characteristics

In the SeqB group, including patients treated in centres b) and c) between 2007 and 2015, the first sequence of treatment included the delivery of 36 Gy in 20 fractions (1.8 Gy daily) given over 4 weeks to the macroscopic primary and nodal tumor and elective volumes including the ischio-anal fossa and mesorectum, the pre-sacral, external and internal iliac nodes, the inguinal regions and the lower part of the common iliac lymphnodes up to the promontorium. After the first sequence a 16-day gap was planned. In the second sequence, an adjunctive dose of 23.4 Gy in 13 fractions was given to the macroscopic disease which finally received a total nominal dose of 59.4 Gy. In the SIB group, including patients treated in centre a) in the period 2007–2015, dose prescription was set according to the RTOG 0529 indications based on clinical stage at presentation [6]. Patients with cT2N0 disease were given 50.4 Gy in 28 fractions (1.8 Gy daily) to the primary anal tumor, while the elective nodal volume was prescribed 42 Gy in 28 fractions (1.5 Gy/daily). Patients presenting cT3-T4/N0-N3 disease were prescribed 54 Gy in 30 fractions (1.8 Gy daily) to the gross tumor volume, while gross nodal disease was prescribed 50.4 Gy in 30 fractions (1.68 Gy daily) if sized ≤ 3 cm or

54 Gy in 30 fractions (1.8 Gy daily) if > 3 cm. Elective nodal volume was prescribed 45 Gy in 30 fractions (1.5 Gy daily) [15, 16] . No brachytherapy boost was given to any patient in either group.

Chemotherapy characteristics

In the SIB group, concomitant chemotherapy (CHT) consisted of 5- fluorouracil (1000 mg/m^2/day) given as continuous infusion for 96 h (days 1–5 and 29–33) combined with mitomycin C (10 mg/m^2) given as bolus (days 1 and 29). A total of 2 concurrent cycles were planned for each patient. In the SeqB group, at day 1 of each sequence, mitomycin C (10 mg/m^2) was associated either with continuous infusion 5- fluorouracil (1000 mg/m^2/day) over 96 h or capecitabine (825 mg/m^2 bid on weekdays). Capecitabine has been used only for patients treated in centres b) and c).

Statistical analysis

The primary study endpoint was CFS defined as the time between RT start and the date of colostomy, death, or last follow-up date on which the patient was known to be colostomy-free. Secondary endpoints were OS and cumulative incidence of colostomy. Overall survival was defined as the time between RT beginning and the date of death from any cause or last follow-up. Cumulative incidence of colostomy was calculated considering death from any cause as competing event. The number of anal cancer cases in the 3 Institutions during the study period determined the sample size. No treated patient was excluded from the present analysis and hence about 200 patients were analysed. For each cohort, the time-to-event functions of CFS and OS were estimated by the Kaplan-Meier product-limit method. Hazard Ratios (HRs) for the treatment group comparison were estimated using univariable and multivariable Cox proportional-hazards models, adjusting in the multivariable analysis for the main prognostic factors. The following variables were included in the multivariate analysis: treatment (SIB vs SeqB), gender, age as continuous variable, clinical stage (stage III vs stage I and II), and grade (G3 vs G1-G2). In order to check for the proportional-hazards assumption, we performed the Grambsch and Therneau test [17]. Although the assumption was satisfied for CFS ($p = 0.37$), we assessed the time-varying effect of treatment in the Cox model, according to 2 follow-up periods: the first 24 months after treatment and the timespan from 24 months to the end of follow-up. Considering the graphical representation of CFS, the two-year time-point was chosen because corresponding to an effect modification of treatments over time. To take into account the occurrence of death as a competing event during time, the cumulative risk of colostomy was estimated using the method described by

Gooley et al. [18]. Difference between cohorts was assessed using univariable and multivariable (adjusting for the same variables used for CFS and OS) Fine & Gray models [19]. For all the endpoints, adjusted analyses were also performed including a propensity score (PS) in the regression models along with the treatment group variable. The PS for the likelihood of receiving the SIB treatment was calculated using a logistic regression model that included the same variables used in the multivariable analysis.

Because of the retrospective nature of the study, no toxicity data were retrieved apart from hematologic toxicity which was considered as reliably exploitable . Hematologic toxicity was scored according to the RTOG scoring scale.

Results

A total of 190 patients were retrieved. The SIB group (center a) included 87 patients, while the SeqB group comprised of 103 cases (centres b and c). Detailed characteristics and comparative evaluation can be found in Table 1. Patients in the SeqB had a significant higher rate of anal margin localization (22.3% vs 16.1%; $p < 0.0001$), positive lymphnodes (48.5% vs 34.5%; $p = 0.0015$), inguinal groin involvement at diagnosis (35.9% vs 20.7%; $p = 0.0187$), and G3 differentiation (24.1% vs 16.5%; $p = 0.0003$). Borderline significant difference was found for advanced global stage (IIIA-IIIB: 54.4% vs 38.0%; $p = 0.0730$) and T-stage (T3-T4: 40.8% vs 31.0%;$p = 0.0725$) between SeqB and SIB groups (Table 1).

Patients in the SIB group had a significantly higher proportion of patients with a longer time between biopsy and RT start (patient with time ≥ 60 days: 66.7% vs 49.5%; $p = 0.0172$). This was due to the inguinal SLNB procedure that was performed in some of the patients in the SIB group, which required extra time for the healing of the surgical scar. Median biopsy-RT time was 74 days (IQR: 54–98) in the SIB and 59 days (IQR: 45–73) in the SeqB groups. Median OTT (time from RT start to end) was 43 days (IQR: 42–45) in the SIB and 60 days (IQR: 58–63) in the SeqB groups. The proportion of patients with OTT ≥ 45 days was significantly higher (95.1% vs 28.7%; $p < 0.0001$) in the SeqB group. In the SeqB, 5 patients received only the first sequence of treatment because of major acute toxicity (OTT range: 28–32 days). Treatment characteristics are shown in Table 2.

Pattern of failure, colostomy rates and survival

Median observation times were 34 (range 9–102) and 31 months (range 2–101) in the SIB and SeqB groups, respectively. However, out of 103 patients, 17 (16.5%) in the SeqB group were lacking of updated observation (last follow up between 1 and 4 years from analysis). In the SeqB group, the pattern of failure comprised 21 (20.4%) local, 8 (7.8%) nodal and 6 (5.8%) distant

Table 1 Patient and tumor characteristics and pattern of failure

Variables	SIB group Pts N (%)	SeqB group Pts N (%)	Total Pts N (%)	p-value
Sex				
Female	64 (73.6)	76 (73.8)	140 (73.7)	0.9722
Male	23 (26.4)	27 (26.2)	50 (26.3)	
Median age (range)	64 (55–70)	62 (53–77)	63 (53–77)	[a]0.4471
Subsite				
Anal canal	73 (83.9)	80 (77.7)	153 (80.5)	<.0001
Anal margin	14 (16.1)	23 (22.3)	37 (19.5)	
Histologic type				
Basaloid	7 (8.0)	7 (6.8)	14 (7.4)	0.7425
Squamous cell	80 (92.0)	96 (93.2)	176 (92.6)	
Grading				
NA	2 (2.4)	19 (18.4)	21 (11.1)	
G1	7 (8.0)	28 (27.2)	35 (18.4)	0.0003
G2	57 (65.5)	39 (37.9)	96 (50.5)	
G3	21 (24.1)	17 (16.5)	38 (20.0)	
T stage				
T1	5 (5.8)	4 (3.9)	9 (4.7)	0.0725
T2	55 (63.2)	57 (55.3)	112 (59.0)	
T3	23 (26.4)	25 (24.3)	48 (25.3)	
T4	4 (4.6)	17 (16.5)	21 (11.0)	
N stage				
N0	57 (65.5)	53 (51.5)	110 (57.9)	0.0015
N1	5 (5.8)	17 (16.5)	22 (11.6)	
N2	21 (24.1)	15 (14.6)	36 (18.9)	
N3	4 (4.6)	18 (17.4)	22 (11.6)	
Global stage				
I	5 (5.7)	3 (2.9)	8 (4.2)	0.0730
II	49 (56.3)	44 (42.7)	93 (48.9)	
IIIA	8 (9.3)	21 (20.4)	29 (15.3)	
IIIB	25 (28.7)	35 (34.0)	60 (31.6)	
Inguinal node involv.				
NA	0 (0%)	1 (1)	1 (0.6)	0.0187
Yes	18 (20.7)	37 (35.9)	55 (28.9)	
No	69 (79.3)	65 (63.1)	134 (70.5)	
Time biopsy-RT (days)				
≥ 60	62 (71.3)	5 (4.9)	67 (35.3)	0.0172
< 60	25 (28.7)	98 (95.1)	123 (64.7)	
OTT (days)				
< 45	62 (71.3)	5 (4.9)	67 (35.3)	<.0001
≥ 45	25 (28.7)	98 (95.1)	123 (64.7)	

[a]U-Mann Whitney Test

Legend: *SIB* simultaneous integrated boost, *SeqB* sequential boost, *pts* patients, *N*: number; *involv.*: Involvement, *RT* radiotherapy; *OTT* overall treatment time

Table 2 Treatment characteristics

Variable	N (%)
Boost approach	
SeqB	103 (54.3)
SIB	87 (45.7)
SIB dose and fractionation	
PTV dose-tumor (Gy)	
54 Gy/30 fractions	57 (65.5)
50.4 Gy/28 fractions	30 (34.5)
PTV dose-positive nodes (Gy) (26 pts)	
50.4 Gy/30 fractions	26 (100.0)
PTV dose-negative nodes (Gy)	
45 Gy/30 fractions	53 (60.9)
42 Gy/28 fractions	34 (39.1)
SeqB dose and fractionation	
PTV dose-first sequence	
36 Gy/20 fractions	103 (100)
PTV dose-sequential boost	
23,4 Gy/13 fractions	103 (100)
Chemotherapy regimens	
5-FU + MMC × 2 cycles	159 (83.7)
5-FU + MMC × 1 cycle	2 (1.0)
Capecitabine + MMC × 2 cycles	26 (13.7)
Capecitabine + MMC × 1 cycle	3 (1.6)

Legend, *SeqB* sequential boost, *SIB* simultaneous integrated boost, *PTV* planning target volume, *Gy* Gray, *pts* patients, *5-FU* 5-fluorouracil, *MMC* mitomycin C

relapses. In the SIB group, local failures were 16 (18.4%), nodal 6 (6.9%) and distant 13 (14.9%). Overall, 12 colostomies (13.8%) were observed in the SIB and 17 (16.5%) in the SeqB groups, respectively. In the SIB group all colostomies were due to salvage surgery done because of local relapse. In the SeqB group all colostomies except one were due to salvage procedures. Only 1 colostomy was performed at 52 months because of functional issues.

The 1- and 2-year cumulative incidence of colostomies were 8.2% (95%CI: 3.6–15.2) and 15.0% (95%CI: 8.1–23.9) in the SIB group and 13.9% (95%CI: 7.8–21.8) and 18.1% (95%CI: 10.8–27.0) in the SeqB group (Fig. 1). Two-year CFS and OS were 78.1% (95%CI: 67.0–85.8) and 87.5% (95%CI: 77.3–93.3) in the SIB group and 73.5% (95%CI: 62.6–81.7) and 85.4% (95%CI: 75.5–91.6) in the SeqB, respectively (Fig. 2). Results from Cox proportional hazards regression models and Fine & Gray models are shown in Table 3. During the whole follow-up, SIB radiotherapy had an adjusted hazard ratio (AdjHR) of 1.18 (95%CI: 0.67–2.09, $p = 0.560$), although AdjHR for the first 24 months was 0.95 (95%CI: 0.49–1.84, $p = 0.877$) (Fig. 2). No significant differences were found between groups for OS (AdjHR = 1.51, 95%CI:

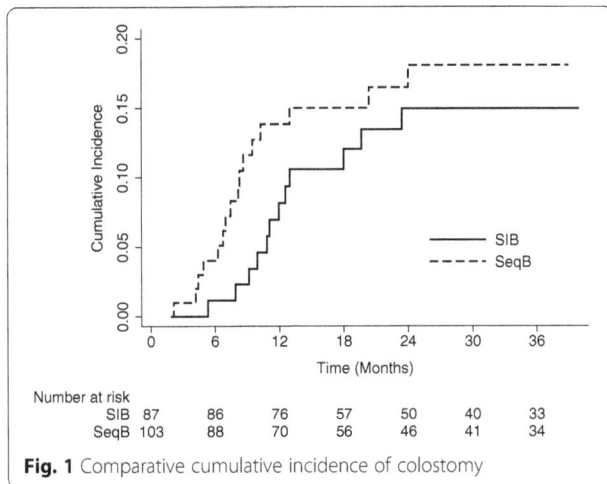

Fig. 1 Comparative cumulative incidence of colostomy

0.77–2.98, p = 0.235) and the cumulative incidence of colostomy (AdjHR = 0.85, 95%CI: 0.39–1.83, p = 0.675). Treatment comparisons adjusted using the PS approach showed results nearly identical to those of multivariable models (Table 3).

No difference (p = 0.65) in terms of ≥G3 hematologic toxicity was found between the SeqB group (22%) and the SIB group (26%).

Discussion

Combined RT-CHT in a concomitant setting is the standard of cancer for anal cancer patients [11]. In Europe, split-course high-dose RT was mostly chosen as a treatment option following established seminal works [20]. A treatment gap was planned between the first large-field phase and the second boost phase on the macroscopic disease. The gap was intended to allow for the resolution of acute skin and mucosa toxicity and for tumor response assessment to better tailor the subsequent overdosage on the residual disease [7]. This approach was set by 2 randomized phase III trials namely

the ACT I and EORTC 22861 trials, which demonstrated the benefit of adding CHT over RT alone, in terms of local control, sphincter preservation rate and overall survival [21, 22]. In these trials, RT was given employing 2 treatment sequences delivered sequentially. In the EORTC 22861 trial, 45 Gy over 5 weeks were given using conventional fractionation to the whole pelvis followed, after a 6-week interval, by a boost dose modulated according to treatment response (20 Gy to partial and 15 Gy to complete responders) and delivered thorough photons, electrons or ^{192}Ir implants [21]. Concomitant CHT (continuously infused 5-FU and bolus MMC) was given only during the first treatment sequence [21]. Similarly, in the ACT I trial, the first phase was made up of 45 Gy in 20 or 25 fraction over 4 to 5 weeks, while the boost (given to complete or > 50% partial responders) employed 15 Gy in 6 fractions with photons or electrons or 25 Gy given at 10 Gy per day given with iridium implants [22]. Mitomycin C was given at the beginning of the first phase and 5-FU at the beginning and end of it. In the US, clinical researches mostly employed a moderate dose and continuously delivered RT course associated to concurrent chemotherapy as in the RTOG 8704-ECOG 1289 trial, in which patients were treated up to 45–50.4 Gy, with field reduction at 30.6–36 Gy, with concurrent 5-FU ± MMC for 2 cycles [23]. Based on the observation that accelerated tumor cell repopulation occurs during RT and may have detrimental effects on clinical outcomes, clinical research started to shorten treatment regimens to decrease overall treatment time [24]. For example the EORTC 22953 phase II trial, investigated the feasibility and toxicity profile of a reduction in the gap period between the whole pelvis phase and the boost to 2 weeks, together with the intensification of the CHT regimen [25]. The compliance to therapy in terms of delivered dose and treatment duration was 93%, with a complete response rate of 90.7% [25]. More recently, SeqB approaches were delivered with no pre-planned interruptions as in the ACT II trial and represent, nowadays, the standard treatment strategy [2]. Neverthelss, compared to the SeqB approach, SIB potentially allows for a further reduction in the OTT, because treatment fractions are continuously delivered and different daily doses to target volumes are given in the same number of fractions [1, 10]. In the attempt to investigate whether SIB may provide a therapeutic gain, we analyzed 2 cohorts of anal cancer patients treated with SIB and SeqB approaches. To the best of our knowledge, this is the first study comparing these 2 treatment strategies in terms of CFS in anal cancer patients. Median follow up was similar for the 2 groups (34 vs 31 months for SIB and SeqB). Focusing on patients characteristics, the 2 cohorts were different since the SeqB group had a significant higher proportion

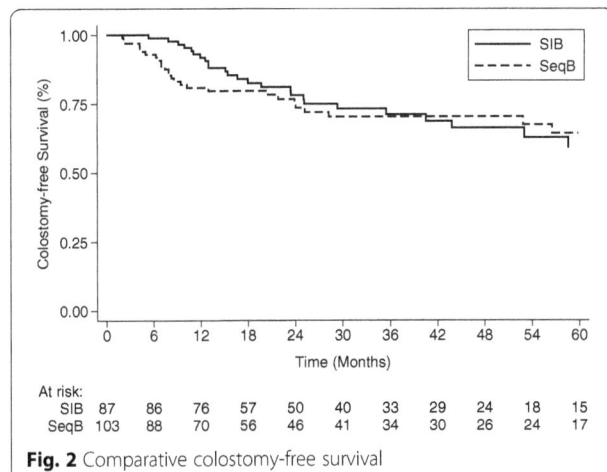

Fig. 2 Comparative colostomy-free survival

Table 3 Clinical factors potentially influencing colostomy-free survival

		Univariable			Multivariable			SIB vs SeqB, Propensity score adjusted		
Endpoint	Parameter	HR	95%CI	p	HR	95%CI	p	HR	95%CI	p
CSF	SIB	0.90	0.53,1.54	0.703	1.18	0.67,2.09	0.560	1.15	0.65,2.04	0.621
	SIB on the first 24 months	0.72	0.38,1.34	0.297	0.95	0.49,1.84	0.877	0.95	0.48,1.85	0.871
	Sex (M vs F)	1.64	0.93,2.90	0.087	1.60	0.90,2.84	0.109			
	Age	1.02	1.00,1.04	0.119	1.02	1.00,1.04	0.124			
	Stage III vs I-II	1.78	1.03,3.05	0.037	1.83	1.04,3.22	0.037			
	G3 vs G2-G1	0.82	0.40,1.71	0.603	0.85	0.41,1.77	0.668			
OS	SIB	1.15	0.61,2.17	0.674	1.71	0.86,3.40	0.127	1.51	0.77,2.98	0.235
	Sex (M vs F)	2.64	1.38,5.07	0.003	2.77	1.43,5.37	0.003			
	Age	1.03	1.00,1.06	0.043	1.03	1.00,1.06	0.031			
	Stage III vs I-II	2.27	1.17,4.38	0.015	2.64	1.30,5.34	0.007			
	G3 vs G2-G1	1.42	0.66,3.06	0.376	1.48	0.68,3.23	0.326			
CIC	SIB	0.71	0.34,1.47	0.352	0.87	0.41,1.85	0.713	0.85	0.39,1.83	0.675
	Sex (M vs F)	0.93	0.39,2.18	0.863	0.83	0.34,2.05	0.690			
	Age	1.00	0.98,1.03	0.765	1.00	0.98,1.02	0.878			
	Stage III vs I-II	2.09	0.99,4.38	0.052	2.13	0.97,4.70	0.061			
	G3 vs G2-G1	0.44	0.13,1.48	0.184	0.43	0.13,1.45	0.173			

Legend *HR* hazard ratio *CI* confidence interval, *M vs F* male vs female, *UFS* colostomy-free survival, *OS* Overall Survival, *CIC* Cumulative Incidence of colostomy

of patients with tumor of the anal margin (22.3% vs 16.1%; $p < 0.0001$), with positive nodes (48.5% vs 34.5%; $p = 0.0015$), inguinal groin localization (35.9% vs 20.7%; $p = 0.0187$), and G3 differentiation (24.1% vs 16.5%; $p = 0.0003$). Borderline significant difference was found for advanced stage (IIIA-IIIB: 54.4% vs 38.0%; $p = 0.0730$). Conversely, patients in the SIB group had a longer time between biopsy and RT start (patient with time ≥ 60 days: 66.7% vs 49.5%; $p = 0.0172$). Median OTTs were 43 and 60 in the SIB and SeqB groups, respectively, due to the different approaches in delivering radiation. Local relapse rate was slightly higher for patients submitted to sequential boost (SeqB: 20.4% vs SIB: 18.4%), as were regional failures (SeqB: 7.8% vs SIB: 6.9%). A higher percentage of distant metastasis was observed in the SIB group (14.9%) compared to the SeqB group (5.8%), even if baseline patients characteristics were more favorable for these patients. A slightly, but non significant, higher colostomy rate was seen in the SeqB group (16.5% vs 13.8%). Noteworthy, in this group, one surgical procedure was performed because of functional issues in this cohort.

After adjusting for known prognostic factors, the effect of undergoing different treatments highlighted an AdjHR with respect to 2-year CFS for the first 24 months of 0.95 (95%CI:0.49–1.84, $p = 0.877$), with an HR supposedly favoring the SIB approach, even if with a confidence interval containing the value 1 and thus not considerable as statistically significant (Fig. 1). We focused on the first 2 years because, for 17 out of 103

patients in the SeqB group, we could not retrieve an updated follow up (last observation time between 1 and 4 years from analysis), which could potentially affect the CFS rates as death from any cause is considered as an event. Interestingly, the cumulative incidence of colostomies at 1 and 2 years was higher in SeqB group (13.9%;95%CI:7.8–21.8 and 18.1%;95%CI: 10.8–27.0, respectively) compared to those of the SIB group (8.2%;95%CI:3.6–15.2 and 15.0%;95%CI: 8.1–23.9, respectively). We can hypothesize that it may suggest an explanation for the observed HR with respect to 2-year CFS when considering the SIB group. This observation may potentially be ascribed to the reduction in OTT given by the SIB strategy, but others clinical factors related to both patient and tumor that were not taken into account in the present analysis might have a consistent role. Given the retrospective nature of the present study and the unbalancement in terms of clinical characteristics between the 2 groups, we could not assess the superiority of one approach over the other nor the equivalence between them. Nevertheless, the clinical results reported within the SIB group are reassuring and strongly suggest the equipoise between the two strategies. Confirmatory prospective randomized trials would be need to prove this hypothesis. It is also interesting to observe that, albeit having a higher proportion of patients with high risk features in the SeqB group, no significant outcome differences were observed. A potential role of stage migration due to the use of inguinal SLNB in the SIB group can be pointed out to partially explain this finding. Several series have shown the detrimental effect of a longer OTT in anal cancer patients submitted to concurrent RT-CHT. Weber et al. have shown the a gap longer that 37.5 days had a significant effect on clinical outcomes in patient treated with split- course radiation [7]. In their series patients with a longer gap had a 75% loco-regional control rate compared to 92.3% for patients with a shorter gap [7]. Graf et al. found that OTT > 41 days significantly affected 5-year local control in anal cancer patients treated with RT-CT, as the rate was 58% for patients having OTT > 41 days and 79% for those with a OTT < 41 days ($p = 0.04$) [14]. This correlation was found regardless of the treatment approach used, either split-course or continuously delivered radiation. Pooled data analysis of patients enrolled in the RTOG 8704 and RTOG 9811 trials have shown a correlation between OTT and local failure, loco-regional failure, colostomy failure and time to failure, but not with CFS or OS [26]. In the RTOG 92–08 trial, dose escalation up to 59.9 Gy concurrent to 5-FU and MMC was investigated with a mandatory 2-week gap after 36 Gy [27]. Clinical outcomes were poor even with a higher dose delivered, suggesting a detrimental effect even of a short gap. Comparison between patients with similar characteristics having a 2-week gap (RTOG 9208) and those without (RTOG 8704) highlighted poorer results for patients with a longer gap [25]. The aforementioned clinical data are explained from a radiobiological point of view by accelerated repopulation that occurs after irradiation and may lead to a loss in tumor control of 1–2% and of 0.4–0.6 Gy for each day of OTT extension [28, 29]. Split-course studies demonstrated that a gap longer than 15 days may consistently affect clinical outcomes [28, 29]. Our study has some limitations including its retrospective nature, the missing of updated follow up for some patients in the SeqB cohort, the lack of the chance to adjust results for all tumor- and patient-related factors potentially affecting clinical outcomes and the maximum reliability of the analysis for the first 24 months of follow up only. Moreover the sample size determination might not be adequate enough to detect a small difference in clinical outcomes. Hence, our data cannot be considered conclusive. Another important limit is the lack of robust data on the toxicity profile that did not allow us to compare the 2 approaches with respect to this endpoint. The only toxicity endpoint analysed in the present study was hematologic toxicity which did not show any difference in the 2 groups with respect to ≥ G3 events. Toxicity data from the RTOG 0529 trial showed a reduction of skin, gastro-intestinal and hematologic toxicity for patients treated with dose-painted IMRT compared to standard treatment. The same treatment schedule was adopted in the SIB group of the present study.

Nevertheless, the comparison between SeqB and SIB approaches seems to suggest that SIB is non-inferior to SeqB in terms of probability of being alive without a colostomy in anal cancer patients, and it could be a valid approach in this clinical setting. A potential advantage in terms of CFS can be hypothesized for SIB due to the shortening in OTT, but this possible finding need to be confirmed with more robust and prospective data.

Conclusions

The present study is the first to report on comparative outcomes of anal cancer patients treated with RT-CHT employing a SIB strategy compared to a SeqB approach. Given its multicenter retrospective frame, potential selection biases due to the different patient and treatment characteristics between the 2 cohorts can be outlined. Different approaches in terms of patient care and follow up modalities, including time to event evaluation, may have had an influence on outcomes. Patients were given different doses to the prophylactic nodal volumes (36 Gy vs 42/45 Gy for the SeqB and SIB group, respectively), even if comparable in terms of biologically equivalent dose since given with diverse dose per fractions (1.8 Gy vs 1.5 Gy daily). Dose to the macroscopic tumor was different (59.4 Gy vs 54 Gy) as delivery technique (3DCRT vs IMRT) for the SeqB and SIB group, respectively. Patients in the SeqB group had, on average, a more advanced stage of disease presentation, while patients in the SeqB had a longer time between biopsy and chemo-radiation start. However, those unbalances were properly adjusted during the analysis to obtain an AdjHR depending mainly on treatment strategy (SIB vs SeqB). One of the pitfall of the study was the lack of toxicity data. We decided not to report on toxicity because of the retrospective nature of the study and the consequent lack of reliability for these outcomes. Thus, we decided to focus on CFS, OS and cumulative incidence of colostomy, since death and colostomy were deemed events whose detection was thought to be sufficiently reliable. With these robust clinical endpoints as comparative parameters, both SIB and SeqB approaches proved to be effective treatment strategies to be included in the combined modality therapy of non-metastatic anal cancer patients.

Abbreviations

5-FU: 5-fluorouracil; AdjHR: Adjusted hazard ratio; CFS: Colostomy-free survival; CT: Computed tomography; DFS: Disease-free survival; HRs: Hazard ratios; LC: Local control; MRI: Magnetic resonance imaging; OS: Overall survival; OTT: Overall treatment time; PET: Positron emission tomography; PS: Propensity score; RT: Radiotherapy; RT-CHT: Concurrent chemo-radiation; SeqB: Sequential boost; SIB: Simultaneous integrated boost; SLNB: Sentinel lymphnode biopsy

Authors' contributions

PF, BD, AL, FA: study conception and design; ET, SM, GCI, MV, AP, ACG: data collection; MC, AE, GF: data analysis; PF; manuscript draft; UR, GC, MM, PC: final revision and approval. All authors read and approved the final manuscript.

Competing interests

The authors declare that they have no competing interests.

Author details

¹Department of Oncology, Radiation Oncology, University of Turin, Via Genova 3, 10126 Turin, Italy. ²Department of Radiation Oncology, Centre Hospitalier Régional Universitaire 'Jean Minjoz', Besançon, France. ³Department of Radiation Oncology, Centre 'Paul Strauss', Strasbourg, France. ⁴Unit of Cancer Epidemiology and CPO Piedmont, AOU Citta' della Salute e della Scienza, Turin, Italy. ⁵Department of Surgical Sciences, University of Turin, Turin, Italy. ⁶Department of Medical Sciences, Pathology Unit, University of Turin, Turin, Italy. ⁷Department of Medical Oncology, Istituto Scientifico Romagnolo per lo Studio e la Cura dei Tumori (IRST) IRCCS, Meldola, Italy. ⁸Department of Radiation Oncology, Centre 'Georges-François-Leclerc', Dijon, France.

References

1. Franco P, Mistrangelo M, Arcadipane F, Munoz F, Sciacero P, Spadi R, et al. Intensity-modulated radiation therapy with simultaneous integrated boost combined with concurrent chemotherapy for the treatment of anal cancer patients: 4-year results of a consecutive case series. Cancer Investig. 2015; 33(6):259–66.

2. James RD, Glynne-Jones R, Meadows HM, Cunningham D, Myint AS, Saunders MP, et al. Mitomycin or cisplatin chemoradiation with or without maintenance chemotherapy for treatment of squamous-cell carcinoma of the anus (ACT II): a randomised, phase 3, open-label, 2 × 2 factorial trial. Lancet Oncol. 2013;14(6):516–24.

3. Franco P, Arcadipane F, Ragona R, Mistrangelo M, Cassoni P, Rondi N, et al. Early-stage node negative (T1-T2N0) anal cancer treated with simultaneous integrated boost radiotherapy and concurrent chemotherapy. Anticancer Res. 2016;36(4):1943–8.

4. Franco P, Arcadipane F, Ragona R, Mistrangelo M, Cassoni P, Rondi N, et al. Locally advanced (T3-T4 or N+) anal cancer treated with simultaneous integrated boost radiotherapy and concurrent chemotherapy. Anticancer Res. 2016;36(4):2027–32.

5. Ajani JA, Winter KA, Gunderson LL, Pedersen J, Benson AB 3rd, Thomas CR Jr, et al. Fluorouracil, mitomycin, and radiotherapy vs fluorouracil, cisplatin, and radiotherapy for carcinoma of the anal canal: a randomized controlled trial. JAMA. 2008;299(6):1914–21.

6. Kachnic LA, Winter K, Myerson RJ, Goodyear MD, Willins J, Esthappan J, et al. RTOG 0529: a phase 2 evaluation of dose-painted intensity modulated radiation therapy in combination with 5-fluorouracil and mitomycin C for the reduction of acute morbidity in carcinoma of the anal canal. Int J Radiat Oncol Biol Phys. 2013;86(1):27–33.

7. Weber D, Kurthz JM, Allal AS. The impact of gap duration on local control of anal cancer treated by split-course radiotherapy and concomitant chemotherapy. Int J Radiat Oncol Biol Phys. 2001;50(3):675–80.

8. Franco P, Ragona R, Arcadipane F, Mistrangelo M, Cassoni P, Rondi N, et al. Dosimetric predictors of acute hematologic toxicity during concurrent intensity-modulated radiotherapy and chemotherapy for anal cancer. Clin Transl Oncol. 2017;19(1):67–75.

9. Call J, Prendergast BM, Jensen LG, Ord CB, Goodman KA, Jacob R, et al. Intensity-modulated radiation therapy for anal cancer. Results from multi-institutional retrospective cohort study. Am J Clin Oncol. 2016;39(1):8–12.

10. Franco P, Arcadipane F, Ragona R, Mistrangelo M, Cassoni P, Munoz F, et al. Volumetric modulated arc therapy (VMAT) in the combined modality treatment of anal cancer patients. Br J Radiol. 2016;89(1060):2015832.

11. Glynne-Jones R, Tan D, Hughes R, Hoskin P. Squamous-cell carcinoma of the anus: progress in radiotherapy treatment. Nat Rev Clin Oncol. 2016;13(7):447–59.

12. Lepinoy A, Lescut N, Puyraveau M, Caubet M, Boustani J, Lakkis Z, et al. Evaluation of a 36 Gy elective node irradiation dose in anal cancer. Radiother Oncol. 2015;116(2):197–201.

13. De Bari B, Jumeau R, Bouchaab H, Vallet V, Matzinger O, Troussier I, et al. Efficacy and safety of helical tomotherapy with daily image guidance in anal cancer patients. Acta Oncol. 2016;55(6):767–73.

14. Graf R, Wust P, Hildebrandt B, Gögler H, Ullrich R, Herrmann R, et al. Impact of overall treatment time on local control of anal cancer treated with radiochemotherapy. Oncology. 2003;65(1):14–22.

15. Franco P, Arcadipane F, Ragona R, et al. Dose to specific subregions of pelvic bone marrow defined with FDG-PET as a predictor of hematologic nadirs during concomitant chemoradiation in anal cancer patients. Med Oncol. 2016;33(7):72.

16. Arcadipane F, Franco P, Ceccarelli M, Furfaro G, Rondi N, Trino E, et al. Image-guided IMRT with simultaneous integrated boost as per RTOG 0529 for the treatment of anal cancer. Asia Pac J Clin Oncol. 2018;14(3):217–23.

17. Grambsch PM, Therneau TM. Proportional hazards test and diagnostic based on weights residuals. Biometrika. 1994;3:515–26.

18. Gooley TA, Leisenring W, Crowley J, Storer BE. Estimation of failure probabilities in the presence of competing risks: new representations of old estimators. Statist Med. 1999;18:695–706.

19. Fine J, Gray R. A proportional hazards model for the subdistribution of a competing risk. J Am Stat Assoc. 1999;94(446):496–7.

20. Papillon J, Montbarbon JF. Epidermoid carcinoma of the anal canal. A series of 276 cases. Dis Colon Rectum. 1987;30(5):324–33.

21. Bartelink H, Roelofsen F, Eschwege F, Rougier P, Bosset JF, Gonzalez DG, et al. Concomitant radiotherapy and chemotherapy is superior to radiotherapy alone in the treatment of locally advanced anal cancer: results of a phase III randomized trial of the European Organization for Research and Treatment of Cancer radiotherapy and gastrointestinal cooperative group. J Clin Oncol. 1997;15(5):2040–9.

22. UKCCCR Anal cancer Trial Working Party. UK co-ordination committee on Cancer research: epidermal anal cancer: results from the UKCCCR randomized trial of radiotherapy alone versus radiotherapy, 5-fluorouracil, and mitomycin. Lancet. 1996;348(9034):1049–54.

23. Flam M, John M, Pajak TF, Petrelli N, Myerson R, Doggett S, et al. Role of mytomicin in combination with fluorouracil and radiotherapy, and of salvage chemoradiation in the definitive nonsurgical treatment of epidermoid carcinoma of the anal canal: results of a phase III randomized intergroup study. J Clin Oncol. 1996;14(9):2527–39.

24. Kim JJ, Tannock IF. Repopulation of cancer cells during therapy: an important cause of treatment failure. Nat Rev Cancer. 2005;5(7):516–25.

25. Bosset JF, Roelofsen F, Morgan DAL, Budach V, Coucke P, Jager JJ, et al. Shortened irradiation scheme, continuous infusion of 5-fluorouracil and fractionation of mitomycin C in locally advanced anal carcinomas. Results of a phase II study of the European Organization for Research and Treatment of Cancer. Radiotherapy and gastrointestinal cooperative groups. Eur J Cancer. 2003;39(1):45–51.

26. Ben-Josef E, Moughan J, Ajani JA, Flam M, Gunderson L, Pollock JD, et al. Impact of overall treatment time on survival and local control in patients with anal cancer: a pooled data analysis of radiation therapy oncology groups trials 87-04 and 98.11. J Clin Oncol. 2010;28(34):5061–6.

27. John M, Pajak T, Flam M, Hoffman J, Markoe A, Wolkov H, et al. Dose escalation in chemoradiation for anal cancer: preliminary results of RTOG 92-08. Cancer J Sci Am. 1996;2(4):205–11.

28. Konski A, Garcia M Jr, Madhu J, Krieg R, Pinover W, Myerson R, et al. Evaluation of planned treatment breaks during radiation therapy for anal cancer: update of RTOG 92-08. Int J Radiation Oncol Biol Phys. 2008;72(1):114–8.

29. Glynne-Jones R, Sebag-Montefiore D, Adams R, McDonald A, Gollins S, James R, et al. "Mind the gap" – The impact of variations in the duration of the treatment gap and overall treatment time in the first UK anal cancer trial (ACT I). Int J Radiation Oncol Biol Phys. 2011;81(5):1488–94.

Molecular signature of response to preoperative radiotherapy in locally advanced breast cancer

Miljana Tanić[1,3]* (iD), Ana Krivokuća[1], Milena Čavić[1], Jasmina Mladenović[2], Vesna Plesinac Karapandžić[2], Stephan Beck[3], Siniša Radulović[1], Snezana Susnjar[4] and Radmila Janković[1]

Abstract

Background: Radiation therapy is an indispensable part of various treatment modalities for breast cancer. Specifically, for non-inflammatory locally advanced breast cancer (LABC) patients, preoperative radiotherapy (pRT) is currently indicated as a second line therapy in the event of lack of response to neoadjuvant chemotherapy. Still approximately one third of patients fails to respond favourably to pRT. The aim of this study was to explore molecular mechanisms underlying differential response to radiotherapy (RT) to identify predictive biomarkers and potential targets for increasing radiosensitivity.

Methods: The study was based on a cohort of 134 LABC patients, treated at the Institute of Oncology and Radiology of Serbia (IORS) with pRT, without previous or concomitant systemic therapy. Baseline transcriptional profiles were established using Agilent 60 K microarray platform in a subset of 23 formalin-fixed paraffin-embedded (FFPE) LABC tumour samples of which 11 radiotherapy naïve and 3 post-radiotherapy samples passed quality control and were used for downstream analysis. Biological networks and signalling pathways underlying differential response to RT were identified using Ingenuity Pathways Analysis software. Predictive value of candidate genes in the preoperative setting was further validated by qRT-PCR in an independent subset of 60 LABC samples of which 42 had sufficient quality for data analysis, and in postoperative setting using microarray data from 344 node-negative breast cancer patients (Erasmus cohort, GSE2034 and GSE5327) treated either with surgery only (20%) or surgery with RT (80%).

Results: We identified 192 significantly differentially expressed genes (FDR < 0.10) between pRT-responsive and non-responsive tumours, related to regulation of cellular development, growth and proliferation, cell cycle control of chromosomal replication, glucose metabolism and NAD biosynthesis II route. *APOA1*, *MAP3K4*, and *MMP14* genes were differentially expressed (FDR < 0.20) between pRT responders and non-responders in preoperative setting, while *MAP3K4* was further validated as RT-specific predictive biomarker of distant metastasis free survival (HR = 2.54, [95%CI:1.42–4.55], p = 0.002) in the postoperative setting.

Conclusions: This study pinpoints *MAP3K4* as a putative biomarker of response to RT in both preoperative and postoperative settings and a potential target for radiosensitising combination therapy, warranting further preclinical studies and prospective clinical validation.

Keywords: Preoperative radiotherapy, Locally advanced breast cancer, Biomarker, Gene expression profiling

* Correspondence: m.tanic@ucl.ac.uk
[1]Laboratory for Molecular Genetics, Institute of Oncology and Radiology of Serbia, Belgrade, Serbia
[3]Medical Genomics, UCL Cancer Institute, University College London, London, UK
Full list of author information is available at the end of the article

Background

Non-inflammatory locally advanced breast carcinoma (LABC) is a late stage breast cancer presented as a bulky primary chest wall tumour and/or extensive adenopathy including patients with large (> 5 cm), usually inoperable tumours and node positive disease [1]. It is a common presentation worldwide but is of special concern in developing countries with limited breast cancer awareness and efficient population screening programs. For instance, in Serbia over 4500 new breast cancer cases are diagnosed each year, with as many as 30% presenting as late stage initially inoperable LABC.

A multimodal approach including systemic therapy, radiotherapy and surgery is usually applied in the treatment of LABC [2]. Currently, neoadjuvant systemic therapy (CHT) is usually administered to downstage the tumour for breast-conserving surgery, while preoperative radiotherapy (pRT) is often indicated if there is no objective reduction of tumour volume after the administration of neoadjuvant (CHT). Radiation therapy (RT) is frequently used in various modalities for treatment of breast cancer of different stages including LABC, and large meta-analyses of multiple randomised trials demonstrated clear long-term benefit both in terms of locoregional control and reduced mortality in breast cancer patients treated with radiotherapy after breast conserving surgery and after radical mastectomy [3–5]. Given the rarity of this treatment modality only a few studies looked into the effects of preoperative radiotherapy (pRT) in combination with breast conserving surgery on locoregional recurrence and overall survival reporting similar results compared to protocols involving neoadjuvant chemotherapy without irradiation [6–9]. However, the molecular basis of tumour sensitivity to radiotherapy is complex, and at present, there are no conclusive biomarkers in clinical use to predict if a patient will, in fact, benefit from radiotherapy.

The concept of personalised medicine has been successfully implemented in medical oncology for over a decade with several biomarkers approved for clinical use. The same principle could be applied to radiation oncology to achieve better clinical responses to radiotherapy, lower radio-toxicity and avoid overtreatment [10, 11]. To achieve this goal there is a clear need to develop biomarkes specific for breast radiotherapy. Hovever, most of the studies in radiation oncology have been limited to the study of biomarkers not necessarily chosen based on their specificity to radiotherapy. Molecular subtypes have shown limited predictive estimation of RT efficacy and have been potentially confounded by adjuvant systemic therapy [11–13]. Several studies aimed to identify a radiosensitivity molecular signature in breast cancer by studying changes in gene and protein expression in response to radiation in cellular and animal model systems. These included determination of cellular radiosensitivity defined by survival fraction at 2 Gy [14], clonogenic doubling time, hypoxic fraction, or clonogenic number [15], with some of these multigene signatures having been validated in retrospective studies in solid tumours including breast cancer [16–18].

Although these studies provided valuable insights into cellular radiation response, the breast tissue has a complex microenvironment composed of several interacting cell types and extracellular molecules that may affect tumour response. The ideal model system for researching the breast tumour response to radiation therapy and evaluating the predictive value of markers is the preoperative setting [19, 20]. Detection and characterization of biomarkers in the patient's tumour biopsies with known clinical response, before and after radiation therapy could select the group of patients with worse response to radiotherapy, to facilitate the choice of more efficient treatment, avoid overtreatment and consequentially reduce associated healthcare costs.

Leveraging a cohort of LABC patients treated with pRT without neoadjuvant or concomitant CHT (IORS LABC cohort) we determined baseline molecular differences between radio-resistant and radio-responsive breast tumours and identified putative predictive biomarkers of response to pRT. In our previous study on this cohort [21] we have shown that the extent of the clinical response to pRT in LABC is predictive of overall survival. Here, we analysed global gene expression patterns and biological pathways associated with differential response to pRT in a discovery subset of the IORS LABC cohort. Selected biomarkers were validated by an orthogonal assay (qPCR) in an independent validation set of pRT IORS LABC samples, and in the postoperative setting using an external microarray dataset (Erasmus cohort) consisting of breast cancer patients treated only with radiotherapy following surgery.

Methods

Patient cohorts

IORS LABC cohort

This retrospective cohort included 134 patients with locally invasive non-inflammatory breast cancer (LABC) (93 patients stage III-a, and 41 patients III-b) treated with pRT between 1997 and 2000, delivering 45Gy in 15 fractions every second day alternately to the breast and regional lymph nodes, followed by radical mastectomy and adjuvant chemo and/or hormonal therapy (Fig. 1a). The median follow-up was 74 months (4–216) counted from the breast cancer diagnosis until last check-up or death from any cause. Five-year overall survival was 56% and 5-year disease free survival was 39.2%. Tumour biopsy was taken both prior to radiation treatment to obtain a radiotherapy-naïve sample (series A), and after RT and radical mastectomy before adjuvant treatment (series B)

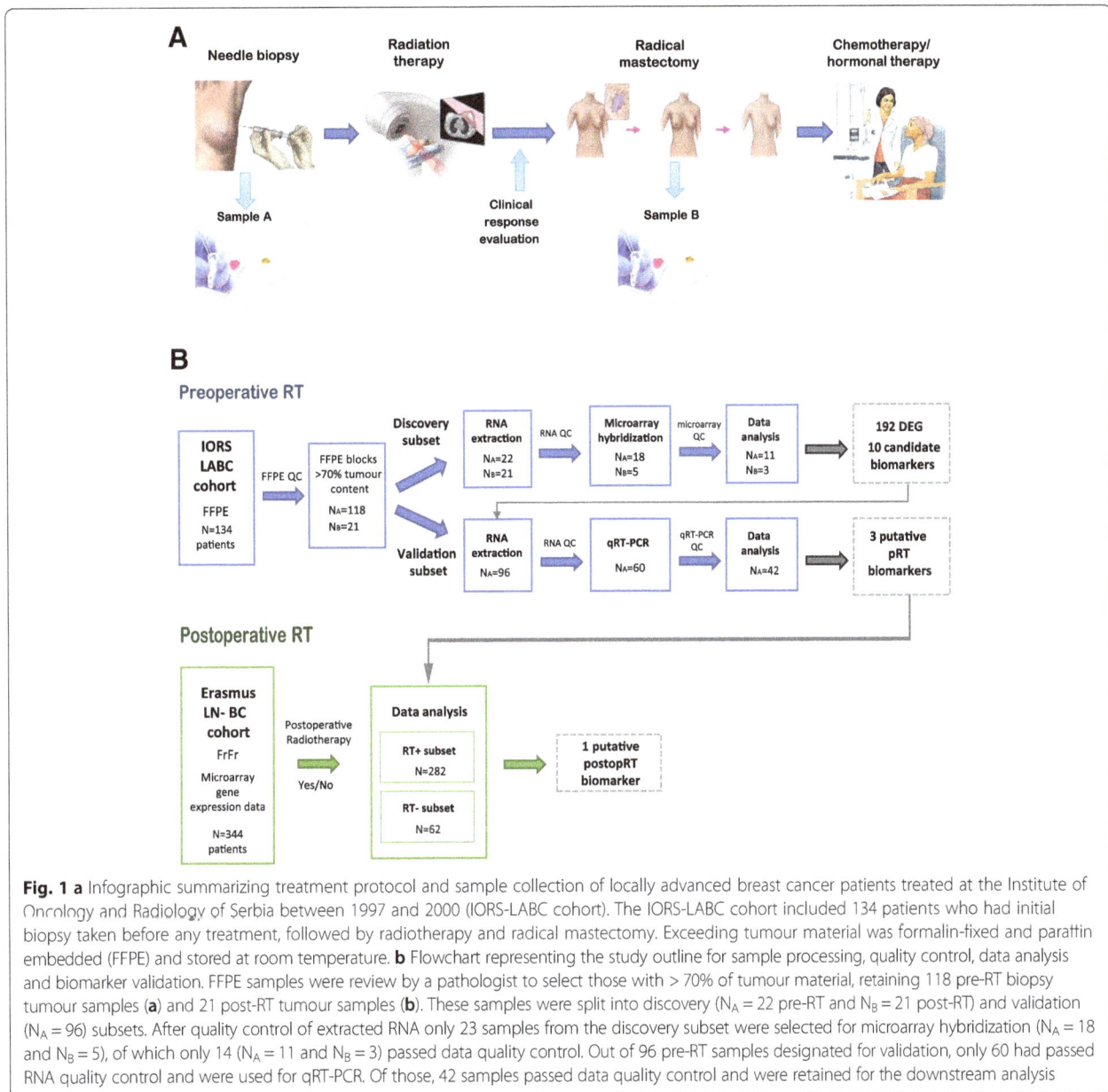

Fig. 1 a Infographic summarizing treatment protocol and sample collection of locally advanced breast cancer patients treated at the Institute of Oncology and Radiology of Serbia between 1997 and 2000 (IORS-LABC cohort). The IORS-LABC cohort included 134 patients who had initial biopsy taken before any treatment, followed by radiotherapy and radical mastectomy. Exceeding tumour material was formalin-fixed and paraffin embedded (FFPE) and stored at room temperature. **b** Flowchart representing the study outline for sample processing, quality control, data analysis and biomarker validation. FFPE samples were review by a pathologist to select those with > 70% of tumour material, retaining 118 pre-RT biopsy tumour samples (**a**) and 21 post-RT tumour samples (**b**). These samples were split into discovery (N_A = 22 pre-RT and N_B = 21 post-RT) and validation (N_A = 96) subsets. After quality control of extracted RNA only 23 samples from the discovery subset were selected for microarray hybridization (N_A = 18 and N_B = 5), of which only 14 (N_A = 11 and N_B = 3) passed data quality control. Out of 96 pre-RT samples designated for validation, only 60 had passed RNA quality control and were used for qRT-PCR. Of those, 42 samples passed data quality control and were retained for the downstream analysis

stored as formalin-fixed paraffin-embedded (FFPE) tissue samples. Clinical response to pRT in the breast was defined per RECIST criteria [22]. All patients gave their informed written consent for the use of residual tissue for research. The study was approved by the Institute of Oncology and Radiology Ethical Review Board for human studies. An overview of the patients' clinicopathological characteristics is summarised in Additional file 1: Table S1.

Erasmus breast cancer cohort

For biomarker validation, we have used a previously published clinical data set from the Erasmus cohort (GSE2034 and GSE5327). This cohort includes 344 lymph-node negative breast cancer patients treated at the Erasmus Medical Center (Rotterdam, Netherlands) from 1980 to 1995, who had not received neoadjuvant nor adjuvant systemic treatment [23]. Primary treatment was breast-conserving surgery or modified radical mastectomy, and 87% of the patients received postoperative RT. Early metastasis was defined as distant recurrence in the first 5 years following completion of primary treatment.

RNA extraction from FFPE tissue

Tumour tissue sections were stained with H&E and examined by a pathologist. Tumour tissue was macrodissected prior to RNA extraction to ensure there was > 70% tumour content. Total RNA was extracted from 3 to 5 10 μm thick FFPE tissue sections using RNeasy

FFPE Kit (Qiagen) with an 18-h Proteinase K tissue digestion step. RNA quantity and purity were assessed by BioSpec-nano (Shimadzu Scientific Instruments).

Microarray hybridization and data analysis

Agilent SurePrint G3-Hmn-GE-v.2-8x60K Microarray platform was used for gene expression profiling following Agilent Gene Expression FFPE Workflow. Raw data pre-processing and quality control was performed using R version 3.0.1 and R/Bioconductor packages 'limma', 'ffpe' and 'ArrayQualityMetrics'. Data were deposited in the GEO database under the GSE101920 accession number. Hierarchical average linkage clustering was performed using Cluster 3.0 and visualised using JavaTreeView [24]. Differential expression analysis was performed using the POMELO II tool applying moderated t-test [25]. The estimated significance levels were corrected for multiple hypotheses testing using Benjamini and Hochberg False Discovery Rate (FDR) adjustment [26]. The ranked target list of the differentially expressed genes was subjected to pathway enrichment analyses using Ingenuity Pathway Analysis software (Ingenuity Systems). Significantly enriched gene networks and canonical pathways based on the curated IPA database KEGG, Biocarta, and Reactome, were identified as previously described [15]. Methods are described in detail in Additional file 2: Supplementary Methods.

Quantitative RT-PCR and statistical analysis

Applied Biosystems High Capacity cDNA Reverse Transcription Kit was used for preparing cDNA from 200 ng RNA. Quantitative RT-PCR was done on an ABI Prism 7300 (Applied Biosystems) using TaqMan® Gene Expression Assays and TaqMan® PreAmp Master Mix Kit (Life Technologies). All qPCR amplicons were designed to be less than 100 bp long and all assays were done in triplicate. Assay ID numbers are shown in Supplementary Table 4. Each plate included a HeLa cell line as inter-plate calibrator (IPC) and a non-template control (NTC). Average Ct values for each gene were standardised to IPC, dCt values were calculated relative to *ACTB* as a reference gene. Genes and samples with over 70% of missing values were excluded from further analysis, retaining 8 genes and 42 samples for further analysis. Undetermined values were set to the number of cycles performed (Ct = 45). Data was log2 transformed and differences in gene expression levels between groups were tested using Student t-test and corrected for multiple testing with FDR set to 20%.

Erasmus dataset processing and statistical analysis

Erasmus dataset was downloaded from GEO database and processed using *affy* R package. Distant metastasis free survival (DMFS) was defined as any distant recurrence within 5 years after the end of treatment. Survival curves were plotted with the Kaplan–Meier method and log-rank test was used to evaluate differences between groups defined by candidate gene expression status. Cutoff Finder was used to determine the optimal cutpoint for gene expression dichotomization based on the log-rank test minimum *P*-value approach [27]. Hazard ratios were estimated using the Cox proportional hazards model, stratified by RT status in a univariable and multivariable analysis. Pearson's χ^2 test was used to check for unbalanced distribution of clinico-pathologcal varables (ER, PR, T-stage and age categories) in subgroup analysis (Additional file 3: Table S2). Measures of biological interaction were determined both on additive scale and multiplicative scale [28, 29]. Stata command icp was used for calculating 3 different measures of interaction contrast on an additive scale: relative excess risk due to interaction [RERI], attributable proportion [AP] and synergy index [S] as described in [30]. Multiplicative interaction was assessed by including an interaction term with main effects in the Cox proportional hazard model. Statistical calculations were performed using STATA version 11.2 (StataCorp). All reported *p*-values were two-sided with a 0.05 significance level.

Results

Molecular signature of radiosensitivity in LABC tumour samples

To gain a better understanding of the molecular response to radiotherapy independently of systemic treatment and to identify a baseline transcriptional signature of radiosensitivity between radio-responsive and non-responsive tumours, we have analysed radiotherapy-naïve LABC tumour biopsies and post radiotherapy mastectomy samples by gene expression profiling. A total of 43 FFPE tumour samples (N_A = 22, N_B = 21) from the patient cohort was randomly selected maintaining balanced group representation of clinical response (CR, PR, SD) and other clinicopathological characteristics (Additional file 4: Table S1). Of those, due to the low concentration or purity of the RNA extracted from FFPE only 23 samples were selected for microarray hybridization. Following stringent microarray quality control 14 samples (N_A = 11, N_B = 3) were included in subsequent data analysis (Additional file 4: Figure S1), comprising of 8 patients with stable disease designated as non-responders (NR) and 6 patients which experienced either complete (2 pts) or partial clinical response (4 pts) to pRT, classified as responders (R) (Fig. 1b).

Although unsupervised clustering analysis over top 20% most variable transcripts revealed separation between non-responders and responders (Additional file 5: Figure S2), not enough post-RT samples were left after QC to draw relevant conclusions regarding changes in pRT response between pre-RT and post-RT biopsies. Therefore, to study intrinsic differences underlying differential response to radiotherapy in the neoadjuvant setting, we have analysed only pre-RT tumour samples (N_A = 11) to look for differences in baseline transcriptional profiles between responders (R) and non-responders-(NR). We identified 192 significantly differentially expressed mRNA transcripts (> 2-fold change and FDR < 0.1), including 89 annotated protein coding genes (PCG) and 78 long non-coding RNAs (lncRNAs) (Additional file 6: Table S3). Of those, only 7 genes were found to be upregulated while the rest of the genes (185) were downregulated in radio-responsive tumours (R) (Fig. 2a). The top 20 differentially expressed PCG are listed in Table 1.

To elucidate which biological processes and signalling pathways are associated with differential response to pRT, we have applied a gene set enrichment analysis using Ingenuity Pathways Analysis software. The bulk of differentially expressed genes were organised in two top scoring gene networks: lipid metabolism, molecular transport and small molecule biochemistry (Network 1)

and cell cycle, DNA replication, recombination, and repair (Network 2) (Additional file 7: Figure S3). Specifically, differentially activated canonical pathways (Fisher's test $p < 0.05$) between pRT responders and non-responders, included cell cycle control of chromosomal replication, and pathways related to glucose metabolism and de novo NAD biosynthesis (Fig. 2b). Similarly, molecular functions significantly enriched within the list of differentially expressed genes included cellular development, cell growth and proliferation, cell cycle and functions related to cell morphology, movement, assembly and organisation in addition to metabolic processes (Fig. 2c).

Candidate gene validation by qRT PCR

Even after controlling for false discovery rate, due to the small size of the discovery cohort and technical challenges related to FFPE-based microarray hybridization, several associations with the outcome of interest may have occurred due to chance alone. Therefore, we

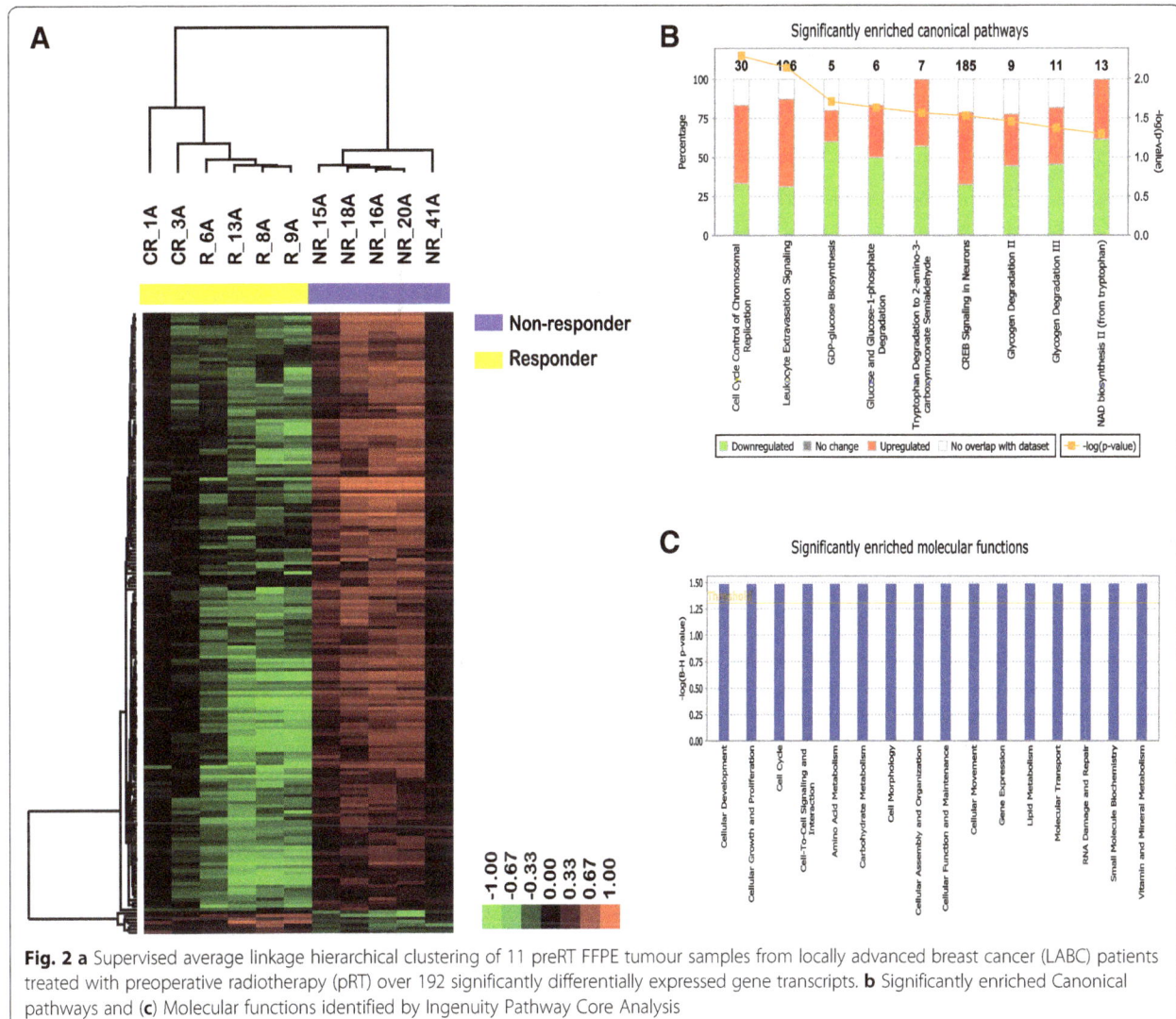

Fig. 2 a Supervised average linkage hierarchical clustering of 11 preRT FFPE tumour samples from locally advanced breast cancer (LABC) patients treated with preoperative radiotherapy (pRT) over 192 significantly differentially expressed gene transcripts. **b** Significantly enriched Canonical pathways and (**c**) Molecular functions identified by Ingenuity Pathway Core Analysis

Table 1 Top 20 significantly differentially expressed protein coding genes between pRT responsive and non-responsive tumor samples

#	Gene Symbol	Gene Name	FDR-adjusted q-value	Fold Change	Super-Pathways
1	ST3GAL4	ST3 beta-galactoside alpha-2, 3-sialyltransferase 4	0.03715[##]	0.10	protein glycosylation
2	C6orf105 (ADTRP)	chromosome 6 open reading frame 105 (Androgen-Dependent TFPI-Regulating Protein)	0.03715[##]	0.17	No Data Available
3	RAP1GAP2	RAP1 GTPase activating protein 2	0.03781[##]	0.18	Immune System
4	A1CF	APOBEC1 complementation factor	0.03874[##]	0.17	mRNA Editing and Processing of Capped Intron-Containing Pre-mRNA
5	MAP3K4	mitogen-activated protein kinase kinase kinase 4	0.03874[##]	0.25	MAPK signaling pathway
6	CHD5	chromodomain helicase DNA binding protein 5	0.05133[#]	0.15	ATP-dependent helicase activity
7	LAS1L	LAS1-like (S. cerevisiae)	0.05209[#]	0.19	biogenesis of the 60S ribosomal subunit.
8	DEFB128	defensin, beta 128	0.05781[#]	0.29	Immune System
9	ENHO	energy homeostasis associated	0.05781[#]	0.23	metabolism
10	CECR9	cat eye syndrome chromosome region, candidate 9 (non-protein coding)	0.05781[#]	0.20	unknown
11	IDO1	indoleamine 2,3-dioxygenase 1	0.05781[#]	0.20	Tryptophan metabolism
12	LRRC55	leucine rich repeat containing 55	0.05788[#]	0.14	ion channel
13	ROGDI	rogdi homolog (Drosophila)	0.05788[#]	0.26	unknown
14	KRT25	keratin 25	0.05796[#]	0.22	cytoskeleton
15	LAMA4	laminin, alpha 4	0.05798[#]	0.25	Focal Adhesion, ECM-receptor interaction
16	PLA2G2C	phospholipase A2, group IIC	0.05798[#]	0.15	alpha-Linolenic acid metabolism and Glycerophospholipid biosynthesis
17	CCDC114	coiled-coil domain containing 114	0.05798[#]	0.25	cell motility
18	CNGB1	cyclic nucleotide gated channel beta 1	0.05798[#]	0.27	cAMP binding and intracellular cAMP activated cation channel activity
19	PRSS53	protease, serine, 53	0.05798[#]	0.30	serine-type endopeptidase activity
20	GSG1	germ cell associated 1	0.05798[#]	0.22	RNA polymerase binding

FDR – false discovery rate; Fold change is shown on a linear scale
[#]q-value < 0.1; [##]q-value < 0.05

proceeded to validate a selected panel of genes in an independent set of pre-RT tumour samples ($N_A = 60$) using an orthogonal assay (qRT-PCR). Ten genes (*CHEK2, XRCC2, MCM6, MAP3K4, MMP14, APOA1, WHSC1L1, IDO1, ST3GAL-4* and *A1CF*) were selected for validation based on the significance threshold, high expression in tumour tissue and plausible biological function. Samples in which over 70% of assays have failed were discarded, retaining 42/60 samples for statistical analysis (Fig. 1b). Considering the cost of missing a potentially interesting gene (false negative) versus the low cost of further external validation to discard any false positive calls, we decided to use a lax False Discovery Rate of 20%. Differential gene expression between responders ($N_R = 30$) and non-responders ($N_{NR} = 12$) was observed for *APOA1, MAP3K4* and *MMP14* genes with over 2-fold down-regulation in pRT-responsive tumours (Table 2).

External validation of candidate gene predictive value for radiotherapy response

To evaluate whether expression of *APOA1, MAP3K4* and *MMP14* genes has an impact on patient survival in the postoperative setting, we analysed distant metastasis-free survival (DMFS) using a well-characterized cohort of 344 lymph node-negative breast patients undergoing surgical treatment, with or without postoperative radiotherapy (Erasmus cohort) (Fig. 1b). The Erasmus cohort was chosen to eliminate potential confounding effects of systemic therapy, and to asses weather these genes are radiation-specific (predictive) or not (simply prognostic) in a stratified analysis. Of the three genes tested in a subgroup analysis, only low *MAP3K4* expression (< 7.94) was significantly associated with better DMFS (HR = 2.41 [95%CI:1.37–4.24], $p = 0.002$) in 282 patients treated with both surgery and RT, but not for those 62 patients

Table 2 Gene expression analysis by qRT-PCR in an independent subset of 42 LABC tumor samples

#	Gene Symbol	Amplicon Length	Responders (R)(n = 30)		Non-responders (NR)(n = 12)		p-value	Fold change
			mean	sd	mean	sd		
1	APOA1	**63**	5.99	1.96	7.55	1.37	**0.0161****	0.34
2	CHEK2	109	−4.63	1.69	−4.18	1.06	0.390	0.73
3	IDO1	**106**	1.06	2.87	0.63	2.82	0.662	1.35
4	MAP3K4	89	−3.00	1.99	−1.78	1.28	**0.0582***	0.43
5	MCM6	**109**	−5.12	1.98	−4.88	2.34	0.741	0.85
6	MMP14	92	7.85	2.85	9.61	2.03	**0.0596***	0.30
7	ST3GAL4	**60**	−3.95	2.68	−3.38	3.32	0.566	0.67
8	WHSC1L1	**67**	−0.98	3.90	−1.16	4.61	0.979	1.13
9	XRCC2	**66**	−4.68	2.08	−4.04	2.13	0.455	0.64

Gene expression was determined by qRT-PCR in independent test set of 60 FFPE breast tumors, of wich 42 were retained for data anlysis. Represented data were interplate calibrated, normalized to B-Actin and log2 transformed. Normality was evaluated using Lilform test. p-values - level of significance according to the Student's t-test or nonparametric Kolmogorov-Smirnov test (WHSC1L1 and ST3GAL4), FC fold change gene expression relative to ACTB between pRT responders (R) to nonresponders (NR) tumors measured by qPR-PCR; Fold change is shown on a linear scale
*p-value < 0.1; **p-value < 0.05

undergoing only surgery (HR = 1.93 [95%CI:0.54–6.84], $p = 0.309$) indicating that the effect is specific for RT-treated patients (Fig. 3). After controlling for age, steroid receptor status, T-stage and menopause status as potential confounders in a multivariable analysis MAP3K4 remained an independent predictor of DMFS (HR = 2.54, [95%CI:1.42–4.55], p = 0.002) in RT-treated patients. (Table 3). To check for the presence of biological interaction between *MAP3K4* levels and radiotherapy, we calculated hazard ratios for each category combination and summary measures of effect modification on both multiplicative and additive scale. There was no evidence of statistical interaction on a multiplicative scale, while the combined effect of *MAP3K4* levels and radiotherapy on additive scale exceeded that of each exposure alone with a 0.91 relative excess risk due to interaction [RERI] (Table 4).

Discussion

Treatment of LABC continues to be challenging with patients being at increased risks of locoregional recurrence, distant metastasis and reduced quality of life. Breast radiotherapy was shown to be effective in the locoregional control and provided benefit in distant metastasis-free survival and for downstaging the tumour in the preoperative treatment of LABC. However, not all patients achieve a satisfying response to radiotherapy. Clinically, a tumour is considered radioresistant when irradiation is unable to reduce its volume or when a recurrence occurs after a possible regression. Thus, it would be beneficial to identify biomarkers predictive of initial response to pRT that could be useful to predict clinical outcome in RT treated patients.

Here we explored gene expression profiles in pre- and post-RT tumour biopsies of LABC samples with

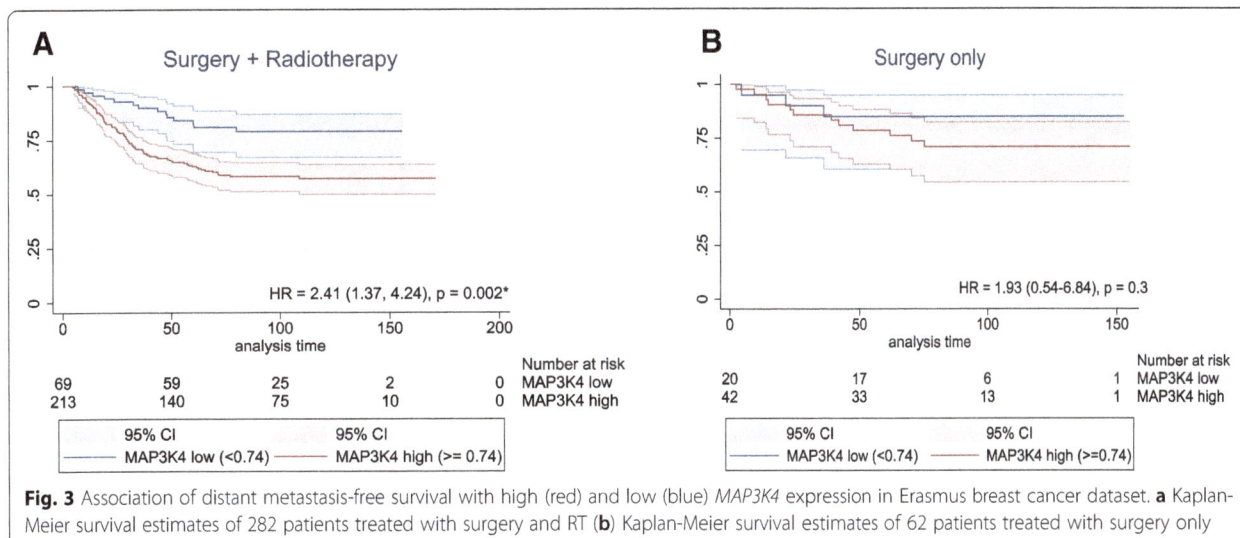

Fig. 3 Association of distant metastasis-free survival with high (red) and low (blue) *MAP3K4* expression in Erasmus breast cancer dataset. **a** Kaplan-Meier survival estimates of 282 patients treated with surgery and RT (**b**) Kaplan-Meier survival estimates of 62 patients treated with surgery only

Table 3 Multivariable Cox regression analysis of distant metastasis free survival in 282 patients treated with radiotherapy and surgery

Variable	Reference vs. level	Hazard Ratio	(95% CI)	p-value
MAP3K4 level	(low vs. high)	2.54	(1.42, 4.55)	0.002*
ER/PR status	(ER+/PR+ vs. ER-/PR+ or ER+/PR-, ER-/PR-)	1.20	(0.94, 1.52)	0.146
Age	(under 40 vs. 40–55, 56–70, over 70)	0.81	(0.53, 1.24)	0.332
Menopause	(pre-menopausal vs. postmenopausal)	1.19	(0.58, 2.42)	0.639
T-stage	(T1 vs. T2, T3, T4)	1.08	(0.75, 1.55)	0.697

*p-value < 0.01

different clinical response to pRT. However, after microarray QC there were too few pre- and post-RT matched samples to be able to draw any statistically significant conclusions regarding changes induced by pRT. Therefore, we focused our further analysis on pre-RT biopsies only, to establish baseline differences in transcriptional profiles between patients achieving either complete or partial clinical response and those who did not respond to pRT. Among 192 significantly differentially expressed transcripts, only 89 corresponded to known protein coding genes and to 78 lncRNA. Although, lncRNAs were shown to have important roles in a broad range of biological processes such as at the level of post-transcriptional processing and transcriptional gene silencing [6, 7] their biological function in breast cancer, and especially in relation to radiation therapy remains unknown.

Using IPA analysis, we explored which gene networks and signalling pathways are conferring radiation resistance/sensitivity in LABC tumour samples. Looking at protein interactions, most of the genes were organised in two major networks, one constituted of genes involved in lipid metabolism, molecular transport and small molecule biochemistry and the second related to cell cycle, DNA replication, recombination, and repair. These results further emphasise the importance of the cell cycle and proliferation state on cellular radiosensitivity, in line with the current body of knowledge [31, 32]. Interestingly, when focusing on specific canonical pathways in addition to cell cycle control of chromosomal

Table 4 Hazard ratios for distant metastasis free survival with 95% CI in 344 lymph node negative breast cancer patients with measures of effect modification

MAP3K4 level	Radiotherapy	Hazard Ratio	(95% CI)	p-value
low	no	Reference = 1		
low	yes	1.33	(0.38, 4.63)	0.652
high	no	1.97	(0.56, 6.97)	0.294
high	yes	3.21	(1.02, 10.15)	0.047*

Measure of effect modification on additive scale: RERI (95% CI) 0.91 (−0.56, 2.39); P = 0.226
Measure of effect modification on multiplicative scale: ratio of HRs (95% CI) 1.23 (0.31, 4.90); P = 0.773

replication, pathways related to glucose metabolism and de novo NAD biosynthesis were significantly overrepresented. This profile potentially reflects a comparatively activated metabolic pathway for de novo synthesis of NAD+ in radio-resistant tumours. In addition to its numerous functions in redox reactions, NAD+ is a sole substrate for the activity of PARP enzyme in the repair of DNA single-strand brakes [33, 34]. Several inhibitors of IDO1 gene, a rate-limiting enzyme for the NAD+ de novo synthesis from tryptophan found to be downregulated in radiosensitive LABC tumours, have shown a radiosensitising effect in in pre-clinical studies, making it an attractive target for drug-radiation combination therapy [35–37].

The second aim of the study was to identify potential biomarkers of response to radiotherapy. To this end, we selected 10 genes to be validated by an orthogonal assay in an independent subset of LABC tumours. Only 3 genes (APOA1, MAP3K4 and MMP14) were confirmed to be downregulated in radiosensitive tumours in the preoperative setting. These markers were further validated in an independent dataset of breast tumours treated only with mastectomy with or without postoperative radiotherapy. Only MAP3K4 gene was found to independently and specifically predict DMFS in radiotherapy-treated patients. Patients with high levels of MAP3K4 treated with RT had shorter DMFS than those with low MAP3K4 levels, due to an adverse interaction of high MAP3K4 expression with RT. MAP3K4 is a member of first layer of kinases of the MAPK signalling pathway that is activated by a variety of stimuli, including ionizing radiation, to mediate activation of transcription factors controlling differentiation, proliferation, cell growth and survival [38]. Increased expression of MAP3K4 in breast tumours may confer radioresistance through augmented signalling for RT-induced DNA damage repair through G2 arrest thus aiding survival of irradiated cancer cells [39]. Therefore, detecting the levels of MAP3K4 expression in breast tumours, may be useful for the prediction of response to RT for tumour downstaging for breast conserving surgery in LABC. Furthermore, inhibition of Ras-Raf-MEK-ERK cascade was shown to increase radiosensitivity both in in vitro as well as in vivo studies rendering MAPK signalling as an attractive radiosensitising target [40–42].

The main limitation of this study is a small sample size of the discovery cohort resulting from suboptimal RNA extracted from FFPE material, that may have led to inflated type I error. To mitigate this effect, we performed validation in larger independent series using an orthogonal assay. However, the limitation of the qPCR method using FFPE tissues is that it is sensitive to degraded DNA thus not all genes could have been detected in all patients' samples. Despite these limitations, the value of these results lies in the use of LABC tumour samples exposed only to RT without systemic therapy administered either previously or concomitantly with RT, and further validation of candidate genes' effect on DMFS in a large independent cohort devoid of any confounding effects of systemic therapy.

Conclusions

In summary, this study provides a novel insight into the underlying biology of intrinsic breast tumour radioresistance and points to genes and pathways that may be targeted to increase radiosensitivity. Additionally, we identified a putative radiotherapy-specific biomarker of response, *MAP3K4* that warrants further mechanistic studies and validation in randomized prospective cohorts to optimise patient selection and treatment planning.

Additional files

Additional file 1: Figure S1. Quality assessment and control for FFPE microarray expression data.

Additional file 2: Figure S2. Unsupervised average linkage hierarchical clustering over top 20% most variable genes of 14 FFPE tumour samples from locally advanced breast cancer (LABC) patients treated with preoperative radiotherapy (pRT).

Additional file 3: Figure S3. Top scoring gene networks identified by Ingenuity Pathway Core Analysis. **A)** Network 1: lipid metabolism, molecular transport and small molecule biochemistry **B)** Network 2: cell cycle, DNA replication, recombination, and repair.

Additional file 4: Table S1. Clinico-pathological characteristics of the pre-radiotherapy LABC sample series included in the study.

Additional file 5: Table S2. List of 192 differentially expressed transcripts between radio-responders and radioresistant pre-operative LABC samples.

Additional file 6: Table S3. List of TaqMan Gene Expression Assays used for validation

Additional file 7: Supplementary Methods. Detailed description of microarray hybridization, microarray data analysis, pathway enrichment analysis, validation of mRNA expression profiles by Q-RT-PCR and statistical analysis.

Abbreviations

cCD: Clinical complete response; CHT: Neoadjuvant systemic therapy; CI: Confidence interval; cPC: Clinical partial responder; cSD: Clinical stable disease; DMFS: Distant metastasis free survival; FDR: False discovery rate; FFPE : Formalin-fixed paraffin-embedded; GEO: Gene expression omnibus; HR: Hazard ratio; IORS: Institute for Oncology and Radiology of Serbia; IPA: Ingenuity Pathway Analysis; IPC: Inter-plate calibrator; LABC: Locally advanced breast cancer; NR: Non-responder; NTC : Non-template control; pRT: Preoperative radiotherapy; qPCR: Quantitative polymerase chain reaction; R: Responder; RT: Radiotherapy

Acknowledgements

We kindly thank Dr. John Foekens for providing RT information for the Erasmus MC cohorts included in GSE2014 and GSE5327.

Funding

This work was supported by the Ministry of Education, Science and Technological Development of Serbia (Grant No. III 41026, OI 172017 and OI 172030. MT was supported by the People Programme (Marie Curie Actions) of the European Union's Seventh Framework Programme (FP7/2007–2013/ 608765) and L'Oreal/UNESCO-Serbia for Women in Science - National Fellowship (2013).

Authors' contributions

MT, RJ, SS conceived and designed the study. MT, AK, MC performed the experimental work. MT analysed the data and drafted the manuscript. JM, SS, SR, JF, VPK, SB, contributed reagents, materials and analysis tools. MT, AK, MC, RJ, JM, SS, SR contributed to the interpretation of results and editing of the final manuscript. All authors read and approved the final manuscript.

Competing interests

The authors declare that they have no competing interests.

Author details

[1]Laboratory for Molecular Genetics, Institute of Oncology and Radiology of Serbia, Belgrade, Serbia. [2]Radiology and Radiotherapy Department, Institute of Oncology and Radiology of Serbia, Belgrade, Serbia. [3]Medical Genomics, UCL Cancer Institute, University College London, London, UK. [4]Medical Oncology Department, Institute of Oncology and Radiology of Serbia, Belgrade, Serbia.

References

1. Lee MC, Newman LA. Management of patients with locally advanced breast cancer. Surg Clin North Am. 2007;87(2):379–98 ix.
2. Tryfonidis K, Senkus E, Cardoso MJ, Cardoso F. Management of locally advanced breast cancer-perspectives and future directions. Nat Rev Clin Oncol. 2015;12(3):147–62.
3. Early Breast Cancer Trialists' Collaborative G, Darby S, McGale P, Correa C, Taylor C, Arriagada R, Clarke M, Cutter D, Davies C, Ewertz M, et al. Effect of radiotherapy after breast-conserving surgery on 10-year recurrence and 15-year breast cancer death: meta-analysis of individual patient data for 10,801 women in 17 randomised trials. Lancet. 2011;378(9804):1707–16.
4. Clarke M, Collins R, Darby S, Davies C, Elphinstone P, Evans V, Godwin J, Gray R, Hicks C, James S, et al. Effects of radiotherapy and of differences in the extent of surgery for early breast cancer on local recurrence and 15-year survival: an overview of the randomised trials. Lancet. 2005;366(9503):2087–106.
5. Le Scodan R, Stevens D, Brain E, Floiras JL, Cohen-Solal C, De La Lande B, Tubiana-Hulin M, Yacoub S, Gutierrez M, Ali D, et al. Breast cancer with synchronous metastases: survival impact of exclusive locoregional radiotherapy. J Clin Oncol. 2009;27(9):1375–81.
6. Darai E, Mosseri V, Hamelin JP, Salmon RJ, Karaitianos I, Bataini P, Mathieu G, Vilcoq RJ, Durand JC. Conservative surgery after radiotherapy with preoperative doses in the treatment of breast cancer. Presse Med. 1991; 20(42):2144–8.
7. Touboul E, Buffat L, Lefranc JP, Blondon J, Deniaud E, Mammar H, Laugier A, Schlienger M. Possibility of conservative local treatment after combined chemotherapy and preoperative irradiation for locally advanced noninflammatory breast cancer. Int J Radiat Oncol Biol Phys. 1996;34(5): 1019–28.

8. Calais G, Berger C, Descamps P, Chapet S, Reynaud-Bougnoux A, Body G, Bougnoux P, Lansac J, Le Floch O. Conservative treatment feasibility with induction chemotherapy, surgery, and radiotherapy for patients with breast carcinoma larger than 3 cm. Cancer. 1994;74(4):1283–8.

9. Calitchi E, Kirova YM, Otmezguine Y, Feuilhade F, Piedbois Y, Le Bourgeois JP. Long-term results of neoadjuvant radiation therapy for breast cancer. Int J Cancer. 2001;96(4):253–9.

10. Ghiam AF, Spayne J, Lee J. Current challenges and future perspectives of radiotherapy for locally advanced breast cancer. Curr Opin Support Palliat Care. 2014;8(1):46–52.

11. Bellon JR. Personalized radiation oncology for breast Cancer: the new frontier. J Clin Oncol. 2015;33(18):1998–2000.

12. Langlands FE, Horgan K, Dodwell DD, Smith L. Breast cancer subtypes: response to radiotherapy and potential radiosensitisation. Br J Radiol. 2013; 86(1023):20120601.

13. Liu FF, Shi W, Done SJ, Miller N, Pintilie M, Voduc D, Nielsen TO, Nofech-Mozes S, Chang MC, Whelan TJ, et al. Identification of a low-risk luminal a breast Cancer cohort that may not benefit from breast radiotherapy. J Clin Oncol. 2015;33(18):2035–40.

14. Eschrich S, Zhang H, Zhao H, Boulware D, Lee JH, Bloom G, Torres-Roca JF. Systems biology modeling of the radiation sensitivity network: a biomarker discovery platform. Int J Radiat Oncol Biol Phys. 2009;75(2):497–505.

15. Tucker SL, Thames HD Jr. The effect of patient-to-patient variability on the accuracy of predictive assays of tumor response to radiotherapy: a theoretical evaluation. Int J Radiat Oncol Biol Phys. 1989;17(1):145–57.

16. Nuyten DS, Kreike B, Hart AA, Chi JT, Sneddon JB, Wessels LF, Peterse HJ, Bartelink H, Brown PO, Chang HY, et al. Predicting a local recurrence after breast-conserving therapy by gene expression profiling. Breast Cancer Res. 2006;8(5):R62.

17. Eschrich SA, Pramana J, Zhang H, Zhao H, Boulware D, Lee JH, Bloom G, Rocha-Lima C, Kelley S, Calvin DP, et al. A gene expression model of intrinsic tumor radiosensitivity: prediction of response and prognosis after chemoradiation. Int J Radiat Oncol Biol Phys. 2009;75(2):489–96.

18. Torres-Roca JF, Fulp WJ, Caudell JJ, Servant N, Bollet MA, van de Vijver M, Naghavi AO, Harris EE, Eschrich SA. Integration of a Radiosensitivity molecular signature into the assessment of local recurrence risk in breast Cancer. Int J Radiat Oncol Biol Phys. 2015;93(3):631–8.

19. Ratain MJ. Bar the windows but open the door to randomization. J Clin Oncol. 2010;28(19):3104–6.

20. Marous M, Bieche I, Paoletti X, Alt M, Razak AR, Stathis A, Kamal M, Le Tourneau C. Designs of preoperative biomarkers trials in oncology: a systematic review of the literature. Ann Oncol. 2015;26(12):2419–28.

21. Mladenovic J, Susnjar S, Tanic M, Jankovic R, Karadzic K, Gavrilovic D, Stojanovic S, Plesinac-Karapandzic V. Tumor response and patient outcome after preoperative radiotherapy in locally advanced non-inflammatory breast cancer patients. J Buon. 2017;22(2):325–33.

22. Therasse P, Arbuck SG, Eisenhauer EA, Wanders J, Kaplan RS, Rubinstein L, Verweij J, Van Glabbeke M, van Oosterom AT, Christian MC, et al. New guidelines to evaluate the response to treatment in solid tumors. European Organization for Research and Treatment of Cancer, National Cancer Institute of the United States, National Cancer Institute of Canada. J Natl Cancer Inst. 2000;92(3):205–16.

23. Wang Y, Klijn JG, Zhang Y, Sieuwerts AM, Look MP, Yang F, Talantov D, Timmermans M, Meijer-van Gelder ME, Yu J, et al. Gene-expression profiles to predict distant metastasis of lymph-node-negative primary breast cancer. Lancet. 2005;365(9460):671–9.

24. Saldanha AJ. Java Treeview--extensible visualization of microarray data. Bioinformatics. 2004;20(17):3246–8.

25. Bignell GR, Warren W, Seal S, Takahashi M, Rapley E, Barfoot R, Green H, Brown C, Biggs PJ, Lakhani SR, et al. Identification of the familial cylindromatosis tumour-suppressor gene. Nat Genet. 2000;25(2):160–5.

26. Benjamini Y, Drai D, Elmer G, Kafkafi N, Golani I. Controlling the false discovery rate in behavior genetics research. Behav Brain Res. 2001;125(1–2):279–84.

27. Budczies J, Klauschen F, Sinn BV, Gyorffy B, Schmitt WD, Darb-Esfahani S, Denkert C. Cutoff finder: a comprehensive and straightforward web application enabling rapid biomarker cutoff optimization. PLoS One. 2012; 7(12):e51862.

28. de Jager DJ, de Mutsert R, Jager KJ, Zoccali C, Dekker FW. Reporting of interaction. Nephron Clin Pract. 2011;119(2):c158–61.

29. Knol MJ, VanderWeele TJ. Recommendations for presenting analyses of effect modification and interaction. Int J Epidemiol. 2012;41(2):514–20.

30. Andersson T, Alfredsson L, Kallberg H, Zdravkovic S, Ahlbom A. Calculating measures of biological interaction. Eur J Epidemiol. 2005;20(7):575–9.

31. West CM, Barnett GC. Genetics and genomics of radiotherapy toxicity: towards prediction. Genome Med. 2011;3(8):52.

32. Barker HE, Paget JT, Khan AA, Harrington KJ. The tumour microenvironment after radiotherapy: mechanisms of resistance and recurrence. Nat Rev Cancer. 2015;15(7):409–25.

33. Lupo B, Trusolino L. Inhibition of poly(ADP-ribosyl)ation in cancer: old and new paradigms revisited. Biochim Biophys Acta. 2014;1846(1):201–15.

34. Hassa PO, Haenni SS, Elser M, Hottiger MO. Nuclear ADP-ribosylation reactions in mammalian cells: where are we today and where are we going? Microbiol Mol Biol Rev. 2006;70(3):789–829.

35. Khan JA, Forouhar F, Tao X, Tong L. Nicotinamide adenine dinucleotide metabolism as an attractive target for drug discovery. Expert Opin Ther Targets. 2007;11(5):695–705.

36. Houtkooper RH, Canto C, Wanders RJ, Auwerx J. The secret life of NAD+: an old metabolite controlling new metabolic signaling pathways. Endocr Rev. 2010;31(2):194–223.

37. Li M, Bolduc AR, Hoda MN, Gamble DN, Dolisca SB, Bolduc AK, Hoang K, Ashley C, McCall D, Rojiani AM, et al. The indoleamine 2,3-dioxygenase pathway controls complement-dependent enhancement of chemo-radiation therapy against murine glioblastoma. J Immunother Cancer. 2014;2:21.

38. Munshi A, Ramesh R. Mitogen-activated protein kinases and their role in radiation response. Genes Cancer. 2013;4(9–10):401–8.

39. Dent P, Yacoub A, Fisher PB, Hagan MP, Grant S. MAPK pathways in radiation responses. Oncogene. 2003;22(37):5885–96.

40. Chung EJ, Urick ME, Kurshan N, Shield W 3rd, Asano H, Smith PD, Scroggins BS, Burkeen J, Citrin DE. MEK1/2 inhibition enhances the radiosensitivity of cancer cells by downregulating survival and growth signals mediated by EGFR ligands. Int J Oncol. 2013;42(6):2028–36.

41. Chung EJ, Brown AP, Asano H, Mandler M, Burgan WE, Carter D, Camphausen K, Citrin D. In vitro and in vivo radiosensitization with AZD6244 (ARRY-142886), an inhibitor of mitogen-activated protein kinase/extracellular signal-regulated kinase 1/2 kinase. Clin Cancer Res. 2009;15(9): 3050–7.

42. Shannon AM, Telfer BA, Smith PD, Babur M, Logie A, Wilkinson RW, Debray C, Stratford IJ, Williams KJ, Wedge SR. The mitogen-activated protein/extracellular signal-regulated kinase kinase 1/2 inhibitor AZD6244 (ARRY-142886) enhances the radiation responsiveness of lung and colorectal tumor xenografts. Clin Cancer Res. 2009;15(21):6619–29.

6

Abdominal organ position variation in children during image-guided radiotherapy

Sophie C. Huijskens[*], Irma W. E. M. van Dijk, Jorrit Visser, Brian V. Balgobind, D. te Lindert, Coen R. N. Rasch, Tanja Alderliesten and Arjan Bel

Abstract

Background: Interfractional organ position variation might differ for abdominal organs and this could have consequences for defining safety margins. Therefore, the purpose of this study is to quantify interfractional position variations of abdominal organs in children in order to investigate possible correlations between abdominal organs and determine whether position variation is location-dependent.

Methods: For 20 children (2.2–17.8 years), we retrospectively analyzed 113 CBCTs acquired during the treatment course, which were registered to the reference CT to assess interfractional position variation of the liver, spleen, kidneys, and both diaphragm domes. Organ position variation was assessed in three orthogonal directions and relative to the bony anatomy. Diaphragm dome position variation was assessed in the cranial-caudal (CC) direction only. We investigated possible correlations between position variations of the organs (Spearman's correlation test, ρ), and tested if organ position variations in the CC direction are related to the diaphragm dome position variations (linear regression analysis, R^2) (both tests: significance level $p < 0.05$). Differences of variations of systematic (Σ) and random errors (σ) between organs were tested (Bonferroni significance level $p < 0.004$).

Results: In all directions, correlations between liver and spleen position variations, and between right and left kidney position variations were weak (ρ ≤ 0.43). In the CC direction, the position variations of the right and left diaphragm domes were significantly, and stronger, correlated with position variations of the liver ($R^2 = 0.55$) and spleen ($R^2 = 0.63$), respectively, compared to the right ($R^2 = 0.00$) and left kidney ($R^2 = 0.25$). Differences in Σ and σ between all organs were small and insignificant.

Conclusions: No (strong) correlations between interfractional position variations of abdominal organs in children were observed. From present results, we concluded that diaphragm dome position variations could be more representative for superiorly located abdominal (liver, spleen) organ position variations than for inferiorly located (kidneys) organ position variations. Differences of systematic and random errors between abdominal organs were small, suggesting that for margin definitions, there was insufficient evidence of a dependence of organ position variation on anatomical location.

Keywords: Interfractional organ position variation, Abdominal organ motion, Pediatric RT, IGRT

Background

Continuous developments in pediatric cancer treatment using multimodality strategies, including surgery, chemotherapy, and radiotherapy have led to increasing numbers of childhood cancer survivors [1]. Inevitably, the occurrence of treatment associated adverse events has also increased. Treatments including radiotherapy significantly contribute to the risk of developing adverse events.

Children are treated with abdominal and thoracic radiotherapy for a wide range of primary cancer diagnoses, including Wilms' tumor, neuroblastoma, and Ewing sarcoma. Moreover, treatment of the craniospinal axis and lung metastasis involve irradiation of the abdominal and thoracic region. The anatomical locations of these tumors and adjacent organs at risk (OARs) vary; target volumes can be in very close proximity to the lungs, diaphragm, liver, spleen, and kidneys. As a result, healthy tissues and OARs are unavoidably exposed to radiation when irradiating the tumor [2, 3]. Although adequate tumor dose coverage is the

* Correspondence: s.c.huijskens@amc.uva.nl
Amsterdam UMC, University of Amsterdam, Department of Radiation Oncology, Cancer Center Amsterdam, Meibergdreef 9, Amsterdam, The Netherlands

primary goal in radiotherapy, sparing the vital and long-term functions of adjacent organs is also of great concern. Especially in children, who have a relative long life expectancy when surviving cancer, organs are still growing and have low tolerance to radiation [4, 5]. To ensure adequate tumor dose coverage while minimizing radiation dose to surrounding healthy tissues, knowledge about the extent of target and organ motion, particularly present in the abdominal and thoracic area, is needed. Thus, quantifying the motion of vital and sensitive organs such as the liver, spleen, and kidneys is essential.

These abdominal organs move with every breathing cycle (intrafraction motion) and from day-to-day (interfraction motion). Intra- and interfractional motion of the tumor and OARs are incorporated by expanding the clinical target volume and OARs volumes to the planning target volume (PTV) and planning risk volumes (PRVs), respectively [6]. In adults, many studies have quantified motion of various organs, enabling to define accurate margins for PTVs and PRVs. Despite the increasing number of publications on pediatric organ motion [7–14], data is still limited and no consensus has been reached in pediatric radiotherapy to define PTV or PRV margins for abdominal tumors or OARs. Therefore, PTV margins for children are currently pragmatically based on available adult data and PRV margins are often not used in pediatric radiotherapy. Due to different anatomical locations (e.g., right vs. left side of the abdomen, (retro)peritoneum, adjacent to the vertebrae), or abdominal processes (e.g., intestinal peristaltic or air pockets), abdominal organ motion might be location-dependent, as was discussed before in Van Dijk et al. [14]. This could lead to differences in PTV and PRV margins depending on the anatomical location.

The most commonly used PTV margin recipe is from van Herk et al. $(2.5\ \Sigma + 0.7\ \sigma)$, where the systematic (Σ) and random (σ) component are based on quadratically adding the systematic/random errors that occur during treatment $(\sqrt{\Sigma^2_{\text{inter}} + \Sigma^2_{\text{intra}}}$ and $\sqrt{\sigma^2_{\text{inter}} + \sigma^2_{\text{intra}}})$ [15]. Previous studies mainly reported on *intra*fractional organ motion, focusing on respiratory-induced abdominal organ motion through various phases of the breathing cycle as measured on a single four-dimensional computed tomography (4DCT) [9, 11, 16] or 4D magnetic resonance imaging (4DMRI) [12, 17]. Although organ motion seems to be more prone to respiratory motion than to day-to-day position variations, Guerreiro et al. showed that in a homogenous group of 15 children, interfractional abdominal organ motion was larger than intrafraction motion $(\Sigma_{\text{inter}}$ and $\sigma_{\text{inter}} > \Sigma_{\text{intra}}$ and $\sigma_{\text{intra}})$ [16]. In addition, Huijskens et al. showed that for respiratory-induced diaphragm motion in children the systematic error was found to be smaller than the random error $(\Sigma_{\text{intra}} < \sigma_{\text{intra}})$ [8]. This seems to indicate that the systematic component of the PTV and PRV margins is predominated by the day-to-day systematic (i.e., interfractional) variations (Σ_{inter}). Moreover, van Herk's margin recipe shows that the systematic component weighs more than the random component [15]. Therefore, quantification and a comprehensive understanding of interfractional abdominal organ motion is essential for high-accuracy image-guided radiotherapy.

Most studies on abdominal organ motion have focused only on the quantification of the *inter*fractional component [7, 10, 16, 18], without investigating location-dependency, or possible correlations between organ position variations. Whenever possible, resection of a tumor takes place before radiation treatment and usually surgical clips are placed to localize the remaining tumor bed. If not, an anatomical structure close to the target could function as a surrogate for localization and position variation. However, such a strategy will only be successful when there is a clear understanding of the correlations between the tumor and the anatomical surrogate. In addition, radiation treatment might also lead in the future towards adaptive strategies in children. However, often, certain organs are not directly visible on daily cone beam CTs (CBCTs), due to artefacts, smaller field of view or, especially in children, low dose imaging protocols. Moreover, markers are rather not placed in children and online evaluation of the positions of organs is thus mostly unfeasible in clinical practice. Here as well, another close anatomical structure might be considered as a surrogate. For instance, when the diaphragm, being very well visible on CBCT images, is used as a surrogate for the assessment of abdominal organ position. Some adult studies have shown reliable correlations of the diaphragm with abdominal organs [19–22], while other studies show weak correlations [20, 23–25]. This is mostly depending on the tumor site and therefore, outcomes cannot be generalized for adults. For children, correlations between the diaphragm and abdominal organs has not been extensively studied. It is therefore crucial to have a clear understanding of the correlation between the tumor or organ and a particular surrogate.

Therefore, the aim of this study was to increase the insight on interfractional position variation of abdominal organs in children. We investigated possible correlations between abdominal organs and determined whether position variation is location-dependent. Additionally, we investigated whether diaphragm position variation could be a surrogate for abdominal organ position variation, by analyzing the right and left diaphragm domes separately.

Methods

Patient population

For this retrospective study, we included 20 patients younger than 18 years, treated for various tumors at our radiation oncology department between December 2010 and

Table 1 Patient characteristics

No.	Sex	Tumor	Age at diagnosis (years)	Height (cm)	Weight (kg)	No. of CBCTs	RT location
1	F	Sarcoma	11.5	155	38	5	Thorax
2	M	Medulloblastoma	6.6	110	18	5	Spinal cord[a]
3	F	Hodgkin lymphoma	16.5	166	49	5	abdomen
4	M	Medulloblastoma	14.1	175	36	5	Spinal cord
5	M	Medulloblastoma	8.3	128	25	5	Spinal cord
6	F	Medulloblastoma	6.7	137	20	2	Spinal cord
7	M	Ewing sarcoma	16.8	184	62	8	Thorax
8	M	Medulloblastoma	6.7	129	24	5	Spinal cord
9	M	Spinal metastesis	2.6	90	12	8	Thorax
10	F	Medulloblastoma	7	118	22	6	Spinal cord
11	M	Anaplastic glioma	7.9	132	31	5	Spinal cord
12[b]	M	Medulloblastoma	5.1	109	17	8	Spinal cord
13	F	Neuroblastoma	5.3	115	24	6	Abdomen
14	M	Sarcoma	10.9	142	37	5	Thorax
15	M	DSRCT	9.9	137	26	5	Abdomen
16	M	Neuroblastoma	4.7	118	22	6	Abdomen
17[b]	M	Medulloblastoma	4.9	105	18	6	Spinal cord
18	M	Ewing sarcoma	17.9	182	81	7	Thorax
19	F	Osteosarcoma	15.1	159	53	5	Thorax
20	M	Neuroblastoma	2.2	90	15	6	Abdomen

Abbreviations: M male, *F* female, *DSRCT* desmoplastic small round cell tumor
[a] Spinal cord was part of craniospinal irradiation
[b] Patients 12 and 17 were treated under general anesthesia.; this did not influence interfractional organ position variations

September 2017 (Table 1). Patients were included if a pre-treatment CT scan and multiple CBCT scans of the abdomen or thorax were available, in which the liver, spleen, kidneys, and right and left diaphragm domes were visible (Fig. 1).

Imaging data

For each patient, a pre-treatment CT scan (120 kV, 2.5- or 5 mm slice thickness) was acquired for planning purposes (LightSpeed RT16; General Electric Company, Waukesha, WI, USA). This scan was considered as the reference CT (refCT) scan and included original organ delineations, as used for clinical practice (Fig. 1). For all patients, CBCT images (1 mm slice thickness, 1 mm in-plane resolution) were routinely acquired using the CBCT scanner mounted on the Elekta Synergy linac (Elekta AB, Stockholm, Sweden) as part of the position verification protocol. This yields CBCT imaging at the first three treatment fractions, followed by daily or weekly CBCT acquisitions, depending on the treatment protocol. To be consistent, we included for all patients the first three CBCTs and thereafter weekly acquired CBCTs. All CBCTs were acquired with 120 kV, 10 mA, and 10 or 40 ms exposure time per projection. The scanning time of the CBCT scan varied between 35–60s, and the degree of circumferential rotation was 200 or 360 degrees. In this study, we retrospectively analyzed the imaging data, including a total of 20 refCTs and 113 CBCTs.

Imaging registration

Elekta X-ray Volume Imaging software (XVI 3.0; Elekta AB, Stockholm, Sweden) was used for a two-step rigid registration for each organ separately (example shown in Fig. 1). First, a region of interest (ROI) was defined in the refCT, including the 12th thoracic through the 4th lumbar vertebra (from the lowest part of the kidneys up to the diaphragm domes). The CBCTs were then registered to the refCT using the automatic chamfer match algorithm [26]. Second, this bony anatomy-based match was followed by registration of each organ separately (i.e., liver, spleen, right kidney, left kidney) with a grey value algorithm [26], based on shaped ROIs defined by the delineated organs including (at least 2/3rd of) the whole organ volume. This enabled the assessment of organ position variation smaller than the slice thickness of the acquired refCT. Automatic registration outcomes (translations and rotations) were visually checked (by SCH/DTL) and manually corrected if necessary. Results were corrected for rotations as follows. First, we assessed the center of mass (COM) coordinates for each organ.

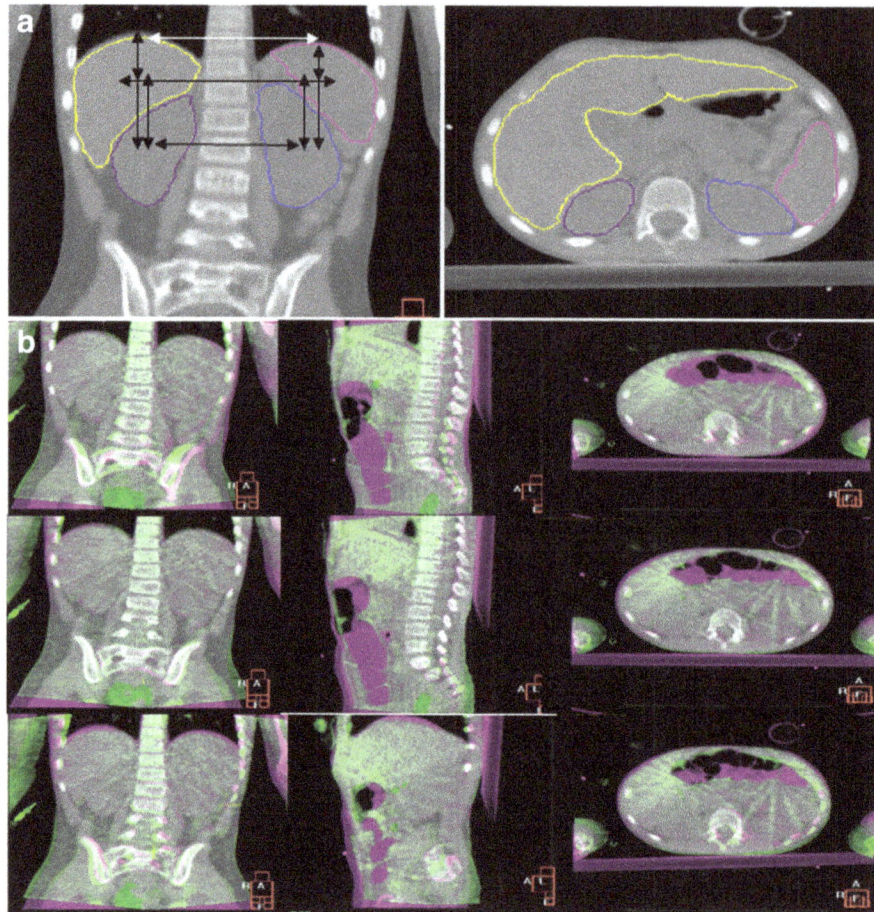

Fig. 1 a Delineated organs (right kidney: purple, left kidney: blue, liver: yellow, spleen: pink) on the reference CT. Diaphragm domes are not delineated. Arrows indicate mutual correlations investigated. **b** Example of the two-step rigid registration (from top to bottom): unaligned overlap of reference CT and CBCT, bones aligned, right kidney aligned (note: bones shifted). (Color figure online only)

Then, we equated these coordinates to the refCT to determine the exact magnitude and direction of the interfractional position variation. By calculating the difference of the magnitude and sign of the COM coordinates of each organ on CBCTs and refCT, registrations resulted in interfractional position variation relative to bony anatomy, expressed as composite vectors in the left-right (LR), cranio-caudal (CC) and anterior-posterior (AP) directions. The + and − signs respectively indicate right/caudal/posterior and left/cranial/anterior directions. For the diaphragm, the bony anatomy-based automatic chamfer match was followed by manual registrations of the right- and left-sided diaphragm dome separately in the CC direction only (by SCH/DTL).

Statistical analysis

For each patient, organ specific mean and standard deviation (SD) of the interfractional position variation relative to the bony anatomy were determined in the three orthogonal directions, and in the CC direction only for the right and left diaphragm domes. Furthermore, over

all patients, we estimated per organ the group mean (i.e., mean of the individual means), the group systematic error (Σ; the SD of the individual means of all patients), and the group random error (σ; the root mean square of the individual SDs of all patients).

To evaluate whether organ position variation is location-dependent, we compared contralateral and superiorly and inferiorly located abdominal organs separately (indicated in Fig. 1). Since not all data fitted a normal distribution (tested with the Shapiro-Wilk's test), differences between contralateral organs' systematic and random errors were separately tested (i.e., right diaphragm dome vs. left diaphragm dome, liver vs. spleen, right kidney vs. left kidney) with the Levene's test (for Σ) and Mann-Whitney U-test (for σ). Also, differences in Σ and σ between superiorly and inferiorly located abdominal organs were tested (i.e., liver vs. right kidney, spleen vs. left kidney). Since differences were tested in 14 combinations (i.e., LR, CC, AP for four organs, and CC only for both diaphragm domes), we adjusted p values according to the Bonferroni correction. Differences were considered to be significant if test outcomes showed a p value< 0.004 (i.e., 0.05/14).

We used the Spearman's correlation test (significance level $p < 0.05$) to investigate the possible correlations in position variations between contralateral organs.

Additionally, to test if right- and left-sided organ position variations in the CC direction are related to the position variations of the superiorly located right- and left-sided diaphragm dome respectively, we used linear regression analysis (significance level $p < 0.05$). Both tests were also performed for each individual patient.

All statistical analyses were done using R version 3.2.1. (R Foundation for Statistical Computing, USA).

Results

Mean organ position variation was smaller than 1.0 mm (range: – 6.9 to 7.4 mm) for the abdominal organs in all orthogonal directions and smaller than 1.8 mm (range: – 4.0 to 7.8 mm) for the diaphragm domes in the CC direction. For all organs and across all fractions, ranges of position variations were largest in the CC direction (varying from 10.6 to 13.0 mm) and smallest in the LR direction (varying from 4.1 to 11.1 mm) (Fig. 2). Overall, kidney position variations were smaller than position variations of the liver and spleen (Fig. 2). Table 2 presents the values of the group mean, systematic and random error per organ in each direction, mainly showing average systematic error in decreasing order of CC (3.2 mm, SD = 0.3 mm), AP (1.9 mm, SD = 0.9 mm), and LR (1.7 mm, SD = 0.5 mm) direction, and average random error also in decreasing order of CC (3.0 mm, SD =0.5 mm), AP (2.1 mm, SD = 0.6 mm), and LR (1.9 mm, SD = 0.7 mm) direction. Differences of the systematic error between right- and left-sided organs were insignificant ($p \geq 0.004$), as were the differences of the random error between right- and left-sided organs ($p \geq 0.004$) (Additional file 1: Table S1). For superiorly and inferiorly located organs, significant but small differences were found between the liver and the right kidney in the AP direction ($p = 0.002$ for Σ), and in the LR direction ($p = 0.000$ for σ). Also, the random error of the spleen and the left kidney was significantly different in the AP direction ($p = 0.001$) (Additional file 1: Table S1).

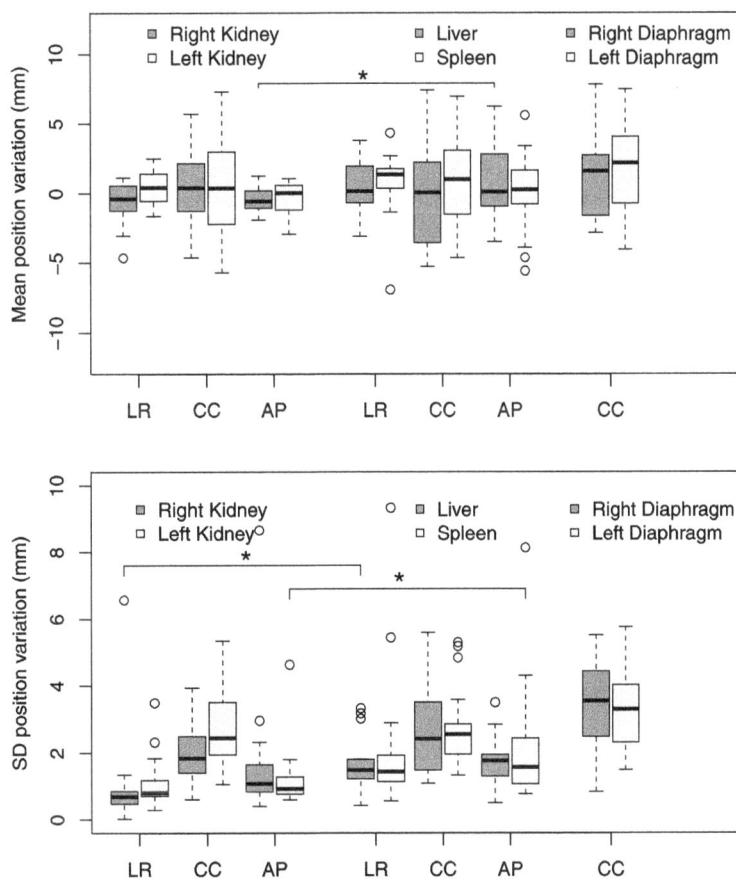

Fig. 2 Boxplots showing the distributions of the individual means (upper panel) and SDs (lower panel) of the interfractional position variations found for right- (light grey) and left-sided (dark grey) organs for all 20 patients. Horizontal bars, boxes, and whiskers represent medians, 50th percentiles (inter quartile range (IQR)), and the highest (lowest) value within 1.5xIQR, respectively. Circles denote outliers. *Significant differences (Bonferroni corrected $p < 0.004$). Abbreviations: LR = left–right; CC = cranial–caudal; AP = anterior–posterior

Table 2 The group systematic (Σ) and group random errors (σ) in mm in the orthogonal directions for the right kidney, left kidney, liver, and spleen and in CC direction for the diaphragm

(mm)	Right Kidney			Left Kidney			Liver			Spleen			Right Diaphragm	Left Diaphragm
	LR	CC	AP	LR	CC	AP	LR	CC	AP	LR	CC	AP	CC	CC
Group mean	−0.6	0.7	−0.4	0.4	0.4	−0.4	0.4	−0.1	1.0	0.8	0.8	0.0	1.2	1.8
Σ	1.4	2.8	0.9	1.1	3.3	1.3	2.1	3.4	2.7	2.2	3.5	2.7	3.0	3.4
σ	1.6	2.2	2.4	1.3	2.9	1.4	1.8	2.8	1.9	2.8	3.0	2.7	3.6	3.4

Abbreviations: *LR* left–right, *CC* cranial–caudal, *AP* anterior–posterior

A moderate and statistically significantly correlation between the position variations of the right and left diaphragm domes was found ($\rho = 0.63$, $p = 0.00$) (Fig. 3a). The position variations of the liver and spleen in the LR and CC direction were weakly, but statistically significantly correlated ($\rho = 0.23$, $p = 0.02$ and $\rho = 0.40$, $p = 0.00$, respectively) (Fig. 3b). Position variations of the right and left kidney were weakly, but statistically significant correlated in the LR and AP directions ($\rho = -0.43$, $p = 0.00$ and $\rho = 0.23$, $p = 0.01$, respectively) (Fig. 3c). Correlations within each individual patient were similar to the overall group outcomes.

Linear regression analysis showed that right and left diaphragm dome position variations in the CC direction were significantly correlated with position variations of the liver ($R^2 = 0.55$, $p = 0.00$) and spleen ($R^2 = 0.63$, $p = 0.00$), respectively. In the CC direction, no (strong) correlation was found between right and left diaphragm dome position variations and the position variations of the right ($R^2 = 0.003$, $p = 0.60$) and left kidney ($R^2 = 0.25$, $p = 0.00$), respectively (Fig. 4).

Discussion

In this study, we quantified interfractional position variation of multiple abdominal organs in 20 children during radiotherapy and evaluated if organ position variation is mutually related and location-dependent. We found weak correlations between the position variations of contralateral organs. In the CC direction, right and left diaphragm dome position variations correlated moderately with the position variations of the liver and spleen, respectively. However, correlations between the position variations of the diaphragm domes and those of both kidneys were negligible. Furthermore, the largest magnitude of organ position variations was observed in the CC direction, followed by the AP and LR directions. We found that differences between group systematic and random errors of abdominal organs were small and insignificant. This comprehensive analysis of organ position variations at different anatomical locations increases the insight in possible consequences for margin definitions, which has not been reported on for children so far.

Nazmy et al. studied interfractional position variation of the liver and kidneys in 9 children (mean age: 4.1 years, SD = 1.6 years) using reference CT and CBCT scans [10]. They also found that, in the CC direction, the liver showed more motion than the kidneys. However, their range of observed position variations of the left kidney was smaller than that of the right kidney. In contrary, when we analyzed patients in our cohort of similar age ($n = 6$; range 2.2–5.3 years) we found slightly

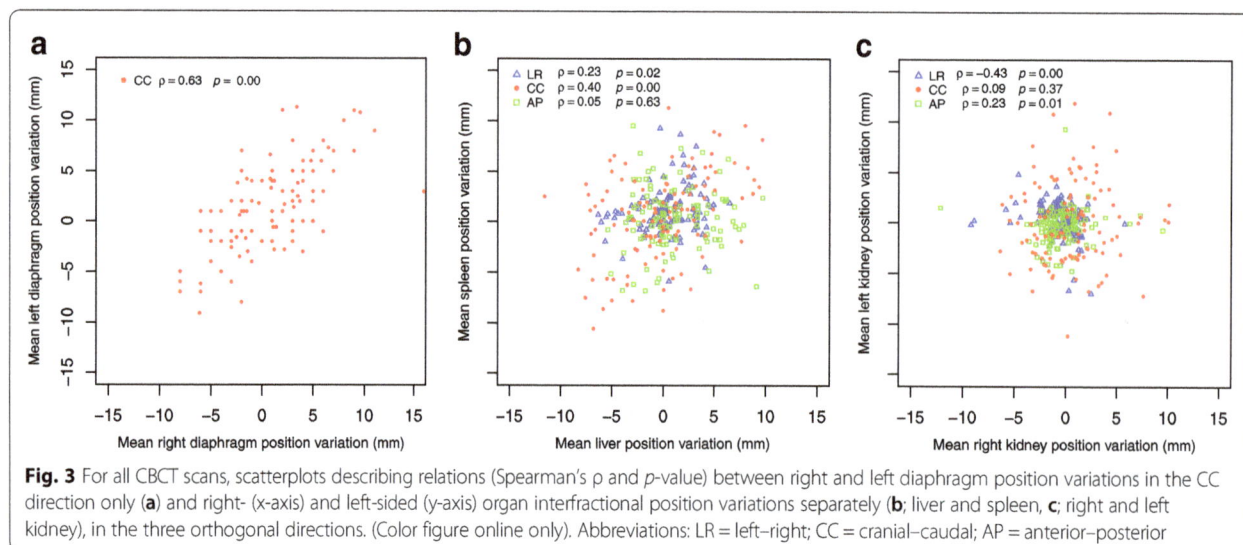

Fig. 3 For all CBCT scans, scatterplots describing relations (Spearman's ρ and *p*-value) between right and left diaphragm position variations in the CC direction only (**a**) and right- (x-axis) and left-sided (y-axis) organ interfractional position variations separately (**b**; liver and spleen, **c**; right and left kidney), in the three orthogonal directions. (Color figure online only). Abbreviations: LR = left–right; CC = cranial–caudal; AP = anterior–posterior

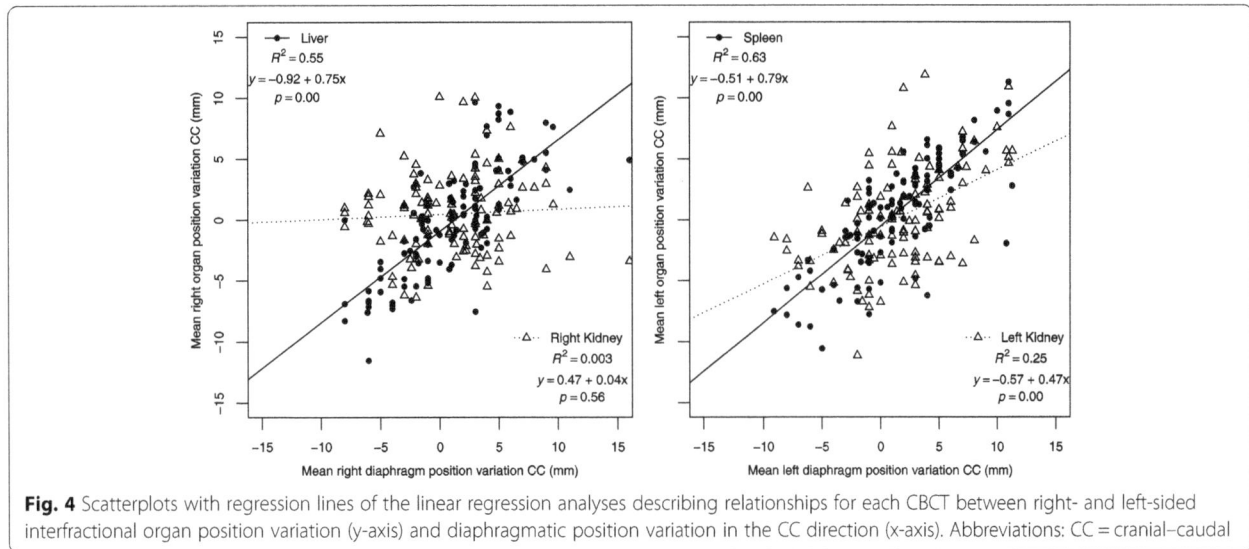

Fig. 4 Scatterplots with regression lines of the linear regression analyses describing relationships for each CBCT between right- and left-sided interfractional organ position variation (y-axis) and diaphragmatic position variation in the CC direction (x-axis). Abbreviations: CC = cranial–caudal

larger position variations of the left kidney compared to the right kidney. Although this comparison involves small sample sizes, a possible explanation might be the different methodology in choosing the point of interest. Nazmy et al. used the upper pole of the kidneys whereby kidney deformations might have been interpreted as translations, resulting in an overestimation of motion. We used the COM as point of interest because it is less sensitive to organ deformations. Although data on organ deformation would provide useful additional information on organ motion characteristics, analyzing organ deformation was outside the scope of the current study.

Our results are comparable to findings of Guerreiro et al. who used a similar methodology as we did [16]. They quantified interfractional position variations of the spleen, liver, and the healthy kidney in patients (n = 15, mean age: 4 years) with Wilms' tumors. Their ranges of interfractional position variation, and the systematic and random errors were generally somewhat smaller than our results, which could be explained by the fact that their cohort consisted of younger patients (age range 1–8 years). However, when we analyzed patients in our cohort of similar age (n = 10; range 2.2–7.8 years), the systematic and random errors for all organs and directions in our cohort remained somewhat larger (for Σ; mean difference 1.0 mm, SD = 0.6 mm, for σ; mean difference 0.7 mm, SD = 0.7 mm).

Using a 3DCT as a reference point to estimate interfractional position variation is arguable. The 3DCT represents 'snapshot' of repeatedly changing organ positions during the respiratory cycle [27]. A CBCT captures in 35–60 s several complete respiratory cycles and averages the motion over the observed breathing phases into one blurred 3D image. To investigate the possible effect of respiratory motion differences on the 3DCT and the CBCTs, we recalculated our measurements using the

first CBCT scan as the reference scan instead of the 3DCT. Differences between the respective calculations based on the refCT and the first CBCT were negligible (< 1 mm). Also, although projection images could enable the quantification of intrafractional motion as well [28], the low dose CBCT protocols that we used for most children [29] unavoidably result in poorer quality of projection images. Therefore, we were not able to distinguish organs on the two-dimensional projection images of these CBCT scans in order to investigate intrafractional motion of the liver, spleen, and kidneys.

The outliers shown in Fig. 2 represent the SD values of the right kidney and spleen position variations of three patients. For one patient, in which the field of view of the CBCT scan was smaller than its refCT, the whole right kidney was visible on the refCT but remained only half visible on the CBCT scan, and registration was performed using an adjusted sub-volume of the kidney. Additionally, in this patient the distance of the COM of the right kidney to the treatment planning isocentre on the refCT was relatively large (> 10 mm), resulting in a large deviation in organ position variation. For two other patients, the two-step rigid registration for the spleen yielded large rotations (> 15 degrees), resulting in large ranges of position variations. However, a sensitivity analysis, excluding these three cases, did not change our results.

The liver and spleen are contralateral organs that substantially differ in tissue composition and function. However, regarding their position variations, differences were small and position variations of both organs were moderately correlated with the position variations of the diaphragm domes. In contrary, the position variations of both kidneys were smaller and showed weak correlations with the diaphragm dome position variations. This might be due to their more inferior and retroperitoneal location.

Further, visual inspection showed that the kidneys seem more prone to deformations than the liver and spleen, probably due to their different tissue composition. Therefore, although in the CC direction only, diaphragm position variations seem to particularly be more representative for position variations of OARs in the upper abdomen than for OAR position variations in the lower abdomen.

The weak to moderate ($\rho < 0.4$), however significant, correlations of position variations between right- and left-sided abdominal organs suggest that organs move only somewhat in similar directions. Therefore, for future online strategies, close located anatomical structures are not recommended as suitable surrogates. However, the overall magnitude of motion is small, and differences of systematic and random errors of the various abdominal organs are small and insignificant, hence negligible. Therefore, regarding margin definitions, there was insufficient evidence of a dependence of organ position variation on anatomical location. Additionally, although differences between abdominal organ position variations were small, overall position variation was largest in the CC direction and smallest in the LR direction. This suggests that margins should be applied anisotropically rather than isotropically. Note, however, that the diaphragm was measured in the CC direction only.

Knowledge about patient's day-to-day anatomical variation is furthermore valuable when (automating) selecting similar patients from a database of patients' CT scans for, e.g., automating treatment planning or dose reconstruction [30–34], because this provides a lower bound on the achievable precision of selection.

Besides, as recommended by the Paediatric Radiation Oncology Society (PROS), consensus needs to be reached regarding appropriate margin definitions in children [35]. With increasing data, knowledge on organ motion during radiotherapy in children is expanding. However, due to generally small patient numbers and different methodologies in separates studies, definitive statements regarding margin definitions cannot be made yet. Therefore, close collaborations between research groups, and pooling of data might contribute to achieving consensus on margin definitions. A summarized all-encompassing overview of all published data so far, including inter- and intrafractional organ motion, could provide a basis for this. Especially, with more proton and carbon therapy facilities in development, aiming for high-precision radiotherapy and the need for the assessment of the anatomical variations in children, induced by organ motion, becomes even more important.

Conclusions

No (strong) correlations between interfractional position variations of abdominal organs in children were observed.

Differences of systematic and random errors between abdominal organs were small, suggesting that for margin definitions, there was insufficient evidence of a dependence of organ position variation on anatomical location. From present results, we concluded that diaphragm dome position variations could be more representative for superiorly located abdominal (liver, spleen) organ position variations than for inferiorly located (kidneys) organ position variations.

Abbreviations
3DCT: 3-Dimensional computed tomography; 4DCT: 4-Dimensional computed tomography; 4DMRI: 4-Dimensional Magnetic Resonance Imaging; AP: Anterior-Posterior; CBCT: Cone Beam Computed Tomography; CC: Cranial-Caudal; COM: Center of Mass; CT: Computed Tomography; LR: Left-Right; OAR: Organ at Risk; PROS: Paediatric Radiation Oncology Society; PRV: Planning Risk Volume; PTV: Planning Target Volume; SD: Standard Deviation

Funding
This work was supported by the Dutch Cancer Society (KWF Kankerbestrijding) project no. 2016–10113.

Authors' contributions
SCH has performed the data analysis and carried out writing of the manuscript. IVD, JV, BVB, TA and AB contributed to the critical interpretation of the results. IVD, DTL and AB contributed to design of the manuscript. CRR and AB provided general supervision. All authors participated in the drafting and revising of the manuscript. All authors read and approved the final manuscript.

Competing interests
Dr. Alderliesten and Dr. Bel are project leaders of several Elekta-sponsored projects outside of this work. Elekta had no involvement in study design, data collection and analysis, or writing of the manuscript. The authors declare that they have no competing interests.

References
1. Curry HL, Parkes SE, Powell JE, Mann JR. Caring for survivors of childhood cancers: the size of the problem. Eur J Cancer. 2006;42:501–8.
2. Bolling T, Konemann S, Ernst I, Willich N. Late effects of thoracic irradiation in children. Strahlenther Onkol. 2008;184:289–95.
3. Bolling T, Willich N, Ernst I. Late effects of abdominal irradiation in children: a review of the literature. Anticancer Res. 2010;30:227–31.
4. Selo N, Bolling T, Ernst I, Pape H, Martini C, Rube C, et al. Acute toxicity profile of radiotherapy in 690 children and adolescents: RiSK data. Radiother Oncol. 2010;97:119–26.
5. Claude L, Laprie A. Which dose constraints on which critical organs in paediatric radiation therapy? Cancer Radiother. 2015;19:484–8.
6. Prescribing, recording and reporting photon beam therapy (supplement to ICRU report 50). ICRU report 62: International Commission on Radiation Units and Measurements; 1999.
7. Huijskens SC, van Dijk IW, de Jong R, Visser J, Fajardo RD, Ronckers CM, et al. Quantification of renal and diaphragmatic interfractional motion in pediatric image-guided radiation therapy: a multicenter study. Radiother Oncol. 2015;117:425–31.
8. Huijskens SC, van Dijk IW, Visser J, Rasch CR, Alderliesten T, Bel A. Magnitude and variability of respiratory-induced diaphragm motion in children during image-guided radiotherapy. Radiother Oncol. 2017;123:263–9.

9. Kannan S, Teo BK, Solberg T, Hill-Kayser C. Organ motion in pediatric high-risk neuroblastoma patients using four-dimensional computed tomography. J Appl Clin Med Phys. 2017;18:107–14.

10. Nazmy MS, Khafaga Y, Mousa A, Khalil E. Cone beam CT for organs motion evaluation in pediatric abdominal neuroblastoma. Radiother Oncol. 2012;102:388–92.

11. Pai Panandiker AS, Sharma S, Naik MH, Wu S, Hua C, Beltran C, et al. Novel assessment of renal motion in children as measured via four-dimensional computed tomography. Int J Radiat Oncol Biol Phys. 2012;82:1771–6.

12. Uh J, Krasin MJ, Li Y, Li X, Tinkle C, Lucas JT Jr, et al. Quantification of pediatric abdominal organ motion with a 4-dimensional magnetic resonance imaging method. Int J Radiat Oncol Biol Phys. 2017;99:227–37.

13. Demoor-Goldschmidt C, Chiavassa S, Josset S, Mahe MA, Supiot S. Respiratory-gated bilateral pulmonary radiotherapy for Ewing's sarcoma and nephroblastoma in children and young adults: Dosimetric and clinical feasibility studies. Cancer Radiother. 2017;21:124–9.

14. van Dijk IW, Huijskens SC, de Jong R, Visser J, Fajardo RD, Rasch CR, et al. Interfractional renal and diaphragmatic position variation during radiotherapy in children and adults: is there a difference? Acta Oncol. 2017:1–7.

15. van Herk M. Errors and margins in radiotherapy. Semin Radiat Oncol 2004; 14:52–64.

16. Guerreiro F, Seravalli E, Janssens GO, van de Ven CP, van den Heuvel-Eibrink MM, Raaymakers BW. Intra- and inter-fraction uncertainties during IGRT for Wilms' tumor. Acta Oncol 2018:1–9.

17. Panandiker AS, Winchell A, Loeffler R, Song R, Rolen M, Hillenbrand C. 4DMRI provides more accurate renal motion estimation in IMRT in young children. Practical radiation oncology. 2013;3:S1

18. Beltran C, Pai Panandiker AS, Krasin MJ, Merchant TE. Daily image-guided localization for neuroblastoma. J Appl Clin Med Phys. 2010;11:3388.

19. Yang J, Cai J, Wang H, Chang Z, Czito BG, Bashir MR, et al. Is diaphragm motion a good surrogate for liver tumor motion? Int J Radiat Oncol Biol Phys. 2014;90:952–8.

20. Xi M, Liu MZ, Li QQ, Cai L, Zhang L, Hu YH. Analysis of abdominal organ motion using four-dimensional CT. Ai Zheng. 2009;28:989–93.

21. Cervino LI, Jiang Y, Sandhu A, Jiang SB. Tumor motion prediction with the diaphragm as a surrogate: a feasibility study. Phys Med Biol. 2010;55:N221–9.

22. Dawson LA, Eccles C, Bissonnette JP, Brock KK. Accuracy of daily image guidance for hypofractionated liver radiotherapy with active breathing control. Int J Radiat Oncol Biol Phys. 2005;62:1247–52.

23. Siva S, Pham D, Gill S, Bressel M, Dang K, Devereux T, et al. An analysis of respiratory induced kidney motion on four-dimensional computed tomography and its implications for stereotactic kidney radiotherapy. Radiat Oncol. 2013;8:248.

24. Lens E, van der Horst A, Versteijne E, Bel A, van Tienhoven G. Considerable pancreatic tumor motion during breath-holding. Acta Oncol. 2016;55:1360–8.

25. Stevens CW, Munden RF, Forster KM, Kelly JF, Liao Z, Starkschall G, et al. Respiratory-driven lung tumor motion is independent of tumor size, tumor location, and pulmonary function. Int J Radiat Oncol Biol Phys. 2001;51:62–8.

26. Roche A, Malandain G, Pennec X, Ayache N. The correlation ratio as a new similarity measure for multimodal image registration. In: Wells WM, Colchester A, Delp S, editors. Medical Image Computing and Computer-Assisted Intervention — MICCAI'98: First International Conference Cambridge, MA, USA, October 11–13, 1998 Proceedings. Berlin, Heidelberg: Springer Berlin Heidelberg; 1998. p. 1115–24.

27. Balter JM, Ten Haken RK, Lawrence TS, Lam KL, Robertson JM. Uncertainties in CT-based radiation therapy treatment planning associated with patient breathing. Int J Radiat Oncol Biol Phys. 1996;36:167–74.

28. Zijp L, Sonke J, van Herk M. Extraction of the respiratory signal from sequential thorax cone-beam X-ray images. Conf Use Comput Radiat Ther (ICCR). 2004:507–9.

29. de Jong RLE, van Herk M, Alderliesten T, Kamphuis M, DF R, Bel A, van Wieringen N. Optimizing cone-beam CT presets for children to reduce imaging dose illustrated with craniospinal axis. In: proceedings of ESTRO 33: Radiother Oncol; 2014. p. S109–S10.

30. Deshpande RR, DeMarco J, Sayre JW, Liu BJ. Knowledge-driven decision support for assessing dose distributions in radiation therapy of head and neck cancer. Int J Comput Assist Radiol Surg. 2016;11:2071–83.

31. Ng A, Nguyen TN, Moseley JL, Hodgson DC, Sharpe MB, Brock KK. Reconstruction of 3D lung models from 2D planning data sets for Hodgkin's lymphoma patients using combined deformable image registration and navigator channels. Med Phys. 2010;37:1017–28.

32. Wang Z, van Dijk I, Wiersma J, Ronckers CM, Oldenburger F, Balgobind BV, et al. Are age and gender suitable matching criteria in organ dose reconstruction using surrogate childhood cancer patients' CT scans? Med Phys. 2018;

33. Schmidt M, Lo JY, Grzetic S, Lutzky C, Brizel DM, Das SK. Semiautomated head-and-neck IMRT planning using dose warping and scaling to robustly adapt plans in a knowledge database containing potentially suboptimal plans. Med Phys. 2015;42:4428–34.

34. Virgolin M, van Dijk I, Wiersma J, Ronckers CM, Witteveen C, Bel A, et al. On the feasibility of automatically selecting similar patients in highly individualized radiotherapy dose reconstruction for historic data of pediatric cancer survivors. Med Phys. 2018;45:1504–17.

35. Kortmann RD, Freeman C, Marcus K, Claude L, Dieckmann K, Halperin E, et al. Paediatric radiation oncology in the care of childhood cancer: a position paper by the international Paediatric radiation oncology society (PROS). Radiother Oncol. 2016;119:357–60.

7

Stereotactic ablative radiotherapy (SABR) as primary, adjuvant, consolidation and re-treatment option in pancreatic cancer: scope for dose escalation and lessons for toxicity

Christy Goldsmith[1]* [ORCID], P. Nicholas Plowman[2,3], Melanie M. Green[4], Roger G. Dale[4] and Patricia M. Price[2,4]

Abstract

Background: Stereotactic ablative radiotherapy (SABR) offers an alternative treatment for pancreatic cancer, with the potential for improved tumour control and reduced toxicity compared with conventional therapies. However, optimal dose planning and delivery strategies are unelucidated and gastro-intestinal (GI) toxicity remains a key concern.

Methods: Patients with inoperable non-metastatic pancreatic cancer who received CyberKnife® SABR (18–36 Gy) in three fractions as primary, adjuvant, consolidation or re-treatment options were studied. Patient individualised planning and delivery variables were collected and their impact on patient outcome examined. Linear-quadratic (LQ) radiobiology modelling methods were applied to assess SABR parameters against a conventional fractionated radiotherapy schedule.

Results: In total 42 patients were included, 37 (88%) of whom had stage T4 disease. SABR was used > 6 months post-primary therapy to re-treat residual disease in 11 (26.2%) patients and relapsed disease in nine (21.4%) patients. SABR was an adjuvant to other primary therapy for 14 (33.3%) patients and was the sole primary therapy for eight (19.0%) patients. The mean (95% CI) planning target volume (PTV), prescription isodose, percentage cover, minimum dose to PTV and biological effective dose (BED) were 76.3(63.8–88.7) cc, 67.3(65.2–69.5)%, 96.6(95.5–97.7)%, 22.3(21.0–23.6) Gy and 50.3(47.7–53.0) Gy, respectively. Only 3/37 (8.1%) patients experienced Grade 3 acute toxicities. Two (4.8%) patients converted to resectable status and median freedom-from-local-progression (FFLP) and overall survival (OS) were 9.8 and 8.4 months, respectively. No late toxicity was experienced in 27/32 (84.4%) patients; however, four (12.5%) patients — of whom two had particularly large PTV, two had sub-optimal number of fiducials and three breached organ-at-risk (OAR) constraints—showed Grade 4 duodenal toxicities. Longer delivery time, extended treatment course and reduced percentage coverage additionally associated with late toxicity, likely reflecting parameters typically applied to riskier patients. Larger PTV size and longer treatment course associated with OS. Comparator regimen LQ modelling analysis indicated 50% of patients received minimum PTV doses less potent than a conventional radiotherapy regimen, indicating scope for dose escalation.

(Continued on next page)

* Correspondence: christy.goldsmith@gstt.nhs.uk
[1]Guys and St Thomas' NHS Foundation Trust, London, UK
Full list of author information is available at the end of the article

(Continued from previous page)

Conclusion: The results demonstrate the value of SABR for a range of indications in pancreatic cancer. Dose escalation to increase BED may improve FFLP and OS in inoperable, non-metastatic disease: however concomitant enhanced stringency for duodenal protection is critical, particularly for patients where SABR is more challenging.

Keywords: Stereotactic ablative radiotherapy (SABR), Cyberknife®, Pancreatic cancer, Radiobiology, Dose escalation, Local control, Toxicity, Survival

Background

Pancreatic cancer is characterised by debilitating symptoms caused by local disease advance, high rates of metastatic progression and dismally close incidence and mortality rates. Median overall survival (OS) from diagnosis for all patients is less than 5 months, ~ 20% of patients overall survive more than 1 year and ~ 5% survive more than 5 years [1–4]. Standard treatment options include single or multi-agent chemotherapy or chemoradiotherapy. For the small minority of patients diagnosed with earlier stage resectable disease, radical surgical resection offers the best chance of long-term survival with reported 5-year survival rates of ~ 20% [5]. However, the disease is typically diagnosed at more advanced stages: ~ 45% of patients present with metastatic disease that has a median OS of ~ 2–5 months, and ~ 30% present with inoperable localized or locally advanced pancreatic cancer (LAPC) that has an intermediate status and prognosis [1–4]. For the latter subset of patients, conversion to resectability currently offers the best outcome [5–7]: nevertheless, median OS reported in LAPC randomised trials remains poor at 7–15 months [8–10].

Modern conformal radiotherapy has a central role in pancreatic cancer disease control to: 1) palliate symptoms and prevent local progression that causes morbidity and may be causal of death [11]; 2) increase the chances of achieving secondary resectability [6, 7]; and 3) extend median survival time [12–15]. However, conventional chemoradiotherapy regimens can be long (~ 5.5 weeks) and arduous with only a modest or no overall survival gain [16]. Furthermore, the radiation doses that can be delivered safely are limited by toxicity to adjacent abdominal structures such that local control rates can be low [8, 15, 17, 18], repeat treatment upon relapse is inhibited, and treatment toxicity may be high and exacerbated by concomitant chemotherapeutics [14, 19–22].

Stereotactic ablative body radiotherapy (SABR) may be used as an alternative, adjunct, consolidation or re-treatment option to conventional therapies in pancreatic cancer. High dose radiotherapy can be delivered in conveniently few fractions, with rapid dose fall-off outside the delineated tumour volume [23, 24]. This offers the potential for increased local tumour control and reduced toxicity, and additionally introduces the valuable possibility of tumour re-irradiation. Due to the highly

conformal target volumes delineated, the high doses delivered and the proximity of adjacent radiosensitive organs-at-risk (OAR — duodenum, stomach, small bowel, liver, kidneys and spinal cord), accurate on-treatment tumour targeting is imperative.

Previous studies have pioneered the use of SABR in pancreatic cancer in various regimens, including as a single boost adjunct to chemotherapy or chemoradiotherapy or for re-treatment following local failure [20–22, 25–37]. The majority have shown relative efficacy for local control with reasonable toxicity, as well as benefits such as convenience and good pain relief [37]. Furthermore, receipt of SBRT compared with conventionally fractionated radiotherapy has shown significantly improved OS for locally advanced disease [38]. However, comparisons, interpretations and treatment optimisation of SABR in pancreatic cancer have been difficult as different planning, delivery and dosimetry methodologies have been used. As a result, local control has been reported as excellent in some studies [22, 25, 29, 31], but not in others [20, 21] and toxicity has been reported to be low in some studies [26, 33], but significant or unacceptable in others [20–22, 25, 28, 36, 39]. With the aim of increasing understanding and enabling treatment improvements for inoperable, non-metastatic pancreatic cancer, in our real-world series of patients we sought to: 1) review patient outcomes following SABR treatment for a range of indications 2) comprehensively examine the contribution of patient, planning, delivery and radiobiological variables upon the toxicity and efficacy of fractionated SABR and 3) use radiobiological modelling to compare SABR treatment to a conventional comparator regimen.

Methods

Patients and data collection

Pancreatic cancer patients referred to The CyberKnife® Centre at The Harley Street Clinic for SABR treatment from March 2009 – October 2012 were included. For comparative radiobiological and outcome purposes, only patients with inoperable status and no detectable metastases (i.e. those with localized or locally advanced disease that was unresectable, who had a prognosis intermediate to resectable and metastatic disease), who were treated in three fractions, were studied. Patient, tumour, treatment planning and delivery parameters were collected at the time of treatment. Patients were longitudinally followed and toxicity and outcome data were acquired at follow-up clinic appointments.

Treatment

SABR was delivered with the CyberKnife™® robotic radio-surgery system (Accuray® Corporation, Sunnyvale, CA, USA) [40]. In the majority of cases, following percutaneous implantation of gold fiducial tumour markers (Cybermark, CIVCO Medical Solutions, Iowa, USA) under computed tomography (CT) or endoscopic ultrasound (EUS) guidance, the Synchrony® (Accuray® Corporation, Sunnyvale, CA, USA) near real-time kilovoltage imaging system was used to achieve dynamic radiation delivery adaptive to patient and tumour movement.

Planning CT scans were performed at least one week after fiducial placement. Patients were advised to drink 300 mls of cold water 30 mins before scanning to promote duodenal filling. Patients were scanned supine in the treatment position and immobilised with an individualised Vac-Lok cushion (Civco Medical Solutions, Iowa, USA) to support the arms and upper torso. Knee and ankle supports were used where needed. A non-contrast CT was performed in all patients and unless contra-indicated by poor renal function, a contrast CT scan was also performed to aid target definition following intravenous administration of 100 mls Omnipaque. Scans were performed in mid-breath hold and were acquired with 1.25 mm slice thickness. The field-of-view encompassed the entire circumference of the body contour with coverage from 15 cm above the most superior fiducial to 15 cm below the most inferior fiducial. Target localisation was performed on the CyberKnife® Multi-Plan® Treatment Planning System (Accuray Inc. Sunnyvale, CA, USA). Treatment was planned on the non-contrast CT scan which was fused with the contrast CT to aid target localisation. Where available, pre-treatment combined 18-fluorodeoxyglucose positron emission tomography and CT (^{18}F-FDG-PET/CT) scan was also fused with the planning CT. Gross tumour volume (GTV) was outlined by the treating clinician, reviewed by a radiologist where appropriate and expanded with an isocentric margin of 2–3 mm to form the planning target volume (PTV).

In two palliative cases where fiducial tracking was not performed, patients were planned and monitored with an internal tumour volume (ITV) and XSight® Spine Tracking (Accuray Corporation, Sunnyvale, CA, USA) approach. Planning CT scans were acquired in free-breathing, maximal inspiration and maximal expiration respiratory phases. An internal target volume (ITV) was constructed to incorporate maximal GTV excursion with respiration

and XSight® Spine tracking was used throughout treatment to assure reproducible patient body anatomy positioning.

For all patients, the duodenum, stomach, small bowel, liver, kidneys and spinal cord were outlined and treated as OAR. The duodenum was considered the primary OAR and constraints were applied as previously published [41, 42]. The preferred OAR dose constraints for three fraction SABR (applied when feasible) are given in Table 1. Tighter constraints were applied if previous radiotherapy had been given. Patients were prescribed 18–36 Gy in three fractions, with total dose influenced by the proximity of dose-limiting OAR (primarily duodenum and stomach) and any prior radiotherapy received. The prescription isodose line was chosen to provide optimum coverage of the target volume whilst respecting OAR constraints. Tumour definition, normal tissue constraints and final treatment plan were approved by the consultant radiation oncologist and attending medical physicist.

Prior to each treatment fraction, patients were premedicated with prophylactic ondansetron 4 mg and metoclopramide 10 mg orally (unless contra-indicated). Patients drank 300 mls of water and set-up was performed as per CT planning. A non-contrast mid-breath hold CT scan was performed on Day 1 for patients with implanted fiducial markers to assess fiducial stability. This scan was fused with the planning CT and was assessed on the MultiPlan® System (Accuray Corporation, Sunnyvale, CA, USA), prior to radiation delivery to ensure that fiducial placement was maintained. Once the CyberKnife® physicist and treating physician were satisfied that the fiducial arrangement on the Day 1 CT matched that of the planning CT, the GTV and PTV contours were overlaid on the Day 1 CT to check contours appropriately covered the tumour target, with no discernible differences to adjacent OAR (e.g. stomach/duodenal filling or tumour growth) impacting target coverage. Following this check, most patients were treated on 3 consecutive weekdays; in all cases treatment was completed within 7 days.

Follow-up

Patients were clinically reviewed 3-months after treatment, then at 6-month intervals thereafter when post-treatment CT scans were acquired. Toxicity was assessed using Common Terminology Criteria for Adverse Events version 3 (CTCAEv3). Local and distant failures were determined by an independent reporting radiologist and the treating physician using radiological information. Local control was defined as stable or decreased tumour size, local failure was defined by an increase in tumour size and distant failure was defined as the appearance of new lesions on CT or PET scan.

Table 1 OAR dose constraints applied for three fraction SABR in this study

	D0.035 cc	D0.1 cc	D10.0 cc	D5.0 cc	V12 Gy	V15 Gy	V21 Gy
Duodenum	≤ 22.2 Gy	–	≤ 11.4 Gy	≤ 16.5 Gy	–	–	–
Stomach	≤ 22.2 Gy	–	≤ 16.5 Gy	–	–	–	–
Small Bowel	≤ 25.2 Gy	–	–	≤ 17.7 Gy	–	–	–
Liver	–	–	–	–	–	≤ 50%	≤ 30%
Kidneys (separate)	–	–	–	–	≤ 25%	–	–
Kidneys (together)	–	–	–	–	–	≤ 35%	–
Spinal cord	≤ 21.0 Gy	≤ 18.0 Gy	–	–	–	–	–

Note: For all pancreatic patients treated with ≤ 30 Gy in three fractions, we have since revised our duodenal D0.035 cc constraint to the higher limit of 24 Gy, but additionally now use D1.0 cc < 31.4 Gy

BED calculation and radiobiological modelling

The biological effective dose (BED) received by each patient was calculated simply as:

$$\mathrm{BED} = \mathrm{D} \times \left[1 + \frac{d}{\frac{\alpha}{\beta}} \right]$$

where D is the total dose delivered, d is the dose per fraction and α/β is the assumed fractionation factor. For pancreatic tumour, the radiobiological assumption was $\alpha/\beta = 10$ Gy. For normal tissues the radiobiological assumption was $\alpha/\beta = 3$ Gy. Comparison between SABR and conventional radiotherapy schedules was carried out using the linear-quadratic (LQ) model modified to account for tumor repopulation. The conventional radiotherapy comparator schedule used was 50.4 Gy in 28 fractions over a total period of 5.5 weeks (37 days). For the calculation of iso-effective SABR schedules a repopulation correction was applied to the BED calculation formula [43, 44], where for pancreatic tumour the radiobiological parameter assumptions used were: doubling time = 42 days, k = 0.5 Gyday^{-1} and repopulation was assumed to be operative throughout the entire treatment. As the majority of SABR treatments were completed within 3 days, a fixed repopulation correction of 3×0.5 Gy = 1.5 Gy was used.

Statistical analysis

The Chi-squared test or ANOVA analysis was used to determine the association between planning and delivery variables and toxicity. Kaplan-Meier analysis was used to calculate freedom-from-local-progression (FFLP), progression-free-survival (PFS) and overall survival (OS), beginning from the start of SBRT treatment and censoring patients lost to follow-up. Log-rank analysis was used to assess the impact of factors on FFLP and OS. The Cox proportional hazard model, adjusted for all variables, was used to assess the impact of multi-variate factors upon FFLP and OS.

Results

Patient, tumour and treatment purpose characteristics (Table 2)

A total of 42 patients were included, with median (range) patient age of 64 (42–85) years. The majority of patients had stage T4 disease located in the head of the pancreas. The reported reasons for SABR as the sole primary treatment (8 patients) were poor performance status (PS), co-morbidity and patient choice. SABR was considered as an adjuvant when it was used within 6 months of standard therapies (14 patients). SABR was used 6 months–3 years after primary therapy as a consolidation or re-treat option for residual or relapsed local disease in 20 patients.

SABR planning and delivery variables (Table 3)

The majority of patients had 3–4 stably implanted fiducials (64%) and received treatment on 3 consecutive days (88%). PTV size ranged from 15.8–193.6 cc, percentage cover ranged from 79.9–99.5%, treatment duration was 3–7 days, treatment delivery time ranged from 36 to 162 mins, BED ranged from 23.4–79.0 Gy and the mean minimum dose to PTV ranged from 11.07–34.45 Gy. Mean and 95% confidence interval (CI) values are given in Table 2. Alternative planning and motion management strategies (ITV and XSight® Spine) were necessary in two palliative patients.

Acute and late treatment toxicity incidence (Table 4)

Acute treatment toxicity information was available in 37 patients. Of these, 11 patients (30%) experienced no adverse effects and 23 patients (62%) experienced Grade 1–2 adverse effects, of which fatigue, nausea and pain were the most common. Only three patients (8%) experienced Grade 3 acute toxicities (pain, fatigue and obstructive jaundice, respectively), which resolved quickly with clinical support. Late toxicity information was available for 32 patients, of whom 27 patients (84%) reported no late adverse events. A total of six patients (19%) experienced late adverse effects. One patient (3%) was diagnosed with Grade 2 pancreatic insufficiency and one patient (3%) experienced Grade 2 pain and nausea. Four

Table 2 Patient, tumour and treatment characteristics (N = 42 patients)

Gender	Male	N = 16 (38.0%)
	Female	N = 26 (62.0%)
Tumour stage	T4	N = 37 (88.1%)
	T3	N = 1 (2.4%)
	T2	N = 3 (7.1%)
	T1	N = 1 (2.4%)
Site	Head	N = 36 (86.0%)
	Body	N = 5 (12.0%)
	Tail	N = 1 (2.0%)
PS (WHO)	0	N = 2 (5.0%)
	1	N = 17 (41.0%)
	2	N = 22 (52.0%)
	3	N = 1 (2.0%)
Previous treatment	None	N = 8 (19.0%)
	Chemotherapy only	N = 23 (54.8%)
	Chemoradiotherapy	N = 4 (9.5%)
	Palliative surgery (gastric/biliary bypass) + chemotherapy	N = 2 (4.8%)
	Curative surgery (Whipples/ Resection) + chemotherapy	N = 1 (2.4%)
	Curative surgery (Whipples/ Resection) + chemoradiotherapy	N = 4 (9.5%)
SABR purpose	PRIMARY	N = 8 (19.0%)
	(no other/prior treatment)	
	ADJUVANT (within 6 months other primary treatment)	N = 14 (33.3%)
	CONSOLIDATION (> 6 months post-primary treatment to residual disease)	N = 11 (26.2%)
	RETREAT	N = 9 (21.4%)
	(> 6 months post-primary treatment to disease relapse)	

patients suffered serious duodenal toxicities attributed to treatment: two patients developed Grade 4 duodenal strictures and two patients suffered Grade 4 gastro-intestinal GI haemorrhage. The patient who experienced Grade 2 pain and nausea also developed Grade 4 GI bleeding at 7 months post-treatment: however, the latter incidence was considered unrelated to treatment as it was concomitant with radiologically confirmed local tumour progression invading the duodenum.

Association of SABR planning and delivery variables with toxicity incidence (Tables 5 and 6)

Treatment factors were examined in relation to post-treatment toxicity incidence (Table 5).

The number of fiducials statistically associated with incidence of acute toxicity ($p = 0.002$). A trend for uneven acute toxicity was observed with treatment purpose: relatively few patients who received only SABR experienced acute toxicity but patients who received SABR for palliative re-treatment of relapsed disease showed increased acute toxicity ($p = 0.064$). SABR variables that associated with late toxicity incidence were number of fiducials, treatment duration, treatment delivery time and percentage coverage (all $p < 0.05$). For the two patients that experienced Grade 2 late toxicity, both had outlying delivery times (58 and 61 mins, respectively). Further, one patient had a very low outlying percentage coverage (79%) and was treated with one implanted fiducial for on-treatment tracking.

Seven patients in total experienced Grade 3+ significant toxicities (Table 6). All three patients who experienced Grade 3 acute toxicities breached preferred duodenal constraints. Of the four patients who experienced late adverse treatment effects of Grade 4 GI bleeding or duodenal stricture, it was noted that all four had T4 tumours, none were planned with PET scan information, and all had outlying or sub-optimal treatment variables. Further, preferred duodenal OAR dose constraints were breached in three of the four patients. The first patient with duodenal toxicity was post-resection (distal pancreatectomy and splenectomy was performed the previous year), had received subsequent adjuvant chemotherapy and was re-treated with SABR with palliative intent for recurrent local disease. The surgery had left the patient with distorted anatomy, an unusually small PTV (20.34 cc) and closely associated OAR. Although the duodenum was within the OAR constraint policy, only one implanted fiducial was possible for tumour tracking and the patient was prescribed treatment in three fractions over a longer treatment duration of 5 days because of anticipated toxicity risk. The second patient with duodenal toxicity also received SABR as a re-treatment with palliative intent for locally relapsed disease, also only had one implanted fiducial for tumour tracking, and was treated in 3 fractions over 5 days. Moreover, retrospective examination of the treatment plan showed that the duodenum was the key OAR, encircling and contacting the PTV more than 270°, and duodenal constraints were considerably exceeded. The third patient with duodenal toxicity received SABR as consolidation treatment for residual disease following chemotherapy > 6 months prior. Their PTV was large (109.3 cc) and although both prescription dose (22 Gy) and BED (38 Gy) were lower than average, preferred duodenal constraints were exceeded. The last patient with duodenal toxicity received SABR adjuvant to primary chemotherapy. The patient had a large PTV (104.5 cc) and again duodenal OAR constraints were exceeded.

Table 3 SABR planning and delivery variables (N = 42 patients)

Number of fiducials	0	N = 2 (5.0%)*
	1	N = 8 (19.0%)
	2	N = 5 (12.0%)
	3	N = 21 (50.0%)
	4	N = 6 (14.0%)
Treatment duration (days)	3	N = 37 (88.1%)
	4	N = 1 (2.4%)
	5	N = 3 (7.1%)
	7	N = 1 (2.4%)
PET scan data used for planning	Yes	N = 11 (26.0%)
	No	N = 31 (74.0%)
PTV size (cc)	Mean (95% CI)	76.25 (63.83–88.67)
Prescription dose (Gy)	Mean (95% CI)	26.77 (19.33–113.39)
Prescription Isodose (%)	Mean (95% CI)	67.3 (65.24–69.35).
Percentage Cover (%)	Mean (95% CI)	96.6 (95.52–97.66)
Min dose to PTV (Gy)	Mean (95% CI)	22.29 (21.0–23.5)
Max dose to PTV (Gy)	Mean (95% CI)	40.2 (38.5–41.9)
Mean dose to PTV (Gy)	Mean (95% CI)	31.5 (30.8–32.3)
Homogeneity Index (HI)	Mean (95% CI)	1.5 (1.45–1.55)
BED (Gy)	Mean (95% CI)	50.3 (47.7–53.0)
Fraction dose (Gy per fraction)	Mean (95% CI)	8.9 (8.6–9.2)
Delivery time (mins)	Mean (95% CI)	71.4 (65.2–77.6)

*alternative planning and delivery strategy used for 2 patients

Table 4 Acute and late toxicity

	Grade 1–2	Grade 3	Grade 4
Acute (≤ 3 months post-treatment) toxicity incidence in N = 37 patients			
NONE	N = 11 (30%)		
Diarrhoea	N = 5 (14%)	0	0
Nausea	N = 8 (22%)	0	0
Vomiting	N = 2 (5%)	0	0
Dyspepsia	N = 2 (5%)	0	0
Anorexia	N = 2 (5%)	0	0
Pain	N = 7 (19%)	N = 1 (3%)	0
Fatigue	N = 11 (30%)	N = 1 (3%)	0
Jaundice	N = 1 (3%)	0	0
Obstructive Jaundice	0	N = 1 (3%)	0
Late (> 3 months post-treatment) toxicity incidence in N = 32			
NONE	N = 27 (84%)		
Pain	N = 1 (3%)*	0	0
Nausea	N = 1 (3%)*	0	0
Pancreatic Insufficiency	N = 1 (3%)	0	0
GI Bleeding	0	0	N = 2 (6%)
Duodenal Stricture	0	0	N = 2 (6%)

*one patient experienced Grade 2 pain and Grade 2 nausea

Survival outcomes (Fig. 1) and association with planning and delivery variables

Post-treatment follow-up information was available for 39/42 (93%) patients. Two patients (5%) converted to resectable status post-treatment: one subsequently underwent complete resection but unfortunately the other was medically unfit for operation. Overall, 15 (36%) patients died with distant progression and no local failure, and two patients (5%) died with local failure and no distant progression. Kaplan-Meier survival analysis showed median FFLP, PFS and OS were 9.8, 5.9 and 8.4 months, respectively. Actuarial 1 year survivor function (95% C.I) for FFLP, PFS and OS were 43.4 (20.8, 64.2)%, 19.8 (7.8, 35.9)%, and 39.0 (22.7, 55.0)%, respectively. Survival plots illustrating FFLP and OS are shown in Fig. 1. Log-rank analysis to test the equality of the Kaplan-Meier survivor function across treatment variables, split by their medians, on FFLP and OS showed no statistical differences. Treatment purpose was also investigated by log-rank analysis, where patients who received SABR > 6 months post-primary therapy as consolidation or re-treat for residual or relapsed disease were compared to patients who received SABR as primary or adjuvant therapy: importantly they showed similar FFLP and OS, indicating SABR may be extending survival outcomes for residual or relapsed disease. When multi-variate Cox proportional hazard regression modelling (adjusted for all treatment variables) was applied to examine the influence of continuous or dichotomous treatment variables on FFLP and OS, both PTV size (cc) and treatment duration (days) significantly associated with OS ($p < 0.05$).

LQ radiobiological modelling: Comparison of calculated parameters (Table 7)

The BED calculated for the reference conventional conformal radiotherapy schedule (50.4 Gy in 28 fractions delivered in 37 days) was 40.5 Gy_{10}. However, as conformal, conventionally fractionated RT is delivered to the minimum 95% isodose within the PTV [45, 46], the minimum dose to the PTV would be 47.88 Gy with the comparator regimen, which equates to a minimum BED of 37.1 Gy_{10}. For the normal tissues, the comparator regimen delivers a minimum BED of 75.2 Gy_3. Using the LQ model, the estimated SABR equivalent to the comparator schedule is 3×7.45 Gy, giving a total dose of 22.35 Gy and associated normal tissue BED of 77.85 Gy_3. For patients in this study who received prescribed dose to optimal individualized isodose (mean = 67.3%), only 21/42 (50%) of patients received a minimum PTV dose of 22.35 Gy.

Discussion

This study was the first to use LQ modelling to assess pancreatic SABR efficacy and to comprehensively

Table 5 Association of treatment factors and treatment toxicity

	Acute toxicity max grade (n = 37)				Late toxicity max grade (n = 32)			
	0	1–2	3	p-value	0	2	4	p-value
Number of fiducials†								
0–1	1	6	0	0.0002*	4	1	2	0.01*
2–4	10	17	3		22	1	2	
Treatment days †								
3	11	20	3	0.37	25	2	2	0.012*
4–7	0	3	0		1	0	2	
Previous surgery†								
Yes	1	5	0	0.47	4	0	1	0.68
No	10	18	3		22	2	3	
Previous irradiation†								
Yes	0	7	1	0.11	6	0	0	0.43
No	11	16	2		20	2	4	
Min dose to PTV†								
< 22.35Gy	5	10	2	0.75	9	2	2	0.17
≥ 22.35Gy	6	11	1		17	0	2	
SABR purpose†								
Sole primary	1	6	0	0.064	6	1	0	0.62
Adjuvant	6	4	1		7	0	1	
Consolidation	4	6	1		8	1	1	
Retreat	0	5	2		5	0	2	
Treatment time (mins)	77.5	69.9	68.3	0.570	67.7	59.5	83.0	0.045*
PTV (cc) ‡	93.5	72.1	67.9	0.355	77.2	61.5	79.3	0.875
PTV min dose (cGy) ‡	2342.6	2227.6	2115.8	0.605	2317.7	1901.5	2332.4	0.396
PTV max dose (cGy) ‡	3951.3	3974.7	4149.2	0.8819	4120.6	3920.5	3861.9	0.622
PTV mean dose (cGy) ‡	3151.9	3118.0	3241.9	0.879	3225.4	3085.6	3015.0	0.493
Prescription dose (cGy) ‡	2736.4	2647.8	2700.0	0.735	2740.4	2700.0	2612.5	0.7067
Prescription isodose (%) ‡	69.6	67.5	65.3	0.554	67.0	69.0	68.3	0.882
Percentage cover (%) ‡	96.1	97.0	97.3	0.771	97.1	88.1	91.1	0.002*
BED (Gy10) ‡	52.3	49.2	52.0	0.650	52.1	51.0	49.0	0.811
HI ‡	1.44	1.50	1.54	0.523	1.51	1.46	1.47	0.833

*Statistically significant at 0.05% level † Numbers are frequencies, tested for association using Chi-squared test; ‡ Numbers are means, tested for association using ANOVA

examine the influence of patient and planning factors on toxicity and outcome. The study was conducted in a 'real--world' patient series, which is crucial for understanding treatment effectiveness and safety in everyday clinical practice. Our results support SABR as an encouraging modality for locally inoperable pancreatic cancer, with particular benefits as a re-treatment, consolidation or salvage boost, or as an alternative treatment for patients with poor PS or co-morbidity. Although toxicity was low and survival was better than expected — especially considering nearly half of patients were treated more than 6-months after primary treatment — both FFLP survival analysis and LQ modelling showed scope to improve local control

through dose escalation. The few serious incidences of late duodenal toxicity indicate that this would need to be approached cautiously with increased stringency on duodenal protection through highly detailed individualised planning.

Low toxicity was obtained that was better than many other SABR studies [20–22, 25, 28, 36], despite larger PTVs and higher prescription doses in this study. This indicates planning methods and on-treatment dynamic targeting with Synchrony® were generally good and consistent with other studies [20, 25, 27–30, 32, 34, 36]. The main limitation when examining patient and treatment factors in relation to toxicity was the low incidence of

Table 6 Duodenal dosimetry and treatment factors for patients with Grade 3+ toxicity

Grade 3+ Toxicity	Treatment Factors				Duodenal Dosimetry					
	Fids	PTV	Prescribed Dose	Dur'n	D0.035 cc	D1.0 cc	D5.0 cc	D10.0 cc	V15 Gy	V20 Gy
ACUTE										
Grade 3 pain	4	39.84 cc	30.0 Gy 3 fractions	3 days	33.9 Gy*	25.4 Gy	15.8 Gy	12.8 Gy*	5.9 cc	2.5 cc
Grade 3 fatigue	3	44.22 cc	30.0 Gy 3 fractions	3 days	34.9 Gy*	27.9 Gy	20.5 Gy*	16.2 Gy*	12.3 cc	5.4 cc
Grade 3 obstructive jaundice	4	119.57 cc	21.0 Gy 3 fractions	3 days	23.8 Gy*	22.6 Gy	21.1 Gy*	19.6 Gy*	32.2 cc	8.6 cc
LATE										
Grade 4 duodenal stricture	1†	20.34 cc	28.5 Gy 3 fractions	5 days	11.2 Gy	8.3 Gy	6.8 Gy	6.2 Gy	0.0 cc	0.0 cc
Grade 4 GI bleed	1†	83.49 cc	27.0 Gy 3 fractions	5 days	29.3 Gy*	28.3 Gy	26.2 Gy*	23.9 Gy*	39.1 cc	19.4 cc
Grade 4 GI bleed	3	109.31 cc	22.0 Gy 3 fractions	3 days	24.2 Gy*	23.2 Gy	22.5 Gy*	21.8 Gy*	63.3 cc	24.3 cc
Grade 4 duodenal stricture	3	104.25 cc	27.0 Gy 3 fractions	3 days	31.6 Gy*	29.1 Gy	26.0 Gy*	21.8 Gy*	24.2 cc	12.8 cc

*Duodenal planning dosimetry exceeded institution preferred 3 fraction constraints. † single fiducial conferring anticipated increased risk of duodenal complications [47]

late and Grade 3+ toxicity events: multiple testing is acknowledged as an additional limitation. The only factors that showed association with acute toxicity were number of fiducials ($p = 0.0002$) and treatment purpose ($p = 0.064$). The former aligns with our previous dose-volume histogram study of duodenal risk in an overlapping cohort of pancreatic SABR patients that showed increased toxicity risk for patients with single or no fiducial [47]. The latter is probably due to the patients who were re-treated who had one or more sub-optimal treatment factors (unusually large or small PTV and/or tightly adjacent OAR and/or only one fiducial and/or breached OAR constraints) and thus a higher risk of treatment toxicity was expected. Number of fiducials also associated with late toxicity [47]. Other variables that associated with late toxicity were increased treatment duration period (> 3 days), treatment delivery time (mins), and coverage: (%): however, we consider these factors to be associative rather than causal for late toxicity for several reasons. First, the main reason for serious duodenal toxicity in three patients was breached duodenal OAR constraints. Second, the uneven distribution noted for treatment delivery time and late treatment toxicities is mainly because two patients who showed Grade 2 late treatment toxicities had lower than average treatment times. Third, the association between treatment duration and percentage coverage likely reflects purposeful selection of these parameters because of recognised increased duodenal toxicity risk due to individual medical, anatomical planning and delivery challenges. For example, SABR is known to be least successful when the treatment volume is large and the 'dose-cloud' is not tightly conformal, and to be sub-optimal when fewer fiducials are used compromising the accuracy of dynamic tumour tracking. As such, it is notable that of the four patients that suffered duodenal toxicity, two had large PTV (> 100 cc), and the other two (who were treated palliatively > 6 months after primary therapy for recurrent disease)

had only one fiducial implanted for on-treatment tumour tracking and were purposefully prescribed treatment over 5 days because of anticipated toxicity risk. Moreover, three of the patients who suffered duodenal toxicity breached the preferred duodenal OAR dose constraints, with the volume of duodenum receiving > 15 Gy considerably exceeding limits correlated with duodenal toxicity [36]. Increased vigilance and stringency to duodenal dose constraints, particularly for patients with large PTV, distorted anatomy, closely adjacent OAR, or fewer fiducials, is therefore appropriate. Indeed, our recent dose-volume histogram duodenal risk map study of duodenal risk in an overlapping cohort of pancreatic SABR patients showed a 10% risk level for Grade 3–4 duodenal haemorrhage or stricture when D1 cc = D31.4 Gy [47]. Furthermore, we found that the use of multiple fiducials showed ~one-fifth of the risk for Grade 3–4 duodenal complications compared with single fiducial or Xsight® Spine tumour tracking. As such, we advocate implanting at least four fiducials and using three or more stable fiducials for optimal tumour tracking during treatment delivery and, based on estimated 10% duodenal risk levels, now impose the stringent duodenal constraint of D1.0 cc < 31.4 Gy for all pancreatic patients treated with ≤30 Gy in three fractions. Concomitantly, in response to collective experience, we have revised our duodenal D0.035 cc constraint to the higher limit of 24 Gy [47]. It is additionally noted that the incorporation of more extensive measures for duodenal assessment during individualised planning/ schedules, such as Lyman modelling for normal tissue complication probability [36], late complications [44] or Red Shell volume calculation [48] may also be helpful in the prevention of duodenal toxicity.

As all patients were inoperable and non-metastatic, they would be expected to have similar prognostic outcomes to intermediate stage patients and may reasonably be compared with similar intermediate stage cohorts in the literature. Overall survival following SABR was good

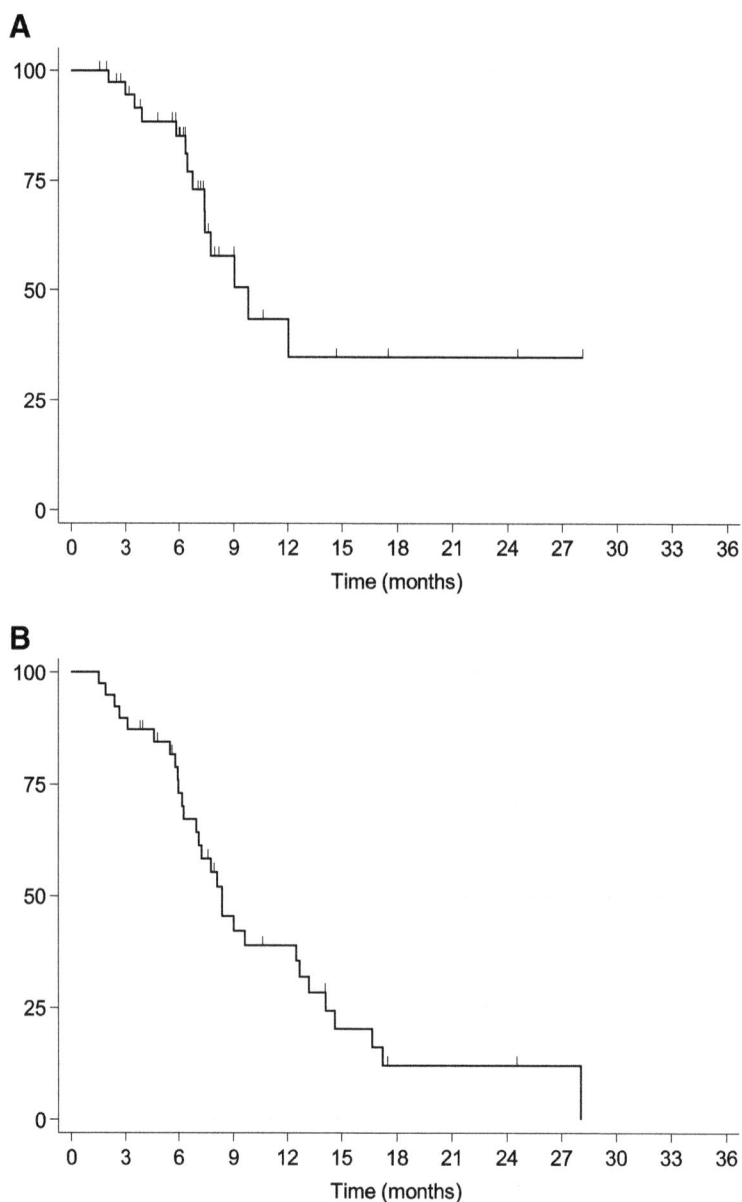

Fig. 1 Kaplan-Meier survival plots illustrating **a**) percentage (%) freedom-from-local-progression (FFLP) in months and **b**) percentage (%) overall survival (OS) in months

Table 7 Radiobiological (LQ) modelling: calculated comparator regimen and SABR equivalent parameters

	Total Dose (D)	Fraction Dose (d)	Fractions (n)	Duration (days)	BED (Gy$_{10}$)	BED (Gy$_3$)
Comparator regimen (100% dose to PTV)	50.4 Gy	1.8 Gy	28	37	40.5 Gy	80.6 Gy
SABR equivalent	23.55 Gy	7.85 Gy	3	3	40.5 Gy	77.0 Gy
Number of patients treated with total dose ≥ 23.55 Gy = 39/42 (92.9%)						
Comparator regimen (min 95% dose to PTV)	47.88 Gy	1.71 Gy	28	37	37.5 Gy	75.27 Gy
SABR equivalent	22.35 Gy	7.45 Gy	3	3	37.5 Gy	77.85 Gy
Number of patients treated with minimum PTV dose ≥ 22.35 Gy = 21/42 (50%)						

considering that 48% of patients were treated > 6 months after primary therapy, indicating that SABR may be extending survival times for patients with residual or relapsed local disease. The median OS of 8.4 months is comparable to that of first line chemoradiotherapy treatments in randomised LAPC trials [9, 10, 49] and the actuarial 1 year OS of 39% is comparable [29–31, 33] or better than [21, 22, 25, 32] other studies of SABR in LAPC. However, the FFLP of 43% at 1 year is lower in comparison to other SABR studies [20–22, 25–35], where some achieved FFLP rates of 70–94% at 1 year [22, 25, 29, 32]. Although the low FFLP rate is likely to have been negatively influenced by the fact that almost half of patients were treated > 6 months after primary therapy to residual or relapsed disease, it also suggests that higher rates of local control may be achievable with SABR. The lack of any association of treatment factors with FFLP in log-rank or multi-variate analysis indicates that neither current planning or delivery methods are contributing to local failure. Both PTV size and treatment course duration (days) associated with OS. The relationship between size and OS is not clear and may be related to disease advance, and the association with treatment days likely reflects purposeful selection of a longer treatment course for re-treat/palliative/relapse patients with more advanced disease and worse PS.

Although there are limitations to LQ modelling when extrapolating from schedules involving conventional fraction sizes to those involving larger fractions, the results indicated that 50% of the patients treated received a minimum PTV dose that was less potent than a comparator standard conformal radiotherapy regimen. The main reason was because prescribed SABR dose was delivered to a patient individualised isodose line to balance target volume coverage with adjacent OAR risk, whereas conformal RT is delivered to the minimum 95% isodose within the PTV. It is additionally notable that the reference schedule of 50.4 Gy in 28 fractions over 5.5 weeks is associated with a tumor BED of ~ 40.5 Gy. This is considered likely to eradicate only the smallest tumour of moderate radiosensitivity, whereas pancreatic tumours are typically moderately sized and relatively radioresistant. Recent analysis of clinical radiation dose response in pancreatic cancer using LQ modelling has indicated that a BED of ~ 40.5 Gy may achieve > 50% local control [18]. A BED > 70 Gy was calculated to achieve significant tumour response (size reduction consistent with complete or partial response) and thus a schedule of three fractions, each delivering 9.2 Gy, was proposed accordingly for SABR [18]. Recent studies have provided support for the feasibility, similar toxicity and potential increased local control with escalated dose [50]. In our study, the lack of association of toxicity with maximum dose to PTV or prescription dose indicates that a higher overall dose is unlikely to affect toxicity if measures to limit duodenal dose are emphasized. Together these data indicate need and scope to escalate SABR doses to achieve minimum PTV doses > 22.5 Gy *and* optimal BED > 70 Gy for improved efficacy. Our revised duodenal D0.035 dose constraint to the higher value of 24 Gy will allow greater scope for dose escalation. The recent adoption of 5–6 fraction SABR regimens are additionally anticipated to improve toxicity profiles. However, given the ongoing risk for serious duodenal toxicity in a proportion of patients, dose escalation would need to be implemented with great care and awareness of risk for individual patients.

Conclusions

CyberKnife® treatment was well tolerated and survival in the cohort was encouraging, supporting SABR as a good treatment option in the primary, adjuvant or re-treatment setting. The LQ modelling results and relatively low FFLP indicate scope for dose escalation to improve local control and survival. However, to avoid serious duodenal toxicity a cautious approach needs to be taken, incorporating careful assessment of individual patients for dose escalation suitability and concomitant enhanced stringency on duodenal protection.

Abbreviations
^{18}F-FDG-PET: 18-fluorodeoxyglucose positron emission tomography; BED: Biological effective dose; CI: Confidence interval; CT: Computed tomography; EUS: Endoscopic ultrasound; FFLP: Freedom-from-local-progression; GI: Gastro-intestinal; GTV: Gross target volume; HI: Homogeneity index; ITV: Internal target volume; LAPC: Locally advanced pancreatic cancer; LQ: Linear-quadratic; OAR: Organs-at-risk; OS: Overall survival; PFS: Progression-free-survival; PS: Performance status; PTV: Planning target volume; SABR: Stereotactic ablative radiotherapy; XSS: XSight Spine

Acknowledgements
Preliminary results of this study were previously presented in Abstract form at the SRS/SBRT Scientific Meeting February 2013, CA, USA. The support of radiographers, medical physicists, dosimetrists and radiation oncologists at The Harley Street Clinic Radiotherapy Department is appreciated for their contributions to the success of treatment and helpful technical discussions. Tim Cross and Gillian Santorelli are gratefully acknowledged for careful data management and efficient statistical analysis, respectively.

Funding
No specific funding source was used for this study as it was carried out as part of research and development within the auspices of HCA International at the CyberKnife Centre, The Harley Street Clinic.

Authors' contributions
CG data acquisition and interpretation, critical revision of manuscript and final approval. NP study conception, data interpretation and manuscript final approval. MG data analysis and interpretation, manuscript preparation and critical revision. RD data analysis and interpretation and final manuscript approval. PP study conception, design and management, data interpretation and manuscript approval. All authors read and approved the final manuscript.

Competing interests

The authors declare that they have no competing interests.

Author details

¹Guys and St Thomas' NHS Foundation Trust, London, UK. ²The London CyberKnife Centre, The Harley Street Clinic, 81 Harley Street, London W1G 8PP, UK. ³St. Bartholomew's Hospital, London, UK. ⁴Department of Surgery and Cancer, Imperial College London, London, UK.

References

1. Carrato A, Falcone A, Ducreux M, Valle JW, Parnaby A, Djazouli K, et al. A systematic review of the burden of pancreatic cancer in Europe: real-world impact on survival, quality of life and costs. J Gastrointest Cancer. 2015;46: 201–11.
2. Siegel R, Naishadham D, Jemal A. Cancer statistics, 2013. CA Cancer J Clin. 2013;63:11–30.
3. Cancer Research UK. Pancreatic Cancer statistics 2018. https://www. cancerresearchuk.org/health-professional/cancer-statistics/statistics-by-cancer-type/pancreatic-cancer. Accessed 06 Sept 2018.
4. Hidalgo M. Pancreatic cancer. N Engl J Med. 2010;362:1605–17.
5. Wagner M, Redaelli C, Lietz M, Seiler CA, Friess H, Buchler MW. Curative resection is the single most important factor determining outcome in patients with pancreatic adenocarcinoma. Br J Surg. 2004;91:586–94.
6. Morganti AG, Massaccesi M, La Torre G, Caravatta L, Piscopo A, Tambaro R, et al. A systematic review of resectability and survival after concurrent chemoradiation in primarily unresectable pancreatic cancer. Ann Surg Oncol. 2010;17:194–205.
7. Truty MJ, Thomas RM, Katz MH, Vauthey JN, Crane C, Varadhachary GR, et al. Multimodality therapy offers a chance for cure in patients with pancreatic adenocarcinoma deemed unresectable at first operative exploration. J Am Coll Surg. 2012;215:41–51 discussion –2.
8. Crane CH, Varadhachary GR, Yordy JS, Staerkel GA, Javle MM, Safran H, et al. Phase II trial of cetuximab, gemcitabine, and oxaliplatin followed by chemoradiation with cetuximab for locally advanced (T4) pancreatic adenocarcinoma: correlation of Smad4(Dpc4) immunostaining with pattern of disease progression. J Clin Oncol. 2011;29:3037–43.
9. Johung K, Saif MW, Chang BW. Treatment of locally advanced pancreatic cancer: the role of radiation therapy. Int J Radiat Oncol Biol Phys. 2012;82: 508–18.
10. Sultana A, Tudur Smith C, Cunningham D, Starling N, Tait D, Neoptolemos JP, et al. Systematic review, including meta-analyses, on the management of locally advanced pancreatic cancer using radiation/combined modality therapy. Br J Cancer. 2007;96:1183–90.
11. Iacobuzio-Donahue CA, Fu B, Yachida S, Luo M, Abe H, Henderson CM, et al. DPC4 gene status of the primary carcinoma correlates with patterns of failure in patients with pancreatic cancer. J Clin Oncol. 2009;27:1806–13.
12. Ben-Josef E, Schipper M, Francis IR, Hadley S, Ten-Haken R, Lawrence T, et al. A phase I/II trial of intensity modulated radiation (IMRT) dose escalation with concurrent fixed-dose rate gemcitabine (FDR-G) in patients with unresectable pancreatic cancer. Int J Radiat Oncol Biol Phys. 2012;84: 1166–71.
13. Chang JS, Wang ML, Koom WS, Yoon HI, Chung Y, Song SY, et al. High-dose helical tomotherapy with concurrent full-dose chemotherapy for locally advanced pancreatic cancer. Int J Radiat Oncol Biol Phys. 2012;83:1448–54.
14. Loehrer PJ Sr, Feng Y, Cardenes H, Wagner L, Brell JM, Cella D, et al. Gemcitabine alone versus gemcitabine plus radiotherapy in patients with locally advanced pancreatic cancer: an eastern cooperative oncology group trial. J Clin Oncol. 2011;29:4105–12.
15. Murphy JD, Adusumilli S, Griffith KA, Ray ME, Zalupski MM, Lawrence TS, et al. Full-dose gemcitabine and concurrent radiotherapy for unresectable pancreatic cancer. Int J Radiat Oncol Biol Phys. 2007;68:801–8.
16. Hammel P, Huguet F, van Laethem JL, Goldstein D, Glimelius B, Artru P, et al. Effect of chemoradiotherapy vs chemotherapy on survival in patients with locally advanced pancreatic cancer controlled after 4 months of gemcitabine with or without erlotinib: the LAP07 randomized clinical trial. JAMA. 2016;315:1844–53.
17. Krishnan S, Rana V, Janjan NA, Varadhachary GR, Abbruzzese JL, Das P, et al. Induction chemotherapy selects patients with locally advanced, unresectable pancreatic cancer for optimal benefit from consolidative chemoradiation therapy. Cancer. 2007;110:47–55.
18. Moraru IC, Tai A, Erickson B, Li XA. Radiation dose responses for chemoradiation therapy of pancreatic cancer: an analysis of compiled clinical data using biophysical models. Pract Radiat Oncol. 2014;4:13–9.
19. Chauffert B, Mornex F, Bonnetain F, Rougier P, Mariette C, Bouche O, et al. Phase III trial comparing intensive induction chemoradiotherapy (60 Gy, infusional 5-FU and intermittent cisplatin) followed by maintenance gemcitabine with gemcitabine alone for locally advanced unresectable pancreatic cancer. Definitive results of the 2000-01 FFCD/SFRO study. Ann Oncol. 2008;19:1592–9.
20. Goyal K, Einstein D, Ibarra RA, Yao M, Kunos C, Ellis R, et al. Stereotactic body radiation therapy for nonresectable tumors of the pancreas. J Surg Res. 2012;174:319–25.
21. Hoyer M, Roed H, Sengelov L, Traberg A, Ohlhuis L, Pedersen J, et al. Phase-II study on stereotactic radiotherapy of locally advanced pancreatic carcinoma. Radiother Oncol. 2005;76:48–53.
22. Koong AC, Christofferson E, Le Q-T, Goodman KA, Ho A, Kuo T, et al. Phase II study to assess the efficacy of conventionally fractionated radiotherapy followed by a stereotactic radiosurgery boost in patients with locally advanced pancreatic cancer. Int J Radiat Oncol Biol Phys. 2005;63:320–3.
23. Chang BK, Timmerman RD. Stereotactic body radiation therapy: a comprehensive review. Am J Clin Oncol. 2007;30:637–44.
24. Martin A, Gaya A. Stereotactic body radiotherapy: a review. Clin Oncol (R Coll Radiol). 2010;22:157–72.
25. Chang DT, Schellenberg D, Shen J, Kim J, Goodman KA, Fisher GA, et al. Stereotactic radiotherapy for unresectable adenocarcinoma of the pancreas. Cancer. 2009;115:665–72.
26. Chuong MD, Springett GM, Freilich JM, Park CK, Weber JM, Mellon EA, et al. Stereotactic body radiation therapy for locally advanced and borderline resectable pancreatic cancer is effective and well tolerated. Int J Radiat Oncol Biol Phys. 2013;86:516–22.
27. Koong AC, Le QT, Ho A, Fong B, Fisher G, Cho C, et al. Phase I study of stereotactic radiosurgery in patients with locally advanced pancreatic cancer. Int J Radiat Oncol Biol Phys. 2004;58:1017–21.
28. Mahadevan A, Jain S, Goldstein M, Miksad R, Pleskow D, Sawhney M, et al. Stereotactic body radiotherapy and gemcitabine for locally advanced pancreatic cancer. Int J Radiat Oncol Biol Phys. 2010;78:735–42.
29. Mahadevan A, Miksad R, Goldstein M, Sullivan R, Bullock A, Buchbinder E, et al. Induction gemcitabine and stereotactic body radiotherapy for locally advanced nonmetastatic pancreas cancer. Int J Radiat Oncol Biol Phys. 2011; 81:e615–e22.
30. Schellenberg D, Goodman KA, Lee F, Chang S, Kuo T, Ford JM, et al. Gemcitabine chemotherapy and single-fraction stereotactic body radiotherapy for locally advanced pancreatic cancer. Int J Radiat Oncol Biol Phys. 2008;72:678–86.
31. Schellenberg D, Kim J, Christman-Skieller C, Chun CL, Columbo LA, Ford JM, et al. Single-fraction stereotactic body radiation therapy and sequential gemcitabine for the treatment of locally advanced pancreatic cancer. Int J Radiat Oncol Biol Phys. 2011;81:181–8.
32. Lominska C, Unger K, Nasr N, Haddad N, Gagnon G. Stereotactic body radiation therapy for reirradiation of localized adenocarcinoma of the pancreas. Radiat Oncol. 2012;7:74.
33. Tozzi A, Comito T, Alongi F, Navarria P, Iftode C, Mancosu P, et al. SBRT in unresectable advanced pancreatic cancer: preliminary results of a mono-institutional experience. Radiat Oncol. 2013;8:148.
34. Gurka M, Collins S, Slack R, Tse G, Charabaty A, Ley L, et al. Stereotactic body radiation therapy with concurrent full-dose gemcitabine for locally advanced pancreatic cancer: a pilot trial demonstrating safety. Radiat Oncol. 2013;8:44.
35. Seo Y, Kim M-S, Yoo S, Cho C, Yang K, Yoo H, et al. Stereotactic body radiation therapy boost in locally advanced pancreatic cancer. Int J Radiat Oncol Biol Phys. 2009;75:1456–61.
36. Murphy JD, Christman-Skieller C, Kim J, Dieterich S, Chang DT, Koong AC. A dosimetric model of duodenal toxicity after stereotactic body radiotherapy for pancreatic cancer. Int J Radiat Oncol Biol Phys. 2010;78:1420–6.
37. Su T-S, Liang P, Lu H-Z, Liang J-N, Liu J-M, Zhou Y, et al. Stereotactic body radiotherapy using CyberKnife for locally advanced unresectable and metastatic pancreatic cancer. World J Gastroenterol. 2015;21:8156–62.

Stereotactic ablative radiotherapy (SABR) as primary, adjuvant, consolidation and re-treatment...

69

38. Zhong J, Patel K, Switchenko J, Cassidy RJ, Hall WA, Gillespie T, et al. Outcomes for patients with locally advanced pancreatic adenocarcinoma treated with stereotactic body radiation therapy versus conventionally fractionated radiation. Cancer. 2017;123:3486–93.

39. Lo SS, Sahgal A, Chang EL, Mayr NA, Teh BS, Huang Z, et al. Serious complications associated with stereotactic ablative radiotherapy and strategies to mitigate the risk. Clin Oncol (R Coll Radiol). 2013;25:378–87.

40. Dieterich S, Gibbs IC. The CyberKnife in clinical use: current roles, future expectations. Front Radiat Ther Oncol. 2011;43:181–94.

41. Benedict SH, Yenice KM, Followill D, Galvin JM, Hinson W, Kavanagh B, et al. Stereotactic body radiation therapy: the report of AAPM task group 101. Med Phys. 2010;37:4078–101.

42. Timmerman RD. An overview of hypofractionation and introduction to this issue of seminars in radiation oncology. Semin Radiat Oncol. 2008;18:215–22.

43. Fowler JF. The linear-quadratic formula and progress in fractionated radiotherapy. Br J Radiol. 1989;62:679–94.

44. Fowler JF. 21 years of biologically effective dose. Br J Radiol. 2010;83:554–68.

45. ICRU Report 50. Prescribing, Recording and Reporting Photon Beam Therapy. Bethesda: International Commission on Radiation Units and Measurements; 1994.

46. ICRU Report 62. Prescribing, Recording and Reporting Photon Beam Therapy. Bethesda: International Commission on Radiation Units and Measurements; 1999.

47. Goldsmith C, Price P, Cross T, Loughlin S, Cowley I, Plowman N. Dose-volume histogram analysis of stereotactic body radiotherapy treatment of pancreatic cancer: a focus on duodenal dose constraints. Semin Radiat Oncol. 2016;26:149–56.

48. Yang J, Fowler JF, Lamond JP, Lanciano R, Feng J, Brady LW. Red shell: defining a high-risk zone of normal tissue damage in stereotactic body radiation therapy. Int J Radiat Oncol Biol Phys. 2010;77:903–9.

49. Crane CH, Varadhachary G, Settle SH, Fleming JB, Evans DB, Wolff RA. The integration of chemoradiation in the care of patient with localized pancreatic cancer. Cancer Radiother. 2009;13:123–43.

50. Rudra S, Jiang N, Rosenberg SA, Olsen JR, Parikh PJ, Bassetti MF, et al. High dose adaptive MRI guided radiation therapy improves overall survival of inoperable pancreatic Cancer. Int J Rad Oncol Biol Phys. 2017;99:E184.

8

Intensity-modulated radiation therapy for definitive treatment of cervical cancer: a meta-analysis

Yanzhu Lin[1†], Kai Chen[1†], Zhiyuan Lu[2], Lei Zhao[1], Yalan Tao[1], Yi Ouyang[1] and Xinping Cao[1*]

Abstract

Background: To compare the efficacies and toxicities of intensity-modulated radiotherapy (IMRT) with three-dimensional conformal radiotherapy (3D-CRT) or conventional two-dimensional radiotherapy (2D-RT) for definitive treatment of cervical cancer.

Methods: A meta-analysis was performed using search engines, including PubMed, Cochrane Library, Web of Science, and Elsevier. In the meta-analysis, odds ratios (ORs) were compared for overall survival (OS), disease-free survival (DFS), and acute and chronic toxicities.

Results: Included data were analysed using RevMan 5.2 software. Six studies encompassing a total of 1008 patients who received definitive treatment (IMRT = 350, 3-DCRT/2D-RT = 658) were included in the analysis. A comparison of 3-year OS and 3-year DFS revealed no significant differences between IMRT and 3D-CRT or 2D-RT (3-year OS: OR = 2.41, 95% confidence interval [CI]: 0.62–9.39, $p = 0.21$; 3-year DFS: OR = 1.44, 95% CI: 0.69–3.01, $p = 0.33$). The incidence of acute gastrointestinal (GI) toxicity and genitourinary (GU) toxicity in patients who received IMRT was significantly lower than that in the control group (GI: Grade 2: OR = 0.5, 95% CI: 0.28–0.89, $p = 0.02$; Grade 3 or higher: OR = 0.55, 95% CI: 0.32–0.95, $p = 0.03$; GU: Grade 2: OR = 0.41, 95% CI: 0.2–0.84; $p = 0.01$; Grade 3 or higher: OR = 0.31, 95% CI: 0.14–0.67, $p = 0.003$). Moreover, the IMRT patients experienced fewer incidences of chronic GU toxicity than did the control group (Grade 3: OR = 0.09, 95% CI: 0.01–0.67, p = 0.02).

Conclusion: IMRT and conventional radiotherapy demonstrated equivalent efficacy in terms of 3-year OS and DFS. Additionally, IMRT significantly reduced acute GI and GU toxicities as well as chronic GU toxicity in patients with cervical cancer.

Keywords: Cervical cancer, IMRT, 3DCRT, 2DRT

Background

Cervical cancer is the second most common malignant tumour in women and is the third leading cause of cancer-related death among women worldwide [1]. Thus, it represents a serious threat to women's health. The incidence and mortality of cervical cancer in China are the highest in the world. Radical surgery and radiotherapy

* Correspondence: caoxp@sysucc.org.cn
†Yanzhu Lin and Kai Chen contributed equally to this work.
[1]Department of Radiation Oncology, Sun Yat-sen University Cancer Center, State Key Laboratory of Oncology in South China, Collaborative Innovation Center for Cancer Medicine, 651 Dongfeng Road East, Guangzhou, Guangdong 510060, People's Republic of China
Full list of author information is available at the end of the article

(RT) are equally efficacious in the treatment of patients with stage I–IIA cervical cancer [2].

External beam radiation combined with intracavitary brachytherapy is the main RT approach for locally advanced cervical carcinoma. In the past few decades, conventional two-dimensional RT (2D-RT) has been widely used in the treatment of cervical cancer, but this treatment option suffers from a high frequency of acute and chronic complications, which affect the treatment efficacy as well as patient quality of life [3]. Three-dimensional conformal RT (3D-CRT) based on computed tomography is becoming a critical part of RT. This approach is relatively favourable in terms of the radiation dose and toxicity to organs in the exposure field [4].

Intensity-modulated RT (IMRT) is a precise RT that has been developed on the basis of 3D-CRT [5]. An advantage of IMRT is that it can deliver a relatively large radiation dose over a target area while minimising the radiation dose to adjacent noncancerous tissue, thereby offering greater locoregional control and leading to fewer side effects. IMRT is associated with lower gastrointestinal and haematological toxicities than is conventional RT (c-RT) in treatment of cervical cancer, and it is therefore used more widely [6, 7]. However, the potential advantages of IMRT for treating cervical cancer remain unclear. Therefore, this meta-analysis evaluated whether IMRT results in more favourable clinical outcomes than 2D-RT or 3D-CRT do in patients with intact cervical cancer in terms of overall survival (OS) and toxicity.

Methods

Search strategy

This analysis strictly followed the guidelines of the Preferred Reporting Items for Systematic Reviews and Meta-Analyses (PRISMA) statement [8]. The analysis was performed on studies with publication dates up to 13 February 2018. Several search engines (PubMed, the Cochrane Library, Web of Science, and Elsevier) were used to identify articles that investigated the relationship between IMRT and conventional RT or 3D conformal RT for treating cervical cancer. The keywords used were as follows: [intensity-modulated OR conformal OR dimensional OR 2D OR 3D] AND [radiotherapy* OR radiation therapy] AND [cervical OR cervix OR uterine] AND [tumour OR cancer OR carcinoma]. Only English-language publications were included.

Inclusion and exclusion criteria

Studies were selected for inclusion in this analysis according to the following selection criteria: 1) Study participants were patients with cervical cancer who were diagnosed by pathological examination. 2) IMRT was compared with 3D-CRT or 2D-RT in previously untreated patients, and the efficacy was reported. 3) Patients were treated with RT and concurrent chemotherapy. 4) The number of participants in the experimental group was ≥10. Exclusion criteria were as follows: 1) Case reports, conference abstracts, comments, and letters to the editors were excluded. 2) Studies based on patients who had received previous surgical treatment for cervical cancer were excluded. 3) Duplicate publications were excluded.

Data extraction

Two reviewers extracted data from each eligible study. Information extracted from eligible studies included the first author's name, year of publication, study design, and number of study participants, as well as participant age, region, cancer stage, RT dose, and major outcomes. Disagreements were resolved through discussion and consensus.

Data analysis and statistical methods

All statistical analyses were performed using RevMan 5.2 (Cochrane Collaboration, Oxford, UK). All survival outcomes and toxicity measurements from the studies were analysed based on odd ratios (ORs) with a 95% confidence interval (CI). The heterogeneity among studies was assessed using chi square or I^2 statistics ($p < 0.1$ indicated significant heterogeneity). If $I^2 > 50\%$ or $p < 0.1$, the results for the chi-squared tests were considered statistically significant, and a random-effects model was chosen. Otherwise, we used a fixed-effects model (the Mantel–Haenszel method) for further evaluations. The pooled effect size was significant if $p < 0.05$.

Results

Literature search

The initial literature search based on the keywords yielded 2808 articles. After examination for and exclusion of duplicate and irrelevant articles, 64 articles remained for full-text review. The full texts of the potentially eligible articles were read, and six publications [9–14] were included in the meta-analysis. The detailed article selection process and exclusion criteria are presented in Fig. 1.

Basic characteristics of the included studies

In total, six articles, encompassing 1008 participants (350 IMRT, 658 CRT), comparing the RT effects of IMRT and 3D-CRT or 2DRT were included in the meta-analysis. The detailed characteristics of the six eligible studies are presented in Table 1. Included studies were published in 2010 or thereafter. Geographically, five trials were conducted in Eastern countries, and one was conducted in the United States. The patients were aged 24–88 years. All the patients were treated with whole pelvis RT in combination with brachytherapy. The range of doses for external beam irradiation was 45–50 Gy. All treated patients were also receiving cisplatin-based chemotherapy at the time of RT treatment.

Clinical outcomes

Four of the included trials, accounting for 678 participants, reported 3-year OS data (Fig. 2a). Heterogeneity existed between the studies, and thus a random-effects model was chosen. The pooled OR for 3-year OS was 2.41, and the 95% CI was 0.62 to 9.39 ($p = 0.21$). The results suggested that patients with cervical cancer in the IMRT group and the 3D-CRT or 2D-RT groups did not exhibit significant differences with respect to 3-year OS.

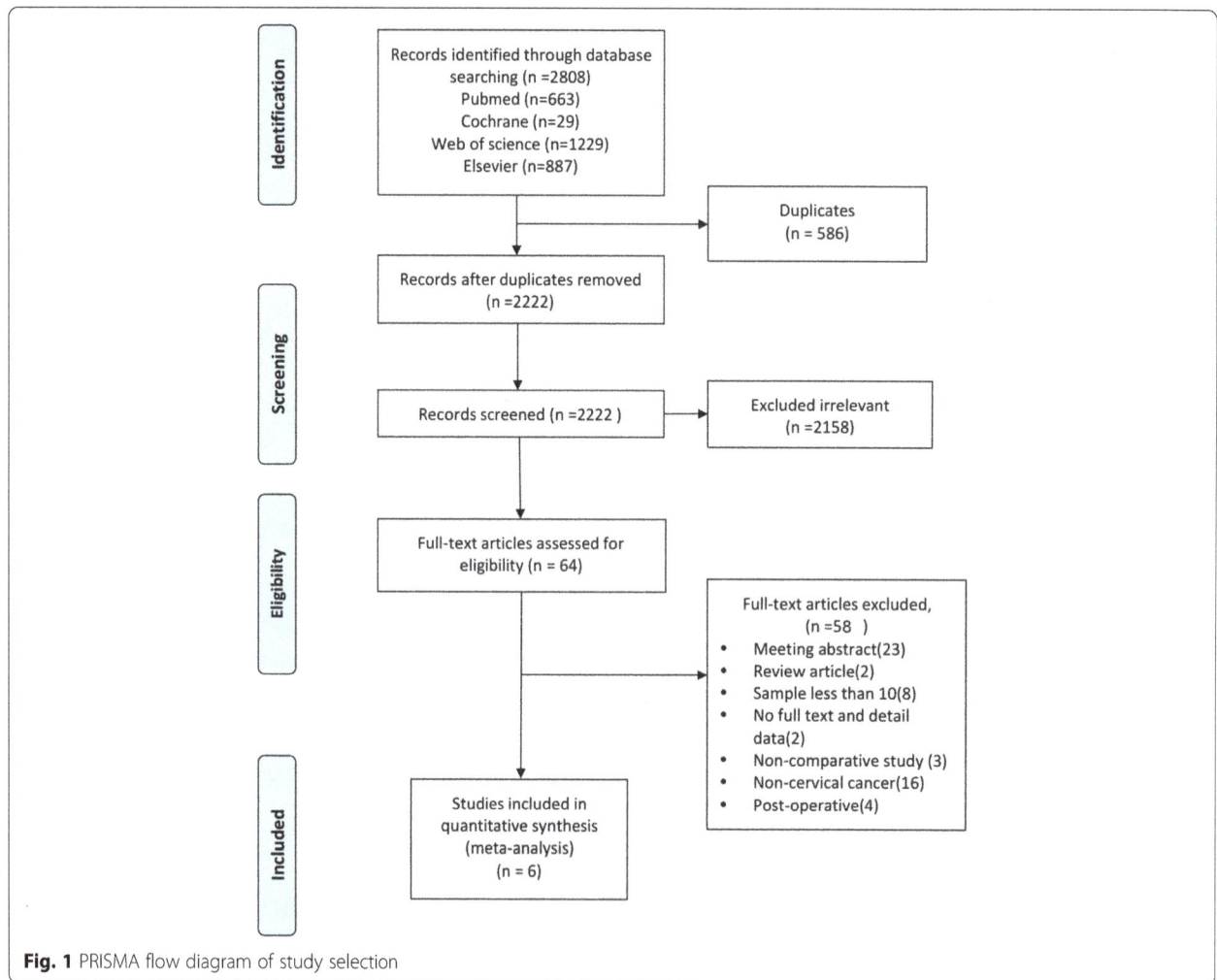

Fig. 1 PRISMA flow diagram of study selection

Data regarding disease-free survival (DFS) were available in four studies. Heterogeneity existed between two of the studies (Chi^2 = 8.47, I^2 = 65%); therefore, a random-effects model was chosen. The pooled estimate of the OR was 1.44, and the 95% CI was 0.69 to 3.01 (p = 0.33). A random-effect meta-analysis indicated no difference between the two groups in terms of 3-year DFS (Fig. 2b).

Acute toxicity

Gastrointestinal (GI) and genitourinary (GU) were the most common side effects for cervical cancer patients treated with RT. A total of five studies reported instances of acute toxicity after patients received treatment, including acute GI and GU side effects. We analysed various grades of GI toxicity to assess the effect of treatment on patients. No statistical difference (OR = 1.05, 95% CI 0.61–1.83, p = 0.85) was evident, indicating that patients who received IMRT therapy exhibited more favourable outcomes than those who received 2D-RT or 3D-CRT therapy in terms of incidence of grade 1 acute GI toxicity. Additionally, the results suggested that

patients in the IMRT group exhibited a lower incidence of grade 2 or higher acute GI toxicity than did those in the 2D-RT or 3D-CRT group (Grade 2: OR = 0.5, 95% CI: 0.28–0.89, p = 0.02; Grade 3 or higher: OR = 0.55, 95% CI: 0.32–0.95, p = 0.03; Fig. 3).

Similarly, overall meta-analysis of the data revealed that the IMRT group was associated with a significantly lower incidence of acute grade 2 GU toxicity compared with the 2D-RT or 3D-CRT group (OR = 0.41, 95% CI: 0.2–0.84; p = 0.01). Pooled analysis revealed that incidence of grade 3 or higher GU toxicity among patients who received IMRT was significantly lower than that among patients who received 2D-RT or 3D-CRT (OR = 0.31; 95% CI: 0.14–0.67; p = 0.003; Fig. 4).

Chronic toxicity

Two studies compared the chronic GI and GU toxicity exhibited by IMRT and control groups. According to our analysis, the trials were heterogeneous, and therefore a random model was chosen. No statistical significance was evident between the two groups in terms of

Table 1 Characteristics of all the included studies

Author	Year	Country	Study design	Stage	Treatment	Patients (n)	Median age (range)	RT doses (Gy)	Chemotherapy
Naik et al.	2016	India	Prospective	IIA–IIIB	IMRT	20	48(28–70)	50	cisplatin
					3D	20	45(30–75)		
Wu et al.	2016	Taiwan.	Retrospective	IB1-IVB	IMRT	30	80.5 (75–88)	45–50.4	cisplatin
					2D/3D	30	77.8 (75–88)		
Ganhdi et al.	2013	India	Prospective	IIB–IIIB	IMRT	22	50(36–65)	50.4	cisplatin
					2D	22	45(36–65)		
Chen et al.	2013	Taiwan	Retrospective	IB2-IIIB	IMRT	83	54	45	cisplatin
					2D/3D	237	54		
Du et al.	2012	China	Retrospective	IIB-IIIB	IMRT	60	52(31–74)	45–50	cisplatin
					2D	62	55(26–77)		
Kidd et al.	2010	USA	Prospective	IA2-IVB	IMRT	135	52	50	cisplatin
					2D/3D	317	52		

n number of patients, *RT* Radiotherapy, *2D* Two-dimensional, *3D* Three-dimensional, *IMRT* Intensity modulated RT

chronic GI (Fig. 5). The incidences of grades 1 and 2 GU toxicity in the two groups were not significantly different (Grade 1: OR = 1.35, 95% CI: 0.6–3.0; *p* = 0.47; Grade 2: OR = 0.44, 95% CI: 0.17–1.14, *p* = 0.09). However, the incidence of grade 3 or higher GU toxicity in the IMRT group was significantly lower than that of the 2D-RT or 3D-CRT group (OR = 0.09, 95% CI: 0.01–0.67; *p* = 0.02; Fig. 6).

Discussion

Pelvic RT combined with brachytherapy plays a critical role in the definitive treatment of patients with cervical cancer. With rapid developments in RT, IMRT has become widely used in treatment of cervical cancer, and it exhibits a dosimetric advantage because it can deliver a high dose of radiation to tumour tissue while restricting dose exposure of adjacent noncancerous tissues [15, 16]. However, because

of the highly specific dose distribution in IMRT, the tumour target may be missed, especially in cases of cervical cancer.

The limitation of current imaging modality is that accurate tumour boundary demarcation cannot be ensured; thus, because of the anatomic specificity of the target location in cases of cervical cancer, organ motion may cause the target to be missed [17]. Therefore, the application of IMRT in cervical cancer treatment is highly controversial. Comparison of the curative effects of IMRT and conventional 2D-RT or 3D-CRT is crucial.

According to a 2012 systematic review and meta-analysis by Yang et al. based on 13 studies [18], IMRT significantly reduced the average proportion of irradiated volume of the rectum and small bowel compared with 3D-CRT in patients with gynaecologic malignancies. However, whether the dosimetric advantage of IMRT leads to more favourable

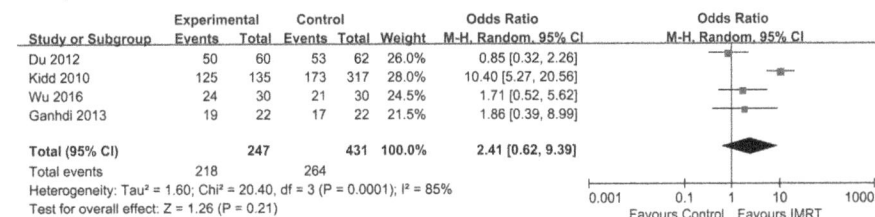

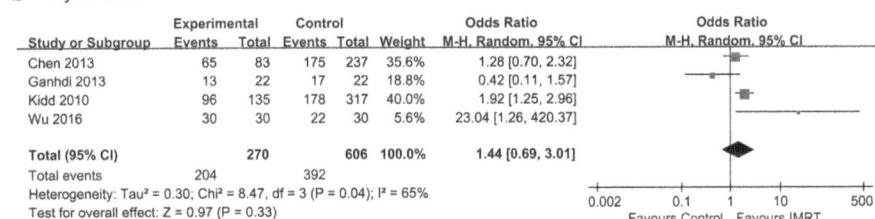

Fig. 2 Comparison between IMRT and 2D-RT/3D-CRT for OS and DFS

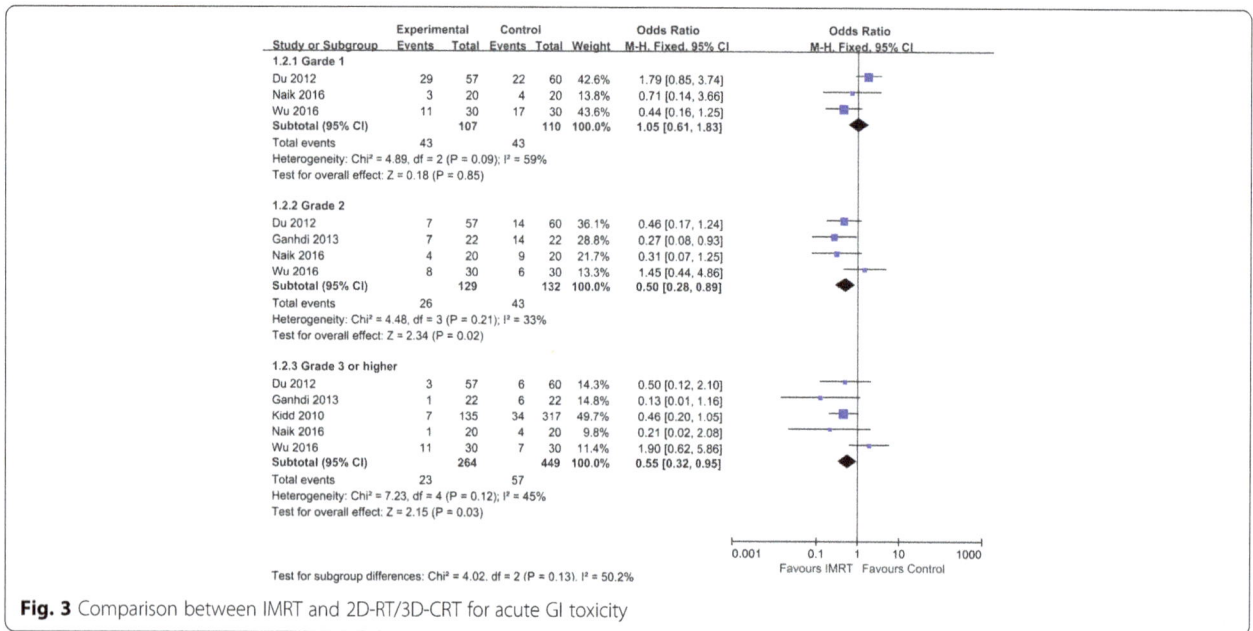

Fig. 3 Comparison between IMRT and 2D-RT/3D-CRT for acute GI toxicity

clinical outcomes than those associated with conventional external beam radiation remains unclear. The pooled results of our meta-analysis indicated that IMRT application was associated with similar clinical outcomes to those of conventional RT (c-RT) in terms of both 3-year OS and 3-year DFS. However, Kidd et al. [13] reported a significantly greater OS for an IMRT group. This may be because the IMRT group had no lymph node involvement, which would have influenced survival rate. Only one relevant study [12] has reported 5-year progression-free survival rates (PFS) and 5-year OS. The results indicated a significantly higher 5-year PFS rate but no improvement in

5-year OS for an IMRT group compared with a c-RT control (5 year PFS: 64.9% vs. 44.3%, $p = 0.03$; 5-year OS: 71.20% vs. 60.30%, $p = 0.064$) for patients with advanced cervical cancer. These data are difficult to analyse and may not represent the true clinical outcomes for patients with cervical cancer. Thus, large-scale randomised trials are required to determine whether IMRT offers long-term survival benefits for women with cervical cancer.

RT exhibits curative effectiveness for cervical cancer in terms of tumour growth control, but the accompanying acute and chronic toxicities, which affect patient life quality, are of concern. Patients' most common acute

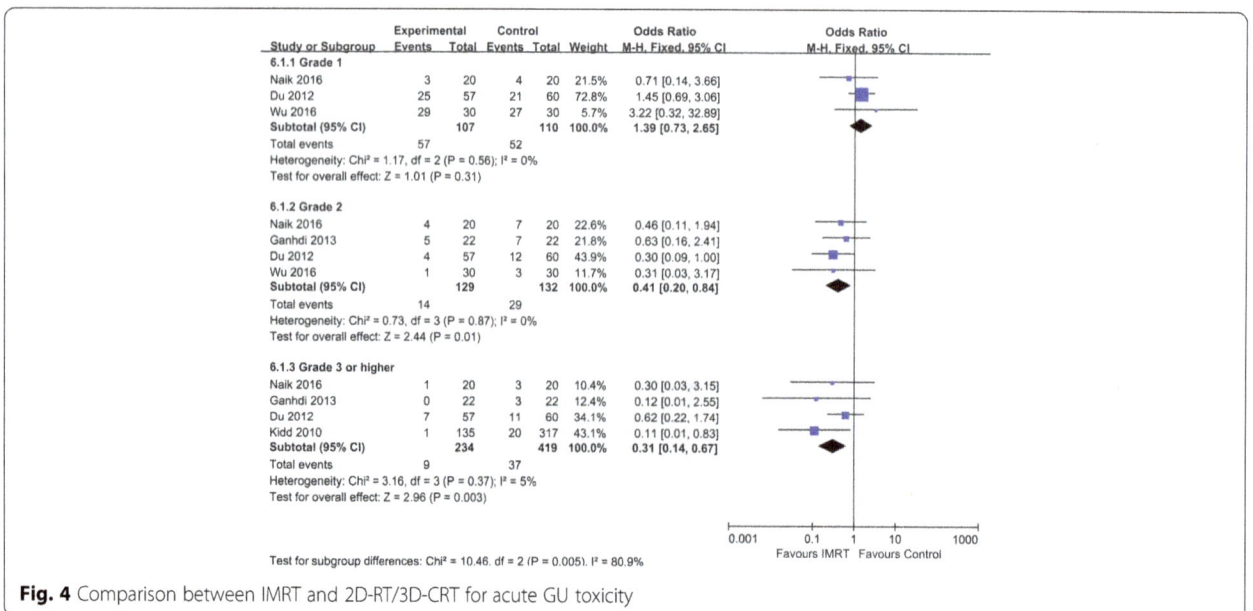

Fig. 4 Comparison between IMRT and 2D-RT/3D-CRT for acute GU toxicity

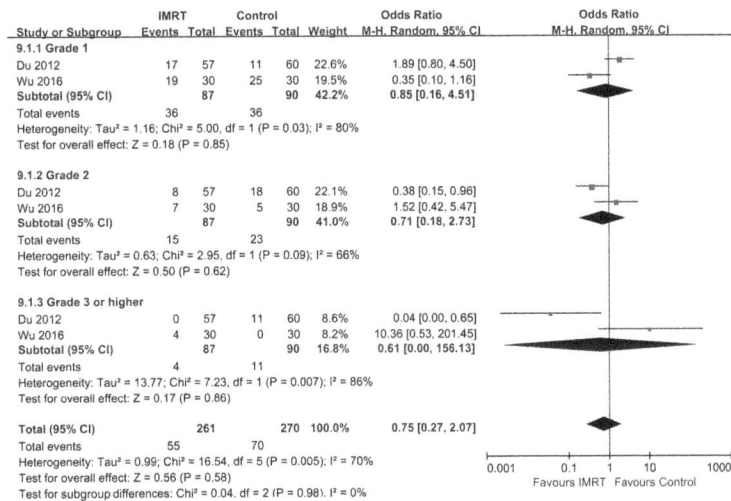

Fig. 5 Comparison between IMRT and 2D-RT/3D-CRT for chronic GI toxicity

adverse reactions to RT are abdominal pain, varying degrees of diarrhoea, haemorrhage, intestinal obstruction, and granulocytopenia, and because of these potential side effects, some patients refuse RT [19]. Late toxicities may arise months to years after whole pelvis RT, and most commonly comprise intermittent diarrhoea; intolerance to certain foods; malabsorption of vitamins, lactose, and bile acids; and severe toxicities such as obstruction and fistulas [20]. Although the reported survival outcomes did not exhibit statistical difference between arms, we did observe a significant benefit with regard to toxicity. Our meta-analysis revealed that the frequency of acute grade 2–4 GI and GU toxicities and of chronic grade 3 GU toxicity was significantly lower in the IMRT group than it was in the control group. One study [10] did not provide the grades of toxicity and thus was not

included in this portion of our analysis. A preliminary study indicated that IMRT was associated with less chronic GI toxicity than c-RT was in patients with gynaecologic malignancies [21]. However, this study involved limited follow-up and was based on patients with endometrial and cervical cancer, including those who had undergone surgery. In the present study, we determined that IMRT and c-RT exhibited no statistically significant difference in terms of chronic GI toxicities. However, in a study by Wu et al. [14], a higher incidence of severe chronic GI toxicities was noted in patients who received IMRT compared with those who received 2D-RT, but the p value was not significant (IMRT vs. 2D-RT: Grade 3 = 13% vs. 0%, p = 0.054). In addition, the number of studies indicating haematological toxicity is limited. In summary, these results indicate that IMRT offers considerable benefit in protecting at-risk

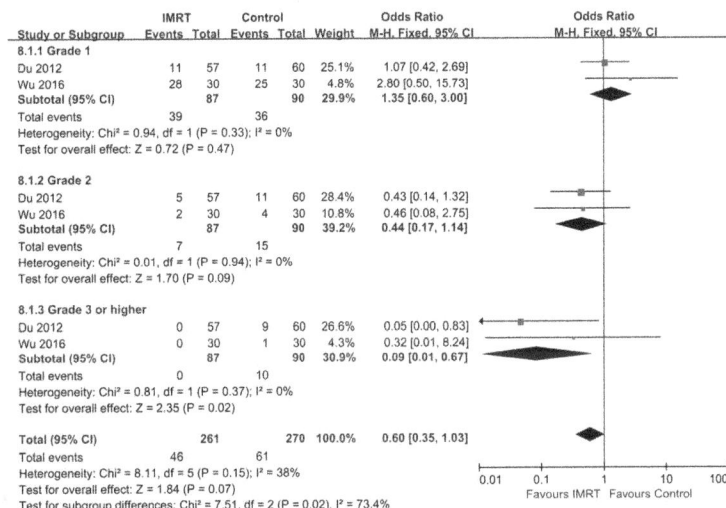

Fig. 6 Comparison between IMRT and 2D-RT/3D-CRT for chronic GU toxicity

organs and improving quality of life among patients with cervical cancer.

Our study involved several limitations. We included both prospective and retrospective studies, which introduced selection bias concerns. Additionally, only English-language publications were included, and thus language bias was probably introduced into the analysis. Moreover, most of the included studies were based on relatively small sample sizes. In addition, not all of the included studies compared clinical outcomes of IMRT groups with control groups, and most of them did not compare locoregional control rate (LRC) and PFS. Only one study provided 5-year PFS, which meant that this factor could not be evaluated in the present meta-analysis. Evidence in the literature was not conclusive enough to determine the efficacy of IMRT in the treatment of cervical cancer based on analysis of only OS, DFS, and toxicity. Additional high-quality clinical trials are warranted to verify the efficacy and benefits of IMRT for cervical cancer.

Conclusion

To our knowledge, this was the first meta-analysis to compare the clinical outcomes and toxicity experienced by patients with cervical cancer who received definitive treatment with IMRT, 3D-CRT, or 2D-RT. This meta-analysis determined that IMRT was not superior to 3D-CRT or 2D-RT in terms of OS, but it was associated with relatively few instances of acute GU and GI toxicities. Regarding cancer control, further studies are required to determine the appropriate role of IMRT in cervical cancer management.

Abbreviations

2D-RT: Two-dimensional radiotherapy; 3D-CRT: Three-dimensional conformal radiotherapy; CI: Confidence interval; DFS: Disease-free survival; GI: Gastrointestinal; GU: gentiourinary; IMRT: Intensity-modulated radiotherapy; LRC: Locoregional control rate; ORs: Odds ratios; OS: Overall survival; PFS: Progression free survival; RT: Conventional radiotherapy

Acknowledgements

The authors would like to thank Shuangyao Wang (University of Tasmania, Hobart, TAS, Australia) for his assistance during this project.

Authors' contributions

YL designed the study, drafted and revised the manuscript. KC and ZL performed the clinical data collection and extraction. LZ performed clinical data collection, extraction and revised the manuscript. YT and YO performed the statistical analysis. XC conceived the study. All authors read and approved the final manuscript.

Competing interests

The authors declare that they have no competing interests.

Author details

[1]Department of Radiation Oncology, Sun Yat-sen University Cancer Center, State Key Laboratory of Oncology in South China, Collaborative Innovation Center for Cancer Medicine, 651 Dongfeng Road East, Guangzhou, Guangdong 510060, People's Republic of China. [2]Department of Oral and Maxillofacial Surgery, First Affiliated Hospital, Sun Yat-sen University, Guangzhou 510080, People's Republic of China.

References

1. Jin J. Screening for cervical cancer. JAMA. 2018;320:732.
2. Vistad I, Fossa SD, Dahl AA. A critical review of patient-rated quality of life studies of long-term survivors of cervical cancer. Gynecol Oncol. 2006;102: 563–72.
3. Gallagher MJ, Brereton HD, Rostock RA, Zero JM, Zekoski DA, Poyss LF, Richter MP, Kligerman MM. A prospective study of treatment techniques to minimize the volume of pelvic small bowel with reduction of acute and late effects associated with pelvic irradiation. Int J Radiat Oncol Biol Phys. 1986;12:1565–73.
4. Bucci MK, Bevan A, Roach MR. Advances in radiation therapy: conventional to 3D, to IMRT, to 4D, and beyond. CA Cancer J Clin. 2005;55:117–34.
5. Bryant AK, Huynh-Le MP, Simpson DR, Mell LK, Gupta S, Murphy JD. Intensity modulated radiation therapy versus conventional radiation for anal cancer in the veterans affairs system. Int J Radiat Oncol Biol Phys. 2018;102:109–15.
6. Hasselle MD, Rose BS, Kochanski JD, Nath SK, Bafana R, Yashar CM, Hasan Y, Roeske JC, Mundt AJ, Mell LK. Clinical outcomes of intensity-modulated pelvic radiation therapy for carcinoma of the cervix. Int J Radiat Oncol Biol Phys. 2011;80:1436–45.
7. Brixey CJ, Roeske JC, Lujan AE, Yamada SD, Rotmensch J, Mundt AJ. Impact of intensity-modulated radiotherapy on acute hematologic toxicity in women with gynecologic malignancies. Int J Radiat Oncol Biol Phys. 2002; 54:1388–96.
8. Moher D, Liberati A, Tetzlaff J, Altman DG. Preferred reporting items for systematic reviews and meta-analyses: the PRISMA statement. PLoS Med. 2009;6:e1000097.
9. Naik A, Gurjar OP, Gupta KL, Singh K, Nag P, Bhandari V. Comparison of dosimetric parameters and acute toxicity of intensity-modulated and three-dimensional radiotherapy in patients with cervix carcinoma: a randomized prospective study. Cancer Radiother. 2016;20:370–6.
10. Chen SW, Liang JA, Hung YC, Yeh LS, Chang WC, Lin WC, Chien CR. Does initial 45Gy of pelvic intensity-modulated radiotherapy reduce late complications in patients with locally advanced cervical cancer? A cohort control study using definitive chemoradiotherapy with high-dose rate brachytherapy. Radiol Oncol. 2013;47:176–84.
11. Gandhi AK, Sharma DN, Rath GK, Julka PK, Subramani V, Sharma S, Manigandan D, Laviraj MA, Kumar S, Thulkar S. Early clinical outcomes and toxicity of intensity modulated versus conventional pelvic radiation therapy for locally advanced cervix carcinoma: a prospective randomized study. Int J Radiat Oncol Biol Phys. 2013;87:542–8.
12. Du XL, Tao J, Sheng XG, Lu CH, Yu H, Wang C, Song QQ, Li QS, Pan CX. Intensity-modulated radiation therapy for advanced cervical cancer: a comparison of dosimetric and clinical outcomes with conventional radiotherapy. Gynecol Oncol. 2012;125:151–7.
13. Kidd EA, Siegel BA, Dehdashti F, Rader JS, Mutic S, Mutch DG, Powell MA, Grigsby PW. Clinical outcomes of definitive intensity-modulated radiation therapy with fluorodeoxyglucose-positron emission tomography simulation in patients with locally advanced cervical cancer. Int J Radiat Oncol Biol Phys. 2010;77:1085–91.
14. Wu M, Chen JC, Tai H, Chang K, Chia P. Intensity-modulated radiotherapy with concurrent chemotherapy for elder cervical cancers: a comparison of clinical outcomes with conventional radiotherapy. Int J Gerontol. 2016;10:159–63.
15. Zukauskaite R, Hansen CR, Grau C, Samsoe E, Johansen J, Petersen J, Andersen E, Brink C, Overgaard J, Eriksen JG. Local recurrences after curative IMRT for HNSCC: effect of different GTV to high-dose CTV margins. Radiother Oncol. 2017;126:48-55.
16. Kam MK, Chau RM, Suen J, Choi PH, Teo PM. Intensity-modulated radiotherapy in nasopharyngeal carcinoma: Dosimetric advantage over conventional plans and feasibility of dose escalation. Int J Radiat Oncol Biol Phys. 2003;56:145–57.

17. Marrazzo L, Arilli C, Pasler M, Kusters M, Canters R, Fedeli L, Calusi S, Casati M, Talamonti C, Simontacchi G, Livi L, Pallotta S. Real-time beam monitoring for error detection in IMRT plans and impact on dose-volume histograms : a multi-center study. Strahlenther Onkol. 2017;194:243-54.

18. Yang B, Zhu L, Cheng H, Li Q, Zhang Y, Zhao Y. Dosimetric comparison of intensity modulated radiotherapy and three-dimensional conformal radiotherapy in patients with gynecologic malignancies: a systematic review and meta-analysis. Radiat Oncol. 2012;7:197.

19. Lee J, Lin JB, Chang CL, Sun FJ, Wu MH, Jan YT, Chen YJ. Impact of para-aortic recurrence risk-guided intensity-modulated radiotherapy in locally advanced cervical cancer with positive pelvic lymph nodes. Gynecol Oncol. 2017;148:291-8.

20. Dang YZ, Li P, Li JP, Bai F, Zhang Y, Mu YF, Li WW, Wei LC, Shi M. The efficacy and late toxicities of computed tomography-based brachytherapy with intracavitary and interstitial technique in advanced cervical cancer. J Cancer. 2018;9:1635–41.

21. Mundt AJ, Mell LK, Roeske JC. Preliminary analysis of chronic gastrointestinal toxicity in gynecology patients treated with intensity-modulated whole pelvic radiation therapy. Int J Radiat Oncol Biol Phys. 2003;56:1354–60.

9

Novel 4D-MRI of tumor infiltrating vasculature: characterizing tumor and vessel volume motion for selective boost volume definition in pancreatic radiotherapy

Wensha Yang[1,2]*, Zhaoyang Fan[2], Zixin Deng[2,3], Jianing Pang[4], Xiaoming Bi[4], Benedick A Fraass[1], Howard Sandler[1], Debiao Li[2] and Richard Tuli[1]

Abstract

Background: Pancreatic ductal adenocarcinoma has dismal prognosis. Most patients receive radiation therapy (RT), which is complicated by respiration induced organ motion in upper abdomen. The purpose of this study is to report our early clinical experience in a novel self-gated k-space sorted four-dimensional magnetic resonance imaging (4D-MRI) with slab-selective (SS) excitation to highlight tumor infiltrating blood vessels for pancreatic RT.

Methods: Ten consecutive patients with borderline resectable or locally advanced pancreatic cancer were recruited to the study. Non-contrast 4D-MRI with and without slab-selective excitation and 4D-CT with delay contrast were performed on all patients. Vessel-tissue CNR were calculated for aorta and critical vessels (superior mesenteric artery or superior mesenteric vein) encompassed by tumor. Respiratory motion trajectories for tumor, as well as involved vessels were analyzed on SS-4D-MRI. Intra-class cross correlation (ICC) between tumor volume and involved vessels were calculated.

Results: Among all 4D imaging modalities evaluated, SS-4D-MRI sampling trajectory results in images with highest vessel-tissue CNR comparing to non-slab-selective 4D-MRI and 4D-CT for all patients studied. Average (±standard deviation) CNR for involved vessels are 13.1 ± 8.4 and 3.2 ± 2.7 for SS-4D-MRI and 4D-CT, respectively. The ICC factors comparing tumor and involved vessels motion trajectories are 0.93 ± 0.10, 0.65 ± 0.31 and 0.77 ± 0.23 for superior-inferior, anterior-posterior and medial-lateral directions respectively.

Conclusions: A novel 4D-MRI sequence based on 3D-radial sampling and slab-selective excitation has been assessed for pancreatic cancer patients. The non-contrast 4D-MRI images showed significantly better contrast to noise ratio for the vessels that limit tumor resectability compared to 4D-CT with delayed contrast. The sequence has great potential in accurately defining both the tumor and boost volume margins for pancreas RT with simultaneous integrated boost.

* Correspondence: wensha.yang@cshs.org
[1]Department of Radiation Oncology, Cedars Sinai Medical Center, 8700 Beverly Blvd., Los Angeles, CA 90048, USA
[2]Department of Biomedical Sciences, Biomedical Imaging Research Institute, Cedars Sinai Medical Center, Los Angeles, CA, USA
Full list of author information is available at the end of the article

Introduction

Pancreatic ductal adenocarcinoma (PDA) has the worst outcome of any solid tumor [1]. Whereas surgical resection remains the mainstay therapy, 80% of patients with non-metastatic disease have unresectable tumors that are unlikely to be down-staged after standard chemo-radiation therapy, due to the geometric relationship of the primary tumor to the surrounding vasculature [2]. Nevertheless, the overall survival rates in the patient group undergoing margin negative resection after neoadjuvant therapy are 2–3 times of the unresectable patient group [3, 4]. Stereotactic body radiation therapy (SBRT) has shown to improve local tumor control rates, yet has disappointing down-staging rates. Alternatively, radiation therapy (RT) with simultaneous integrated boost (SIB) to cancerous tissue surrounding tumor infiltrating vasculature has the potential to sterilize tumor around the vessels that have precluded resectability [5, 6]. However there are significant technical challenges associated with accurately escalating (boosting) radiation dose to the vessel/tumor interface due to substantial internal organ motion in the upper abdominal region. [7–10] SBRT with SIB to tumor/vessel interface is further complicated by the fact that the motion of the cancerous tissue surrounding the tumor infiltrating vessels may be different from center of the pancreas tumor [11]. Per standard clinical practice in our institution, a free-breathing (FB) contrast enhanced helical CT and a four dimensional CT (4D-CT) are performed to quantify the motion. Depending on patient compliance, 4D-CT can either be performed right after FB-CT with a sufficient amount of contrast left over in the blood vessels to enhance vasculature visibility, or after a long breathing coaching session to reach a stable respiration pattern required for a successful 4D-CT acquisition, when the contrast in the region of interest has already diminished. Risks associated with radiation dose and contrast agents also prevent this procedure from being repetitively performed on patients. [12, 13] The problem is further compounded by poor CT soft tissue contrast and 4D-CT stitching artifacts [14]. For these reasons, 4D-CT with delayed intravenous and oral contrasts often has limited value to evaluate soft tissue and blood vessel respiratory motion.

Recently the interest in using magnetic resonance imaging (MRI) in pancreas radiotherapy has increased. The superior soft tissue contrast and versatile imaging sequences of MRI can facilitate margin definitions in SBRT-SIB. Frequent imaging procedures necessary for organ motion characterization are also impeded by radiation dose from 4D-CT while not an issue in MRI. Since current MRI speed is insufficient to capture the three-dimensional motion of upper abdominal organs in real time, four dimensional MRI (4D-MRI) was developed to reconstruct motion encoded images from multiple breathing cycles. Early 4D-MRI was reconstructed by sorting 2D cine images from consecutive slices, thus its quality was degraded by severe stitching artifacts [15–17]. The artifacts were eliminated with new 4D-MRI techniques based on 3D acquisition sequences [18] and k-space sorting such as the recently developed self-gated 4D-MRI technique with 3D radial sampling and k-space sorting [16, 19]. The new class of 4D-MRI sequences also provides high isotropic resolution that was unachievable with 2D cine based 4D-MRI.

Recently, slab-selective excitation was proposed to improve vessel-tissue contrast and overall image quality in 3D radial-sampling-based 4D-MRI [20]. This approach exploits the in-flow effect. As fresh blood first enters the imaging volume of interest and experiences fewer RF-pulses than stationary tissues, blood signal is markedly higher than that of tissue, creating appreciable vessel-tissue contrast for various types of cancers including the pancreatic cancer. However, its ability of quantifying the pancreatic tumor and tumor infiltrating vessel motion has not been studied and compared with the current state of the art method 4D-CT.

To quantify this ability, the current study aims to exploit the technological potential of contrast free vessel highlighting in combination with the high resolution 4D-MRI method for a pancreatic patient cohort. The goal is to show the reproducibility and consistency of this novel 4D-MR method. Through the comparison with 4D-CT, we specifically evaluate the respiratory motion trajectories for both the tumor and the tumor infiltrating blood vessels that used to define potential boost volumes in the pancreas SIB treatment.

Methods and materials

Patients

Ten consecutive patients (seven males and three females, average age of 65) diagnosed with locally advanced, borderline resectable or locally recurrent PDA were recruited for the study under a protocol approved by the institutional review board. Gross tumor volumes range from 14 to 220 cc (mean $\pm \sigma = 86 \pm 56$ cc).

Imaging studies

The 4D-MRI sequence was described in details in previous publications [16]. In short, an in-house developed, RF and spoiled gradient recalled echo (GRE) sequence with Koosh-Ball (KB) 3D k-space radial-sampling trajectory, 1D self-gating and slab-selective (SS) excitation was implemented at 3 T (Biograph mMR, Siemens Healthineers. USA). Amplitude based sorting was applied in k-space before image reconstruction. This sequence is denoted as SS-4D-MRI. KB 4D-MRI with non-selective excitation was also performed and denoted as NS-4D-MRI. The shared imaging protocol for SS and NS were as follows: field of view (FOV) = (400 mm) [3];

prescribed spatial resolution =1.56 mm; flip angle = 12°; repetition time (TR)/echo time (TE) = 5.5/2.68 ms; readout bandwidth = 429 Hz/pixel; fat suppression with water excitation on; total scan time = 5 min. Patients were lying on the imaging couch in the head first supine position, with arms placed on the side for the comfort. No special immobilization was used.

During the patient's clinical CT simulation visit, a standard contrast enhanced FB-CT scan was first performed on a 16-slice scanner (Optima CT580; GE Healthcare, Milwaukee, WI), followed by a 4D-CT scan. Cine mode was used for the 4D-CT with the following parameters: 120 kV, variable mA, gantry rotation period of 1 s, and slice thickness of 2.5 mm. The cine duration was set to be the patient's breathing period plus 1.5 s. A total of 3000 images were set as the limit, which typically covers the region from above the diaphragm down to below the distal portion of the kidneys. 4D-CT images were then retrospectively binned using phase based sorting method in AdvantageSim™ 4D software (GE Healthcare, Milwaukee, WI). Variable time gaps ranging from 5 min to 30 min between the first contrast FB-CT scan and the following 4D-CT scan had to be used depending on the individual patient's compliance with the audio coaching of the respiration. Patients were immobilized in a vacuum lock bag and simulated in a head-first supine position with both arms raised above the head.

Image analysis

Pancreatic tumor and the involving blood vessels were delineated on the end-of-exhalation image bin by a single radiation oncologist. A B-spline based image registration was performed on both the 4D-MRI and 4D-CT using VelocityAI™ (Varian Medical System, Palo Alto, CA). Contours were mapped to the other bins. Motion trajectories for both the tumor and the tumor infiltrating blood vessels were extracted by the coordinates of the geometric centers from each respiration bin. The correlation coefficient (CC) was calculated from the tumor and the involved vessel motion trajectories for each patient.

Vessel-tissue contrast to noise ratio (CNR) is defined as $CNR = \frac{|S_V - S_P|}{\sigma_L}$ in which S_V is the average intensity of a selected region in the vessel, S_P is the average intensity of the adjacent region in the pancreas tumor and σ_L is the standard deviation of a relatively homogeneous region in the liver. Two CNRs, the aorta (CNR_{aorta}) and tumor infiltration blood vessel (CNR_{IV}), were calculated on both the 4D-MRI and 4D-CT.

Results

SS-4D-MRI was successfully implemented on 10 pancreatic cancer patients. All scans resulted consistent and satisfactory imaging quality.

Figure 1 shows an example patient's SS-4D-MRI in three cardinal planes (coronal, sagittal and axial). Excellent image quality and high isotropic image resolution (1.6 mm) are achieved in all planes. Fine image features such as blood vessels in the liver, stomach wall, diaphragm and bifurcation of the blood vessels from the great vessels are all visible in 4D-MRI images. Red circles show the tumor region and green arrows show the tumor infiltrating blood vessels. Excellent vessel contrast was also observed in all three planes.

Figure 2 shows an example patient's SS-4D-MRI in the coronal plane at end-of-inhalation (EOI), mid-ventilation and end-of-exhalation (EOE) bins (Fig. 2a-c), respectively. The patient's diaphragm motion is readily visible using a white dashed straight line as the reference. Motion trajectories extracted from the center of mass coordinates for both the tumor and involved vessel contours were plotted for the superior-interior (SI), anterior-posterior (AP) and medial-lateral (ML) directions (Fig. 2d-f). For this patient, tumor and involved vessel movements correlate well in the SI direction, but less well in the AP and ML directions, possibly due to the small motion amplitudes (< 1.6 mm, the image resolution) observed in these two directions.

Figure 3 shows the comparisons of SS-4D-MRI (a) to NS-4D-MRI (b) and 4D-CT (c) for an example patient. 4D-MRI with slab selective excitation clearly enhances the imaging signal and improved the vessel CNR, compared to NS-4D-MRI. SS-4D-MRI also results in visually improved vessel CNR compared to 4D-CT. Relative image intensity profiles (as shown in Fig. 3d, normalized to the starting of the profile for each imaging technique), also present the CNR enhancement in a quantitative manner. The white straight line on the CT (3c) shows the image region for the plotted profiles.

Table 1 summarizes basic clinical information, the vessel-tissue CNR and correlation coefficients calculated from motion trajectories of involved vessel and from tumor for the patient cohort. Quantitative analysis showed significantly improved CNR_{aorta} of 23.0 ± 18.3 (mean ± SD) on SS-4D-MRI from 2.1 ± 2.0 on 4D-CT with delayed contrast with a p value of 0.002. CNR_{IV} also significantly improved from 3.2 ± 2.7 on 4D-CT to 13.1 ± 8.4 on SS-4D-MRI with a p value of 0.001. The mean correlation coefficients (mean ± SD) calculated from tumor and vessel motion trajectories were 0.93 ± 0.10, 0.65 ± 0.31 and 0.77 ± 0.23 in the SI, AP and ML directions respectively. Correlation coefficients for the SI direction are greater than 0.9 for all patients except two (CC = 0.81 and 0.69), which might be a result of local anatomical deformation of the tumor in the vessel regions or small motion amplitudes for these two patients. For this patient cohort, tumor moves more than involved vessels, with SI motion range of 3.6 ± 1.5 mm

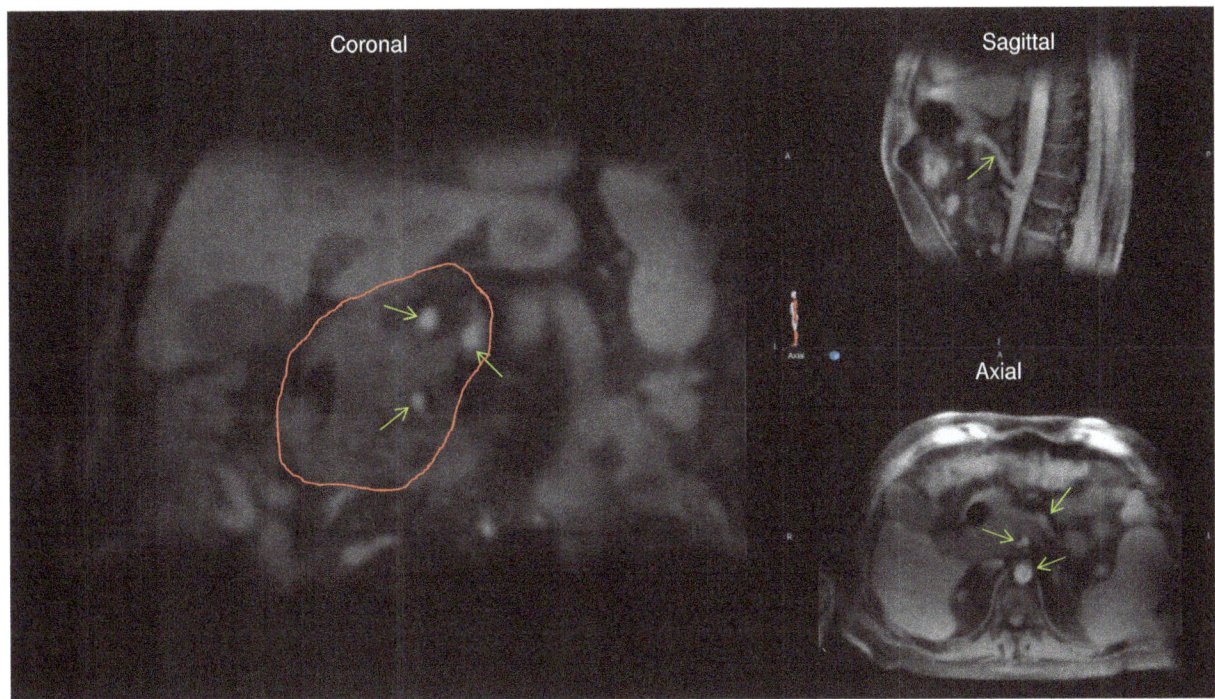

Fig. 1 Example 4D-MRI images in coronal, sagittal and axial planes showing the tumor (red circle) and infiltrated blood vessels (green arrows)

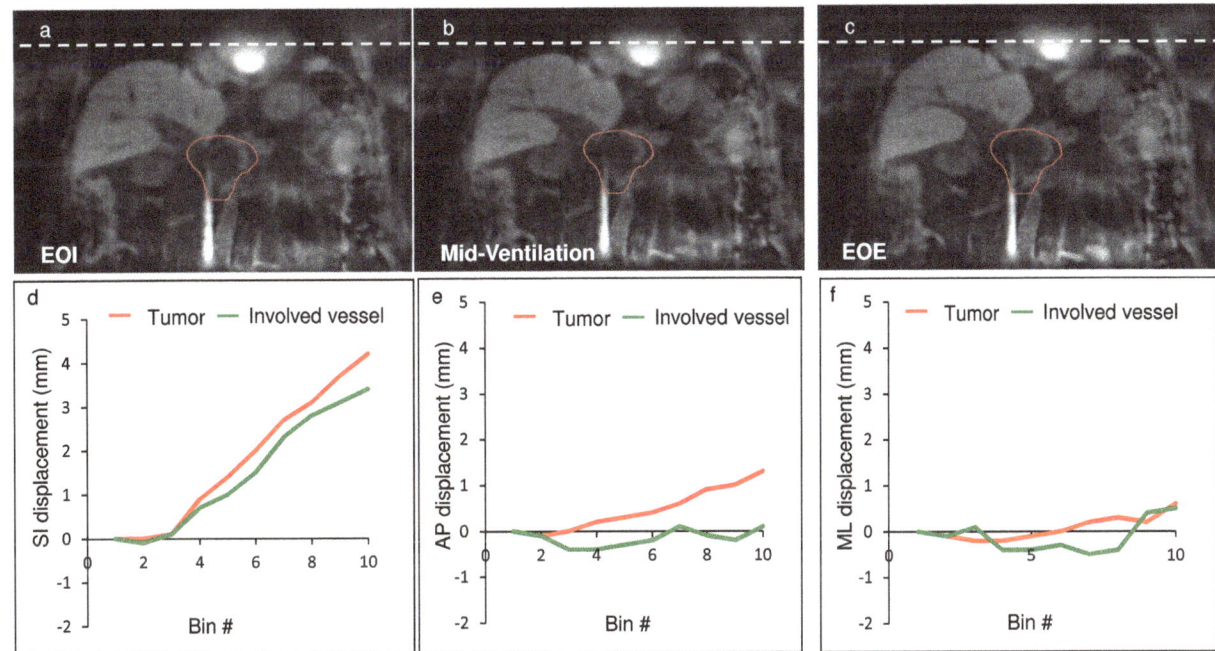

Fig. 2 Example 4D-MRI coronal images at (**a**). end-of-inhalation (EOI), (**b**). mid-ventilation, and (**c**). end-of-exhalation (EOE) bins; (**d-f**) show the motion trajectories derived from the tumor (red) and involved vessel (green) in the superior-inferior, anterior-posterior and medial-lateral directions

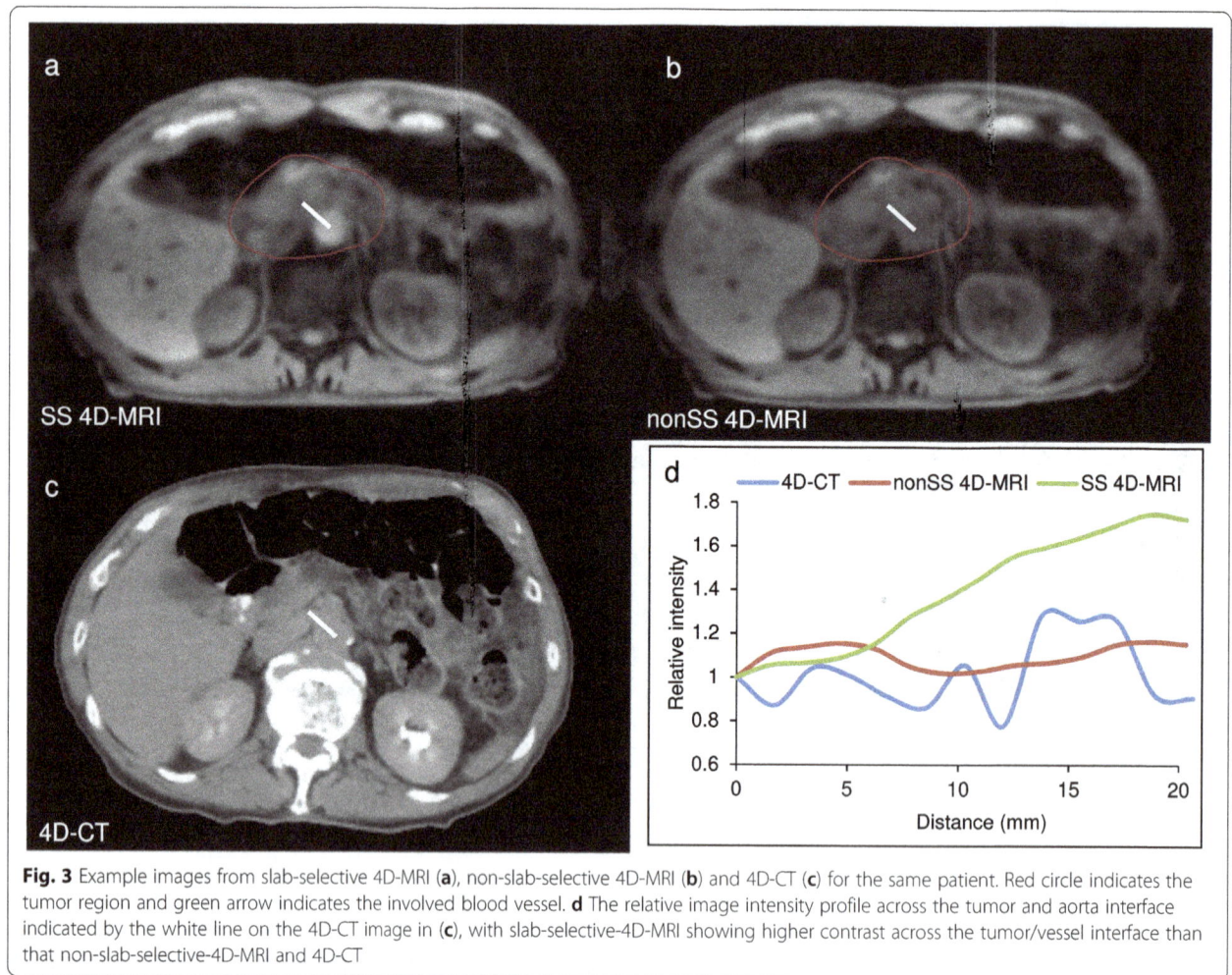

Fig. 3 Example images from slab-selective 4D-MRI (**a**), non-slab-selective 4D-MRI (**b**) and 4D-CT (**c**) for the same patient. Red circle indicates the tumor region and green arrow indicates the involved blood vessel. **d** The relative image intensity profile across the tumor and aorta interface indicated by the white line on the 4D-CT image in (**c**), with slab-selective-4D-MRI showing higher contrast across the tumor/vessel interface than that non-slab-selective-4D-MRI and 4D-CT

Table 1 Patient characteristics, motion range, comparison of contrast to noise ratio, and correlation coefficient of tumor and vessel motion trajectories

Patient ID	Gender	Age	GTV (cc)	GTV SI motion (mm)	IV SI motion (mm)	SS-4D-MRI / 4D-CT		ICC (PTV vs. involved vessels) on SS-4D-MRI		
						CNR aorta	CNR IV	SI	AP	ML
1	M	54	220	3.7	3.2	13.2 / 0.7	11.2 / 2.9	0.99	0.18	0.97
2	M	79	53	4.2	3.5	13.5 / 0.3	4.6 / 0.7	1.00	0.44	0.42
3	M	69	100	3.3	2.5	43.8 / 7.3	27.5 / 5.8	0.96	0.88	0.96
4	M	79	38	3.8	2.4	14.5 / 1.0	4.7 / 1.6	0.99	0.93	0.87
5	F	48	58	1.5	1.1	32.0 / 0.8	23.1 / 0.8	0.81	0.44	0.94
6	M	69	48	2.3	1.5	6.2 / 2.0	6.9 / 0.3	0.93	0.72	0.44
7	M	67	87	4.8	4.6	14.8 / 1.4	9.1 / 1.4	0.99	0.98	0.63
8	F	79	125	2.3	0.1	18.7 / 1.7	11.9 / 6.5	0.69	0.11	1.00
9	M	34	112	7.3	7.6	64.2 / 1.9	23.5 / 7.6	1.00	0.92	0.93
10	F	72	14	3.0	2.3	9.5 / 3.8	8.7 / 4.4	0.97	0.85	0.52
Average	n/a	65	86	3.6	2.9	23.0 / 2.1	13.1 / 3.2	0.93	0.65	0.77
Stdev	n/a	14.3	55.8	1.5	2.1	18.3 / 2.0	8.4 / 2.7	0.10	0.31	0.23
p	n/a	n/a	n/a	n/a	n/a	0.002*	0.001*	n/a	n/a	n/a

(mean ± SD) vs. 2.9 ± 2.1 mm for tumor and vessels respectively.

Discussion

Despite the poor prognosis, evidence suggests that pancreas tumor respond to sufficiently high radiation dose [21]. The dose is often excluded by sensitive nearby organs. As shown in Fig. 4, pancreas is surrounded by major blood vessels that supply nutrients and oxygen to the organs nearby. Tumors grown on the pancreas head and/or body usually wrap around these vessels such as superior mesenteric artery and superior mesenteric vein that prevent the surgical procedures. SBRT with SIB to the cancerous regions around the vessels can be designed to specifically sterilize the tumor non-invasively, although the complete control of the whole tumor is limited by the radiation dose tolerable by the normal critical organs nearby. Down-staging the patients after controlling the tumor around the vessels is the key to the success of the margin negative resection post radiation therapy. Therefore, radiation therapy with simultaneously integrated boost to the infiltrated blood vessels has attracted increasing interest for its potential to improve the resectability conversion rate and long-term disease free survival for the pancreas cancer patients who did receive subsequent margin negative resection. However, SIB of a moving target is challenging even with image guided radiation therapy (IGRT). Lack of image quality to differentiate soft tissue tumor and involved blood vessels in current clinical IGRT practice, which uses 4D-CT to evaluate pancreas tumor motion, calls for novel and advanced imaging strategies with high isotropic resolution, reduced imaging artifacts and improved soft tissue contrast. To our knowledge, this study is the first one that implements such a 4D-MRI sequence with the intent of characterizing not only the tumor motion, but also the motion of tumor infiltrating blood vessels. The key feature of this novel non-contrast 4D-MRI sequence is the fact that it can distinguish between motion of the vessels and the rest of the tumor. Another key feature is the ability to significantly improve the vessel conspicuity, which was extremely poor in non-vessel highlighting 4D-MRI or non-contrast 4D-CT images. The remarkable improvement in vessel contrast

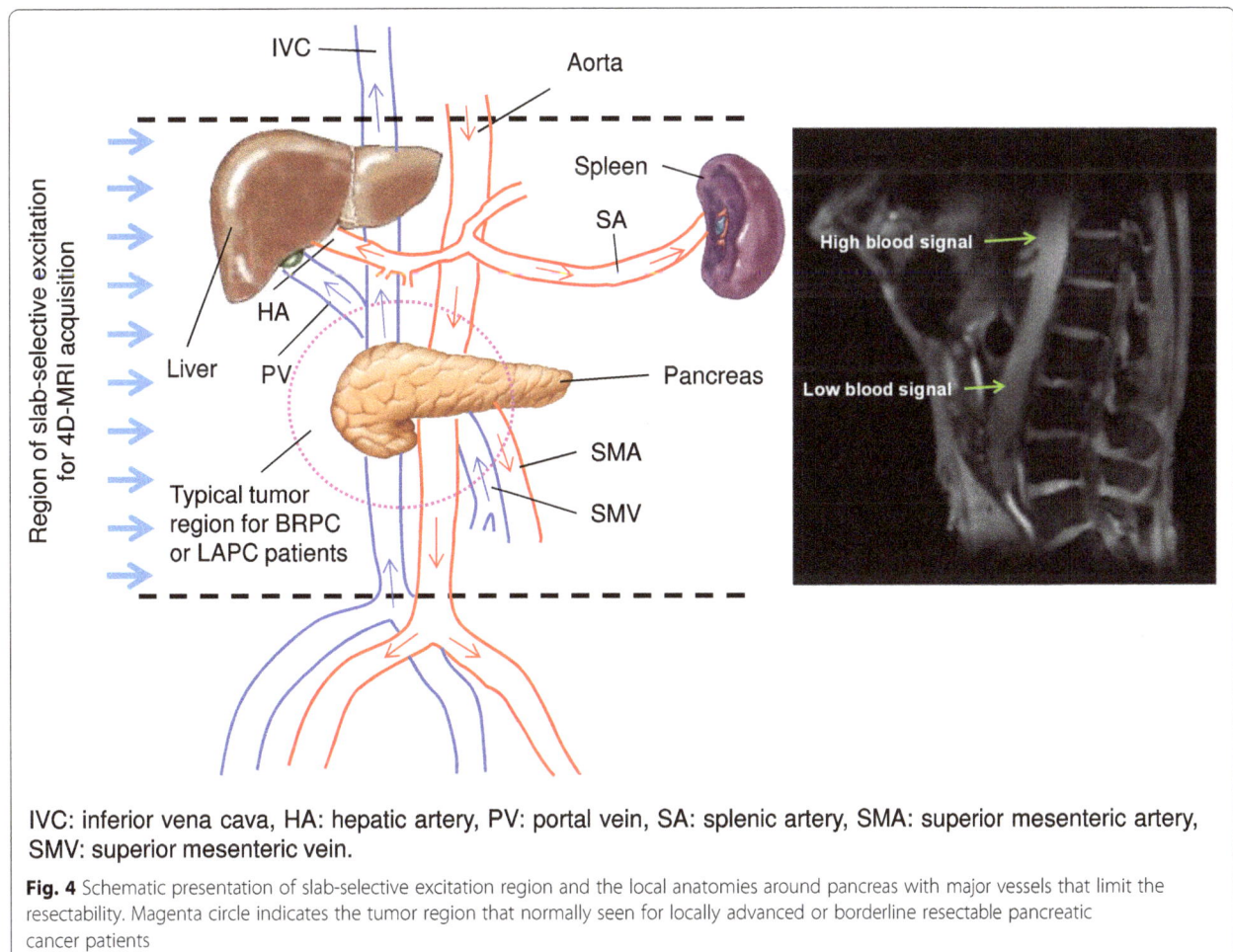

IVC: inferior vena cava, HA: hepatic artery, PV: portal vein, SA: splenic artery, SMA: superior mesenteric artery, SMV: superior mesenteric vein.

Fig. 4 Schematic presentation of slab-selective excitation region and the local anatomies around pancreas with major vessels that limit the resectability. Magenta circle indicates the tumor region that normally seen for locally advanced or borderline resectable pancreatic cancer patients

can help clinicians better identify and analyze the boost volume margin in the pancreas SBRT-SIB. The sequence uses slab-selective excitation during image acquisition with a 3D radial Koosh-Ball like sampling trajectory, which takes advantage of the fresh in-flow blood to enhance the blood signal. The vessel contrast enhancement only relies on the natural blood flow of the patients, so no additional contrast agent is needed. This feature makes frequent imaging possible for treatment strategies such as adaptive radiation therapy in which fast daily motion assessments prior to radiation dose delivery are preferred. Recent development in tumor response assessment using 4D imaging modalities potentially can also benefit from this novel 4D-MRI sequence with more frequent longitudinal 4D imaging data becoming available.

This study also contributes to the recent emergence of MRI-only simulation for radiotherapy treatment planning. Besides its superior soft-tissue contrast as compared to CT, other benefits of MRI including functional and dynamic imaging for tumor delineation and motion assessment without radiation dose are well acknowledged by the radiation therapy society. Both the tumor and involved Advancement in 4D-MRI sequence including our vessel highlighting 4D-MRI will facilitate the MR-only simulation being implemented in radiation therapy.

One drawback of this study is the imaging reconstruction speed. It takes around 8 h for our in-house developed program to reconstruct and post-process a KB 4D-MRI data set on a server equipped with 12-core Intel (Beaverton, OR) Xeon central processing unit and 96 GB of memory. The speed of image reconstruction and imaging processing needs to be significantly improved for wide clinical adaptation. There are several methods that can be implemented to speed up the image reconstruction. One example is to use fast iterative shrinkage-thresholding algorithm (FISTA), which preserves the computational simplicity of iterative shrinkage-thresholding algorithms but with a global rate of convergence which is proven to be significantly better theoretically and practically [22]. Working closely with the MRI vendors to implement the sequence will also help adapting the sequence with more practical reconstruction time in a real clinical setting.

Conclusion

A novel 4D-MRI sequence based on 3D-radial sampling and slab-selective excitation has been assessed on pancreas cancer patients. The non-contrast 4D-MRI images showed significantly better contrast to noise ratio for the vessels that limit tumor resectability compared to 4D-CT with delayed contrast. The sequence has great potential in accurately defining both the tumor and boost volume margins for pancreas SBRT-SIB.

Abbreviations
4D-CT: Four dimensional computed tomography; AP: Anterior-posterior; CNR: Contrast to noise ratio; EOE: End-of-exhalation; EOI: End-of-inhalation; FB-CT: Free breathing computed tomography; GRE: Gradient recalled echo; ML: Medial-lateral; MRI: Magnetic resonance imaging; NS: Non-selective; PDA: Pancreatic ductal adenocarcinoma; RT: Radiation therapy; SBRT: Stereotactic body radiation therapy; SI: Superior-inferior; SIB: Simultaneous integrated boost; SS: Slab-selective

Funding
This work is supported by NCI grant 1R03CA173273 and CTSI core voucher V095.

Authors' contributions
WY, ZF, ZD, JP, and XB carried out the study (MR imaging acquisition, image reconstruction and analysis), and prepared the manuscript. BF, HS and DL helped with manuscript preparation. RT recruited patients and helped with the manuscript preparation. All authors read and approved the final manuscript.

Competing interests
Xiaoming Bi and Jianing Pang are MR scientists at Siemens, the vendor of the MR scanner.

Author details
[1]Department of Radiation Oncology, Cedars Sinai Medical Center, 8700 Beverly Blvd., Los Angeles, CA 90048, USA. [2]Department of Biomedical Sciences, Biomedical Imaging Research Institute, Cedars Sinai Medical Center, Los Angeles, CA, USA. [3]Department of Bioengineering, University of California, Los Angeles, Los Angeles, CA, USA. [4]Siemens Healthineers, Los Angeles, USA.

References
1. Corbo V, Tortora G, Scarpa A. Molecular pathology of pancreatic cancer: from bench-to-bedside translation. Curr Drug Targets. 2012;13:744–52.
2. Mian OY, Ram AN, Tuli R, Herman JM. Management options in locally advanced pancreatic cancer. Curr Oncol Rep. 2014;16:388.
3. Katz MH, Fleming JB, Bhosale P, et al. Response of borderline resectable pancreatic cancer to neoadjuvant therapy is not reflected by radiographic indicators. Cancer. 2012;118:5749–56.
4. Springett GM, Hoffe SE. Borderline resectable pancreatic cancer: on the edge of survival. Cancer Control. 2008;15:295–307.
5. Chuong MD, Springett GM, Freilich JM, et al. Stereotactic body radiation therapy for locally advanced and borderline resectable pancreatic cancer is effective and well tolerated. Int J Radiat Oncol Biol Phys. 2013;86:516–22.
6. Passoni P, Reni M, Cattaneo GM, et al. Hypofractionated image-guided IMRT in advanced pancreatic Cancer with simultaneous integrated boost to infiltrated vessels concomitant with Capecitabine: a phase I study. Int J Radiat Oncol Biol Phys. 2013;87:1000–6.
7. Herman JM, Chang DT, Goodman KA, et al. A phase II multi-institutional study to evaluate gemcitabine and fractionated stereotactic body radiotherapy for unresectable, locally advanced pancreatic adenocarcinoma. ASCO Annual Meeting. Vol 30: ASC University; 2012:abstr 4045.
8. Pollom EL, Alagappan M, von Eyben R, et al. Single- versus multifraction stereotactic body radiation therapy for pancreatic adenocarcinoma: outcomes and toxicity. Int J Radiat Oncol Biol Phys. 2014;90:918–25.
9. Tai A, Liang Z, Erickson B, Li XA. Management of respiration-induced motion with 4-dimensional computed tomography (4DCT) for pancreas irradiation. Int J Radiat Oncol Biol Phys. 2013;86:908–13.
10. Ge J, Santanam L, Noel C, Parikh PJ. Planning 4-dimensional computed tomography (4DCT) cannot adequately represent daily intrafractional motion of abdominal tumors. Int J Radiat Oncol Biol Phys. 2013;85:999–1005.
11. Liu F, Erickson B, Peng C, Li XA. Characterization and management of interfractional anatomic changes for pancreatic cancer radiotherapy. Int J Radiat Oncol Biol Phys. 2012;83:e423–9.

12. McDonald JS, Leake CB, McDonald RJ, et al. Acute kidney injury after intravenous versus intra-arterial contrast material Administration in a Paired Cohort. Investig Radiol. 2016;51(12):804–9.

13. Pearce MS, Salotti JA, Little MP, et al. Radiation exposure from CT scans in childhood and subsequent risk of leukaemia and brain tumours: a retrospective cohort study. Lancet. 2012;380:499–505.

14. Castillo SJ, Castillo R, Castillo E, et al. Evaluation of 4D CT acquisition methods designed to reduce artifacts. J Appl Clin Med Phys. 2015;16:4949.

15. Yue Y, Fan Z, Yang W, et al. Geometric validation of self-gating k-space-sorted 4D-MRI vs 4D-CT using a respiratory motion phantom. Med Phys. 2015;42:5787–97.

16. Deng Z, Pang J, Yang W, et al. Four-dimensional MRI using three-dimensional radial sampling with respiratory self-gating to characterize temporal phase-resolved respiratory motion in the abdomen. Magn Reson Med. 2016;75:1574–85.

17. Yang W, Fan Z, Tuli R, et al. Four-dimensional magnetic resonance imaging with 3-dimensional radial sampling and self-gating-based K-space sorting: early clinical experience on pancreatic Cancer patients. Int J Radiat Oncol Biol Phys. 2015;93:1136–43.

18. Stemkens B, Tijssen RH, de Senneville BD, et al. Optimizing 4-dimensional magnetic resonance imaging data sampling for respiratory motion analysis of pancreatic tumors. Int J Radiat Oncol Biol Phys. 2015. https://doi.org/10.1016/j.ijrobp.2014.10.050.

19. Han F, Zhou Z, Cao M, Yang Y, Sheng K, Hu P. Respiratory motion-resolved, self-gated 4D-MRI using rotating cartesian k-space (ROCK). Med Phys. 2017;44:1359–68.

20. Deng Z, Yang W, Pang J, et al. Improved vessel-tissue contrast and image quality in 3D radial sampling-based 4D-MRI. J Appl Clin Med Phys. 2017. https://doi.org/10.1002/acm2.12194.

21. Nagakawa Y, Hosokawa Y, Nakayama H, et al. A phase II trial of neoadjuvant chemoradiotherapy with intensity-modulated radiotherapy combined with gemcitabine and S-1 for borderline-resectable pancreatic cancer with arterial involvement. Cancer Chemother Pharmacol. 2017. https://doi.org/10.1007/s00280-017-3288-7.

22. Beck A, Teboulle M. A fast iterative shrinkage-Thresholding algorithm for linear inverse problems. Siam J Imaging Sci. 2009;2:183–202.

10

Worth a local treatment? – Analysis of modern radiotherapy concepts for oligometastatic prostate cancer

M. Oertel[1*†] (ORCID), S. Scobioala[1†], K. Kroeger[1], A. Baehr[1], L. Stegger[2], U. Haverkamp[1], M. Schäfers[2] and H.-T. Eich[1]

Abstract

Background: Prostate cancer (PCA) is the most-prevalent non-skin cancer in men worldwide. Nevertheless, the treatment of oligometastatic, especially lymph-node (ln) recurrent, PCA remains elusive. The aim of our study was to provide insights in radiotherapy (RT)-treatment of recurrent PCA exhibiting ln- or osseous (oss)-oligometastases.

Methods: Between April 2012 and April 2017, 27 oligometastatic PCA patients (19 ln and 8 single oss) were treated with RT at our institution.

Results: The metastasis-free survival (MFS) was 24.8 m (22.0–36.0 m) and 25.4 m (23.9–28.1 m) for the ln- and oss-subgroup resulting in 1-year MFS of 75.4 and 100% and 2-year MFS of 58.7 and 83.3% for ln- and oss-metastatic patients, respectively. Of notice, none of the recurrences for ln-patients was in the RT-field, constituting a local control of 100%.
Within the ln-group, pre-RT median-PSA was 2.6 ng/ml, median post-RT PSA was 0.3 ng/ml, which was significant ($p = 0.003$). Median biochemical-free survival (bfS) was 12.2 m. PCA that was initially confined to the prostate had a better bfS ($p < 0.001$) and MFS ($p = 0.013$). The oss-group had a median PSA of 4.9 ng/ml pre-treatment which dropped to a median value of 0.14 ng/ml ($p = 0.004$).
Toxicities were moderate, with only 1 case of III° toxicity. There were no deaths in the ln-group, thus overall survial was 100% here.

Conclusion: Our study points out the feasibility of RT as a treatment option in recurrent PCA and demonstrates an excellent local control with a low-toxicity profile.

Keywords: Prostate cancer, Lymph-node recurrence, IMRT, Salvage therapy

Background

Prostate cancer (PCA) is the most prevalent non-skin cancer worldwide in men with over 63,000 newly diagnosed men each year in Germany and around 13,000 dying from it annually [1, 2]. It is biologically heterogenous with aggressive subtypes being contrasted by slow growing carcinoma with a long latency to diagnosis [3]. Histological carcinomas are found in autopsy-series from the 4th decade of life, whereas the diagnosis is at 71 of age (median) [2, 4]. In vivo diagnosis is achieved via digital-rectal exam (DRE), measurement of the prostate-specific antigen (PSA), transrectal ultrasound and systematic biopsy [5, 6] although even a combined approach with PSA-value and DRE may fail in detecting the disease [7]. After primary therapy (radical prostatectomy, radiotherapy (RT) as teletherapy or brachytherapy) PSA is recommended as a follow-up parameter [5, 6].

In case of recurrent PCA, functional imaging like PET-CT, has shown its value in identification or exclusion of localized tumor manifestations and may give guidance for directing RT and surgical therapy [5, 6, 8–14]. Also MRI may offer the possibility of precise and accurate cancer detection and target volume delineation in the PSA-relapse or metastatic situation [15].

---
* Correspondence: Michael.oertel@ukmuenster.de
†Michael Oertel and S. Scobiouted equally to this work.
[1]Department of Radiation Oncology, Albert-Schweitzer Campus 1 A1, 48149 Muenster, Germany
Full list of author information is available at the end of the article

National and international guidelines struggle to standardize treatment strategies in case of lymph-node (ln) metastasis after primary therapy [5, 6] focusing on systemic androgen-deprivation-therapy (ADT), although this treatment is known to be associated with considerable side effects such as diabetes, cardiovascular morbidity, decrease in bone density with danger of fracture, sexual dysfunctions and onset of depression [16, 17].

Anyhow, RT has shown promising results and may efficiently prolong the time till the initiation of ADT [8–11, 13, 18–25]. These studies included only limited patient numbers and were partly conducted retrospectively, calling for further investigation. In a more broad definition, these patients reveal an "oligometastatic state", a term coined by Hellmann and Weichselbaum defining a disease state in which a low number of metastases with limited malignant potential exist, putatively without microscopic ubiquitous dissemination, forming an intermediate state between localized and generalized form of disease [26]. This concept implies a limitation of metastatic spread to one or a only some organs due to an impaired/undeveloped ability for further progression and highlights a continuum of biologic behavior in the development of cancer [26]. In the setting of oligometastases, local therapy (RT, operation) may be of use [23, 24, 27].

In the present study, we have analyzed the use of RT as an individual treatment approach for men with ln recurrent PCA. As a control group, we established a subcollective of single osseous metastasis (oss), thus also being oligometastatic. We demonstrate use and feasibility of image-guided RT with modern RT techniques and could present an effective treatment with high local control and tolerable toxicity.

Methods

Patients

Between April 2012 and April 2017, 19 patients with ln recurrent PCA were treated with RT at our institution. Median age at initial diagnosis was 60.6 years (y) (48.1–79.1 y) and 66.5 y (57.7–78.3 y) for ln- and oss-group, respectively. Further tumor characteristics are provided in Table 1. Primary therapy consisted of radical prostatectomy followed by post-operative or salvage RT in all but 1 case.

At a median time of 5.4 y (0.5–15.6 y) or 6.7 y (2.2–16.6 y) after primary therapy, at a median age of 67.9 y (49.9–83.3 y) or 74.4 y (64.8–82 y) for ln- or oss-metastatic patients respectively, metastatic spread was diagnosed. The ln recurrence occurred in regionary (8), distant (5) or both ln-stations (6) (Table 2). Regionary lymph nodes were defined as pelvic ln below lumbal vertebra 5, marking the field border of a potential whole pelvic RT. We further simplified categories to distinguish between patients with regionary and distant (also involving combined occurrence of regionary ln) ln-regions. In the majority of patients 1–2

Table 1 Initial characteristics of the study patients. A: ln-metastatic patients; B: osseous metastases

A)			B)		
Age at inital diagnosis	median	60.6	Age at inital diagnosis	median	66.5
	maximum	79.1		maximum	78.3
	minimum	48.1		minimum	57.7
T	T2b	1	T	T2c	2
	T2c	5		T3a	1
	T3a	9		T3b	5
	T3b	4	N	N0	5
N	N0	16		N1	2
	N1	3		missing	1
M	M0	13	M	M0	4
	MX	1		missing	4
	missing	5	Gleason	7	3
Gleason	6	1		8	2
	7	10		9	3
	9	6	R-status	R0	2
	10	1		R1	3
	missing	1		missing	3
R-Status	R0	11			
	R1	6			
	missing	2			

ln were involved. In the case of ≥3 metastases, a localized distribution was essential to define a RT volume, a disseminated metastatic situation being an exclusion criterion of our study. Diagnosis was achieved with functional imaging in 17/19 patients (17 PET-CT (2 C^{11}-Choline; 15 Ga^{68}-prostate-specific membrane antigen (PSMA)) and morphological via CT/MRI in 2 cases.

All patients were reviewed interdisciplinary and were counseled about RT as an individual treatment approach in their oncological situation. Informed consent was given.

Twenty patients received an ADT during treatment (13 in the ln-group, 7 in the oss-group).

Radiotherapy

Overall, 37 RT-series were conducted in the 29 ln-group and 8 in the oss-subgroup patients with the anatomic regions shown in Table 1. Concentrating on the ln-group, a salvage RT of the prostate bed was part of the treatment in two cases, 4 series were extended to adjacent ln stations and 3 series consisted of an extended ln RT with a sequential boost. The other series were localized treatments of involved ln. For RT-planning, the gross tumor volume (GTV) was delineated via image fusion with functional imaging and a margin of 2 mm- 25 mm was applied to receive the planning target volume (PTV). The PTV was covered by the 100% isodose and dose prescriptions were

Table 2 Characteristic of diagnosis for the ln-recurrences (A) and single-osseous (B) metastases

A)

Age at ln diagnosis	
median	67.9
maximum	49.9
minimum	83.3
region	
regionary	8
distant	5
regionary and distant	6
number of ln	
1	8
2	2
≥3	9
imaging	
PET-CT (Ga^{68}-PSMA)	15
PET-CT (C^{11}-Cholin)	2
CT/MRT	2

B)

Age at metastases diagnosis	
median	74.4
maximum	82.0
minimum	64.8
imaging	
PET-CT (Ga^{68}-PSMA)	4
PET-CT (C^{11}-Cholin)	1
SPECT (Tc^{99m})	1
CT/MRT	1
CT	1

according to ICRU 83 [28]. Median PTV size was 29.3 ml (Maximum 674.7 ml, Minimum 3.7 ml). In the oss-group PTV size differed between 56.2 ml and 351.9 ml (median: 72.6 ml) and was located in the pelvis (4 patients), thoracic vertebrae (2), scapula (1) or humerus (1).

RT was delivered as intensity-modulated and image-guided RT with a TrueBeam linear accelerator (Varian Medical Systems, Palo Alto, USA) or in helical VMAT with a tomotherapy (Tomotherapy Hi-Art II, Accuray, Sunnyvale, USA) with the usual immobilisation equipment (see Fig. 1 for an example).

In the ln-group, doses varied between 35 and 66 Gy in daily fractions of 1.8 Gy (with one exception of 7 Gy daily fraction). In 6 cases, subsequent boosts up to 70.2 Gy were applied. Median dose was 63 Gy (30.6–70.2 Gy). Comparably, doses in the oss-group were 30–66.6 Gy (median: 54 Gy) in daily normofractionated regimes of 1.8–2 Gy.

Follow-up

Patients were seen on regular basis at their treating urologist and in the radiation oncology department with regular PSA-measurements and clinical examinations. Last follow-up was at the end of February 2018. Toxicities were graded according to the Common Terminology Criteria for Adverse Events – Score [29].

We evaluated PSA-behavior after therapy and registered a nadir, if existent, and biochemical-free survival (bfS), defined as the period of time without PSA-elevation. In addition, we evaluated metastasis-free survival (MFS) which is defined as the time after treatment without evidence of disease recurrence (on morphological/functional imaging). Overall survival (OS) was also analyzed.

Statistics

All statistics were done with SPSS version 22 (IBM, Armok, USA). PSA-values were compared with a 1-sided Mann-Whitney-U test as a decrease in PSA was expected. OS, MFS and bfS were examined with a Kaplan-Meier-analysis, factors were compared using a log-rank-test. Correlation between RT-dose and bfS or MFS respectively were examined, using a two-sided Pearson correlation coefficient.

Results

Follow-up data was available for all of the aforementioned ln-patients and mean MFS was 24.8 m (22.0–36.0 m) with a 1-year MFS of 75.4% and a 2-year MFS of 58.7% (Fig. 2a). The initial T-status (initial T2 vs. T3 carcinoma 29.3 m vs. 13.6 m; $p = 0.013$) showed an association with MFS. Neither Gleason-Score (gleason-score: 6,7 vs. higher: $p = 0.693$), number of involved ln (1–2 vs. > 2 ln; $p = 0.544$), ln-region (regionary vs. distant $p = 0.2$), initial N-status (N0 vs. N1 $p = 0.827$) or the application of concomitant ADT ($p = 0.363$) had a significant impact on MFS. There was a trend towards longer survival for R0-resected patients ($p = 0.332$) which did not reach significance. RT dose showed no linear correlation with MFS (coefficient: – 0.005; significance: 0.981).

Further analysis revealed, that morphological recurrence occurred after a mean time of 13.9 m (1.7–35.1 m). Of notice, none of these recurrences were in the RT-field, with two recurrences being adjacent to past treatment (field border), constituting a local control of 100%. There was one distant metastasis in thoracic vertebra 8, one in the 9th costa and 6 cases of additional ln-metastases, which were addressed by local RT in some cases. Four patients suffered another local recurrence after a median time of 10.7 m (3.9–41 m) with ln-metastases in 3 cases and 1 case of ln- and oss metastases.

PSA-values were available for 17 of the 19 patients, enabling an examination of PSA-dynamics. Pre-RT median-PSA was 2.6 ng/ml (range: 0.35 ng/ml - 41.9 ng/ml), median

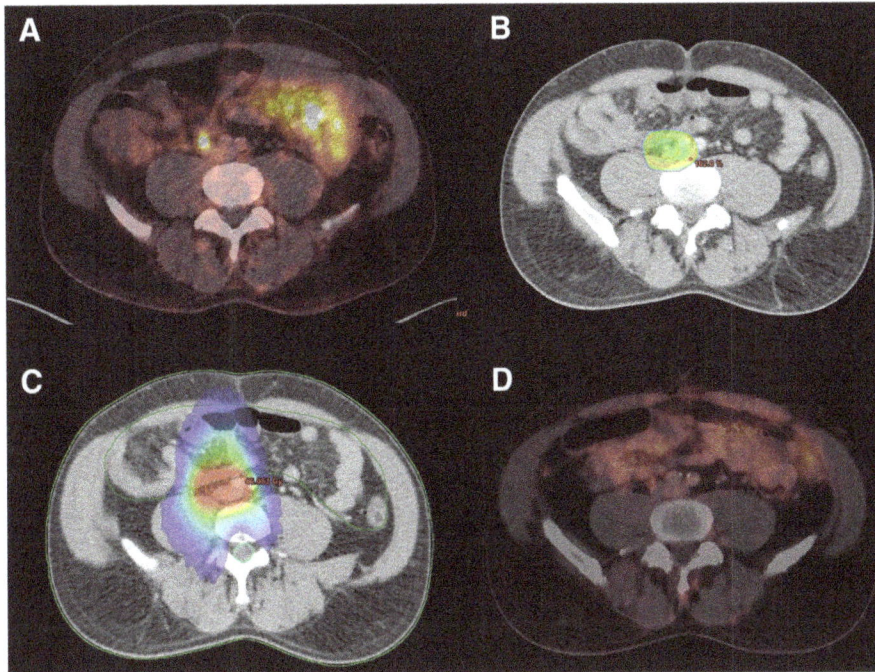

Fig. 1 Example for ln-RT. **a** ^{68}Ga-PSMA-PET-CT positive left iliacal lymph node was treated by radiation therapy up to 45 Gy and subsequent boost to 63 Gy. **b** 95%-isodose in colour-wash covering the PTV. **c** Excellent organs-at-risk sparing radiotherapy via helical tomotherapy (15 Gy isodose shown blue in colour wash). **d** No relevant tracer uptake 6 months after radiotherapy

post-RT PSA was 0.3 ng/ml (0.01–6.26 ng/ml), which was significant ($p = 0.003$). 2/17 Patients (11.8%) showed an increase in PSA, resulting in a response rate of 88.2% (see Fig. 3). Median bfS was 12.2 m (6.2–18.2 m) with a 1-year bfS of 52.4% and 2-year bfS of 22.4% (Fig. 2b). PCA which was initially confined to the prostate had a better bfS (median T2: 16.9 m, T3: 5.3 m), which was significant ($p > 0.001$; Fig. 2c). Neither the number of ln (1–2 vs. > 2; $p = 0.955$), nor the application of ADT ($p = 0.954$) had a significant impact. Pelvic ln-metastases showed a trend towards better bfS (16.9 m vs. 8.8 m), which did not reach significance ($p = 0.082$). Again, R0-resected patients tended to have a longer bfS without significance ($p = 0.054$). No significant dose-response-correlation was demonstrated between RT-dose and bfS (coefficient: – 0.074; significance: 0.385).

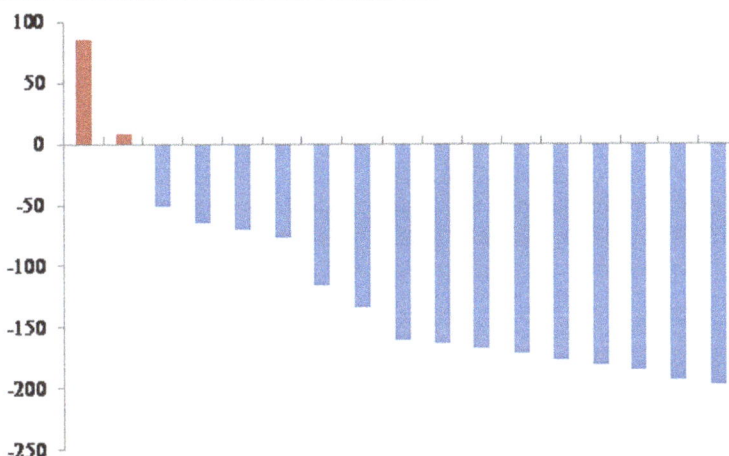

Fig. 2 Waterfall-plot showing PSA-response to ln-RT. Each bar depicts an individual patient, the blue ones being decreases, while the two red ones indicate increase in PSA. Overall, response to therapy was > 88%

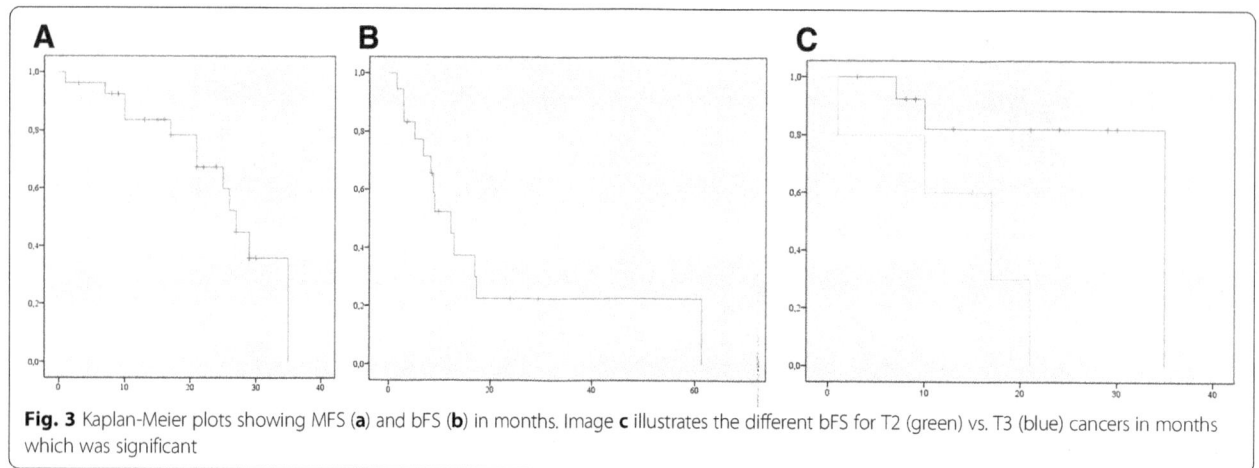

Fig. 3 Kaplan-Meier plots showing MFS (**a**) and bFS (**b**) in months. Image **c** illustrates the different bFS for T2 (green) vs. T3 (blue) cancers in months which was significant

No patient died within the ln-group, thus overall survial (OS) was 100% with a median OS of 21.2 m (3.7–67.7 m). One patient developed secondary rectal cancer 26 m after ln-irradiation. With 3 deaths in the oss-group, mortality was higher with a median survival of 28.1 m (16.7–46.5 m).

In the oss-subgroup, all patients received ADT (1 unknown) so its impact could not be evaluated. MFS was 26 m (23.9–28.1 m) with a 1-year MFS of 100% and 2-year MFS of 83.3%. Neither T-stage (T2 vs. T3; $p = 0.736$), gleason score (6 or 7 vs. higher $p = 0.732$), tumor-free resection margin (R0 vs. R1 $p = 0.221$) had a significant impact on MFS. For PSA-follow up values were available for 6/8 patients with a median bfS of 15 m (1-year bfS 66.7%, 2-year bfS 16.7%) which was not influenced significantly by T-stage (T2 vs. T3; $p = 0.951$), gleason score (6 or 7 vs. higher $p = 0.207$), initial nodal status (N0 vs. N1 $p = 0.277$) or tumor-free resection margin (R0 vs. R1 $p = 0.157$).

There was no dose-response correlation for MFS and bfS (MFS: coefficient: − 0.234; significance: 0.288; bfS: coefficient: − 0.471; significance: 0.173). In this subcollective, 3 patients died, the mean overall survival (OS) being 38.8 m (28.8–48.9 m). Four patients revealed recurrences after a median time of 26.2 m (21.6–27.6 m) which included skeletal structures again in 4 cases with additional ln-metastasis in 1 case.

Follow-up PSA-values were available for 6 patients and revealed a median PSA-value of 4.9 ng/ml pre-treatment (range: 0.34 ng/ml – 24.8 ng/ml) which dropped to a median value of 0.14 ng/ml (0.01 ng/ml-0.68 ng/ml; $p = 0.004$). Responses were observed in 5/6 patients, thus constituting a response rate of 83.3%.

Comparing MFS and bfS between the two subcollectives, we could not find a significant difference (MFS: 26 m vs. 29 m $p = 0.883$; bfS: 15 vs. 12.2 m; $p = 0.748$).

Toxicities

Acute toxicities were fatigue, diarrhea and increased urinary frequency. Overall, toxicities in the ln-group were tolerable

with one III° toxicity of urinary incontinence, 7 II° toxicites (3 urinary incontinence, 1 urethral stricture, 1 flatulence, 1 urinary spasmus, 1 fatigue) and 7 I° toxicities (3 increased urinary frequency/nycturia, 1 diarrhea, 2 fatigue, 1 rectal bleeding). In the oss-group, toxicities were mild, as no III° toxicities or higher occurred (1 erythema I°, 1 erythema II°, 1 nausea I°, 1 fatigue, 2 increased urinary frequency/nycturia).

Discussion

The presented study demonstrates the application of RT for oligometastatic (ln-reccurent and single oss) PCA, highlights its significant impact on PSA and identified the initial T-stadium as a significant predictor for bfS and MFS in the ln-subgroup.

To our knowledge, this was the first report of initial T-stadium as a predictor for biochemical aggressivity and treatment outcome in this clinical setting. The bfS is reduced to 5.3 m for locally advanced PCA. These PCA bear a worse prognosis à priori, although some studies showed 10-year disease-free survival of > 90% after surgical interventions [5, 6]. They also have an increased risk of ln-reccurence [30]. A possible explanation for this finding may be the distinctive and more aggressive tumor biology of advanced PCA which may be indicated by marker profile, as e.g. some isoforms of insulin-growth factor, a central signaling molecule for cellular processes, show an overexpression more frequently in advanced stages of PCA [31, 32].

Comparing different studies on RT for ln-recurrent PCA, RT-doses and -field definitions are very heterogenous. Doses may reach 74 Gy with daily fractions of up to 12 Gy [8, 9, 11, 19, 21, 23]. Hypofractionated regimes may have the potential to enhance local control [11, 19], but might not be suitable for every patient. Anyhow, RT confers a high local control of > 90% in most studies with in-field recurrences being rare events [8, 11, 21, 23]. Consistently, our study collective did not reveal in-field recurrences further encouraging the use of RT. A cut-off dosage value has been defined by Schlick et at., recommending a RT > 64 Gy for improved biochemical control [13]. Our study did not prove a significant dose-response correlation, although the biology of PCA suggests the use of high-dose regimes.

We demonstrated a 1-year MFS of 75.4% and a 2-year MFS of 58.7% while other RT-studies revealed a disease-free or clinical failure-free survival ranging from 50% after 2 y up to 61.8% after 3 y or 63.5% after 30 m respectively [8–10, 13].

Due to its retrospective nature, our patient collective includes various RT field definitions ranging from limited stereotactic setups to ln-chains with the inclusion of the former prostate bed in 2 cases, which also reflects the various concepts described by other authors [8–11, 13, 20]. Of importance, even an extended whole-pelvic RT does not exclude further metastatic spread [8] while the idea of limited toxicity with a small field delineation is not necessarily corroborated by the literature [10, 11, 13]. Thus, the field and dose decisions demand further investigation.

Local RT directed towards ln metastases also influence PSA significantly, a known effect [8–11, 13]. The use of ADT in the literature as well as in the majority of our study patients prompts the evaluation of PSA-dynamics rather than absolute values. Overall, PSA-response rate to treatment was 88.2%, which is comparable to previous studies (81–91.4%) [9, 11, 20]. Anyhow, some studies point out a possible "delay" of ADT up to 44 m till the beginning of ADT by treating oligometastases with RT [21, 25].

During and after treatment, we could demonstrate an excellent toxicity profile with expected side effects for pelvic irradiation withour any III° or higher toxicites. Of notice, the patients in our collective were extensively pretreated and were in a (re-)salvage situation.

The location of ln-metastases may have a prognostic impact as suggested by the study of Fodor et al. who identified extrapelvic ln metastases as a significant factor for worse OS [9]. As no patient died in our study, we could not examine this parameter, but MFS may be a suitable surrogate. Although not being significant, there was a trend towards better MFS and bfS for regionary metastases. This finding may encourage the use of local therapies like pelvic radiation or ln-dissection for PCA confined to pelvis as they may enable a long disease-free survival. In contrast, distant-ln metastases warrant an intensified, systemic therapy. Interestingly, a tumor positive resection margin may herald a worse MFS, which may be explained by the lack of local control in the pelvis.

A deterioration in prognosis is found with increasing number of metastases, the cutoff number being controversial (1–3) [33–36]. In our study collective, the number of ln was not a significant predictor for MFS or bfS in comparison between 1 and 2 or > 2 ln. Nevertheless, our patients

had a maximum of 5 ln-metastases (thus making them suitable candidates for RT) and true polymetastatic patients were not included. Importantly, the analysis by Schweitzer et al. was not limited to ln-metastases and Briganti et al. focused on patients with ln-metastases in the primary therapy [33, 36], which contrasts the initially predominant N0-patients in our study. These studies underline a superiority in prognosis for mono- or oligometastatic disease.

The lack of a significant impact of R-status and ln-number on bfS may be caused by the small study collective as both parameters showed a trend towards better bfS in the more limited categories. This may reflect the increased risk of local and biochemical failure for positive resection margins in the primary therapy [37, 38].

It has to be emphasized, that diagnosis relies essentially on functional imaging. With the advent of Gallium as a PMSA PET-Tracer, sensitivity especially at low PSA-levels has increased remarkably [39]. Most studies in the literature were conducted with a choline-tracer [9, 11, 12, 20, 35] which demonstrates inferiority in PCA detection, especially at a PSA < 2 ng/ml [39]. The meta-analysis by von Eyben et al. revealed a detection rate of 50% for recurrent PCA in men with a PSA as low as 0.2 ng/ml [22], thus enabling an image-guided therapy as in our study. A recent study on ^{68}Ga-PSMA PET-scans used in patients with biochemical-relapse after radical prostatectomy demonstrated that metastases were confined to the prostate bed in only 30.3% independent of PSA-value, whereas a PSA > 1 ng/ml was significantly associated with extrapelvic recurrence [40]. Despite increasing sensitivity, false-negative patients who do not undergo a "targeted" local approach via surgery or RT but only receive ADT have to be considered. In case of serious doubts, repetitive imaging in the short-term follow-up may be suitable.

RT has an established role in the treatment of oss-metastases [5, 6] but may experience a renaissance in the context of oligometastases with putative curative intent, an indication not covered by national and international guidelines so far [23, 27]. We decided to include only patients with solitary bony metastases as increasing number of metastases may herald a worse survival [41]. In a study with 15 patients (20 lesions) using hypofractionated concepts (5 fractions 5–7 Gy with additional simultaneous boost in some cases) progression-free survival was 7.4 m with a high local control (only 1 failure) and a slight increase in the time till ADT onset/intensification of systemic therapy [18]. PSA-progression-free survival was 6.9 m but only 3 patients in this study received ADT [18], hampering a direct comparison with our data.

The hereby presented study is the first to demonstrate the equality of MFS and bFS for ln- and oss-category. In a comparative study including ln- as well as oss-oligometastases, Schick et al. found a 3-year bfS of

54.5% and an OS of 91.7% taking both categories alltogether [13]. In accordance with that, a Belgian study group investigated the subject with no direct oss- and ln- comparison [23]. Interestingly, it could be demonstrated that relapses of ln-metastases are found mainly in ln, while oss-metastatic patients relapse predominantly in the bone [23], a finding also corroborated in the hereby presented study. The same research group conducted a prospective phase II-trial in which metastases-directed therapy (mostly RT) showed a clear advantage in bFS further postponing ADT-onset in comparison to the observation group while maintaining an excellent toxicity profile without II°-toxicities [24].

Our study bears several shortcomings as patient number and follow-up are yet limited. Furthermore, it is retrospective and monocentric, but already points out important aspects for the use of RT in this clinical setting.

Further studies are warranted: As ADT was utilized in most cases of our study, its precise impact may not be evaluated and it remains state-of-the art treatment for ln-recurrent PCA. Notwithstanding this fact, RT and ADT are not to be seen as mere competitors but may have synergistic effects encouraging a combined use, with ADT controlling PCA systemically and RT conferring a high local control, a possibility pointed out by the literature [13] and our study. Another combined modality treatment is the combination of a ln-dissection and RT for ln-recurrences further enhancing local control and relapse free-survival [42]. Ongoing studies (www.clinicaltrials.gov, search on: 6th august 2017: NCT01859221, NCT02274779, NCT02563691, NCT02680587, NCT02685397, NCT0275 9783, NCT02816983) investigate the role of RT in an oligometastatic setting. The prospective phase II trial NCT022 74779 (OLIGOPELVIS – GETUG P07) evaluates the use of RT for 1–5 pelvic nodal metastases in combination with an ADT concerning bfS and relapse-free survival [43]. Patient enrollment has ended and final results are expected in autumn/winter 2018 [43]. New insights into the biology of PCA and its possible and necessary treatment options are expected.

Conclusions

Our study points out the feasibility of RT as a treatment option in ln recurrent PCA. It has demonstrated an excellent local control with a low-toxicity profile and may complement androgen-deprivation therapy as a local treatment option.

Abbreviations
ADT: Androgen-deprivation-therapy; bfS: Biochemical-free survival; DRE: Digital-rectal exam; GTV: Gross tumor volume; Ln: Lymph node; m: Month; MFS: Metastasis-free survival; OS: Overall survival; oss: Single-osseous; PCA: Prostate cancer; PSA: Prostate-specific antigen; PSMA: Prostate-specific membrane antigen; PTV: Planning target volume; RT: Radiotherapy; VMAT: Volumetric arc therapy; y: year

Authors' contributions
All authors participated in the patient treatment and were involved in the preparation of the manuscript. All authors reviewed and approved the final manuscript.

Competing interests
The authors declare that they have no competing interests.

Author details
[1]Department of Radiation Oncology, Albert-Schweitzer Campus 1 A1, 48149 Muenster, Germany. [2]Department of Nuclear Medicine, Albert-Schweitzer Campus 1 A1, 48149 Muenster, Germany.

References
1. Haas GP, Delongchamps N, Brawley OW, et al. The worldwide epidemiology of prostate cancer: perspectives from autopsy studies. Can J Urol. 2008;15: 3866–71.
2. Koch-Institut R (2015) Krebs in Deutschland 2011/2012. Gesundheitsberichterstattung des Bundes. 10 Ausg. 2015. RKI-Bib1 (Robert Koch-Institut).
3. Sheldon CA, Williams RD, Fraley EE. Incidental carcinoma of the prostate: a review of the literature and critical reappraisal of classification. J Urol. 1980; 124:626–31.
4. Sakr WA, Haas GP, Cassin BF, et al. The frequency of carcinoma and intraepithelial neoplasia of the prostate in young male patients. J Urol. 1993;150:379–85.
5. Leitlinienprogramm Onkologie (Deutsche Krebsgesellschaft, Deutsche Krebshilfe, AWMF). Konsultationsfassung: Interdisziplinäre Leitlinie der Qualität S3 zur Früherken-nung, Diagnose und Therapie der verschiedenen Stadien des Prostatakarzinoms, Lang-version 4.0, 2016 AWMF Registernummer: 043/022OL. http://leitlinienprogramm-onkologie.de/ Prostatakarzinom.58.0.html. Accessed 6 Aug 2017.
6. Mottet N, Bellmunt J, Briers E, Bolla M, Bourke L, Cornford P, De Santis M, Henry AM, Joniau S, Lam TB, Mason MD, van der Poel HG, van der Kwast TH, Rouvière O, Wiegel T, Guidelines Associates: Arfi N, van den Bergh RCN, van den Broeck T, Cumberbatch M, Fossati N, Gross T, Lardas M, Liew M, Moldovan P, Schoots IG, Willemse PM. EAU-ESTRO-ESUR-SIOG Guidelines on Prostate Cancer (Version March 2017). https://uroweb.org/wp-content/ uploads/09-Prostate-Cancer_2017_web.pdf. Accessed 6 Aug 2017.
7. Thompson IM, Pauler DK, Goodman PJ, et al. Prevalence of prostate cancer among men with a prostate-specific antigen level ≤4.0 ng per milliliter. N Engl J Med. 2004;350:2239–46. https://doi.org/10.1056/NEJMoa031918.
8. Casamassima F, Masi L, Menichelli C, et al. Efficacy of eradicative radiotherapy for limited nodal metastases detected with choline PET scan in prostate cancer patients. Tumori. 2011;97:49–55.
9. Fodor A, Berardi G, Fiorino C, et al. Toxicity and efficacy of salvage carbon 11-choline positron emission tomography/computed tomography-guided radiation therapy in patients with lymph node recurrence of prostate cancer. BJU Int. 2017;119:406–13. https://doi.org/10.1111/bju.13510.
10. Henkenberens C, von Klot CA, Ross TL, et al. 68Ga-PSMA ligand PET/CT-based radiotherapy in locally recurrent and recurrent oligometastatic prostate cancer. Strahlenther Onkol. 2016;192:431–9. https://doi.org/10.1007/s00066-016-0982-z.
11. Jereczek-Fossa BA, Beltramo G, Fariselli L, et al. Robotic image-guided stereotactic radiotherapy, for isolated recurrent primary, lymph node or metastatic prostate cancer. Int J Radiat Oncol Biol Phys. 2012;82:889–97. https://doi.org/10.1016/j. ijrobp.2010.11.031.
12. Jilg CA, Rischke HC, Reske SN, et al. Salvage lymph node dissection with adjuvant radiotherapy for nodal recurrence of prostate cancer. J Urol. 2012; 188:2190–7. https://doi.org/10.1016/j.juro.2012.08.041.
13. Schick U, Jorcano S, Nouet P, et al. Androgen deprivation and high-dose radiotherapy for oligometastatic prostate cancer patients with less than five regional and/or distant metastases. Acta Oncol. 2013;52:1622–8. https://doi. org/10.3109/0284186X.2013.764010.
14. von Eyben FE, Picchio M, von Eyben R, et al (2016) (68)Ga-labeled prostate-specific membrane antigen ligand positron emission tomography/ computed tomography for prostate cancer: a systematic review and meta-analysis. Eur Urol Focus. doi: https://doi.org/10.1016/j.euf.2016.11.002.

15. Parra NA, Orman A, Padgett K, et al. Dynamic contrast-enhanced MRI for automatic detection of foci of residual or recurrent disease after prostatectomy. Strahlenther Onkol. 2017;193:13–21. https://doi.org/10.1007/s00066-016-1055-z.

16. Donovan KA, Walker LM, Wassersug RJ, et al. Psychological effects of androgen-deprivation therapy on men with prostate cancer and their partners. Cancer. 2015;121:4286–99. https://doi.org/10.1002/cncr.29672.

17. Taylor LG, Canfield SE, Du XL. Review of major adverse effects of androgen-deprivation therapy in men with prostate cancer. Cancer. 2009;115:2388–99. https://doi.org/10.1002/cncr.24283.

18. Habl G, Straube C, Schiller K, et al. Oligometastases from prostate cancer: local treatment with stereotactic body radiotherapy (SBRT). BMC Cancer. 2017;17 https://doi.org/10.1186/s12885-017-3341-2.

19. Baumann R, Koncz M, Luetzen U, et al. Oligometastases in prostate cancer : metabolic response in follow-up PSMA-PET-CTs after hypofractionated IGRT. Strahlenther Onkol. 2018;194:318–24. https://doi.org/10.1007/s00066-017-1239-1.

20. Picchio M, Berardi G, Fodor A, et al. 11C-Choline PET/CT as a guide to radiation treatment planning of lymph-node relapses in prostate cancer patients. Eur J Nucl Med Mol Imaging. 2014;41:1270–9. https://doi.org/10.1007/s00259-014-2734-6.

21. Ponti E, Ingrosso G, Carosi A, et al. Salvage stereotactic body radiotherapy for patients with prostate cancer with isolated lymph node metastasis: a single-center experience. Clin Genitourin Cancer. 2015;13:e279–84. https://doi.org/10.1016/j.clgc.2014.12.014.

22. von Eyben FE, Kangasmäki A, Kiljunen T, Joensuu T (2017) Volumetric-modulated arc therapy for a pelvic lymph node metastasis from prostate cancer: a case report. Tumori J 99:0. doi: https://doi.org/10.1700/1334.14819.

23. Decaestecker K, De Meerleer G, Lambert B, et al. Repeated stereotactic body radiotherapy for oligometastatic prostate cancer recurrence. Radiat Oncol. 2014;9:135. https://doi.org/10.1186/1748-717X-9-135.

24. Ost P, Reynders D, Decaestecker K, et al. Surveillance or metastasis-directed therapy for oligometastatic prostate cancer recurrence: a prospective, randomized, multicenter phase II trial. J Clin Oncol. 2018;36:446–53. https://doi.org/10.1200/JCO.2017.75.4853.

25. Ost P, Jereczek-Fossa BA, Van As N, et al. Pattern of progression after stereotactic body radiotherapy for oligometastatic prostate cancer nodal recurrences. Clin Oncol R Coll Radiol G B. 2016;28:e115–20. https://doi.org/10.1016/j.clon.2016.04.040.

26. Hellman S, Weichselbaum RR. Oligometastases. J Clin Oncol. 1995;13:8–10. https://doi.org/10.1200/JCO.1995.13.1.8.

27. Dunst J, Baumann R. Lokale Metastasentherapie bei oligometatasierten Karzinomen: Ein spannendes Thema auch beim Prostatakarzinom. Strahlenther Onkol. 2018; https://doi.org/10.1007/s00066-018-1284-4.

28. Grégoire V, Mackie TR. State of the art on dose prescription, reporting and recording in intensity-modulated radiation therapy (ICRU report no. 83). Cancer Radiother. 2011;15:555–9. https://doi.org/10.1016/j.canrad.2011.04.003.

29. National Institutes of Health Common Terminology Criteria for Adverse Events (CTCAE) Version 4.0 Published: May 28, 2009 (v4.03: June 14, 2010), NIH Publication No. 09-5410 Revised June 2010, Reprinted June 2010. http://www.hrc.govt.nz/sites/default/files/CTCAE%20manual%20-%20DMCC.pdf. Accessed 6 Aug 2017.

30. Wang Y-J, Huang C-Y, Hou W-H, et al. The outcome and prognostic factors for lymph node recurrence after node-sparing definitive external beam radiotherapy for localized prostate cancer. World J Surg Oncol. 2015;13:312. https://doi.org/10.1186/s12957-015-0721-4.

31. Mita K, Nakahara M, Usui T. Expression of the insulin-like growth factor system and cancer progression in hormone-treated prostate cancer patients. Int J Urol. 2000;7:321–9.

32. Savvani A, Petraki C, Msaouel P, et al. IGF-IEc expression is associated with advanced clinical and pathological stage of prostate cancer. Anticancer Res. 2013;33:2441–5.

33. Briganti A, Karnes JR, Da Pozzo LF, et al. Two positive nodes represent a significant cut-off value for cancer specific survival in patients with node positive prostate cancer. A new proposal based on a two-institution experience on 703 consecutive N+ patients treated with radical prostatectomy, extended pelvic lymph node dissection and adjuvant therapy. Eur Urol. 2009;55:261–70. https://doi.org/10.1016/j.eururo.2008.09.043.

34. Ost P, Decaestecker K, Lambert B, et al. Prognostic factors influencing prostate cancer-specific survival in non-castrate patients with metastatic prostate cancer. Prostate. 2014;74:297–305. https://doi.org/10.1002/pros.22750.

35. Rischke HC, Eiberger A-K, Volegova-Neher N, et al. PET/CT and MRI directed extended salvage radiotherapy in recurrent prostate cancer with lymph node metastases. Adv Med Sci. 2016;61:212–8. https://doi.org/10.1016/j.advms.2016.01.003.

36. Schweizer MT, Zhou XC, Wang H, et al. Metastasis-free survival is associated with overall survival in men with PSA-recurrent prostate cancer treated with deferred androgen deprivation therapy. Ann Oncol. 2013;24:2881–6. https://doi.org/10.1093/annonc/mdt335.

37. Kumar A, Samavedi S, Mouraviev V, et al. Predictive factors and oncological outcomes of persistently elevated prostate-specific antigen in patients following robot-assisted radical prostatectomy. J Robot Surg. 2017;11:37–45. https://doi.org/10.1007/s11701-016-0606-8.

38. Kupelian PA, Katcher J, Levin HS, Klein EA. Stage T1-2 prostate cancer: a multivariate analysis of factors affecting biochemical and clinical failures after radical prostatectomy. Int J Radiat Oncol Biol Phys. 1997;37:1043–52.

39. Morigi JJ, Stricker PD, van Leeuwen PJ, et al. Prospective comparison of 18F-Fluoromethylcholine versus 68Ga-PSMA PET/CT in prostate cancer patients who have rising PSA after curative treatment and are being considered for targeted therapy. J Nucl Med Off Publ Soc Nucl Med. 2015;56:1185–90. https://doi.org/10.2967/jnumed.115.160382.

40. Henkenberens C, Derlin T, Bengel FM, et al. Patterns of relapse as determined by 68Ga-PSMA ligand PET/CT after radical prostatectomy: importance for tailoring and individualizing treatment. Strahlenther Onkol. 2018;194:303–10. https://doi.org/10.1007/s00066-017-1231-9.

41. Sridharan S, Steigler A, Spry NA, et al. Oligometastatic bone disease in prostate cancer patients treated on the TROG 03.04 RADAR trial. Radiother Oncol. 2016;121:98–102. https://doi.org/10.1016/j.radonc.2016.07.021.

42. Rischke HC, Schultze-Seemann W, Wieser G, et al. Adjuvant radiotherapy after salvage lymph node dissection because of nodal relapse of prostate cancer versus salvage lymph node dissection only. Strahlenther Onkol. 2015; 191:310–20. https://doi.org/10.1007/s00066-014-0763-5.

43. Supiot S, Rio E, Pacteau V, et al. OLIGOPELVIS - GETUG P07: a multicentre phase II trial of combined salvage radiotherapy and hormone therapy in oligometastatic pelvic node relapses of prostate cancer. BMC Cancer. 2015; 15:646. https://doi.org/10.1186/s12885-015-1579-0.

11

Effect of radiochemotherapy on T2* MRI in HNSCC and its relation to FMISO PET derived hypoxia and FDG PET

Nicole Wiedenmann[1,4,5*] , Hatice Bunea[1,4,5], Hans C. Rischke[1,3,4,5], Andrei Bunea[1,4,5], Liette Majerus[1,4,5], Lars Bielak[2], Alexey Protopopov[2], Ute Ludwig[2], Martin Büchert[2], Christian Stoykow[3,4,5], Nils H. Nicolay[1,4,5], Wolfgang A. Weber[6], Michael Mix[3,4,5], Philipp T. Meyer[3,4,5], Jürgen Hennig[2,4,5], Michael Bock[2,4,5] and Anca L. Grosu[1,4,5]

Abstract

Background: To assess the effect of radiochemotherapy (RCT) on proposed tumour hypoxia marker transverse relaxation time (T2*) and to analyse the relation between T2* and ^{18}F-misonidazole PET/CT (FMISO-PET) and ^{18}F-fluorodeoxyglucose PET/CT (FDG-PET).

Methods: Ten patients undergoing definitive RCT for squamous cell head-and-neck cancer (HNSCC) received repeat FMISO- and 3 Tesla T2*-weighted MRI at weeks 0, 2 and 5 during treatment and FDG-PET at baseline. Gross tumour volumes (GTV) of tumour (T), lymph nodes (LN) and hypoxic subvolumes (HSV, based on FMISO-PET) and complementary non-hypoxic subvolumes (nonHSV) were generated. Mean values for T2* and SUVmean FDG were determined.

Results: During RCT, marked reduction of tumour hypoxia on FMISO-PET was observed (T, LN), while mean T2* did not change significantly. At baseline, mean T2* values within HSV-T (15 ± 5 ms) were smaller compared to nonHSV-T (18 ± 3 ms; $p = 0.051$), whereas FDG SUVmean (12 ± 6) was significantly higher for HSV-T (12 ± 6) than for nonHSV-T (6 ± 3; $p = 0.026$) and higher for HSV-LN (10 ± 4) than for nonHSV-LN (5 ± 2; $p \leq 0.011$). Correlation between FMISO PET and FDG PET was higher than between FMSIO PET and T2* (R^2 for GTV-T (FMISO/FDG) = 0.81, R^2 for GTV-T (FMISO/T2*) = 0.32).

Conclusions: Marked reduction of tumour hypoxia between week 0, 2 and 5 found on FMISO PET was not accompanied by a significant T2*change within GTVs over time. These results suggest a relation between tumour oxygenation status and T2* at baseline, but no simple correlation over time. Therefore, caution is warranted when using T2* as a substitute for FMISO-PET to monitor tumour hypoxia during RCT in HNSCC patients.

Trial registration: *DRKS, DRKS00003830. Registered 23.04.2012.*

Keywords: Tumour hypoxia, T2*, Multiparametric MRI, FMISO PET, FDG PET, HNSCC

Background

In squamous cell carcinoma of the head and neck (HNSCC) assessment of the extent of tumour hypoxia under primary radiochemotherapy (RCT) is warranted to obtain an early prognostic marker and to define potential dose escalation volumes [1–14]. Positron emission tomography (PET) can be considered the gold standard method

for hypoxia imaging using hypoxia-associated tracers such as [^{18}F]-fluoromisonidazole (FMISO) and [^{18}F]-fluoroazomycinarabinoside (FAZA) [15–18]. Magnetic resonance imaging (MRI) can be used to characterize tumour function in several ways: Gadolinium(Gd)-perfusion MRI analyzes the tumour perfusion using the dynamic signal change after contrast medium injection, while Blood Oxygen Level Dependent (BOLD) MRI aims at assessing oxygen consumption. The MRI apparent transverse relaxation time T2*, respectively its reciprocal the relaxation rate R2*, obtained from T2*-weighted MRI, have been proposed as a potential imaging biomarker and surrogate

---

* Correspondence: nicole.wiedenmann@uniklinik-freiburg.de
[1]Department of Radiation Oncology, Medical Center University of Freiburg, Faculty of Medicine, University of Freiburg, Freiburg, Germany
[4]German Cancer Consortium (DKTK), Partner Site Freiburg, Freiburg, Germany
Full list of author information is available at the end of the article

for hypoxia PET [19–34]. A change in regional concentration of oxy- vs. deoxyhaemoglobin can result in a change in magnetic field homogeneity, which is leading to a signal change in T2*-weighted MR acquisitions.

In the literature, controversial findings are reported for T2* at baseline and during RCT: T2*-weighted MRI has recently been compared to FMISO-PET in glioma patients [32] where it provided complementary information rather than spatial correlation. In cervix cancer patients Kim et al. studied BOLD MRI before and after RCT, and they report a correlation between tumour R2* pre-RCT with tumour size response but not with tumour volume response [29]. Li et al. identified tumour R2* before RCT as a significant prognostic factor for progression-free and overall survival [30]. In HNSCC patients undergoing RCT, Panek et al. examined T2* signal stability and reproducibility pre-RCT, and they found that T2* measurements are highly reproducible [23]. Min et al. and Wong et al. evaluated serial functional imaging including R2*/T2*-weighted MRI in HNSCC during RCT and found no clear pattern for changes in R2* [33, 34].

Here, we assessed hypoxia by analyzing T2* as a measure of the deoxyhaemoglobin concentration and used T2-weighted sequences and Gd-contrast enhanced T1 sequences for morphological characterization and delineation of tumours and lymph node metastasis. The aim of our study was to examine the effect of RCT on T2* in HNSCC at an early and late time point during RCT and to analyse the relation between T2* and FMISO-PET. Serial imaging was scheduled before RCT and at week 2 and week 5 during RCT. Baseline ^{18}F-fluorodeoxyglucose-PET/CT (FDG-PET) was included to optimize pretherapy staging and considered for image analysis. To our knowledge, this is the first study to combine T2*-weighted MRI with FMISO-PET in HNSCC.

Methods

Patients, imaging schedule and treatment

Thirty two patients (T2–4 N+) were enrolled for this prospective functional MRI and hypoxia PET/CT imaging study during definitive RCT for HNSCC. Patients were recruited from 08/2014 to 11/2015. RCT was administered for 7 weeks in daily fractions of 2 Gy to a total dose of 70 Gy to the primary tumour and macroscopic lymph node metastases and 50 Gy to the elective lymphatic drainage. Concurrent chemotherapy was administered once in weeks 1, 4, and 7 with cisplatin (100 mg/kg/d or adjusted to lower dose) or carboplatin in case of chronic renal insufficiency.

Patients underwent serial FMISO-PET as previously described [7, 8] and MRI in weeks 0, 2 and 5. FDG-PET was conducted in week 0. From the total patient cohort, 10 patients (Additional file 1: Table S1) met inclusion criteria for functional MRI image analysis, i.e. imaging

with repeat 3 Tesla MRI and presence of a complete set of serial FMISO-PET data.

PET/CT imaging

[18F]-FMISO and [18F]-FDG production met standard quality criteria (tracer synthesis: Euro-PET GmbH, Freiburg, Germany). All patients received an injection of 243–332 MBq (6.6–9.0 mCi) ^{18}F-MISO and of 303–471 MBq (8.2–12.7 mCi) ^{18}F-FDG, respectively. In case of ^{18}F-FDG whole body PET/CT scans were performed 1 h p.i. (2 min per bed position, 288×288 matrix) with contrast-enhanced diagnostic CT (120 keV, 100–250 mAs, dose modulation, 600 mm data collection diameter, 512×512 matrix) and 2 mm slice thickness from the base of the skull to the proximal femur (Gemini TF Big Bore, Philips Healthcare, Cleveland, USA). A subsequent low-dose PET/CT scan was performed in one bed position (10 min) covering the head and neck region. Static ^{18}F-MISO PET/CT was executed in one bed position (20 min) covering the head and neck region 160 min p.i., following our previous study [7]. PET data were corrected for scatter, attenuation, randoms and decay and expressed as standardized uptake value (SUV; i.e. local radioactivity concentration normalized to injected dose per body weight). Head and neck FDG SUV images were normalized to mean uptake in normal tissue, defined as spherical volume within the contralateral sternocleidomastoid muscle.

MRI imaging and calculation of T2* parameter maps

As part of a multi-parameter MR imaging protocol consisting of T1w-MRI, T2w-MRI, dynamic contrast enhanced (DCE-MRI) perfusion measurements and diffusion weighted measurements (DWI-MRI), and multi-echo fast spoiled gradient echo (FLASH) data were acquired on a clinical 3 Tesla MRI system (Tim Trio, Siemens). For this, patients were positioned on the MR system table in the MR-compatible immobilization mask, an anterior 4-element flexible radiofrequency receiver coil (Flex Loop Large) was wrapped around the head-and-neck region, and data were acquired in combination with the posterior spine coil elements within the patient table to maximize the local signal-to-noise ratio at the tumour. The multi-echo acquisition for T2* measurements was acquired prior to the DCE measurements, and imaging slices were defined in transverse orientation. The following imaging parameters were used: 22 slices, spatial resolution: 3 (slice thickness) × 1.1×1.1 mm^3, matrix size: 256^2, 12 echoes, monopolar readout gradients, echo times TE = 4.83–33.0 ms, echo spacing ΔTE = 2.55 ms, repetition time TR = 400 ms, flip angle α = 60°, readout bandwidth = 815 Hz/pixel, total acquisition time = 1:42 min:s.

From the multi-echo FLASH image series, a T2* map was calculated for each slice position by a pixel-wise mono-exponential $(S(TE) = S_0 \exp.(-TE/T2^*))$ fit to the signal. To avoid noise bias, signal intensities in later echoes that were smaller than 5 times the noise level were not used for fitting.

For all image acquisitions (FDG-PET, FMISO-PET, MRI) patients were immobilized identical to the radiation position with individually casted head and neck masks.

Contouring and image analysis

Image data were transferred to iplan net planning software (BrainLAB) and co-registered. The GTV for primary tumour (GTV-T) and pathological lymph nodes (GTV-LN) for weeks 0, 2, and 5 were contoured within MRI images based on contrast-enhanced T1w-MRI Gd (Gadolinium) and T2 sequences as consensus volumes between a board certified radiologist and radiation oncologist. At week 0, the FDG-PET additional information was considered for GTV contouring. A representative normal tissue volume (NT) was contoured as a sphere within the contralateral sternocleidomastoid muscle. Hypoxic tumour subvolumes (HSV-T), hypoxic lymph node subvolumes (HSV-LN), and complementary non-hypoxic tumour subvolumes and non-hypoxic lymph node subvolumes (nonHSV-T, nonHSV-LN) were generated for a threshold level of 1.4 times the FMISO SUVmean within the NT. Volumes were contoured for all time points (week 0, 2 and 5) individually. Average values and standard deviation for T2* values and FDG SUVmean were obtained within the volumes NT, GTV-T, GTV-LN, and hypoxic subvolumes HSV-T, HSV-LN and complementary non-hypoxic subvolumes nonHSV-T and nonHSV-LN, respectively (Additional file 2: Figure S1).For statistical analysis IBM SPSS Statistics version 24.0.0.1 and SigmaPlot Version 8.02 were used. A paired samples t-test was applied to compare mean values and test for statistical significance (95% confidence interval). For correlation analysis, R^2 was calculated using linear regression analysis (SigmaPlot). For week 0, correlations between FMISO uptake, FDG uptake and T2* were analysed by correlating SUVmax tumour/SUVmean muscle for FMISO and FDG with each other and with mean T2* signal: within GTV-T (respectively within GTV-LN), R^2 (FMISO to T2*) was calculated for FMISO SUVmax GTV-T/SUVmean NT to T2* mean GTV-T and R^2 (FMISO to FDG) was calculated for FMISO SUVmax GTV-T/SUVmean NT to FDG SUVmax GTV-T/SUVmean NT. For weeks 2 and 5, correlations between FMISO uptake and T2* were analysed.

Legal issues

The study was approved by the Federal Office for Radiation Protection, the Federal Institute for Drugs and Medical Devices, and the local ethical committee. Production and use of PET radiopharmaceutical [18F]-FMISO was approved and registered at the appropriate authority.

Results

GTV and HSV under RCT

10/32 patients met inclusion criteria for image analysis by presenting a complete set of serial FMISO-PET and at least two serial 3 Tesla MRI image sets. Images were co-registered and volumes for GTV-T, GTV-LN, and NT were delineated within T1w-MRI Gd, with T2 and FDG-PET being co-registered. The number of lymph nodes present in the GTV-LN is shown in Additional file 3: Table S2. HSV were obtained within FMISO-PET as described and are shown in Table 1. GTV-T and GTV-LN more than halved from week 0 to 5. Hypoxic subvolumes HSV-T and HSV-LN decreased over time and nearly completely resolved (see Table 1, Fig. 1). A representative example of imaging modalities (T1w-MRI, T2* MRI and FMISO-PET) showing reduction of GTV during RCT and location of HSV is demonstrated in Fig. 2.

Mean T2*

Mean values for T2* were obtained within designated volumes for each patient (Fig. 3, Additional file 4: Table S3 and Additional file 5: Figure S2). For mean T2* no significant difference was seen between GTV-T and NT for all time points ($p = 0.239$ to 0.879). GTV-LN showed significantly higher mean T2* at week 2 compared to NT and GTV-T: 27.6 ms for GTV-LN compared to 21.0 ms for NT ($p = 0.021$) and 19.1 ms for GTV-T ($p = 0.009$). Mean T2* showed no significant change over time for GTV-T while for GTV-LN a slight decrease week 2 to 5 was seen ($p = 0.049$). GTV and HSV contours in MRI T2* as well as the range of T2* values are visualized in Additional file 6: Figure S3.

Hypoxic vs. non-hypoxic subvolumes

Hypoxic and complementary non-hypoxic tumour and lymph node subvolumes derived from FMISO-PET were compared for T2* signal and FDG SUVmean. HSV-T showed smaller mean T2* values compared to nonHSV-T for all time points, reaching borderline significance level at week 0 (15.0 ± 4.6 ms for HSV-T versus 18.3 ± 2.9 ms for nonHSV-T, $p = 0.051$), see

Table 1 Tumour and lymph node volumes, hypoxic subvolumes

week	GTV-T [ml]	GTV-LN [ml]	HSV-T [ml]	HSV-LN [ml]
0	37 ± 22	16 ± 14	4 ± 7	2.1 ± 3.3
2	24 ± 15	14 ± 14	1 ± 2	0.8 ± 1.4
5	16 ± 11	7 ± 6	0.001 ± 0.004	0.19 ± 0.59
Δ 0–5	- 57%	- 56%	- 100%	- 91%

Mean volumes (± STD) for tumour (GTV-T), lymph nodes (GTV-LN) and hypoxic subvolumes delineated on FMISO-PET (HSV-T, HSV-LN) before (week 0) and during radiochemotherapy (week 2 and 5)

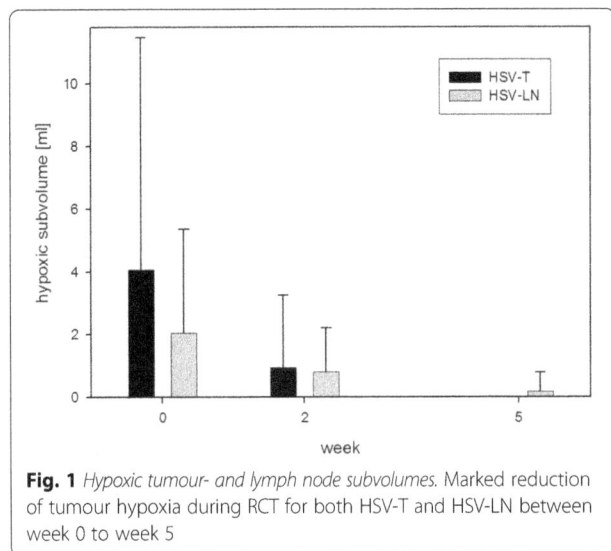

Fig. 1 *Hypoxic tumour- and lymph node subvolumes.* Marked reduction of tumour hypoxia during RCT for both HSV-T and HSV-LN between week 0 to week 5

Fig. 4. T2* values within HSV-LN and nonHSV-LN were not significantly different for all time points ($p = 0.895$, $p = 0.545$, Additional file 4: Table S3). FDG SUVmean was significantly higher within hypoxic regions of both tumour and lymph nodes: HSV-T 12.1 ± 5.5 as compared to nonHSV-T 6.1 ± 2.6 and HSV-LN of 10.2 ± 3.9 as compared to nonHSV-LN of 4.7 ± 1.9 ($p = 0.026$ and $p = 0.011$). By definition, FMISO uptake was higher within hypoxic tumour subvolumes as compared to non-hypoxic tumour subvolumes. See Fig. 4 for GTV-T FMISO SUVmean and FMISO SUVmax. Within HSV-T, T2* steadily increased from week 0 to 5, while within HSV-LN a slight decrease was seen. Neither of these changes reached significance level on a paired t-test ($p = 0.53$ and $p = 0.94$).

Correlation analysis

For GTV-T at week 0, the linear regression coefficient R^2 between FMISO and FDG was 0.81 ($p = 0.0054$), and 0.32 between FMISO and T2* ($p = 0.1157$). For GTV-LN, the comparison between FMISO and FDG yielded an R^2 of 0.30 ($p = 0.2057$), and an R^2 of 0.51 ($p = 0.0459$) between FMISO and T2*. At weeks 2 and 5, R^2 between FMISO and T2* was 0.37 ($p = 0.1073$) and 0.12 ($p = 0.3663$) for GTV-T, and 0.04 ($p = 0.6334$) and 0.01 ($p = 0.8089$) for GTV-LN. Correlation plots for GTV-T at baseline are shown in Fig. 5.

Discussion

T2* measurements are being considered a novel non-invasive MRI imaging marker for tumour oxygenation [19–34] whereas FMISO-PET is among the most commonly used imaging modalities for non-invasive hypoxia imaging [1–13, 35–38] and could be considered the gold standard. In this prospective longitudinal imaging study

we investigated the effect of RCT on T2* values of primary tumours and lymph node metastasis of HNSCC. The imaging protocol included serial MR measurements of T2* and FMISO-PET imaging at 3 time points during definitive RCT. This study is among the first to analyse the effect of radiation on T2* and the first to combine FMISO imaging with T2* measurements in HNSCC.

The more than 50% reduction of GTV-T and GTV-LN up to week 5 and the marked reduction of tumour hypoxia on FMISO-PET (i.e. HSV) in this study are in line with previous findings [4, 7, 8]. Specifically, the pronounced reduction of HSV for both tumour and lymph node metastasis at week 2 and nearly complete resolution at week 5 can be interpreted as tumour reoxygenation. Contrary to the time course of FMISO, we did not see significant changes for T2* over time: A significant difference was only seen for GTV-LN between week 2 and 5, possibly a statistical artefact due to a slight T2* increase from week 0 and 2, as between weeks 0 to 5 there was no significant change. The absence of significant changes for T2* over time is in contrast to the dynamic changes seen with FMISO-PET. While it is possible to stratify patients according to their reoxygenation pattern found on FMISO-PET, this is currently not possible with T2*. For methodological reasons, different endpoints had to be used for FMISO-PET derived hypoxia (hypoxic volumes) and T2* MRI derived oxygenation status (average value within volumes).

It is of note that for GTV-LN higher T2* values were found than for GTV-T for all time points (reaching significance level at week 2). In line with this finding, Panek et al. [23] also described higher T2* values for lymph node metastasis than for primary tumours. Possible explanations might be local magnetic field inhomogeneity caused by air–tissue interfaces that affects T2* values at the outer rim of primary tumours more than that of lymph nodes, as the primary tumours are closer to the air-filled structures of the pharynx and the airways. In addition, T2* is also affected by the T2 value of the tissue which is different for tumour and lymph node.

The comparison between FMISO-PET derived hypoxic tumour subvolumes to complementary non-hypoxic tumour subvolumes showed smaller T2* values for HSV as compared to non-HSV for all time points. This might indicate a correlation between oxygenation status and T2* before therapy. Statistical significance was not reached, however a borderline significance level ($p = 0.051$). Our findings on T2* values within HSV over time were opposed for GTV-T and GTV-LN: within hypoxic tumour volumes, T2* steadily increased from week 0 to 5, supportive for improved tumour oxygenation over time, whereas within hypoxic lymph node subvolumes a slight decrease was seen (none of these changes were significant).

FDG-PET was conducted only once (week 0) and not at later time points for patient convenience. FDG uptake

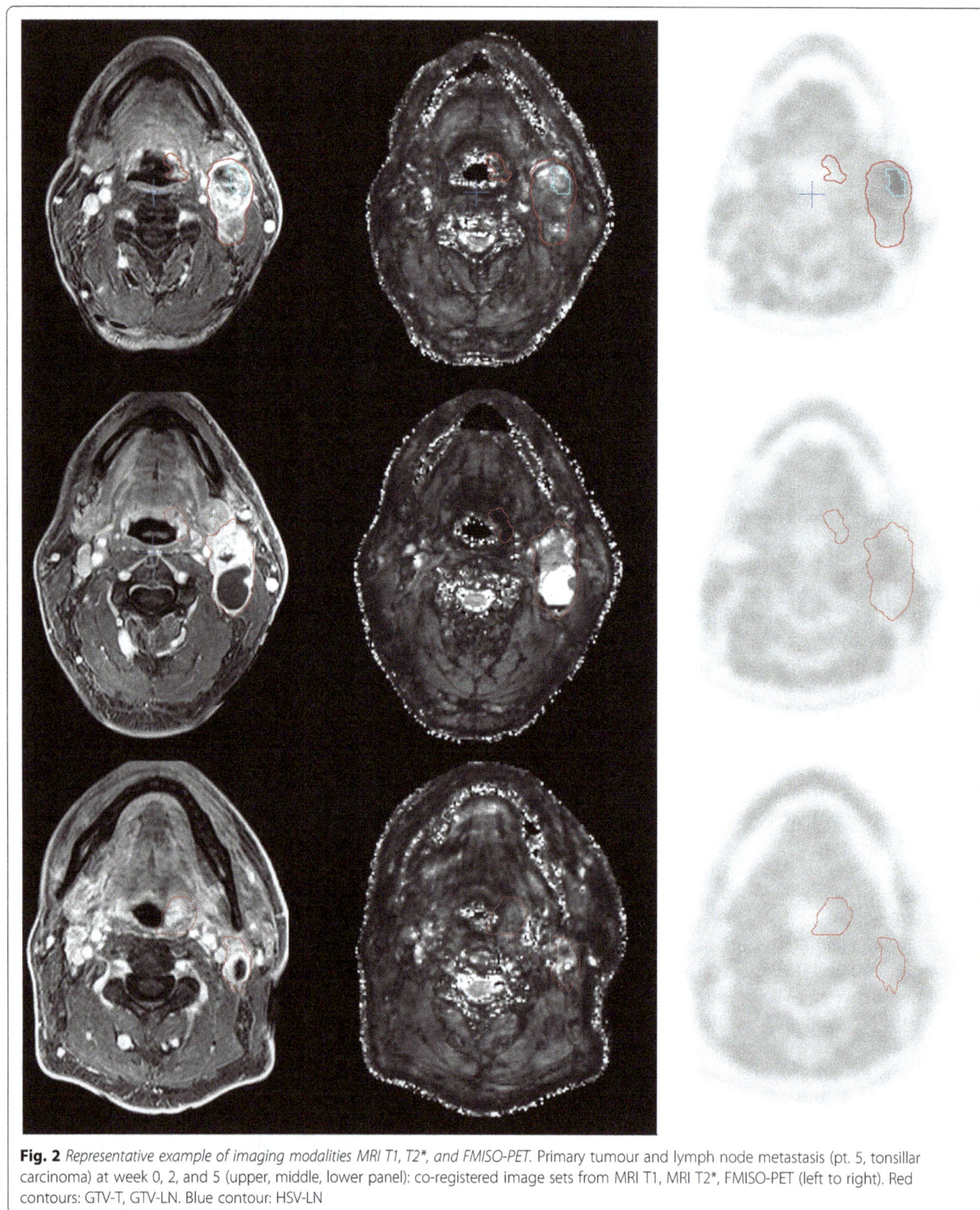

Fig. 2 *Representative example of imaging modalities MRI T1, T2*, and FMISO-PET.* Primary tumour and lymph node metastasis (pt. 5, tonsillar carcinoma) at week 0, 2, and 5 (upper, middle, lower panel): co-registered image sets from MRI T1, MRI T2*, FMISO-PET (left to right). Red contours: GTV-T, GTV-LN. Blue contour: HSV-LN

within hypoxic subvolumes was significantly higher than within complementary non-hypoxic subvolumes for both tumour and lymph nodes. Accordingly, within GTV-T the correlation between FMISO uptake and FDG uptake was strong ($R^2 = 0.81$) whereas only a weak correlation ($R^2 = 0.32$) was found between FMISO uptake and mean T2*. Interestingly, for lymph nodes the correlation between FMISO and T2* was moderate ($R^2 = 0.51$) while

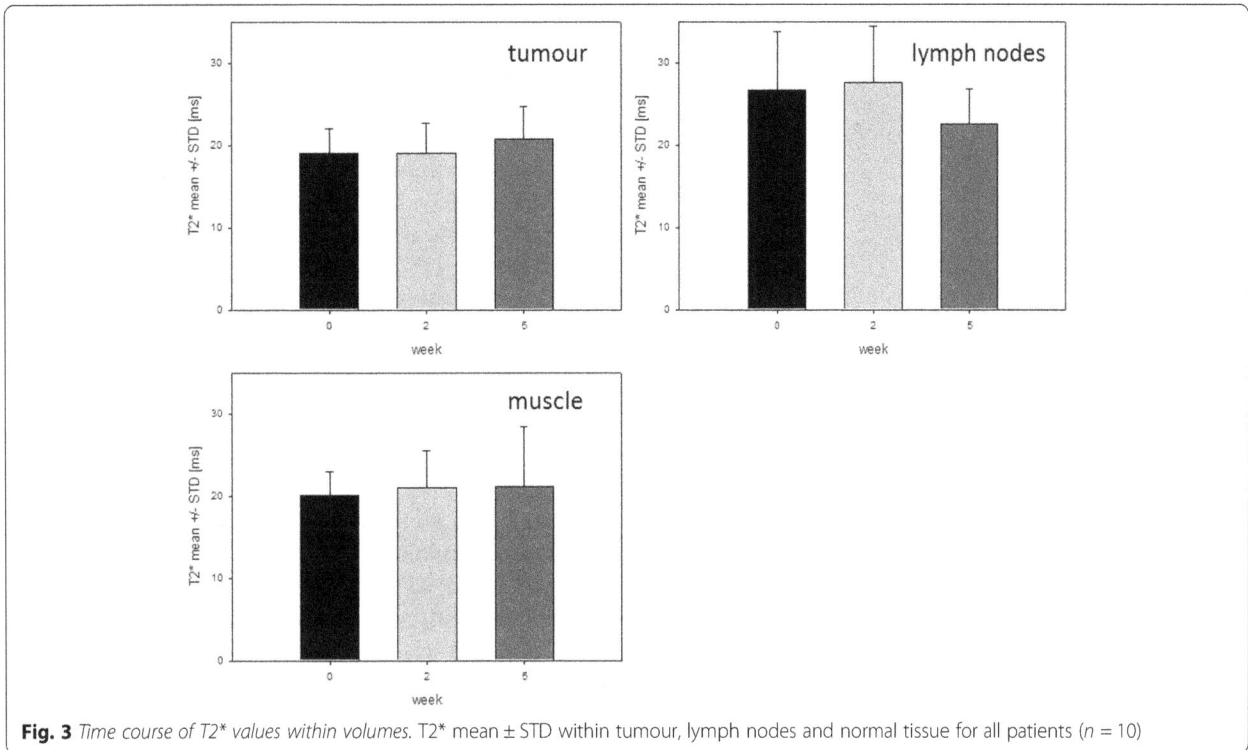

Fig. 3 *Time course of T2* values within volumes.* T2* mean ± STD within tumour, lymph nodes and normal tissue for all patients (*n* = 10)

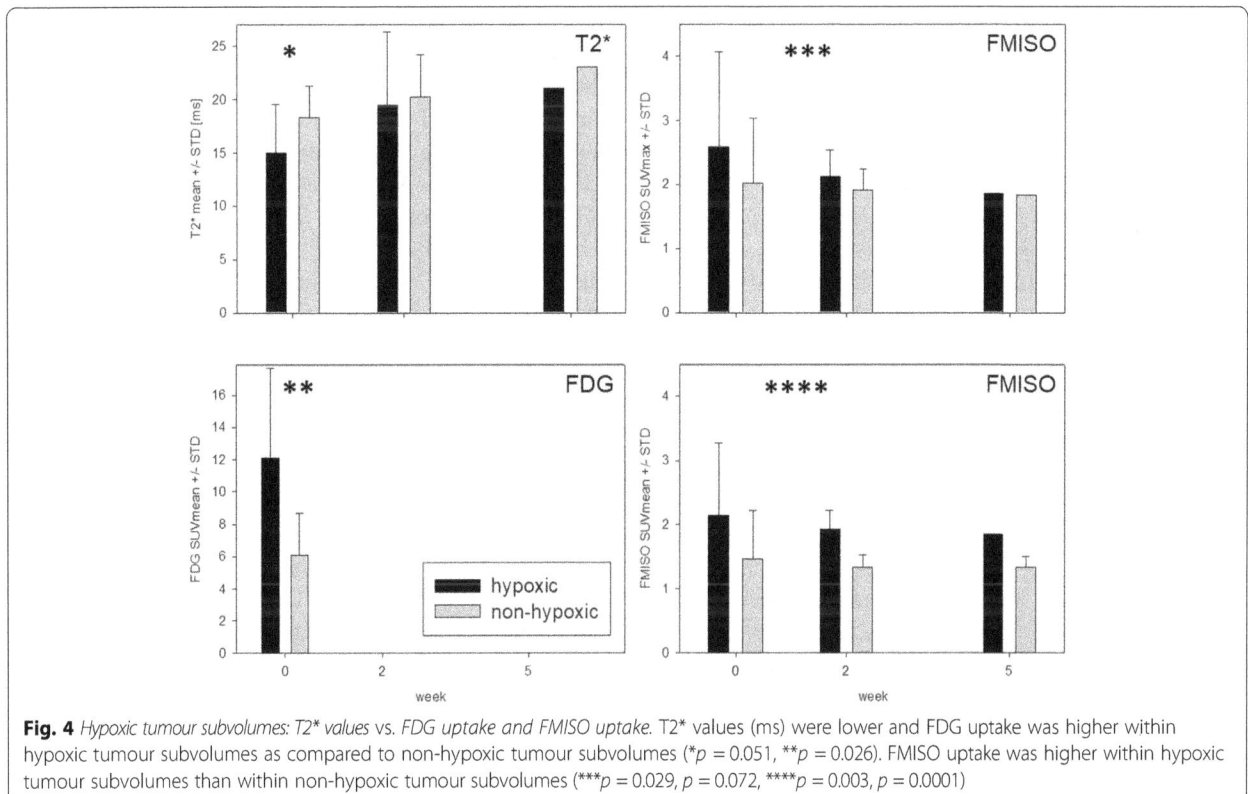

Fig. 4 *Hypoxic tumour subvolumes: T2* values* vs. *FDG uptake and FMISO uptake.* T2* values (ms) were lower and FDG uptake was higher within hypoxic tumour subvolumes as compared to non-hypoxic tumour subvolumes (*p = 0.051, **p = 0.026). FMISO uptake was higher within hypoxic tumour subvolumes than within non-hypoxic tumour subvolumes (***p = 0.029, p = 0.072, ****p = 0.003, p = 0.0001)

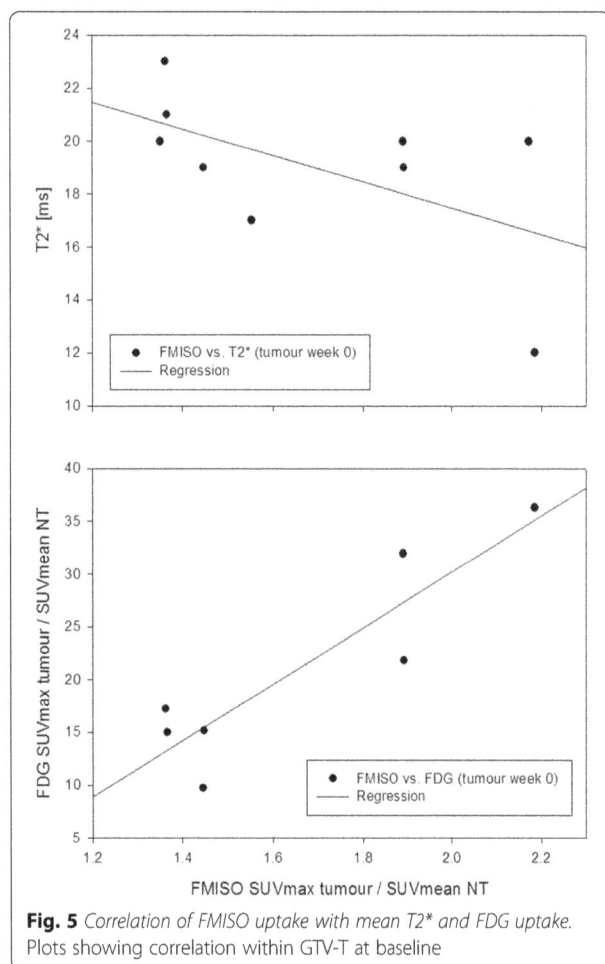

Fig. 5 *Correlation of FMISO uptake with mean T2* and FDG uptake.* Plots showing correlation within GTV-T at baseline

the correlation between FMISO and FDG was weak ($R^2 = 0.30$).

Due to the overlap between FDG avid regions and hypoxic regions on FMISO-PET [8, 39], FDG-PET has been discussed as a potential surrogate for FMISO-PET for the definition of a dose escalation volume. Based on our data of primary tumours, we can support the finding of a correlation between FDG uptake and FMISO uptake. The correlation between T2* and FMISO uptake was less pronounced.

The effective transverse relaxation time, T2*, and its inverse, the transverse relaxation rate, $R2^* = 1/T2^*$, are influenced by the presence of paramagnetic deoxyhaemoglobin in venous blood. Thus, deoxyhaemoglobin serves as a naturally occuring contrast agent that allows quantification of oxygenation [20, 22, 25]. Changes in T2* are stronger in large vessels than in microvasculature. For brain imaging at 1.5 Tesla, short T2* down to 10 ms were reported in the sagittal sinus compared with 25–50 ms in larger arterioles and venules [24, 40].

Punwani et al. measured T2* in the brain of neonatal piglets and found a strong correlation between R2* and the absolute deoxyhaemoglobin concentration [25].

Panek et al. investigated T2* at baseline before onset of radiation therapy in ten HNSCC patients and found T2* at 3 Tesla applicable to assess clinically relevant changes in tumour oxygenation [23]. Additionally, T2* measurements were applied in a mouse tumour model and R2* fluctuations were described by the authors in both xenografts and patient tumours [41]. The same group used T2* to assess the effect of blood transfusions on tumour oxygenation in HNSCC patients, revealing no change in tumour oxygenation after transfusion [42]. Spontaneous fluctuations of T2* signal were also reported by Baudelet et al. in a mouse tumour model [19]. This observation was found within regions of functional vasculature and therefore interpreted as spontaneous fluctuations in blood flow and oxygenation associated with the pathophysiology of acute hypoxia in tumours [19]. Li et al. investigated R2* for predicting the prognosis of cervical squamous carcinoma treated with RCT and found significantly lower R2* values for responders compared to the non-responders [30]. Contrarily in HNSCC during RCT, Wong et al. found no significant difference between R2* for responders and non-responders [34] and Min et al. found no clear pattern for changes in R2* by analyzing intra-tumour ROIs [33]. For cervical cancer patients, Kim et al. reported significantly lower R2* values pre-RCT than post-RCT, indicating increased tumour hypoxia after treatment - a finding that was interpreted as caused by increased deoxyhaemoglobin concentration through reduction in vascular permeability and blood flow after treatment [29]. In a preclinical rat tumour model, Hallac et al. was able to correlate R2* obtained by blood oxygen level dependent (BOLD) MRI with pO_2 [43]. In our study, no distinct correlation between hypoxia as derived from FMISO-PET and T2* was found. As tumour size in HNSCC during RCT is rapidly changing, the change in tumour size and composition might be a possible explanation for this discrepancy. In addition, T2* measurements are strongly affected by the amount of blood supply (perfusion, vascular permeability) and deoxyhaemoglobin concentration, which might change during RCT. Appropriately, in a recent study in prostate cancer patients undergoing neoadjuvant androgen deprivation therapy, assessment of hypoxia by FMISO-PET and MRI-based perfusion showed a correlation at baseline only but not following therapy [44].

There are some limitations to the present study: 1. optimal image fusion is crucial for correlation analysis. MRI and PET/CT images (both with identical mask fixation of the head and neck region) were fused by a treatment planning software with validated image registration algorithm. However, image fusion within the head and neck region is more critical than intracranial image fusion due to anatomical and physiological reasons. 2. The hypoxic subvolumes used for analysis of average T2* values were representative at baseline but became very small at later time points. 3. The study evaluates a relatively small number of patients. Including a higher number of patients however would raise an ethical problem due to the burden imposed on patients by frequent imaging sessions and long imaging protocols. In the current study, 11 of 32 patients could not be considered as they were included before availability of the 3 Tesla MRI. For the remaining 21 patients, a high dropout rate was found, as only 10 fulfilled inclusion criteria due to missing image sets.

Nevertheless, this prospective trial demonstrated that clinically, T2* may not be suitable to replace FMISO PET as a valuable surrogate imaging marker to monitor tumour oxygenation and hypoxic areas during the course of radiotherapy. Future analyses are planned to further examine the role of T2* imaging in the context of tumour hypoxia.

Conclusions

In summary, marked reduction of tumour hypoxia between week 0, 2 and 5 found on FMISO-PET was not accompanied by a significant T2*change within GTVs over time. Our results suggest a relation between tumour oxygenation status and T2* at baseline, but no simple correlation during the course of radiotherapy. Therefore, caution is warranted when using T2* as a substitute for FMISO-PET to monitor tumour hypoxia during RCT in HNSCC patients.

Additional files

Additional file 1: Table S1. Patient characteristics.

Additional file 2: Figure S1. *Volumes analysed.* FMISO-PET with volumes used for analysis: GTV-T, GTV-LN, HSV-T, nonHSV-T, HSV-LN, nonHSV-LN.

Additional file 3: Table S2. T2* values within volumes. Mean, median, and STD for T2*mean (ms) measurements for all patients ($n = 10$).

Additional file 4: Table S3. Number of lymph nodes within GTV-LN.

Additional file 5: Figure S2. *Individual plots of T2*.* Plots of T2*mean for individual patients over time.

Additional file 6: Figure S3. *Hypoxic subvolume HSV-LN and GTVs on MRI T2*.* MRI T2* (ms) showing GTV-T, GTV-LN (red contours) and HSV-LN (green contour) at week 0.

Abbreviations

Δ: Delta; BOLD: Blood oxygenation level-dependent; CT: Computed tomography; DCE-MRI: Dynamic contrast enhanced MRI; DWI-MRI: Diffusion weighted MRI; FAZA : ^{18}F-fluoroazomycinarabinoside; FDG: ^{18}F-fluorodeoxyglucose; FDG-PET: ^{18}F-fluorodeoxyglucose PET/CT; FLASH: Multi-echo fast spoiled gradient echo; FMISO: ^{18}F-misonidazole; FMISO-PET: ^{18}F-misonidazole PET/CT; Gd: Gadolinium; GTV: Gross tumour volume; GTV-LN: Gross tumour volume of metastatic lymph nodes; GTV-T: Gross tumour volume of primary tumour; HNSCC: Squamous cell head-and-neck cancer; HSV: Hypoxic subvolume; HSV-LN: Hypoxic subvolume of lymph node metastasis; HSV-T: Hypoxic subvolume of primary tumour; LN: Lymph nodes; MRI: Magnetic resonance imaging; nonHSV-LN: Non-hypoxic subvolume of lymph node metastasis; nonHSV-T: Non-hypoxic subvolume of primary tumour; NT: Normal tissue; p.i.: Post injection; PET: Positron emission tomography; PET/CT: Positron emission tomography/computed tomography;

R2*: Relaxation rate; RCT: Radiochemotherapy; STD: Standard deviation; SUV: Standardized uptake value; SUVmax: Maximum standardized uptake value; SUVmean: Mean standardized uptake value; T: Primary tumour; T1w-MRI: T1-weighted MRI; T2*: Transverse relaxation time; T2w-MRI: T2-weighted MRI; TE: Echo time; TR: Repetition time

Acknowledgements

We thank Eva Hermann, Christopher Schmitt, Carmen Meffle, Erika Lübke and Hans-Jürgen Koth for technical and administrative support. We thank Jeffrey and Tanja Davis for proofreading.

Funding

This trial was supported by the *German Cancer Consortium (DKTK)*.

Authors' contributions

The manuscript was written by NW. MB, ALG, MM, CS, MBü, NHN and LB were contributors in writing the manuscript. HB and AB were concerned with patient treatment. LM and HB prepared image analysis. NW, HB and LM generated hypoxic subvolumes. HCR and NW delineated GTVs. PTM, MM, CS were concerned with PET/CT imaging (acquisition and protocol definition), analysis and interpretation of PET/CT data. MB, MBü, UL, LB, and AP were concerned with the MRI sequences. NW, MB, ALG analysed and interpreted the data. NW performed the statistical analysis. ALG, JH and PTM supervised the project. The concept was established by ALG and WW. All authors read and approved the final manuscript.

Competing interests

The authors declare that they have no competing interests.

Author details

[1]Department of Radiation Oncology, Medical Center University of Freiburg, Faculty of Medicine, University of Freiburg, Freiburg, Germany. [2]Department of Radiology, Medical Physics, Medical Center University of Freiburg, Faculty of Medicine, University of Freiburg, Freiburg, Germany. [3]Department of Nuclear Medicine, Medical Center University of Freiburg, Faculty of Medicine, University of Freiburg, Freiburg, Germany. [4]German Cancer Consortium (DKTK), Partner Site Freiburg, Freiburg, Germany. [5]German Cancer Research Center (DKFZ), Heidelberg, Germany. [6]Clinic for Nuclear Medicine, Technische Universität München, Munich, Germany.

References

1. Thorwarth D, Eschmann SM, Scheiderbauer J, Paulsen F, Alber M. Kinetic analysis of dynamic 18F-fluoromisonidazole PET correlates with radiation treatment outcome in head-and-neck cancer. BMC Cancer. 2005;5:152.
2. Rajendran JG, Schwartz DL, O'Sullivan J, Peterson LM, Ng P, Scharnhorst J, et al. Tumor hypoxia imaging with [F-18] fluoromisonidazole positron emission tomography in head and neck cancer. Clin Cancer Res. 2006;12:5435–41.
3. Padhani AR, Krohn KA, Lewis JS, Alber M. Imaging oxygenation of human tumours. Eur Radiol. 2007;17:861–72.
4. Zips D, Zophel K, Abolmaali N, Perrin R, Abramyuk A, Haase R, et al. Exploratory prospective trial of hypoxia-specific PET imaging during radiochemotherapy in patients with locally advanced head-and-neck cancer. Radiother Oncol. 2012;105:21–8.
5. Alber M, Thorwarth D. Multi-modality functional image guided dose escalation in the presence of uncertainties. Radiother Oncol. 2014;111:354–9.
6. Schutze C, Bergmann R, Bruchner K, Mosch B, Yaromina A, Zips D, et al. Effect of [(18)F]FMISO stratified dose-escalation on local control in FaDu hSCC in nude mice. Radiother Oncol. 2014;111:81–7.

7.   Wiedenmann NE, Bucher S, Hentschel M, Mix M, Vach W, Bittner MI, et al. Serial [18F]-fluoromisonidazole PET during radiochemotherapy for locally advanced head and neck cancer and its correlation with outcome. Radiother Oncol. 2015;117:113–7.

8.   Bittner MI, Wiedenmann N, Bucher S, Hentschel M, Mix M, Weber WA, et al. Exploratory geographical analysis of hypoxic subvolumes using 18F-MISO-PET imaging in patients with head and neck cancer in the course of primary chemoradiotherapy. Radiotherapy Oncol. 2013;108:511–6.

9.   Thorwarth D. Biologically adapted radiation therapy. Z Med Phys. 2018;28(3): 177–83.

10. Welz S, Monnich D, Pfannenberg C, Nikolaou K, Reimold M, La Fougere C, et al. Prognostic value of dynamic hypoxia PET in head and neck cancer: results from a planned interim analysis of a randomized phase II hypoxia-image guided dose escalation trial. RadiotherOncol. 2017;124:526–32.

11. Boeke S, Thorwarth D, Monnich D, Pfannenberg C, Reischl G, La Fougere C, et al. Geometric analysis of loco-regional recurrences in relation to pre-treatment hypoxia in patients with head and neck cancer. Acta oncologica (Stockholm, Sweden). 2017;56:1571–6.

12. Lock S, Perrin R, Seidlitz A, Bandurska-Luque A, Zschaeck S, Zophel K, et al. Residual tumour hypoxia in head-and-neck cancer patients undergoing primary radiochemotherapy, final results of a prospective trial on repeat FMISO-PET imaging. Radiother Oncol. 2017;124:533–40.

13. Grkovski M, Schoder H, Lee NY, Carlin SD, Beattie BJ, Riaz N, et al. Multiparametric imaging of tumor hypoxia and perfusion with 18F-Fluoromisonidazole dynamic PET in head and neck Cancer. J Nucl Med. 2017;58:1072–80.

14. Linge A, Lohaus F, Lock S, Nowak A, Gudziol V, Valentini C, et al. HPV status, cancer stem cell marker expression, hypoxia gene signatures and tumour volume identify good prognosis subgroups in patients with HNSCC after primary radiochemotherapy: a multicentre retrospective study of the German Cancer consortium radiation oncology group (DKTK-ROG). Radiother Oncol. 2016;121:364–73.

15. Peeters SG, Zegers CM, Lieuwes NG, van Elmpt W, Eriksson J, van Dongen GA, et al. A comparative study of the hypoxia PET tracers [(1)(8)F]HX4, [(1)(8)F]FAZA, and [(1)(8)F]FMISO in a preclinical tumor model. Int J Radiat Oncol Biol Phys. 2015;91:351–9.

16. Carlin S, Zhang H, Reese M, Ramos NN, Chen Q, Ricketts SA. A comparison of the imaging characteristics and microregional distribution of 4 hypoxia PET tracers. J Nucl Med. 2014;55:515–21.

17. Wack LJ, Monnich D, van Elmpt W, Zegers CM, Troost EG, Zips D, et al. Comparison of [18F]-FMISO, [18F]-FAZA and [18F]-HX4 for PET imaging of hypoxia–a simulation study. Acta oncologica (Stockholm, Sweden). 2015;54:1370–7.

18. Grosu AL, Souvatzoglou M, Roper B, Dobritz M, Wiedenmann N, Jacob V, et al. Hypoxia imaging with FAZA-PET and theoretical considerations with regard to dose painting for individualization of radiotherapy in patients with head and neck cancer. Int J Radiat Oncol Biol Phys. 2007;69:541–51.

19. Baudelet C, Ansiaux R, Jordan BF, Havaux X, Macq B, Gallez B. Physiological noise in murine solid tumours using T2*-weighted gradient-echo imaging: a marker of tumour acute hypoxia? Phys Med Biol. 2004;49:3389–411.

20. Chavhan GB, Babyn PS, Thomas B, Shroff MM, Haacke EM. Principles, techniques, and applications of T2*-based MR imaging and its special applications. Radiographics. 2009;29:1433–49.

21. Christen T, Lemasson B, Pannetier N, Farion R, Remy C, Zaharchuk G, et al. Is T2* enough to assess oxygenation? Quantitative blood oxygen level-dependent analysis in brain tumor. Radiology. 2012;262:495–502.

22. Ogawa S, Lee TM, Kay AR, Tank DW. Brain magnetic resonance imaging with contrast dependent on blood oxygenation. Proc Natl Acad Sci U S A. 1990;87:9868–72.

23. Panek R, Welsh L, Dunlop A, Wong KH, Riddell AM, Koh DM, et al. Repeatability and sensitivity of T2* measurements in patients with head and neck squamous cell carcinoma at 3T. J Magn Reson Imaging. 2016;44:72–80.

24. Prielmeier F, Nagatomo Y, Frahm J. Cerebral blood oxygenation in rat brain during hypoxic hypoxia. Quantitative MRI of effective transverse relaxation rates. Magn Reson Med. 1994;31:678–81.

25. Punwani S, Ordidge RJ, Cooper CE, Amess P, Clemence M. MRI measurements of cerebral deoxyhaemoglobin concentration [dHb]–correlation with near infrared spectroscopy (NIRS). NMR Biomed. 1998;11:281–9.

26. Taylor NJ, Baddeley H, Goodchild KA, Powell ME, Thoumine M, Culver LA, et al. BOLD MRI of human tumor oxygenation during carbogen breathing. J Magn Reson Imaging. 2001;14:156–63.

27. Hallac RR, Ding Y, Yuan Q, McColl RW, Lea J, Sims RD, et al. Oxygenation in cervical cancer and normal uterine cervix assessed using blood oxygenation level-dependent (BOLD) MRI at 3T. NMR Biomed. 2012;25:1321–30.

28. Zhou H, Zhang Z, Denney R, Williams JS, Gerberich J, Stojadinovic S, et al. Tumor physiological changes during hypofractionated stereotactic body radiation therapy assessed using multi-parametric magnetic resonance imaging. Oncotarget. 2017;8:37464–77.

29. Kim CK, Park SY, Park BK, Park W, Huh SJ. Blood oxygenation level-dependent MR imaging as a predictor of therapeutic response to concurrent chemoradiotherapy in cervical cancer: a preliminary experience. Eur Radiol. 2014;24:1514–20.

30. Li XS, Fan HX, Fang H, Song YL, Zhou CW. Value of R2* obtained from T2*-weighted imaging in predicting the prognosis of advanced cervical squamous carcinoma treated with concurrent chemoradiotherapy. J Magn Reson Imaging. 2015;42:681–8.

31. Wacker CM, Bock M, Hartlep AW, Beck G, van Kaick G, Ertl G, et al. Changes in myocardial oxygenation and perfusion under pharmacological stress with dipyridamole: assessment using T*2 and T1 measurements. Magn Reson Med. 1999;41:686–95.

32. Preibisch C, Shi K, Kluge A, Lukas M, Wiestler B, Göttler J, et al. Characterizing hypoxia in human glioma: A simultaneous multimodal MRI and PET study. NMR Biomed. 2017;30(11). https://doi.org/10.1002/nbm.3775

33. Min M, Lee MT, Lin P, Holloway L, Wijesekera D, Gooneratne D, et al. Assessment of serial multi-parametric functional MRI (diffusion-weighted imaging and R2*) with (18)F-FDG-PET in patients with head and neck cancer treated with radiation therapy. Br J Radiol. 2016;89:20150530.

34. Wong KH, Panek R, Dunlop A, Mcquaid D, Riddell A, Welsh LC, et al. Changes in multimodality functional imaging parameters early during chemoradiation predict treatment response in patients with locally advanced head and neck cancer. Eur J Nucl Med Mol Imaging. 2018;45(5):759–67.

35. Thorwarth D, Monnich D, Zips D. Methodological aspects on hypoxia PET acquisition and image processing. Q J Nucl Med Mol Imaging. 2013;57:235–43.

36. Bittner MI, Wiedenmann N, Bucher S, Hentschel M, Mix M, Rucker G, et al. Analysis of relation between hypoxia PET imaging and tissue-based biomarkers during head and neck radiochemotherapy. Acta oncologica (Stockholm, Sweden). 2016;55:1299–304.

37. Leibfarth S, Simoncic U, Monnich D, Welz S, Schmidt H, Schwenzer N, et al. Analysis of pairwise correlations in multi-parametric PET/MR data for biological tumor characterization and treatment individualization strategies. Eur J Nucl Med Mol Imaging. 2016;43:1199–208.

38. Simoncic U, Leibfarth S, Welz S, Schwenzer N, Schmidt H, Reischl G, et al. Comparison of DCE-MRI kinetic parameters and FMISO-PET uptake parameters in head and neck cancer patients. Med Phys. 2017;44:2358–68.

39. Monnich D, Thorwarth D, Leibfarth S, Pfannenberg C, Reischl G, Mauz PS, et al. Overlap of highly FDG-avid and FMISO hypoxic tumor subvolumes in patients with head and neck cancer. Acta oncologica (Stockholm, Sweden). 2017;56:1577–82.

40. Wedegartner U, Kooijman H, Andreas T, Beindorff N, Hecher K, Adam G. T2 and T2* measurements of fetal brain oxygenation during hypoxia with MRI at 3T: correlation with fetal arterial blood oxygen saturation. Eur Radiol. 2010;20:121–7.

41. Panek R, Welsh L, Baker LCJ, Schmidt MA, Wong KH, Riddell AM, et al. Noninvasive imaging of cycling hypoxia in head and neck Cancer using intrinsic susceptibility MRI. Clin Cancer Res. 2017;23:4233–41.

42. Welsh L, Panek R, Riddell A, Wong K, Leach MO, Tavassoli M, et al. Blood transfusion during radical chemo-radiotherapy does not reduce tumour hypoxia in squamous cell cancer of the head and neck. Br J Cancer. 2017;116:28–35.

43. Hallac RR, Zhou H, Pidikiti R, Song K, Stojadinovic S, Zhao D, et al. Correlations of noninvasive BOLD and TOLD MRI with pO2 and relevance to tumor radiation response. Magn Reson Med. 2014;71:1863–73.

44. Mainta IC, Zilli T, Tille JC, De Perrot T, Vallée JP, Buchegger F, Garibotto V, Miralbell R. The effect of neoadjuvant androgen deprivation therapy on tumor hypoxia in high-grade prostate cancer: an (18)F-MISO PET-MRI study. Int J Radiat Oncol Biol Phys. 2018. https://doi.org/10.1016/j.ijrobp.2018.02.170.

12

Effect of machine learning methods on predicting NSCLC overall survival time based on Radiomics analysis

Wenzheng Sun[1,2], Mingyan Jiang[1*], Jun Dang[3], Panchun Chang[4] and Fang-Fang Yin[2]

Abstract

Background: To investigate the effect of machine learning methods on predicting the Overall Survival (OS) for non-small cell lung cancer based on radiomics features analysis.

Methods: A total of 339 radiomic features were extracted from the segmented tumor volumes of pretreatment computed tomography (CT) images. These radiomic features quantify the tumor phenotypic characteristics on the medical images using tumor shape and size, the intensity statistics and the textures. The performance of 5 feature selection methods and 8 machine learning methods were investigated for OS prediction. The predicted performance was evaluated with concordance index between predicted and true OS for the non-small cell lung cancer patients. The survival curves were evaluated by the Kaplan-Meier algorithm and compared by the log-rank tests.

Results: The gradient boosting linear models based on Cox's partial likelihood method using the concordance index feature selection method obtained the best performance (Concordance Index: 0.68, 95% Confidence Interval: 0.62~0.74).

Conclusions: The preliminary results demonstrated that certain machine learning and radiomics analysis method could predict OS of non-small cell lung cancer accuracy.

Keywords: Overall survival, Non-small cell lung cancer, Machine learning, Radiomics analysis

Background

Lung cancer is the leading cause of cancer-related deaths worldwide [1]. Lung cancer could be clinically divided into several groups: 1) the non-small cell lung cancer (NSCLC, 83.4%), 2) the small cell lung cancer (SCLC, 13.3%), 3) not otherwise specified lung cancer (NOS, 3.1%), 4) Sarcoma lung cancer (0.2%), and 5) other specified lung cancer (0.1%) [2]. The ability to predict clinical outcomes accurately is crucial for it allows clinicians to judge the most appropriate therapies for patients.

Radiomics analysis can extract a large number of imaging features quantitatively, which could offer a cost-effective and non-invasive approach for individual medicine [3–5]. Several studies have shown the predictive and diagnostic ability of radiomics features in different kinds of cancers using various medical imaging modalities, such as PET [6–8], MRI [9] and CT [4, 10, 11]. It is also demonstrated that the radiomic features are associated with the overall survival. Besides, these associations can be used to establish positive predictive models.

Machine-learning (ML) can be resumptively defined as the computational methods utilizing data/experience to obtain precise predictions [12]. The ML method can first learn laws from the data and then establish accuracy and efficiency prediction model based on these laws automatically. Moreover, an appropriate model is essential for the success use of radiomics. Hence, it is crucial to compare the performance of different ML models for clinical biomarkers based on radiomics analysis. Besides, appropriate feature selection methods should be applied first for the high-throughput radiomics features who may cause serious overfitting problems.

In this study, we investigated the effect of 8 ML and 5 feature selection methods on predicting OS for non-small cell lung cancer based on radiomics analysis. The effectiveness of ML and feature selection methods

* Correspondence: jiangmingyan@sdu.edu.cn
[1]School of Information Science and Engineering, Shandong University, Qingdao, Shandong 266237, People's Republic of China
Full list of author information is available at the end of the article

on the prediction of OS were evaluated utilizing the concordance index (CI) [6, 13–16].

Methods

Data acquisition

The data used in this study was obtained from the 'NSCLC-Radiomics' collection [4, 17, 18] in the Cancer Imaging Archive which was an open access resource [19]. All the NSCLC patients in this data set were treated at MAASTRO Clinic, the Netherlands. For each patient, manual region of interest (ROI), CT scans and survival time (including survival status) were available. All the ROIs in this data set were the 3D volume of the gross tumor volume (GTV) delineated by a radiation oncologist.

Prediction process

The flow chart of the prediction process [20, 21] for all the ML methods in this study was outlined in Fig. 1. The performance of each ML and feature selection methods for the 283 NSCLC patients were evaluated using the cross-validation (CV) method (3-CV in this study). For each CV process, the total patients were divided into three folds, in which two folds (training fold) for training the machine learning model and the third (validation fold) for evaluating the model.

For each training fold, the training algorithm required both the training inputs (for prediction) and the prediction targets (for validation) data. The training inputs referred to the selected radiomics features, while the prediction targets referred to the OS of the patients. The radiomics features were first extracted from the images and then selected (dimension reduction) using the filter based feature selection methods to reduce the risk of overfitting. Finally, the selected features would be used to optimize and train all the ML models. In this study, the Bayesian optimization method was applied to determine the optimal parameters [22].

For each validation fold, the corresponding selected radiomics features were first extracted from the images and then transferred into the trained model. Finally, the prediction OS would be used to evaluate the goodness of each model.

Image pre-processing and Radiomics features extraction

Prior to extracting the radiomics features, we fixed the bin number (32 bins) of all the pre-treatment CT scans to discretize the image intensities. It should be noted that the original voxels for the images were used in this study. Then, the radiomics features were automatically extracted from the GTV region of the CT images by our in-house developed radiomics image analysis software and the Wavelet toolbox based on the Matlab R2017a (The Mathworks, Natick, MA). Total 43 unique quantitative features in 4 categories (Fig. 2) were extracted:

1) Intensity features: to describe the shape characteristics of the CT volume's gray-level intensity histogram, i.e., a probability density function (PDF) of gray-level distribution.

2) Fine texture features: to describe the high-resolution heterogeneity in the ROI. These features were derived from the ROI's Gray-Level Co-Occurrence Matrix (GLCOM), a joint PDF that measures the frequency of co-occurring adjacent voxel pairs having the same gray-scale intensity at a given direction [23].

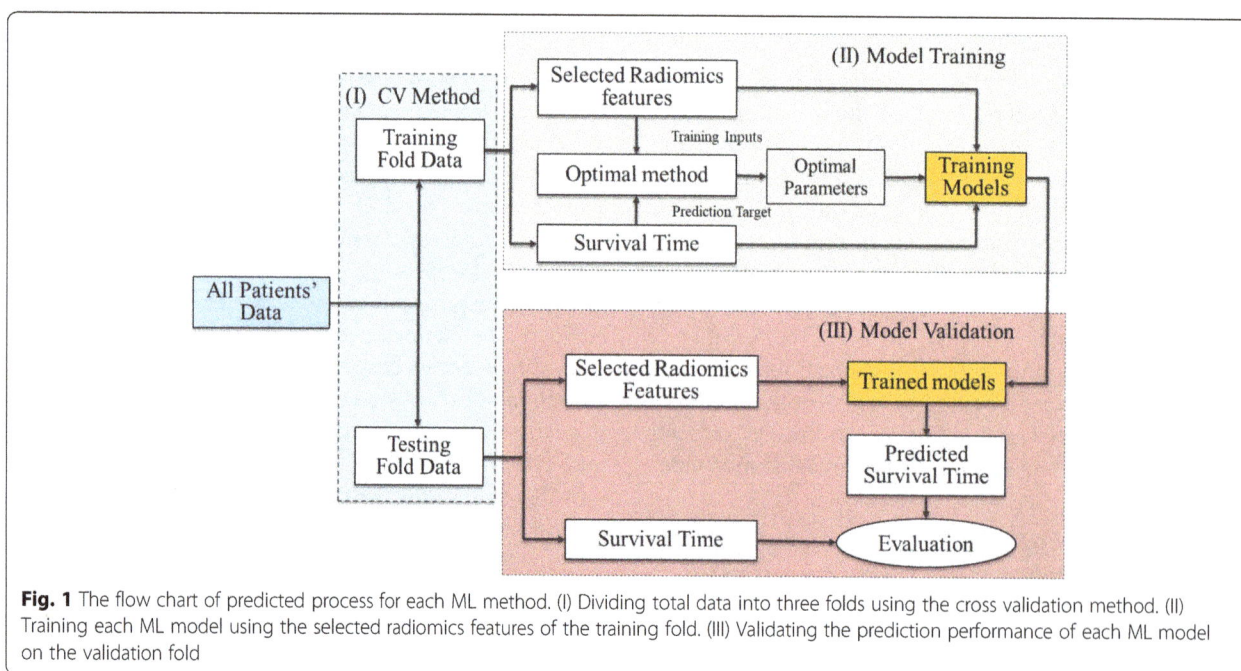

Fig. 1 The flow chart of predicted process for each ML method. (I) Dividing total data into three folds using the cross validation method. (II) Training each ML model using the selected radiomics features of the training fold. (III) Validating the prediction performance of each ML model on the validation fold

#	Feature Name	#	Feature Name
1	Intensity Histogram Energy	27	Short Run Emphasis
2	Intensity Histogram Entropy	28	Long Run Emphasis
3	Intensity Histogram Kurtosis	29	Gray Level Non-uniformity
4	Intensity Histogram Skewness	30	Run Length Non-uniformity
5	Autocorrelation	31	Run Percentage
6	Cluster Prominence	32	Low Gray Level Run Emphasis
7	Cluster Shade	33	High Gray Level Run Emphasis
8	Cluster Tendency	34	Short Run Low Gray Level Emphasis
9	Contrast	35	Short Run High Gray Level Emphasis
10	Correlation	36	Long Run Low Gray Level Emphasis
11	Difference Entropy	37	Long Run High Gray Level Emphasis
12	Dissimilarity	38	Shape Size Compactness 1
13	Energy	39	Shape Size Compactness 2
14	Entropy	40	Shape Size Sphericity
15	Homogeneity 1	41	Shape Size Sphericity Disproportion
16	Homogeneity 2	42	Shape Size Surface Area
17	Informational Measure of Correlation 1	43	Shape Size Volume
18	Informational Measure of Correlation 2		
19	Inverse Difference Moment Normalized		**Intensity Features**
20	Inverse Difference Normalized		
21	Inverse Variance		**Fine Texture Features**
22	Maximum Probability		
23	Sum Average		**Coarse Texture Features**
24	Sum Entropy		
25	Sum Variance		**Morphological Features**
26	Variance		

Fig. 2 Radiomics features used in this study. The definitions of radiomics features could be found in the IBSI document [26]. (I) Intensity features (1–4): 3.4.19, 3.4.18, 3.3.4 and 3.3.3 sections; (II) Fine texture features (5–26): 3.6.20, 3.6.23, 3.6.22, 3.6.21, 3.6.12, 3.6.19, 3.6.7, 3.6.5, 3.6.11, 3.6.4, 3.6.14, 3.6.16, 3.6.24, 3.6.25, 3.6.17, 3.6.15, 3.6.18, 3.6.1, 3.6.8, 3.6.10, 3.6.9 and 3.6.3 sections; (III) Coarse texture features (27–37): 3.7.1, 3.7.2, 3.7.9, 3.7.11, 3.7.13 and 3.7.3–3.7.8 sections; (IV) Morphological feature: 3.1.5, 3.1.6, 3.1.8, 3.1.7, 3.1.3 and 3.1.1 sections

3) Coarse texture features: to describe the low-resolution heterogeneity in the ROI. These features were calculated from the ROI's Gray-Level Run Length Matrix (GLRLM), a joint PDF that measures the size of a set of consecutive voxels with the same grayscale intensity at a given direction [24].

4) Morphological features: to describe the morphological characteristics of the ROI [25].

Here, the first category and the following two (second and third) categories required the intensity histogram and textural image processing steps, respectively. Both the above two image processing steps and the 43 radiomics features used in this study matched benchmarks of the Image Biomarker Standardization Initiative (IBSI) [26].

Moreover, these radiomics features were also extracted from different wavelet decompositions of the original CT image by a three levels wavelet transformation [27, 28]. However, the morphological features weren't extracted from the images with the wavelet decompositions for the wavelet transformation didn't have effect on these features. Hence in total, 339 features were extracted for each patient in this study.

Features selection and machine learning methods
Pearson's (PCC) [29], Kendall's (KCC), [30] Spearman's linear correlation coefficient (SCC) [31], Mutual information (MI) [32] and CI [15] were used as the filter based feature selection methods to reduce the dimensions of radiomics features in this study. In order to make sure the reliability of the selected features, we repeated each feature selection process 100 times using the bootstrap samples of each training fold and recorded the selected feature subset each time. Then, we selected the most frequently selected radiomics features as the final features which were used to train the ML models [6]. In this study, the first four feature selected methods (PCC, KCC, SCC and MI) were implemented using the Matlab R2017a and the following one method (CI) was implemented using the R software 3.5.1. All the feature selection methods would be performed on each training fold.

The effect of 8 ML methods were investigated in this study, including: Cox proportional hazards model (Cox) [33], gradient boosting linear models based on Cox's partial likelihood (GB-Cox) [34], gradient boosting linear models based on CI's partial likelihood (GB-Cindex) [34], Cox model by likelihood based boosting (CoxBooxt) [35], bagging survival tree (BST) [36], random forests for survival model (RFS) [37], survival regression model (SR) [38] and support vector regression for censored data model (SVCR) [39, 40]. All the machine learning methods were implemented on each training fold using the R software 3.5.1. The specifics of the packages for each feature selection and ML method were showed in the Table 1. Besides, the descriptions of each feature selection and ML method could be found in the Additional file 1: Supplementary A and B, respectively.

Parameters tuning

For each ML method, the parameters were selected from the combination of parameters that produced the best performance using the three-fold CV on each training fold. Similar procedures were implemented in Brungard et al. [41] and Heung B et al [42].

The range of parameters used in this study was showed in Table 1. The GB-Cox, GB-Cindex, SVCR and SR methods just required one parameter to tune while the Cox method did not require parameterization. The complex models, such as the BTS and RFS, were time consuming for tuning parameters. The parameters from all of these models, such as the average terminal node size of forest and the number of trees for the RFS model, the minimum number of observations that must exist in a node (Minsplit) and the number of trees for BST, made up a large range of parameter permutation and combination choices. It should be noted that the feature number selected by the feature selection methods were also used as a tuning parameter (range [3, 29]) for all the ML methods.

Evaluation methods

CI with confidence interval (CFI) based on bootstrapping technique (the number of bootstrap samples was

2000 in this study) was used to assess the performance of difference ML methods on the merged validation fold (merged all the three validation folds). The percentage of CFI was 95% in this study. A nonparametric analytical approach method proposed by Kang L et al. [43] and the z-score test method were used to compare the significance between pairs of machine learning algorithms for each validation fold. Besides, the survival curves were evaluated by the Kaplan-Meier algorithm and compared by the log-rank tests [44] for each validation fold.

Results

Figure 3 depicted the performance of ML (in rows) and feature selection methods (in columns) on the merged validation fold. Besides, the maximum CI with confidence interval for each ML method on the merged validation fold was showed in Table 2. The GB-Cox method using the CI feature selection method obtained the best performance (CI: 0.682, 95% CFI: [0.620, 0.744]). However, the CoxBoost method using CI feature selection method also obtained a favorable performance (CI: 0.674, 95% CFI: [0.615, 0.731]). We found only the above mentioned two prediction method's CIs were close. Hence, we just calculated the p-value using the z-test between the above two methods. The p-value of CI between these two methods was 0.5, indicating that the difference of prediction performance between these two methods wasn't significant. The values selected for the hyper-parameters mentioned in Table 3, as well as the number of selected features on each validation fold could be found in the Additional file 1: Supplementary C.

Patients on each validation fold were divided into two groups (low- and high- risk group) based on the

Table 1 The specifics of the packages for each feature selection and machine learning method

Methods	Software	Packages	Website Links
PCC	SML toolbox	corr	https://ww2.mathworks.cn/help/stats/corr.html
KCC			
SCC			
MI	MIToolbox	mi	https://github.com/Craigacp/MIToolbox
CI	Hisc	rcorr.cens	https://github.com/harrelfe/Hmisc
Cox	survival	coxph	https://github.com/therneau/survival
GB-Cox	mboost	mboost	https://github.com/boost-R/mboost
GB-Cindex	mboost	mboost	https://github.com/boost-R/mboost
CoxBoost	CoxBoost	CoxBoost	https://github.com/binderh/CoxBoost
BST	ipred	bagging	https://github.com/cran/ipred
RFS	randomForestSRC	rfsrc	https://github.com/kogalur/randomForestSRC
SR	survival	survreg	https://github.com/therneau/survival
SVCR	survivalsvm	survivalsvm	https://git-hub.com/imbs-hl/survivalsvm

SML statistics and machine learning

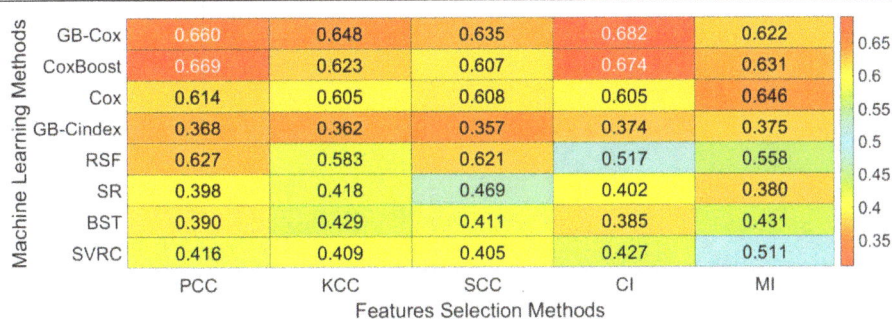

Fig. 3 The performance of feature selection and machine learning methods on the merged validation fold

predicted risk of each radiomics model at the cut-off value. The cut-off value utilized for stratification was the median of each training fold which would be applied to the corresponding validation fold unchanged. Then, the Kaplan-Meier and log-rank tests methods were used to evaluate and compare the survival curves for each validation fold, respectively. Among all the ML methods, the GB-Cox method with the CI feature selection method obtained the best stratified result on the 3 CV folds (Fig. 4). Besides, the p-value of the CoxBoost method with the PCC feature selection method was also significant for each validation fold. The heatmap of p-values on each validation fold for all the ML methods was showed in the Additional file 1: Supplementary D.

Discussion

Several previous studies have compared the prediction performance of the ML models based on the radiomics analysis. Parmar C et al. [11] identified that three classifiers, included Bayesian, random forest (RF) and nearest neighbor, showed high OS prediction performance for the head and neck squamous cell carcinoma (HNSCC). Parmar C et al. [17] also evaluated the effect of ML models (classifiers) on the OS prediction for NSCLC patients and found that the random forest method with Wilcoxon test feature

selection method obtained the highest prediction performance. However, the outcome of interest in these two studies explored by Parmar C et al. was transformed into a dichotomized endpoint. This may lead to the bias of prediction accuracy [13]. Hence, Leger S et al. [13] assessed the prediction performance (OS and loco-regional tumor control) of ML models which could dealt with continuous time-to-event data for HNSCC. His study found that the random forest using maximally selected rank statistics and the model based on boosting trees using CI methods with Spearman feature selection method got the best prediction performance for the loco-regional tumor control. Besides, the survival regression model based on the Weibull distribution, the GB-Cox and the GB-Cindex methods with the random feature selection method achieved the highest prediction performance for the OS. In this study, the effect of 8 ML models and five feature selection methods based on radiomics feature analysis were investigated to predict the time-to-event data (OS) of non-small cell lung cancer. In general, the GB-Cox method obtained the best predictive performance in the systematic evaluation on the merged validation

Table 2 Maximum CI with confidence interval for each machine learning method on the merged validation fold

Methods	FS	Maximum CI	CFI of Maximum CI
GB-Cox	CI	0.682	[0.620, 0.744]
CoxBoost	CI	0.674	[0.615, 0.731]
Cox	MI	0.646	[0.578, 0.714]
GB-Cindex	SCC	0.357	[0.290, 0.423]
RFS	PCC	0.627	[0.558, 0.695]
SR	MI	0.380	[0.310, 0.452]
BST	SCC	0.385	[0.318, 0.450]
SVCR	KCC	0.405	[0.341, 0.470]

FS feature selection method

Table 3 The range of parameter tuning

Methods	Parameters	Range of Parameters
Cox		
GB-Cox	Number of boosting steps	[1, 500]
GB-Cindex	Number of boosting steps	[1, 500]
Coxboost	Number of boosting steps	[1, 500]
BST	Minsplit	[1, 10]
	Number of trees	[1, 500]
RFS	Average terminal node size of forest	[1, 10]
	Number of trees	[1, 500]
SR	Assumed distribution	Weibull, Gaussian, Exponential
SVCR	Parameter of regularization	[0.01, 1]

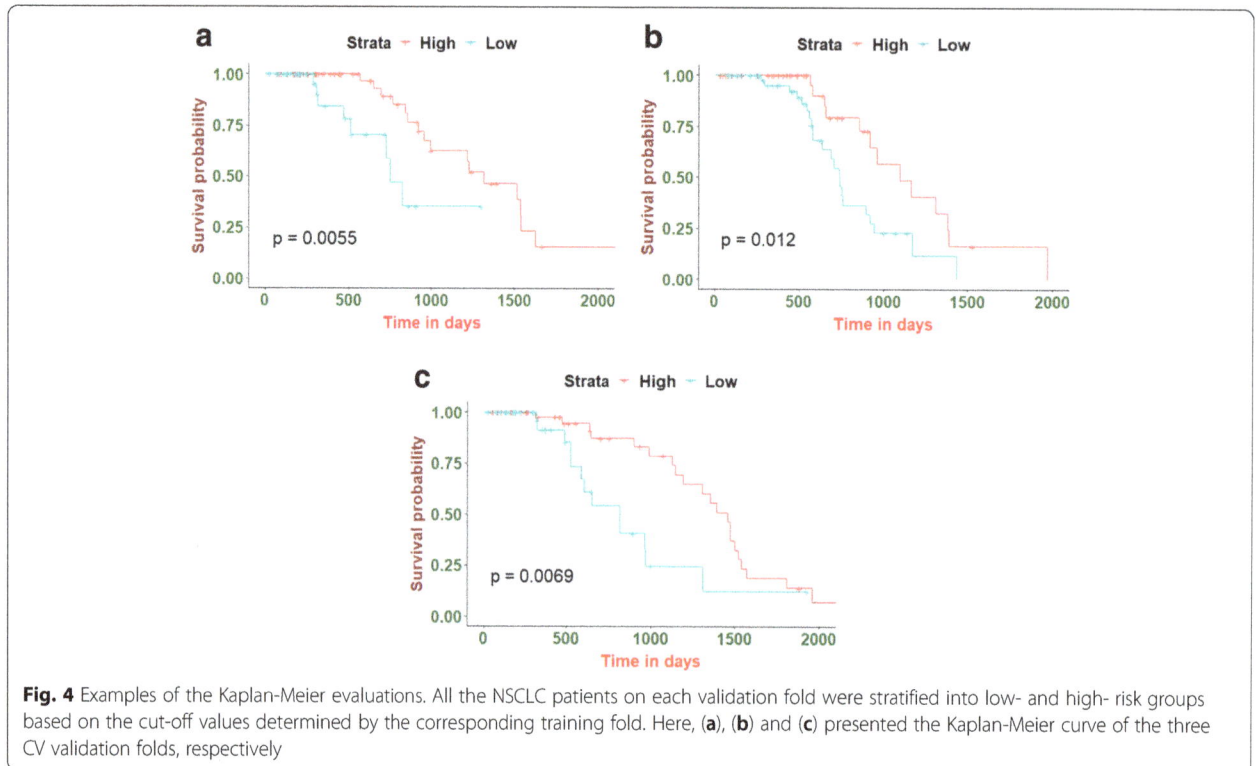

Fig. 4 Examples of the Kaplan-Meier evaluations. All the NSCLC patients on each validation fold were stratified into low- and high- risk groups based on the cut-off values determined by the corresponding training fold. Here, (**a**), (**b**) and (**c**) presented the Kaplan-Meier curve of the three CV validation folds, respectively

fold. However, the CoxBoost methods with certain feature selection method also showed comparable positive performance compared with the GB-Cox method. Hence, we thought a wide range of ML methods have the potential to be effective radiomics analysis tools. Besides, a significant difference for OS prediction on each validation fold was found between the low- and high- risk groups using the GB-Cox and CoxBoost methods, which showed the clinical potential of ML methods on the OS prediction.

As shown in Fig. 3, almost all of the ML methods using the KCC feature selection method didn't obtain a positive result. This indicated that the feature selection method was also important for the performance of OS prediction. Sometimes, the effect of feature selection methods was even more obvious than the ML models. A large panel of feature selection methods had been used for data mining of high-throughput problems [45, 46]. In general, the feature selection methods would be divided into three categories: the filter based, the wrapper based and the embedded methods. In this study, we only investigated five different filter based methods because this kind of methods were not only less prone to overfitting but also more efficient in computation than other two methods [45, 46]. Moreover, the filter based methods were more independent than the wrapper and embedded methods, which could increase the fairness of ML methods comparison.

Some previous studies [4, 5] have shown the potential clinical utility of the prognostic models based on radiomics analysis. This study could be a crucial supplementary reference for the use of prognostic models based on radiomics analysis because we compared a large number of machine-learning methods for the OS prediction of the NSCLC cancer. Such a comparison would be helpful in the selection of the optimal ML methods for OS prediction based on radiomics analysis.

Conclusion

The preliminary results demonstrated that certain machine learning and radiomics analysis method could predict OS of non-small cell lung cancer accuracy.

Abbreviations

BST: Bagging survival tree; CFI: Confidence interval; CI: Concordance index; Cox: Cox proportional hazards model; CoxBoost: Cox model by likelihood based boosting; CT: Computed tomography; CV: Cross-validation; GB-Cindex: gradient boosting linear models based on concordance index; GB-GB-Cox: gradient boosting linear models based on Cox's partial likelihood; GLCOM: Gray-level co-occurrence matrix; GLRLM: Gray-level run length matrix; GTV: Gross tumor volume; HNSCC: head and neck squamous cell carcinoma; KCC: Kendall's correlation coefficient; MI: Mutual information; ML: Machine-learning; NSCLC: Non-small cell lung cancer; OS: Overall survival; PCC: Pearson's correlation coefficient; PDF: Probability density function; RFS: Random forests for survival model; ROI: Region of interest; SCC: Spearman' linear correlation coefficient; SCLC: Small cell lung cancer; SR: Survival regression model; SVCR: Support vector regression for censored data model

Funding
This work was supported in part by the National Natural Science Foundation of China, P. R. China (No.61771293).

Authors' contributions
WS and MJ designed the methodology. WS and PC written the program. WS written the manuscript. DJ, MJ and FY reviewed the manuscript. All authors read and approved the final manuscript.

Competing interests
The authors have no competing interests.

Author details
[1]School of Information Science and Engineering, Shandong University, Qingdao, Shandong 266237, People's Republic of China. [2]Department of Radiation Oncology, Duke University Cancer Center, Durham, NC 27710, USA. [3]Department of Oncology, The First Affiliate Hospital of Chongqing Medical University, Chongqing 400016, People's Republic of China. [4]School of Electrical and Information Engineering, Qilu Institute of Technology, Jinan, Shandong 250200, People's Republic of China.

References
1. Bhattacharjee A, Richards WG, Staunton J, Li C, Monti S, Vasa P, et al. Classification of human lung carcinomas by mRNA expression profiling reveals distinct adenocarcinoma subclasses. Proc Natl Acad Sci U S A. 2001; 98(24):13790–5.
2. Howlader N, Noone AM, Krapcho M, et al. SEER Cancer statistics review, 1975–2012. Seer.cancer.gov/csr/1975_2012/ Bethesda. MD: National Cancer Institute; 2015.
3. Gillies RJ, Kinahan PE, Hricak H. Radiomics: images are more than pictures, they are data. Radiology. 2015;278(2):563–77.
4. Aerts HJ, Velazquez ER, Leijenaar RT, et al. Decoding tumour phenotype by noninvasive imaging using a quantitative radiomics approach. Nat Commun. 2014;5:4006.
5. Vallières M, Zwanenburg A, et al. Responsible radiomics research for faster clinical translation. J Nucl Med. 2018;59:189–93.
6. Cui Y, Song J, Pollom E, et al. Quantitative analysis of 18F-Fluorodeoxyglucose positron emission tomography identifies novel prognostic imaging biomarkers in locally advanced pancreatic cancer patients treated with stereotactic body radiation therapy. Int J Radiat Oncol Biol Phys. 2016;96(1):102–9.
7. Lambin P, van Stiphout RG, Starmans MH, et al. Predicting outcomes in radiation oncology–multifactorial decision support systems. Nat Rev Clin Oncol. 2013;10(1):27–40.
8. Chen HH, Su W, Hsueh W, Wu Y, Lin F. Summation of F18-FDG uptakes on PET/CT images predicts disease progression in non-small cell lung cancer. Int J Radiat Oncol. 2010;78((3):S504.
9. Tiwari P, Kurhanewicz J, Madabhushi A. Multi-kernel graph embedding for detection, Gleason grading of prostate cancer via MRI/MRS. Med Image Anal. 2013;17(2):219–35.
10. Ahmad C, Christian D, Matthew T, Bassam A. Predicting survival time of lung cancer patients using radiomic analysis. Oncotarget. 2017;8(61): 104393–407.
11. Parmar C, Grossmann P, et al. Radiomic machine-learning classifiers for prognostic biomarkers of head and neck cancer. Front Oncol. 2015;5:272.
12. Mohri M, Rostamizadeh A, Talwalkar A. Foundations of machine learning. Ch. 1, 1–3, MIT press, 2012.
13. Leger S, Zwanenburg A, et al. A comparative study of machine learning methods for time-to-event survival data for radiomics risk modelling. Sci Rep. 2017;7:13206.
14. Harrel FE Jr, Lee KL, Mark DB. Tutorial in biostatistics: multivariable prognostic models: issues in developing models, evaluating assumptions and adequacy, and measuring and reducing error. Stat Med. 1996;15(4):361–87.
15. Newson R. Confidence intervals for rank statistics: Somers' D and extensions. Stata J. 2006;6(3):309–34.
16. Harrell FE. Regression modeling strategies: with applications to linear models, logistic regression, and survival analysis. New York: springer science & business media; 2001.
17. Parmar C, Grossmann P, et al. Machine learning methods for quantitative Radiomic biomarkers. Sci Rep. 2015;5:13087.
18. Aerts HJ, Rios V, et al. Data from NSCLC-Radiomics. Cancer Imaging Archive. 2015.
19. Clark K, Vendt B, Smith K, et al. The Cancer imaging archive (TCIA): maintaining and operating a public information repository. J Digit Imaging. 2013;26(6):1045–57.
20. Collins GS, Reitsma JB, et al. Transparent reporting of a multivariable prediction model for individual prognosis or diagnosis (TRIPOD): the TRIPOD statement. Ann Intern Med. 2015;162:55.
21. Moons KGM, Altman DG, et al. Transparent reporting of a multivariable prediction model for individual prognosis or diagnosis (TRIPOD): explanation and elaboration. Ann Intern Med. 2015;162:W1.
22. Snoek J, Larochelle H, Adams RP. Practical Bayesian optimization of machine learning algorithms. Adv Neural Inf Proces Syst. 2012;2:2951–9.
23. Haralick RM Shanmugam K. Textural features for image classification. IEEE Trans Syst Man Cybern. 1973;3(6):610–21.
24. Tang X. Texture information in run-length matrices. IEEE Trans Image Process. 1998;7(11):1602–9.
25. Guo W, et al. Prediction of clinical phenotypes in invasive breast carcinomas from the integration of radiomics and genomics data. J Med Imaging (Bellingham). 2015;2(4):041007.
26. Zwanenburg A, Leger S, Vallie'res M, Löck S. Image biomarker standardization initiative arXiv161207003. 2016.
27. Selesnick I. The double density DWT wavelets in signal and image analysis: from theory to practice. Norwell: Kluwer Academic Publishers; 2001.
28. Selesnick I, Baraniuk RG, Kingsbury NG. The dual-tree complex wavelet transform. IEEE Signal Processing Mag. 2005;22(6):123–51.
29. Karl P. Notes on regression and inheritance in the case of two parents. Proc R Soc London. 1895;58(1895):240–2.
30. Kendall M. A new measure of rank vorrelation. Biometrika. 1991;30(1–2):81–9.
31. Jerome LM, Arnold DW. Research design and statistical analysis 2nd. Mahwah: Lawrence Erlbaum; 2003.
32. Pocock A, Zhao MJ, Luján M. Conditional likelihood mximisation: a unifying framework for information theoretic feature selection gavin brown. J Mach Learn Res. 2012;13:27–66.
33. Andersen P, Gill R. Cox's regression model for counting processes, a large sample study. Ann Stat. 1982;10:1100–20.
34. Hofner B, Mayr A, Robinzonov N, Schmid M. Model-based boosting in R: a hands-on tutorial using the R package mboost. Comput Stat. 2014;29:3–35.
35. Binder H, Allignol A, Schumacher M, Beyersmann J. Boosting for high-dimensional time-to-event data with competing risks. Bioinformatics. 2009; 25:890–6.
36. Hothorn T, Lausen B, Benner A, Radespiel-Troeger M. Bagging survival trees. Stat in Med. 2004;23(1):77–91.
37. Ishwaran H, Kogalur UB, Blackstone EH, Lauer MS. Random survival forests. Ann Appl Stat. 2008;2:841–60.
38. Kalbfleisch JD, Prentice RL. The statistical analysis of failure time data. New York: Wiley; 2002.
39. Van Belle V, Pelcmans K, et al. Improved performance on high-dimensional survival data by application of survival-SVM. Bioinformatics (Oxford). 2011;27:87–94.
40. Van Belle V, Pelcmans K, et al. Support vector methods for survival analysis: a comparison between ranking and regression approaches. Artif Intell Med. 2011;53:107–18.
41. Brungard CW, Boettinger JL, et al. Machine learning for predicting soil classes in three semi-arid landscapes. Geoderma. 2015;239-240:8–83.
42. Heung B, Bulmer CE, Schmidt MG. Predictive soil parent material mapping at a regional-scale: a random forest approach. Geoderma. 2014;214-215:41–154.
43. Kang L, Chen W, Petrick NA, Gallas BD. Comparing two correlated C indices with right-censored survival outcome: a one-shot nonparametric approach. Stat Med. 2014;34(4):685–703.
44. Royston P, Altman DG. External validation of a cox prognostic model: principles and methods. BMC Med Res Methodol. 2013;13:33.
45. Bolón-Canedo V, Sánchez-Maroño N, et al. Review of microarray datasets and applied feature selection methods. Inform Sciences. 2014;282(20):111–35.
46. Guyon I, Elisseeff A. An introduction to variable and feature selection. J Mach Learn Res. 2003;3(6):1157–82.

13

Survival benefit of re-irradiation in esophageal Cancer patients with Locoregional recurrence: a propensity score-matched analysis

Liang Hong[1†], Yun-xia Huang[1†], Qing-yang Zhuang[1], Xue-qing Zhang[1], Li-rui Tang[1], Kai-xin Du[2], Xiao-yi Lin[2], Bu-hong Zheng[1], Shao-li Cai[3], Jun-xin Wu[1] and Jin-luan Li[1*] ⓘ

Abstract

Background: To investigate the treatment failure pattern and factors influencing locoregional recurrence of esophageal squamous cell carcinoma (ESCC) and examine patient survival with re-irradiation (re-RT) after primary radiotherapy.

Methods: We retrospectively analyzed 87 ESCC patients treated initially with radiotherapy. Failure patterns were classified into regional lymph node recurrence only (LN) and primary failure with/without regional lymph node recurrence (PF). Patients received either re-RT or other treatments (non-re-RT group). Baseline covariates were balanced by a propensity score model. Overall survival (OS) and toxicities were assessed as outcomes.

Results: The median follow-up time was 87 months. Thirty-nine patients received re-RT. Failure pattern and re-RT were independent prognostic factors for OS ($P = 0.040$ and 0.015) by Cox multivariate analysis. Re-RT with concomitant chemotherapy showed no survival benefit over re-RT alone ($P = 0.70$). No differences in characteristics were found between the groups by Chi-square tests after propensity score matching. The Cox model showed that failure pattern and re-RT were prognostic factors with hazard ratios (HR) of 0.319 ($P = 0.025$) and 0.375 ($P = 0.002$), respectively, in the matched cohort. Significant differences in OS were observed according to failure pattern ($P = 0.004$) and re-RT ($P < 0.001$). In the re-RT and non-re-RT groups, 9.09% and 3.03% of patients experienced tracheoesophageal fistulas, and 15.15% and 3.03% of patients developed pericardial/pleural effusion, respectively ($P > 0.05$). The incidence of radiation pneumonitis was higher in the re-RT group (24.24% vs. 6.06%, $P = 0.039$), but no cases of pneumonia-related death occurred.

Conclusions: Re-RT improved long-term survival in patients with locoregional recurrent ESCC. Despite a high incidence of radiation pneumonitis, toxicities were tolerable.

Keywords: Esophageal squamous cell carcinoma, Locoregional recurrence, Re-irradiation, Propensity score-matched analysis, Overall survival

Background

Locoregional recurrence is the most common mode of failure in esophageal cancer treated initially with chemoradiotherapy (CRT) and/or surgery [1]. The local recurrence rate after definitive CRT has ranged from 40 to 60% with a low 5-year survival rate upon recurrence [2, 3]. To date,

there is no consensus regarding a curative treatment, leaving limited treatment options for patients with locoregional recurrence esophageal squamous cell carcinoma (ESCC) after CRT.

Chemotherapy is preferred as a systemic treatment for multiple-site recurrence or distant metastasis, whereas definitive local therapy is suitable for locoregional recurrent ESCC with the goal of improving prognosis. Although salvage surgery has curative potential, studies have reported high rates of pulmonary complications (17–30%), anastomotic leakage (17–39%), intensive care

* Correspondence: lijinluan@pku.org.cn
Accepted by ASTRO Annual Meeting, 2018, San Antonio, abstract #23681
†Liang Hong and Yun-xia Huang contributed equally to this work.
¹Department of Radiation Oncology, Fujian Medical University Cancer Hospital, Fujian Cancer Hospital, Fuzhou 350014, China
Full list of author information is available at the end of the article

unit admission (17–22%), and postoperative mortality (3–15%) with salvage surgery for locoregional recurrent ESCC after definitive CRT [4, 5]. These limit the number of patients who are candidates for salvage surgery.

Advancements in radiotherapy have allowed conformal radiation dose distribution with delivery of incremental doses to tumors and a minimal dose to adjacent critical structures. Re-irradiation has shown satisfactory clinical outcome in certain recurrent tumors such as lung cancer, head and neck cancer, high-grade glioma, and rectal cancer [6–11]. In the present study, we evaluated the clinical prognostic factors associated with overall survival (OS) in recurrent ESCC. Propensity score-matched (PSM) analysis was applied to assess clinical outcomes and toxicities of re-RT for locoregional recurrent ESCC to correct for the baseline covariates.

Methods

Patients

In the current study, we retrospectively examined 87 consecutive ESCC patients with locoregional recurrence who were admitted to Fujian Cancer Hospital between June 2000 and June 2014. All included patients met the following criteria: a) pathological confirmation of primary ESCC at initial diagnosis; b) a history of initial radiation; c) histological and/or PET-CT confirmation of locoregional recurrence including regional lymph node recurrence only (LN) or primary failure with/without regional lymph node recurrence (PF); d) no evidence of esophageal perforation or ulcer; and e) adequate liver, kidney, and bone marrow functioning with a Karnofsky performance status (KPS) score ≥ 70. The exclusion criteria were as follows: a) history of other malignancies; b) distant metastases; and c) confirmation of recurrence within 3 months of initial treatment.

Clinical staging at first diagnosis was determined by chest computed tomography (CT) and barium esophagram and/or endoscopic ultrasound (EUS). Re-staging of initial ESCC was done according to the 8th edition of American Joint Committee on Cancer (AJCC). The current study was approved by the Ethics Committee of Fujian Medical University Cancer Hospital, Fuzhou, China (KT2018–006-01). Because this was a retrospective study involving patient medical records, the requirement of patients' consent was waived.

Treatment

For initial treatment, 11 (12.6%) patients received radical resection with adjuvant radio (chemo) therapy (median dose = 52 Gy, range 40–56 Gy). Thirty-nine (44.8%) and 37 (42.6%) patients received CRT and RT, respectively. Among the 43 (49.4%) cases initially treated with chemotherapy (median of 3 cycles, range 1–6 cycles), 30

(34.5%) received cisplatin and paclitaxel, whereas the remaining 13 (14.9%) received cisplatin or oxaliplatin.

Patients were treated with 6- or 10-MV linear accelerators for initial radiotherapy with 1.8–2.2 Gy/fraction and 5 fractions/week. Initial RT was conventional two-dimensional (36.8%) or conformal three-dimensional (63.2%) RT with a median dose of 62 Gy (range 40–76 Gy). The median dose of re-RT was 50 Gy (ranged 21–70 Gy) with 2Gy (range 1.8–4 Gy) per fraction. Intensity-modulated RT (56.4%; 22/39) and conformal three-dimensional RT (43.6%; 17/39) were employed for re-RT. Among the 39 patients treated with re-RT, 19 patients (48.7%) received concomitant chemotherapy, of which 6 received cisplatin, 4 received 5-flurouracil (5-FU), and 9 received cisplatin combined with 5-FU. The remaining 20 (51.3%) patients received RT alone.

The biological effectiveness of radiation schedule was calculated by the biologically effective dose (BED) formula: BED = n × d $(1 + d/(\alpha/\beta))$, d for the dose per fraction (Gy) and n for the number of fractions. Assuming an α/β ratio of 10 Gy for ESCC (BED_{10}) [12]. For re-RT patients, the cumulative dose was calculated.

For patients without re-RT, 7 (8.0%) patients received chemotherapy alone with cisplatin combined with 5-FU, whereas 3 (3.4%) patients underwent salvage total esophagectomy with gastric pull-through. The remaining 38 (43.7%) patients received supportive care including esophageal stenting, dilation or percutaneous endoscopic gastrostomy to relieve dysphagia.

Follow-up

The primary endpoint was OS, which was defined as the time duration from recurrence diagnosis to death or last follow-up. The recurrence-free interval (RFI) was defined as the time interval from the end of initial treatment to the recurrence diagnosis. According to the National Cancer Institute Common Terminology Criteria for Adverse Events (CTCAE) version 4.0, toxicities recorded in the patients' medical records were retrospectively graded [13]. Tracheoesophageal fistula (TEF), pericardial/pleural effusion, and radiation pneumonitis (RP) were recorded.

Statistical analysis

All statistical tests were performed using SPSS version 22.0 (IBM Corporation, Armonk, NY, USA). The propensity score matching ratio was set to 1:1 to minimize differences due to age, gender, primary tumor location, and initial clinical stage. Chi-square (χ^2) and Fisher's exact tests were applied to compare unmatched background factors. Survival curves were constructed and compared by the Kaplan-Meier method and log-rank tests. The Cox regression model was employed for the univariate analysis and multivariate analysis. P-values < 0.05 were considered statistically significant.

Table 1 Characteristics of 87 patients with locoregional recurrent esophageal cancer

Variables	Number	Percent
Age (years)		
< 65	58	66.7
≥ 65	29	33.3
KPS		
70–80	32	36.8
> 80	55	63.2
Gender		
Male	65	74.7
Female	22	25.3
Smoking		
Yes	31	35.6
No	56	64.4
Alcohol consumption		
Yes	15	17.2
No	72	82.8
Primary tumor location		
Upper thoracic	34	39.1
Middle and lower thoracic	53	60.9
Initial clinical stage		
I + II	23	32.9
III	47	67.1
Initial treatment		
Surgery + adjuvant radio(chemo)therapy	11	12.6
Definitive chemoradiotherapy	39	44.8
Definitive radiotherapy	37	42.6
Pattern of recurrence		
Regional lymph node recurrence only	14	16.1
Local failure	62	71.3
Both	11	12.6
Radiation dose in the initial treatment (Gy)		
≤ 50	12	13.8
> 50	75	86.2
Recurrence-free interval (months)		
≤ 12	38	43.7
> 12	49	56.3
Chemotherapy after recurrence		
Yes	26	29.9
No	61	70.1
Re-RT after recurrence		
Yes	39	44.8
No	48	55.2

Table 1 Characteristics of 87 patients with locoregional recurrent esophageal cancer (Continued)

Variables	Number	Percent
Treatment modility after recurrence		
Re-RT only	20	23.0
CRT only	7	8.0
Re-RT concomitant chemotherapy	19	21.8
Best supportive care	39	43.7
Salvage total esophagectomy	3	3.4

Abbreviation: *Re-RT* Re-irradiation, *KPS* Karnofsky performance status

Results
Patient characteristics

The patient characteristics are summarized in Table 1. The median age was 62 years (range 39–86 years), and the study population included 65 (74.7%) males and 22 (25.3%) females. Considering KPS at recurrence diagnosis, 32 (36.8%) of patients were 70–80, while 55 (63.2%) were ≥ 80. Eight (9.2%) patients had stage I disease, 18 (20.7%) had stage II, and 61 (70.1%) had stage III at the initial diagnosis. The primary tumor location was the upper thoracic esophagus in 34 (39.1%) patients and the middle and lower thoracic esophagus in 53 (60.9%) patients. The median RFI was 16 months (range 3–168 months), and the RFI was ≤12 months in 38 (43.7%) patients and > 12 months in 49 (56.3%) patients. The failure pattern of 62 (71.3%) patients was primary recurrence, 14 (16.1%) cases of regional LN recurrence alone and 11 (12.6%) cases of combined sites. All patients were divided into two groups, 14 patients with regional LN recurrence and the remaining 73 patients with PF. For re-RT patients, 36 of 39 cases received in-field re-irradiation, while the other three cases experienced out-field locoregional failure.

For re-RT patients, the median BED_{10} of 74.11 Gy (range 48–86.32 Gy) and 60 Gy (range 25.41–84.87 Gy) were delivered in the initial radiation and re-RT,

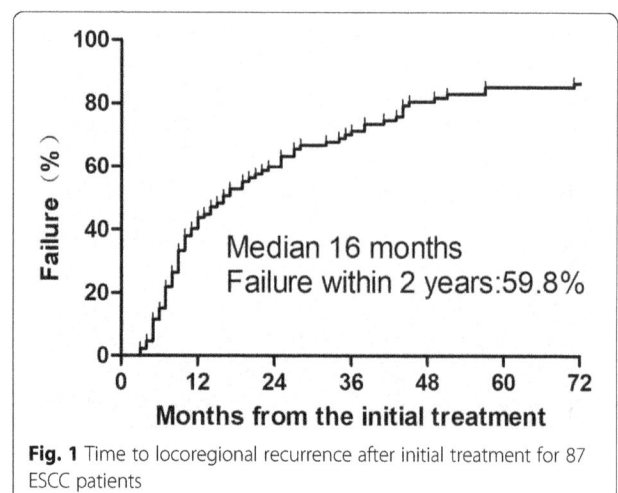

Fig. 1 Time to locoregional recurrence after initial treatment for 87 ESCC patients

respectively. The median cumulative BED_{10} was 135.53 Gy (range 96–168 Gy). The median Dmax of spinal cord was 25 Gy (range 9–39 Gy), the median V20 of the total lung and V30 of the heart was 10% (range 0–24%) and 9% (range 0–25%), respectively.

OS for the total study population

The median follow-up was 87 months (range 2–206 months). The follow-up rate was 96.6% (84/87). One patient without re-RT and 7 patients with re-RT remained alive at the last follow-up. For re-RT, 82.1% (32/39) patients were dead at last follow up, among which, 84.4% (27/32) patients were cancer-related death. After re-RT, 89.7% (35/39) suffered from failure, with 24 (68.6%) cases of distant metastasis alone, 5 (14.3%) cases of local failure alone and 6 (17.1%) cases of both. The median survival time (MST) was 10 months (range 1–85 months). The median RFI was 16 months (range 3–168 months). Fifty-two (59.8%) patients were diagnosed with recurrence within 2 years after initial treatment (Fig. 1).

Propensity score matching and χ^2 tests

Significant differences in the clinical stage of initial cancer were observed for patients with re-RT ($n = 39$) and without re-RT ($n = 48$) before matching ($P = 0.003$) (Table 2). A nearest neighbor and 1:1 matching algorithm was applied within a default caliper (0.2) [14]. After matching, baseline covariates of the clinicopathological characteristics were corrected, with characteristics being evenly distributed between the re-RT group ($n = 33$) and the non-re-RT group ($n = 33$, all $P > 0.1$).

Cox regression analysis for overall sample

The results of univariate and multivariate analyses for OS are summarized in Table 3. LN recurrence alone and re-RT were associated with better OS ($P = 0.006$ and $P < 0.001$) by Cox univariate analysis. The 1-, 3-, and 5-year OS rates in the LN group were 84.62%, 30.77%, and 23.01%, respectively, and the 1-, 3-, and 5-year OS rates in the PF group were 37.86%, 10.29%, and 2.57%, respectively. The MST in the LN group was 23 months, whereas the MST in the PF group was 9 months ($P = 0.004$, Fig. 2a). The 1-, 3-, and 5-year OS rates in the re-RT group were 67.94%, 22.89%, and 13.08%, respectively, and the 1-, 3-, and 5-year OS rates for patients without re-RT were 28.52%, 6.58%, and 2.19%, respectively. Their MSTs were 21 months and 8 months, respectively ($P < 0.001$, Fig. 2b).

Initial clinical stage (I + II vs. III), failure pattern (LN vs. PF), re-RT (with vs. without), and chemotherapy for both courses of treatment (with vs. without) were possible prognostic factors in the Cox multivariate model. The failure pattern and re-RT were independent prognostic factors for OS ($P = 0.040$ and $P = 0.015$, respectively). However, no statistical difference in OS was observed between the re-RT alone and re-RT with concomitant chemotherapy groups (18 vs. 19, $P = 0.70$, Fig. 3) in the subgroup analysis.

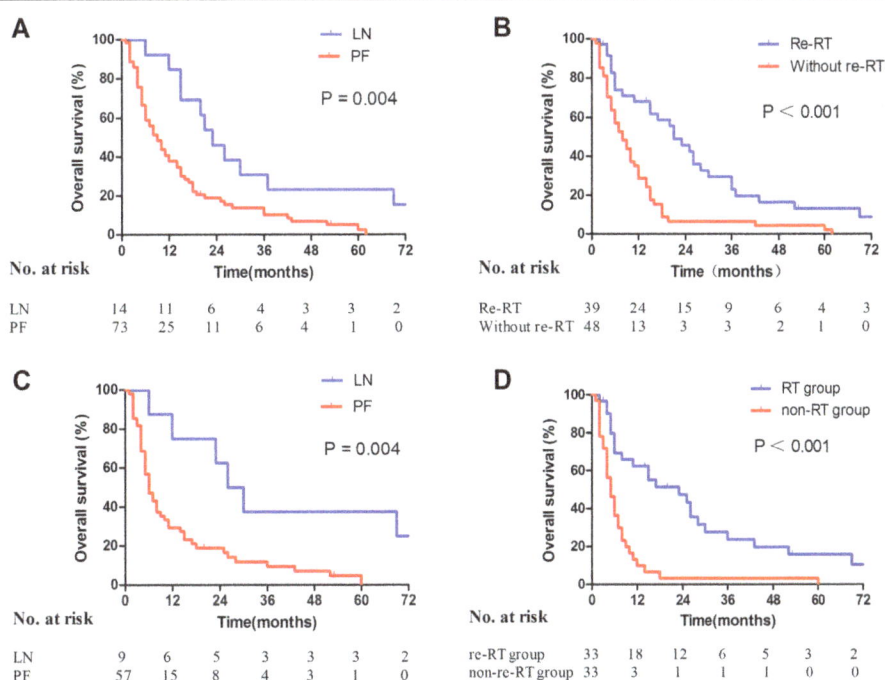

Fig. 2 Kaplan–Meier analysis of OS according to (**a**) failure pattern (LN vs. PF, $P = 0.004$) before matching; (**b**) re-irradiation (re-RT vs. without re-RT, $P < 0.001$) before matching; (**c**) failure pattern (LN vs. PF, $P = 0.004$) after matching; and (**d**) re-irradiation (re-RT group vs. non-re-RT group, $P < 0.001$) after matching

Table 2 Chi-square test of re-RT and without re-RT for locoregional recurrent ESCC before and after matching

Variables	Before matching			After matching		
	With re-RT (n)	Without re-RT (n)	P	With re-RT (n)	Without re-RT (n)	P
Age (years)			1.000			1.000
< 65/≥65	26/13	32/16		21/12	21/12	
KPS			0.770			0.802
70–80/>80	15/24	17/31		13/20	14/19	
Gender			0.572			0.580
Male/Female	28/11	37/11		23/10	25/8	
Smoking			0.619			0.796
Yes/No	15/24	16/32		12/21	11/22	
Alcohol consumption			0.679			1.000
Yes/No	6/33	9/39		5/28	5/28	
Primary tumor location			0.583			0.802
Upper/Middle and lower thoracic	14/25	20/28		14/19	13/20	
Initial clinical stage			0.003			0.284
I + II/III	18/21	8/40		12/21	8/25	
Surgery in the initial treatment			0.488			0.392
Yes/No	6/33	5/43		2/31	4/29	
Chemotherapy in the initial treatment			0.582			0.806
Yes/No	18/21	25/23		16/17	17/16	
Radiation dose in the initial treatment (Gy)			0.101			0.213*
≤ 50/> 50	8/31	4/44		5/28	2/31	
Recurrence-free interval (months)			0.187			0.215
Median (range)	27(4163)	12.5(3168)		27(5163)	12(3144)	
≤ 12/> 12	14/25	24/24		12/21	17/16	

Abbreviation: *Re-RT* Re-irradiation, *KPS* Karnofsky performance status. *:Fisher's exact tests

Cox regression analysis for matched cohort

In the matched cohort, failure pattern and re-RT were independently associated with OS for recurrent ESCC ($P = 0.025$ and $P = 0.002$, respectively; Table 4). For the two failure patterns (LN vs. PF), the comparative 1-, 3-, and 5-year OS rates were 75.00% vs. 29.49%, 37.50% vs. 9.53%, and 37.50% vs. 0%, respectively. The MSTs in the LN and PF groups were 28 months and 6 months, respectively ($P = 0.004$, Fig. 2c). For treatment with re-RT or no re-RT (with or without), the comparative 1-, 3-, and 5-year OS rates were 62.38% vs. 9.93%, 23.71% vs. 3.31%, and 15.81% vs. 0%, respectively. The MSTs in the re-RT and without re-RT groups were 23 months and 5 months, respectively ($P < 0.001$, Fig. 2d).

Toxicity

In the re-RT and non-re-RT groups of the matched cohort, 9.09% (3/33) and 3.03% (1/33) of cases experienced TEF, 15.15% (5/33) and 3.03% (1/33) of cases experienced pericardial/pleural effusion ($P = 0.613$ and $P = 0.197$, respectively). The rates of grade 3 RP were 24.24% (8/33) and 6.06% (2/33) in the re-RT and

non-re-RT groups, respectively ($P = 0.039$). No case of grade 5 RP was observed. The median age of the 10 patients who developed RP was 61 years (range 43–83 years). The radiation doses for primary RT in 2 patients not treated with re-RT were 63 Gy and 70 Gy. The median doses for primary RT and re-RT in the other eight patients were 62.2 Gy (range 41–64 Gy) and 50.3 Gy (range 36–60 Gy), respectively. No significant correlation was found between RP and the V20 of the total lungs in re-RT ($P = 0.25$). No treatment-related deaths were recorded.

Discussion

Locoregional recurrence occurs frequently after primary definitive RT or multimodal therapy for ESCC. Yet, therapeutic options remain limited, and no consensus regarding the optimal treatment has been reached. Re-RT for the management of recurrent ESCC is one of the options, and in the present study, the effectiveness and toxicity of re-RT were retrospectively analyzed via PSM analysis. In the whole cohort, the failure pattern and re-RT were found to be independent prognostic

Survival benefit of re-irradiation in esophageal Cancer patients with Locoregional...

115

Table 3 Cox model analysis for 87 ESCC patients with locoregional recurrence before matching

Variable	n	Univariate			Multivariate		
		HR	95%CI	P	HR	95%CI	P
Age (years)							
< 65/≥65	58/29	0.786	0.467–1.322	0.364			
KPS							
70–80/>80	32/55	0.752	0.467–1.212	0.243			
Gender							
Male/Female	65/22	1.008	0.607–1.673	0.976			
Smoking							
Yes/No	31/56	1.438	0.893–2.317	0.135			
Alcohol consumption							
Yes/No	15/72	1.229	0.668–2.261	0.507			
Primary tumor location							
Upper/Middle and lower thoracic	34/53	1.241	0.779–1.977	0.364			
Clinical stage							
I + II/III	26/61	1.083	0.645–1.820	0.763	1.027	0.599–1.761	0.923
Surgery in the initial treatment							
Yes/No	11/76	1.161	0.608–2.216	0.652			
Chemotherapy in the initial treatment							
Yes/No	43/44	0.954	0.601–1.514	0.842			
Recurrence-free interval (months)							
≤12/> 12	38/49	0.884	0.558–1.402	0.601			
Pattern of recurrence							
LN/PF	14/73	0.385	0.195–0.762	0.006	0.461	0.221–0.964	0.040
Re-RT after recurrence							
Yes/No	39/48	0.392	0.239–0.642	< 0.001	0.513	0.299–0.878	0.015
Chemotherapy after recurrence							
Yes/No	26/61	0.799	0.478–1.335	0.391			
Chemotherapy for both course treatment							
Yes/No	13/74	0.540	0.274–1.063	0.074	0.520	0.257–1.051	0.069

Abbreviations: *HR* Hazard ratio, *95%CI* 95% confidence interval, *Re-RT* Re-irradiation, *LN* Regional lymph node recurrence only, *PF* Primary failure with/without regional lymph node recurrence, *KPS* Karnofsky performance status

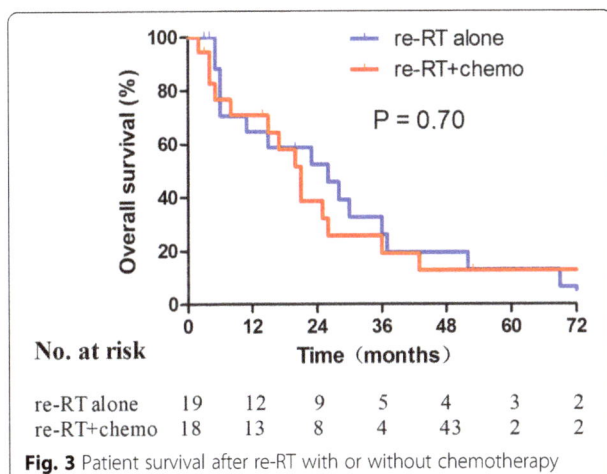

Fig. 3 Patient survival after re-RT with or without chemotherapy

factors for OS ($P = 0.040$ and $P = 0.015$, respectively), and these results were also verified in the two well-balanced groups after propensity score matching. Furthermore, significant differences in OS and MST were observed for different failure patterns (LN vs. PF, MST 28 months vs. 6 months, $P = 0.004$) as well as for re-RT (re-RT vs. non-re-RT, MST 23 months vs. 5 months, $P < 0.001$).

The current study showed that in the majority of cases (59.8%), locoregional recurrence occurred within 2 years after initial treatment. The median RFI was 16 months (range 3–168 months), which was similar to the results of Chen et al. [15]. PF was the most common (71.3%) failure pattern, followed by regional LN alone (16.1%)

Table 4 Cox model analysis for 66 ESCC patients with locoregional recurrence after matching

Variable	n	Univariate			Multivariate		
		HR	95%CI	P	HR	95%CI	P
Age (years)							
< 65/≥65	42/24	0.736	0.407–1.330	0.310			
KPS							
70–80/>80	27/39	0.843	0.491–1.447	0.535			
Gender							
Male/Female	48/18	0.942	0.530–1.674	0.838			
Smoking							
Yes/No	23/43	1.486	0.857–2.577	0.159			
Alcohol consumption							
Yes/No	10/56	1.083	0.526–2.233	0.828			
Primary tumor location							
Upper/Middle and lower thoracic	27/39	1.265	0.733–2.183	0.398			
Clinical stage							
I + II/III	20/46	1.021	0.561–1.858	0.946	1.541	0.814–2.916	0.184
Surgery in the initial treatment							
Yes/No	6/60	2.258	0.942–5.414	0.068			
Chemotherapy in the initial treatment							
Yes/No	33/33	1.005	0.585–1.729	0.984			
Recurrence-free interval (months)							
≤12/> 12	29/37	0.739	0.433–1.262	0.268			
Pattern of recurrence							
LN/PF	9/57	0.277	0.108–0.714	0.008	0.319	0.117–0.869	0.025
Re-RT after recurrence							
Yes/No	33/33	0.299	0.167–0.535	< 0.001	0.375	0.201–0.701	0.002
Chemotherapy after recurrence							
Yes/No	20/46	0.817	0.456–1.463	0.497			
Chemotherapy for both course treatment							
Yes/No	10/56	0.621	0.291–1.323	0.217	0.710	0.323–1.562	0.395

Abbreviations: HR Hazard ratio, 95%CI 95% confidence interval, Re-RT Re-irradiation, LN Regional lymph node recurrence alone, PF Primary failure with/without regional lymph node recurrence, KPS Karnofsky performance status

and both (12.6%). This distribution deviated slightly from that in a previous study by Versteijne et al., which was 57%, 14% and 29% respectively [16]. This might be attributed to differences in the pathological composition of the tumors or radiation doses given for initial treatment. Also, in the current study, failure pattern (LN vs. PF) was an independent prognostic factor for OS. PF indicated a worse OS compared to LN ($P = 0.004$, HR = 0.3754, 95% confidence interval [CI] 0.1939–0.7266), which emphasized that good control of the primary tumor plays a vital role in ESCC management.

Patients with recurrent ESCC previously treated with RT who are in good clinical condition could be selected for potentially curative treatment. Previous study had

reported encouraging outcomes of re-RT for symptoms relief [17], in which 4 had complete resolution and 4 had diminished or stable symptoms among the 10 patients who presented with symptomatic disease. Moreover, Zhou et al. [18] reported that the 3-years OS for primary tumor recurrent ESCC was 21.8% with a MST of 20 months upon salvage RT group. Similarly, the 3-years OS was 22.89% among our re-RT patients with a MST of 21 months. The re-RT group had a significantly higher OS compared to the non-re-RT group in the current matched cohort ($P < 0.001$, HR = 0.2426, 95% CI 0.1294–0.4547). Yamashita et al. [19] reported a MST of 13.8 months for locoregional recurrent ESCC patients with re-RT. This inferior MST might be related to

Survival benefit of re-irradiation in esophageal Cancer patients with Locoregional...

117

differences in the recurrent tumor location and initial treatment baseline characteristics. Salvage doses of re-irradiation should be delivered to patients with localized disease to improve local control and OS.

Concurrent CRT is the standard treatment for ESCC patients who decline or cannot tolerate surgery. However, no evidence of survival benefits from concurrent CRT was found. Concurrent CRT was shown to cause severe acute esophagitis in 15–25% of thoracic radiotherapy cases [20]. In addition, most cases of recurrent ESCC occurred in older patients for whom concurrent CRT might be sub-optimal. In the current subgroup analysis, no statistical difference in OS was found between the groups treated with re-RT alone and re-RT combined with chemotherapy ($P = 0.70$). Also, two of three cases suffered from TEF upon concurrent CRT. Thus, concurrent CRT might increase toxicity without a survival benefit.

Concerning the potentially serious complications, re-RT was performed in a small and highly selected group of patients in clinical practice. In a prospective and randomized study, which included 34 patients who received re-RT and 35 patients who received dilatation alone, 6 cases of TEF were observed in the non-re-RT group, while no case of TEF was found in the re-RT group [21]. In the current study, no statistical differences were found in the incidence of TEF ($P = 0.613$) and pericardial/pleural effusion ($P = 0.197$) between re-RT and non-re-RT groups. As reported by Yamaguchi et al. [19], advanced T stage (T3 or T4) at the recurrence diagnosis was significantly associated with grade 3 or above toxicities. This might imply that TEF might associated with tumor progression. However, the impact of repair disability for re-irradiated tissues should also be considered.

RP is another concern in thoracic re-RT. Sumita et al. [22] had retrospectively analyzed 21 lung cancer patients who underwent X-ray beam re-RT and only one grade 3 RP was observed. The incidence of grade 3 RP was 24.24% for re-RT group in our study, but even with this high incidence of RP, no pneumonia-related deaths occurred. There was no correlation between RP and the V20 of the total lungs in the present study, which might relate to the limited sample, the different initial radiation schedules and interval. In addition, Ren et al. [23] showed that both re-RT and initial-RT influenced the incidence of grade 3 or above RP. However, further studies concerning the toxicities of the OARs are required.

As a retrospective study, records for symptoms such as dysphagia, weight loss, hoarseness, and cough were not available, and thus, symptom control was not evaluated in the present study. Moreover, because this was a single-center study, the number of cases was limited due to the rarity of re-RT treatment. Therefore, the implications of the findings could be limited.

Conclusions

Re-RT was feasible and beneficial for locoregional recurrent ESCC patients after primary RT. Compared to CRT, re-RT alone is more appropriate. Long-term survival was improved with re-RT. Despite a high incidence of RP, toxicities were tolerable.

Abbreviations
5-FU: 5-flurouracil; AJCC: American Joint Committee on Cancer; CRT: Chemoradiotherapy; CT: Computed tomography; CTCAE: National Cancer Institute Common Terminology Criteria for Adverse Events; ESCC: Esophageal squamous cell carcinoma; EUS: Endoscopic ultrasound; HR: Hazard ratios; KPS: Karnofsky performance status; LN: Regional lymph node recurrence only; MST: Median survival time; OS: Overall survival; PF: Primary failure with/without regional lymph node recurrence; PSM: Propensity score-matched; Re-RT: Re-irradiation; RFI: Recurrence-free interval; RP: Radiation pneumonitis; TEF: Tracheoesophageal fistula

Funding
This study was supported by The Fujian Province Natural Science Foundation (2016 J01437 and 2017 J01260), The Fujian Medical Innovation Project (2015-CX-8), Joint Funds for the Innovation of Science and Technology, Fujian province (2017Y9074) and Peking University Cancer Hospital & Institute, Key Laboratory of Carcinogenesis and Translational Research, Ministry of Education/Beijing (2017 Open Project-9).

Authors' contributions
All authors helped to perform the research; LH manuscript writing and performing procedures; YXH manuscript writing and data analysis; QYZ, XQZ and LRT contribution to drafting conception and design; KXD, XYL and BHZ contribution to writing the manuscript, JXW and SLC participated in data analysis; JLL contribution to writing the manuscript, drafting conception and design. All authors approved the final manuscript.

Competing interests
The authors declare that they have no competing interests.

Author details
[1]Department of Radiation Oncology, Fujian Medical University Cancer Hospital, Fujian Cancer Hospital, Fuzhou 350014, China. [2]Department of Radiation Oncology, Xiamen Humanity Hospital, Xiamen, China. [3]Biomedical Research Center of South China, Fujian Normal University, Fuzhou, China.

References
1. Welsh J, Settle SH, Amini A, Xiao L, Suzuki A, Hayashi Y, et al. Failure patterns in patients with esophageal cancer treated with definitive chemoradiation. Cancer. 2012;118(10):2632–40. [PMID:PMC3747650 10.1002/cncr.26586]
2. Pennathur A, Gibson MK, Jobe BA, Luketich JD. Oesophageal carcinoma. Lancet. 2013;381(9864):400–12. 10.1016/S0140-6736(12)60643-6]
3. Shioyama Y, Nakamura K, Ohga S, Nomoto S, Sasaki T, Yamaguchi T, et al. Radiation therapy for recurrent esophageal cancer after surgery: clinical results and prognostic factors. Jpn J Clin Oncol. 2007;37(12):918–23. 10.1093/jjco/hym138]
4. Markar SR, Karthikesalingam A, Penna M, Low DE. Assessment of short-term clinical outcomes following salvage esophagectomy for the treatment of esophageal malignancy: systematic review and pooled analysis. Ann Surg Oncol. 2014;21(3):922–31. 10.1245/s10434-013-3364-0]

5. Swisher SG, Wynn P, Putnam JB, Mosheim MB, Correa AM, Komaki RR, et al. Salvage esophagectomy for recurrent tumors after definitive chemotherapy and radiotherapy. J Thorac Cardiovasc Surg. 2002;123(1):175–83.

6. Bots WTC, van den Bosch S, Zwijnenburg EM, Dijkema T, van den Broek GB, Weijs WLJ, et al. Reirradiation of head and neck cancer: Long-term disease control and toxicity. Head Neck. 2017;39(6):1122–30. [PMID:PMC5485062 10.1002/hed.24733]

7. Chao HH, Berman AT, Simone CB 2nd, Ciunci C, Gabriel P, Lin H, et al. Multi-institutional prospective study of Reirradiation with proton beam radiotherapy for Locoregionally recurrent non-small cell lung Cancer. J Thorac Oncol. 2017;12(2):281–92. 10.1016/j.jtho.2016.10.018]

8. Zemlin A, Martens B, Wiese B, Merten R, Steinmann D. Timing of re-irradiation in recurrent high-grade gliomas: a single institution study. J Neurooncol. 2018;138(3):571-9. https://doi.org/10.1007/s11060-018-2824-6.

9. Kim YS. Reirradiation of head and neck cancer in the era of intensity-modulated radiotherapy: patient selection, practical aspects, and current evidence. Radiat Oncol J. 2017;35(1):1–15. [PMID:PMC5398346 10.3857/roj.2017.00122]

10. Nieder C, De Ruysscher D, Gaspar LE, Guckenberger M, Mehta MP, Cheung P, et al. Reirradiation of recurrent node-positive non-small cell lung cancer after previous stereotactic radiotherapy for stage I disease : a multi-institutional treatment recommendation. Strahlenther Onkol. 2017;193(7):515–24. 10.1007/s00066-017-1130-0]

11. Tao R, Tsai CJ, Jensen G, Eng C, Kopetz S, Overman MJ, et al. Hyperfractionated accelerated reirradiation for rectal cancer: an analysis of outcomes and toxicity. Radiother Oncol. 2017;122(1):146–51. 10.1016/j.radonc.2016.12.015]

12. Chen HY, Ma XM, Ye M, Hou YL, Xie HY, Bai YR. Esophageal perforation during or after conformal radiotherapy for esophageal carcinoma. J Radiat Res. 2014;55(5):940–7. [PMID:PMC4202289 10.1093/jrr/rru031]

13. Graves PR, Siddiqui F, Anscher MS, Movsas B. Radiation pulmonary toxicity: from mechanisms to management. Semin Radiat Oncol. 2010;20(3):201–7. 10.1016/j.semradonc.2010.01.010]

14. Huang F, Du C, Sun M, Ning B, Luo Y, An S. Propensity score matching in SPSS. Nan Fang Yi Ke Da Xue Xue Bao. 2015;35(11):1597–601.

15. Chen Y, Lu Y, Wang Y, Yang H, Xia Y, Chen M, et al. Comparison of salvage chemoradiation versus salvage surgery for recurrent esophageal squamous cell carcinoma after definitive radiochemotherapy or radiotherapy alone. Dis Esophagus : official journal of the International Society for Diseases of the Esophagus. 2014;27(2):134–40. 10.1111/j.1442-2050.2012.01440.x]

16. Versteijne E, van Laarhoven HW, van Hooft JE, van Os RM, Geijsen ED, van Berge Henegouwen MI, et al. Definitive chemoradiation for patients with inoperable and/or unresectable esophageal cancer: locoregional recurrence pattern. Dis Esophagus : official journal of the International Society for Diseases of the Esophagus. 2015;28(5):453–9. 10.1111/dote.12215]10.1111/dote.12215]

17. Fernandes A, Berman AT, Mick R, Both S, Lelionis K, Lukens JN, et al. A prospective study of proton beam Reirradiation for esophageal Cancer. Int J Radiat Oncol Biol Phys. 2016;95(1):483–7. 10.1016/j.ijrobp.2015.12.005]

18. Zhou ZG, Zhen CJ, Bai WW, Zhang P, Qiao XY, Liang JL, et al. Salvage radiotherapy in patients with local recurrent esophageal cancer after radical radiochemotherapy. Radiat Oncol. 2015;10:54. [PMID:PMC4351944 10.1186/s13014-015-0358-z]

19. Yamaguchi S, Ohguri T, Imada H, Yahara K, Moon SD, Higure A, et al. Multimodal approaches including three-dimensional conformal re-irradiation for recurrent or persistent esophageal cancer: preliminary results. J Radiat Res. 2011;52(6):812–20.

20. Werner-Wasik M, Pequignot E, Leeper D, Hauck W, Curran W. Predictors of severe esophagitis include use of concurrent chemotherapy, but not the length of irradiated esophagus: a multivariate analysis of patients with lung cancer treated with nonoperative therapy. Int J Radiat Oncol Biol Phys. 2000;48(3):689–96.

21. Teli MA, Mushood GN, Zargar SA, Andrabi WH. Comparative evaluation between re-irradiation and demand endoscopic dilatation vs endoscopic dilatation alone in patients with recurrent/reactivated residual in-field esophageal malignancies. J Cancer Res Ther. 2008;4(3):121–5.

22. Sumita K, Harada H, Asakura H, Ogawa H, Onoe T, Murayama S, et al. Re-irradiation for locoregionally recurrent tumors of the thorax: a single-institution, retrospective study. Radiat Oncol. 2016;11:104. [PMID: PMC4971641 10.1186/s13014-016-0673-z]

23. Ren C, Ji T, Liu T, Dang J, Li G. The risk and predictors for severe radiation pneumonitis in lung cancer patients treated with thoracic reirradiation. Radiat Oncol. 2018;13(1):69. [PMID:PMC5902864 10.1186/s13014-018-1016-z]

14

Technical and dosimetric implications of respiratory induced density variations in a heterogeneous lung phantom

Dennis J. Mohatt[1,2]* , Tianjun Ma[1,2], David B. Wiant[3], Naveed M. Islam[1,2], Jorge Gomez[2], Anurag K. Singh[2] and Harish K. Malhotra[1,2]

Abstract

Background: Stereotactic Body Radiotherapy (SBRT) is an ablative dose delivery technique which requires the highest levels of precision and accuracy. Modeling dose to a lung treatment volume has remained a complex and challenging endeavor due to target motion and the low density of the surrounding media. When coupled together, these factors give rise to pulmonary induced tissue heterogeneities which can lead to inaccuracies in dose computation. This investigation aims to determine which combination of imaging techniques and computational algorithms best compensates for time dependent lung target displacements.

Methods: A Quasar phantom was employed to simulate respiratory motion for target ranges up to 3 cm. 4DCT imaging was used to generate Average Intensity Projection (AIP), Free Breathing (FB), and Maximum Intensity Projection (MIP) image sets. In addition, we introduce and compare a fourth dataset for dose computation based on a novel phase weighted density (PWD) technique. All plans were created using Eclipse version 13.6 treatment planning system and calculated using the Analytical Anisotropic Algorithm and Acuros XB. Dose delivery was performed using Truebeam STx linear accelerator where radiochromic film measurements were accessed using gamma analysis to compare planned versus delivered dose.

Results: In the most extreme case scenario, the mean CT difference between FB and MIP datasets was found to be greater than 200 HU. The near maximum dose discrepancies between AAA and AXB algorithms were determined to be marginal ($< 2.2\%$), with a greater variability occurring within the near minimum dose regime ($< 7\%$). Radiochromatic film verification demonstrated all AIP and FB based computations exceeded 98% passing rates under conventional radiotherapy tolerances (gamma 3%, 3 mm). Under more stringent SBRT tolerances (gamma 3%, 1 mm), the AIP and FB based treatment plans exhibited higher pass rates ($> 85\%$) when compared to MIP and PWD ($< 85\%$) for AAA computations. For AXB, however, the delivery accuracy for all datasets were greater than 85% (gamma 3%,1 mm), with a corresponding reduction in overall lung irradiation.

(Continued on next page)

* Correspondence: djmohatt@buffalo.edu
[1]Medical Physics Program, Jacobs School of Medicine and Biomedical Sciences, University at Buffalo, Buffalo, NY 14214-3005, USA
[2]Department of Radiation Medicine, Roswell Park Cancer Institute, Buffalo, NY 14293, USA
Full list of author information is available at the end of the article

(Continued from previous page)

Conclusions: Despite the substantial density variations between computational datasets over an extensive range of target movement, the dose difference between CT datasets is small and could not be quantified with ion chamber. Radiochromatic film analysis suggests the optimal CT dataset is dependent on the dose algorithm used for evaluation. With AAA, AIP and FB resulted in the best conformance between measured versus calculated dose for target motion ranging up to 3 cm under both conventional and SBRT tolerance criteria. With AXB, pass rates improved for all datasets with the PWD technique demonstrating slightly better conformity over AIP and FB based computations (gamma 3%, 1 mm). As verified in previous studies, our results confirm a clear advantage in delivery accuracy along with a relative decrease in calculated dose to the lung when using Acuros XB over AAA.

Keywords: Lung SBRT, Acuros XB, Respiratory induced tissue heterogeneity, Phase weighted density,

Background

Stereotactic Body Radiotherapy (SBRT) is an ablative dose delivery technique which requires the highest levels of precision and accuracy [1, 2]. Modeling dose to a lung treatment volume has remained a complex and challenging endeavor for two major reasons. First, the gross tumor volume (GTV) is typically surrounded by lung tissue approximately 75% less dense than the tumor itself [3]. Second, the actual density of the treatment volume is further complicated by the movement of GTV due to patient respiratory motion. Even though certain motion management techniques [4] such as deep inspirational breath hold [5], abdominal compression [6], tumor tracking [7] and respiratory gating [8] have been incorporated with lung SBRT to restrict the size of the irradiated target volume, an additional margin to account for set-up errors is still required which encompasses a substantial portion of low density lung tissue [9]. When coupled together these factors give rise to pulmonary induced tissue heterogeneities which could possibly lead to inaccuracies in dose computation [10].

The accuracy of the dose distributions predicted by the treatment planning system is of critical importance in maximizing the tumor control probability in lung SBRT [11, 12]. Tissue heterogeneity is of particular interest for dose computation in the lung due to the relative low electron density which requires greater photon fluence to achieve a similar build-up equilibrium equivalent to that of soft tissue. Compared to homogeneous media, where modeling of high energy photon beams is a relatively straight forward process, energy transport in heterogeneous media involves an intricate extrapolation of various density-dependent correction factors. To date, the most accurate dose computational algorithm for handling highly heterogeneous media is Monte Carlo (MC) simulation [13] –unfortunately it requires the greatest processing time [14]. For enhanced computational performance, alternative algorithms [15] such as Analytical Anisotropic Algorithm (AAA) [16]

and Acuros External Beam (AXB) [17] have been commercially developed which implement various levels of simplifications and assumptions to allow calculations to be completed within clinically acceptable time frames. Fundamentally, material density with AAA is accounted for anisotropically by the implementation of Gaussian weighted photon scattering kernels [18]. In contrast, AXB seeks a more direct approach in solving the linear Boltzmann transfer equation by taking into consideration the specific chemical composition of the surrounding media [19]. Still, dose computational accuracy in all respects is ultimately governed by the actual target density as defined by the CT dataset.

Model based algorithms provide a realistic generation of absorbed dose in heterogeneous media by sampling CT values (Hounsfield Units –HU). This information is then used to scale high energy particle interactions with respect to actual physical density. In modern radiology, 4D computed tomography (4DCT) has become the standard to account for changes in patient anatomy during respiration [20, 21]. Generally, the most common CT datasets used for dose computation for lung SBRT are average intensity projection (AIP) and free breathing (FB). However, FB is essentially a single phase snapshot of the GTV at a given location in time which does not capture the effects of target movement, whereas AIP will compress all temporal motion information into a single 3DCT image. While AIP imaging assigns the average pixel value to a specific location, we also considered the maximum intensity projection (MIP) in this study which assigns only the greatest point pixel value to represent our highest target density scenario. In addition, we introduced a fourth dataset based on a novel phase weighted density (PWD) technique. With the PWD approach, sub-regions generated by 10 individual phased GTV structures were overridden with specific CT values based on the temporal dependence of the GTV overlap.

Despite all state-of-the-art advances in radiological imaging, the medical physics community has yet to reach a consensus to best account for dynamic target motion in heterogeneous media. To date, a limited number of studies have been conducted to compare different image generated datasets [22–27]. However, no systematic study exists to determine which is better for dose computation. Although Monte Carlo simulation is recognized as the gold standard for handling tissue heterogeneity, its use in the clinical environment has been very limited. This investigation aims to determine which combination of imaging techniques and algorithms yields the most accurate dose distributions, under extreme lung density variations, that are experimentally achievable within a clinical environment.

In this study, we evaluate the physical properties associated with motion-induced lung target densities by comparing representative image sets. In addition, we introduce an innovative PWD dataset based on the time dependent location of the GTV structure over the course of one respiratory cycle. We compared each plan calculated for AAA and AXB, and evaluated these dose distributions with respect to the actual dose delivered using radiochromatic film. To ensure our assessment certainty, end-to-end testing of all plans was generated using one treatment planning system, and then delivered using a single Truebeam STx linear accelerator.

Methods

Lung tumor motion was simulated using a Quasar Respiratory Motion Phantom (Modus, London, Ontario, CA) as shown in Fig. 1. To replicate clinically relevant tissue properties, the phantom contains a low density cedar wood insert that mimics lung tissue (HU = − 750 − -600). This encapsulates an offset spherical polystyrene target (HU = − 100 − 0) 3.0 cm in diameter. The Quasar apparatus provided simple harmonic motion along the superior-inferior direction for which the target range was adjusted to ±0.5, ±1.0, and ± 1.5 cm translational increments at 15 cycles per minute.

Calculations in anthropomorphic phantom

Heterogeneous density calculations were performed using the Quasar Phantom in a static configuration. A single anterior field (3.0×3.0 cm^2) was aligned perpendicular to the phantom and prescribed with fixed monitor units of 500 MU for photon energy of 6 MV flattening filter free as shown in Fig. 2a. Dose distributions along the beam central axis, as function of depth, were then calculated using AAA and AXB algorithms with 0.2 cm^3 grid size. As illustrated in Fig. 2b, points of interest were selected along the central axis where P1 is located 3 cm anterior to the target, P2 at the target isocenter, P3 is 3 cm posterior to the target center, and P4 beyond the lung cavity located 2 cm below P3. To mimic density variation effects caused by tumor movement, the CT values of the target structure were systematically overridden from − 200 to + 200 in increments of 25 HU. Due to the density variation of the target structure, a relationship between the dose errors was represented as percentage dose change relative to nominal HU value of the target for each point of interest.

4DCT imaging and target delineations

4DCT image sets were acquired using a GE Lightspeed Pro 16 slice scanner (General Electric, Milwaukee, WI), with a slice width setting of 1.25 mm. Respiratory cycle information was subsequently recorded using a Real-time Position Management (RPM) system (Varian, Palo Alto, CA). In general, the external movement of the phantom was synchronized to the internal movement of the target via an illuminated infrared signal reflected from a marker block and directed to a CCD camera. The recorded respiratory waveform was then referenced in the binning process to coordinated projected image sets, with respect to their appropriate anatomical locations, over the course of one respiratory period. Reconstructed images and respiratory data were then transferred to Advantage 4D workstation (General Electric, Milwaukee, WI). These images were sorted and binned with respect to couch position and corresponding respiratory phase at ten uniformly spaced intervals within the respiratory cycle, with CT$_{0\%}$ indicating the max-inhalation phase and CT$_{50\%}$ the max exhalation phase. From these bins, AIP and MIP image sets were automatically generated by selecting

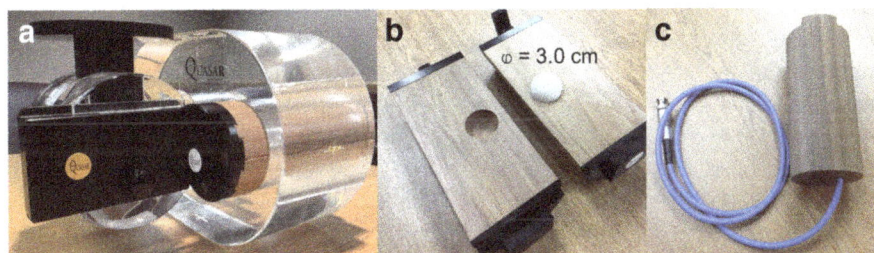

Fig. 1 **a** Quasar phantom with (**b**) cedar lung insert encapsulating an offset polystyrene target 3.0 cm diameter. **c** Shows an identical cedar insert with imbedded 3.0 cm target bored out to fit a 0.125 cc ion chamber at isocenter

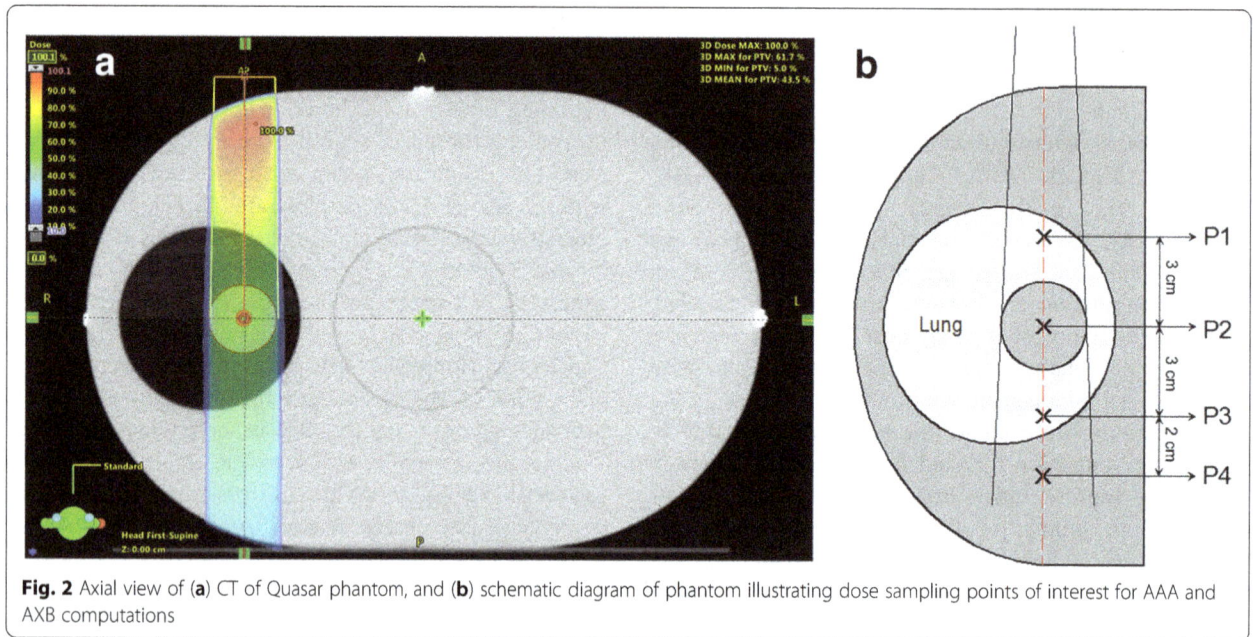

Fig. 2 Axial view of (**a**) CT of Quasar phantom, and (**b**) schematic diagram of phantom illustrating dose sampling points of interest for AAA and AXB computations

the average and the maximum pixel densities across all respiratory phases of the 4DCT dataset, respectively. A subsequent helical image was also taken immediately after the 4DCT acquisitions and was designated as the corresponding free-breathing (FB) scan. This procedure was repeated for target amplitudes ranging from ±0.5 to ±1.5 cm at ±0.5 cm increments, for which the processed images were imported into Eclipse (version 13.6) treatment planning system (TPS). Furthermore, an additional FB scan was taken with the no phantom motion and planned accordingly for verification of image registration and dose calibration process.

In order to infer the motion information using Eclipse, manual contouring of individual GTVs was performed on individual CT image sets within multiple respiratory phases ($CT_{0\%}$ - $CT_{90\%}$). To avoid any interplanner differences, all contours were segmented by one individual using the same lung window setting in all image sets. The internal target volume (ITV) structure was then generated using Boolean "OR" operation to union all 10 GTV phased structures from individual CT image sets corresponding to set motion amplitude. In accordance with RTOG 0915 protocol, the planned treatment volume (PTV) was then created by expanding a uniformly isotropic 0.5 cm margin from the ITV [9]. All ITV and PTV structures were initially created in the FB image set and subsequently copied to the AIP, MIP and PWD datasets.

It is noted in a similar study, the Mid-Ventilation ($CT_{50\%}$) image set was included for comparative analysis [25]. With the exception of target location, the target density associated with $CT_{50\%}$ is very similar to that represented by the FB image set. Therefore, since the

central focus of this current study is to evaluate the extreme density variations between datasets, examination of $CT_{50\%}$ was not taken into consideration in order to circumvent redundancy.

Defining the phased weighted density structure

In addition to the FB, AIP and MIP CT datasets, we created a hybrid phase weighted density (PWD) structure for comparison. In principle, the changing density of the target region over time can be generalized by the following relation:

$$d\rho = \left(\rho_{GTV} + \rho_{lung}\right)dt \tag{1}$$

where ρ_{GTV} is the target density, and ρ_{lung} represents the density of the lung. It follows that a solution for the density for a PWD structure (ρ_{PWD}) yields the following expression

$$\rho_{PWD} = \left(\frac{t}{T}\right)\rho_{GTV} + \left(\frac{(T-t)}{T}\right)\rho_{lung} \tag{2}$$

where t is the occupational time of the GTV at one location, and T is the period of the respiratory cycle. In practice, the duration of t occurs at discrete increments of 1/10th of the respiratory period in association with the phase binning process. Thus, as illustrated in Fig. 3, the final t value reflects how many times the GTV has overlapped with itself during the period of oscillation, giving rise to higher density within a particular sub-region.

Discrete sub-regions within the ITV were created by the addition and/or subtraction of the 10 individually defined GTV phase binned structures, using Boolean

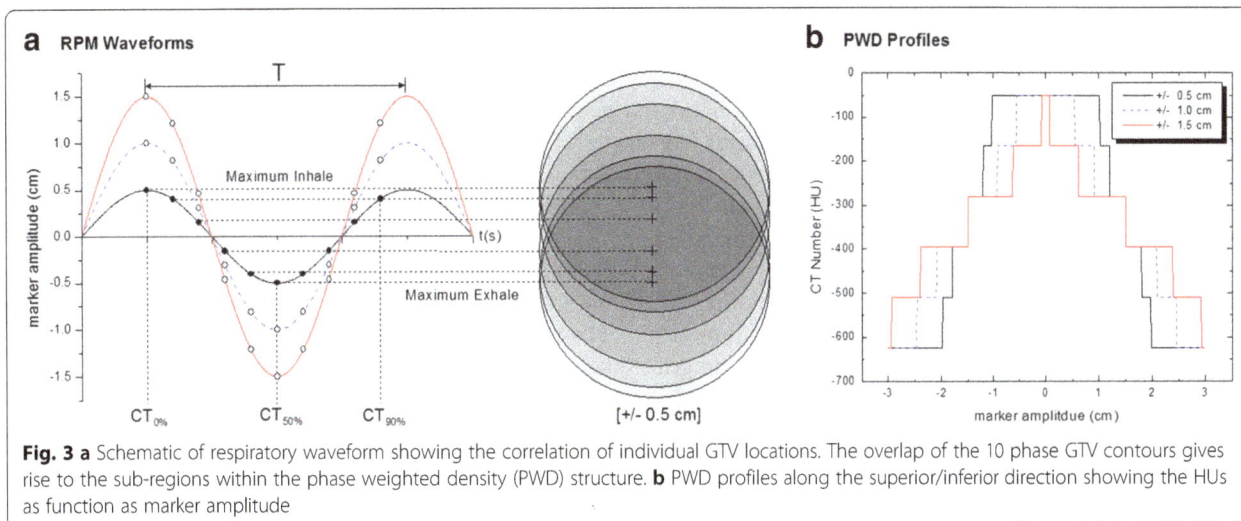

Fig. 3 a Schematic of respiratory waveform showing the correlation of individual GTV locations. The overlap of the 10 phase GTV contours gives rise to the sub-regions within the phase weighted density (PWD) structure. **b** PWD profiles along the superior/inferior direction showing the HUs as function as marker amplitude

operations within the TPS. CT values for each sub-region were then overridden and weighted accordingly to the mean GTV (− 50 HU) and lung (− 625 HU) density value as defined by the FB image set.

HU density extraction

HU voxel values for each PTV structure were extracted using an in-house program written in Matlab (MATLAB, The MathWorks Inc., Natick, MA, 2017). For FB, AIP and MIP data set, original DICOM CT images and RT structures were directly imported into Matlab software. Based on the corresponding contoured structure set, a binary mask was created to segment out the region of interest (ROI) for HU data export. The output of all HU values inside the ROI for each image set were then analyzed as a histogram format ranging from CT numbers − 850 to 50 HU with bin size of 20. Plotting and statistical analysis was performed using Origin (version 6.0) software. Using the HU density extraction method, Fig. 4 shows the histogram representations for the (a) cedar insert, (b) polystyrene target, and (c) PTV structure.

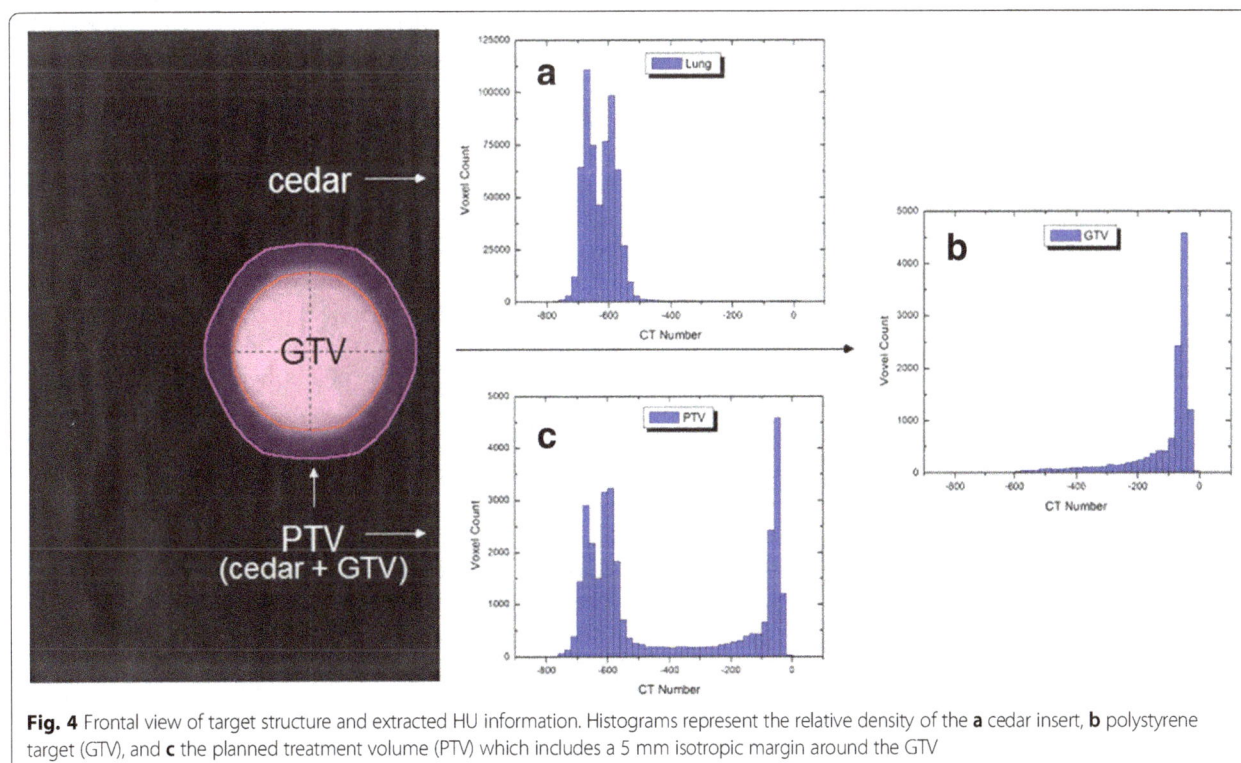

Fig. 4 Frontal view of target structure and extracted HU information. Histograms represent the relative density of the **a** cedar insert, **b** polystyrene target (GTV), and **c** the planned treatment volume (PTV) which includes a 5 mm isotropic margin around the GTV

Treatment planning

Individual treatment plans were created from FB, AIP, MIP and PWD datasets in Eclipse. Irradiation of the target structure was planned for a photon 6 MV flattening filter free beam using simple Anterior-Posterior (AP) and Posterior-Anterior field configurations. The MLC was fitted to the shape of the PTV and collimator jaws were set to the recommended position determined by the TPS, with width spacing no less than 3.5 cm as dictated by RTOG protocol [9]. Dose calculations for each plan were executed using AAA and AXB algorithms at a predetermined value of 500 MU per field for 0.2 cm grid size. The initial parameters for segmented ITV and PTV structures for each range of motion are summarized in Table 1.

Radiochromatic film measurements

Phantom set up was done using the same simulation positions for dose delivery by means of a TrueBeam STx. The dose from the treatment planning system was verified using an identical cedar insert phantom (Modus, Model No. 500–3332) specifically designed to house a PTW 0.125 cc ion chamber (Fig. 1c). Gafchromic EBT3 film (International Specialty Products, Wayne, NJ, Lot #: 03311401) was used for both film calibration and phantom measurements. The film was positioned inside the cedar insert, central to the target location and marked at the time of irradiation. Each phantom irradiation measurement was repeated 3 times for which subsequent measurements were taken to reference machine output and scaled to film response. The film was then stored in a dry, dark environment for 24 h and later scanned using Epson Perfection V700 flatbed scanner (Epson America, Inc. Long Beach, Ca) with 48 bit color and 150 dpi resolution. RIT113 (Radiological Imaging Technology, Inc., Colorado Springs, CO) version 5.1 software was used to analyze the film using the red channel. A dose calibration curve for the red channel was generated by irradiating individual films for known doses from 0 to 10 Gy.

Due to phantom motion, the center of film does not remain in the center of dose distribution over the time of delivery. Hence, dose generated from a static CT by the TPS cannot be directly compared to the dose measured on moving film (consult Ref [26] for an excellent review of the dose smearing effect and compensation). Film motion was accounted for by convolving the TPS

dose using a custom script written in MATLAB developed by Wiant et al. [26]. Convolved dose plane distributions were then imported into RIT113 software for gamma analysis. As formulated by Low, the standard criterion for "measured" versus "calculated" dose was evaluated for a particular dose threshold within an acceptance radius (i.e. 3%, 3 mm) [28].

Results

Anthropomorphic lung phantom calculations

The results of our phantom calculations in a static configuration are shown in Fig. 5a, b. For a single AP field as shown in Fig. 2a, the percent depth dose (PDD) profiles for AAA and AXB are plotted in Fig. 5a. When compared to calculations with no heterogeneity, both the AAA and AXB profiles are virtually identical as indicated by the dashed line. The algorithms reveal a subtle distinction between lung versus tumor media, which is unnoticeable when heterogeneity is turned off. Interestingly, the first time these curves intersect after the build-up region, is near isocenter of the target. This is where the target density is roughly equivalent to that of water.

Figure 5b shows the trend in dose errors at particular points of interest in reference to Fig. 2b. For each point, the percentage dose error is defined relative to the nominal CT value of the GTV structure, which was overridden spanning from – 200 to 200 HU. For the fixed point located just above the target (P1), both AAA and AXB traces are flat lined and unaffected by the downstream change of target density. At isocenter (P2), the negative slope associated with AXB calculation indicates the relative increase in target density, or photon attenuation. This attenuation is compensated for by the decrease of photon fluence. On the other hand, the slightly positive slope associated with the AAA algorithm indicates an opposing effect caused by secondary electron transport. As interpreted in a related study by Liu, the density variation of the target when using AAA makes a larger impact on electron fluence over photon attenuation, where electron fluence becomes the dominating factor for compensation [29]. For points beyond the target structure, both algorithms show a similar attenuation response to the target density variation within the lung (P3), and beyond (P4) where electron equilibrium is re-established.

Extracted PTV density formations

The wide range of density variations for each PTV structure is illustrated in Fig. 6. As shown from left to right, each column represents an additional 1 cm increase in target movement. Each row displays voxel count versus CT number as defined by the AIP, FB, MIP and PWD data sets. Due to the 5 mm isotropic margin expansion

Table 1 A summary of the initial parameters for all ranges of target motion

Range of motion (cm)	ITV (cc)	PTV (cc)	Rx Dose (MU)
1 [± 0.5]	21.87	48.41	500
2 [± 1.0]	27.36	58.33	500
3 [± 1.5]	34.64	71.13	500

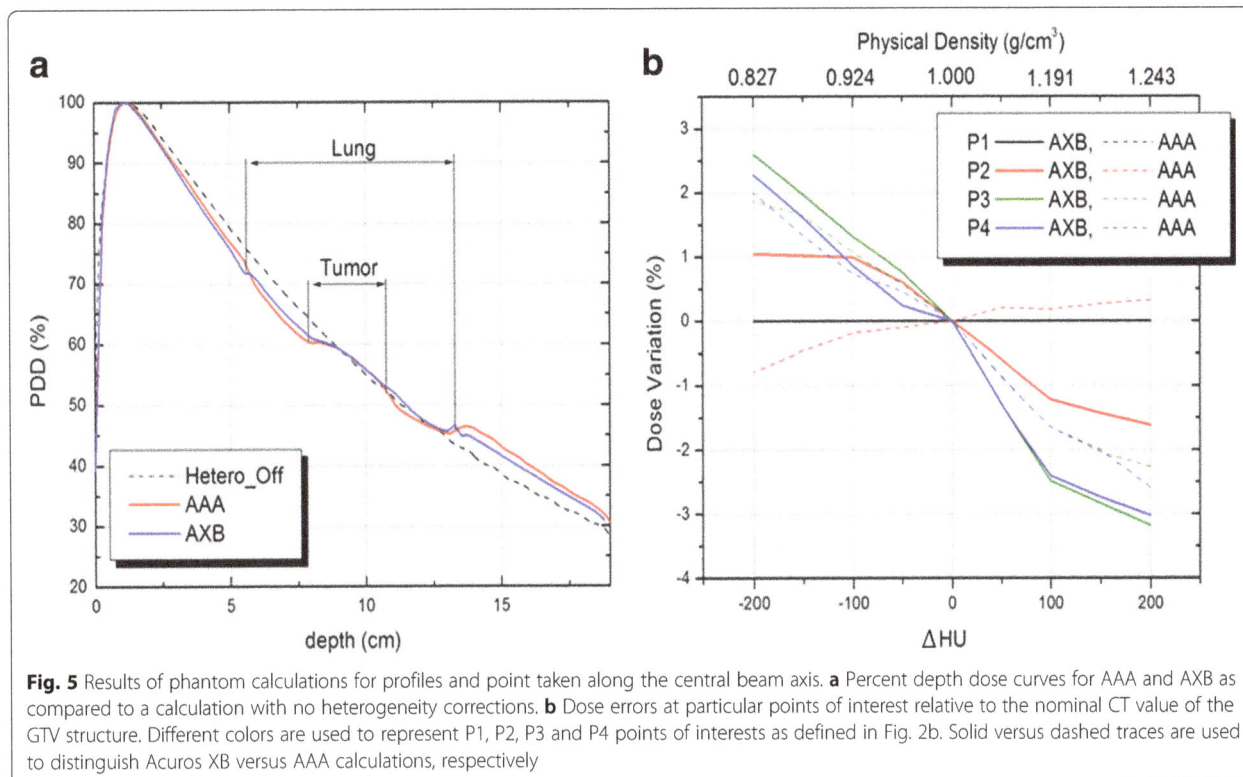

Fig. 5 Results of phantom calculations for profiles and point taken along the central beam axis. **a** Percent depth dose curves for AAA and AXB as compared to a calculation with no heterogeneity corrections. **b** Dose errors at particular points of interest relative to the nominal CT value of the GTV structure. Different colors are used to represent P1, P2, P3 and P4 points of interests as defined in Fig. 2b. Solid versus dashed traces are used to distinguish Acuros XB versus AAA calculations, respectively

from the ITV, the PTV will include a significant portion of low density media concentrated at approximately – 625 HU. In general, as the range of target movement increases, the GTV peak (center around – 50 HU) will essentially become absorbed into the lower density media. This effect is most pronounced for FB data sets, where the average CT number decreases from – 479 to – 569 HU, versus AIP – 473 to – 524 HU, and PWD – 472 to – 507. For MIP data sets, the average CT number remains fairly consistent ranging from – 352 to – 370 HU. Thus, in our most extreme case scenario, the difference between low density FB and high density MIP data sets is greater than 200 HU. The PTV average CT values extracted from each dataset are listed in Table 2.

AAA vs. AXB Dosimetric impact

Results for mean PTV HU values and dosimetric differences between AXB versus AAA are listed in Table 2. In this analysis we considered the dosimetric parameters (D_{max}, $D_{2\%}$, D_{mean}, $D_{95\%}$, $D_{98\%}$) as evaluated from dose volume histograms (DVH). When compared with AXB, AAA will consistently overestimate the dose to the treatment volume. This is indicated by a negative sign for a predominant portion of the analysis with exceptions occurring at D_{mean} ($D_{50\%}$) –the approximate location of where the two curves may intersect. In general, the near maximum dose ($D_{2\%}$) discrepancies are marginal (< 2.2%), with a greater variability occurring

within the near minimum ($D_{98\%}$) dose regime (< 7.0%). Considering that the size of the PTV structure increases as range of motion increases (see Table 1), the resulting widening of collimator jaws will yield a slight increase in dose at target isocenter. This can be depicted by the standard deviation. Thus, even for extended range of target motion, the dose discrepancies between the two algorithms near target isocenter are still small, with the greatest differences observed for MIP (2.1 ± 0.1%), followed by PWD (1.9 ± 0.6%), AIP (1.3 ± 0.1%), and least with FB (0.9 ± 0.4%).

A direct comparison of AAA versus AXB calculated planner dose distributions are illustrated in Fig. 7. Plans generated using the AIP, FB, MIP and PWD image sets for all ranges of motion are benchmarked with respect to AXB-based computations. Using nominal gamma criteria of 3%, 3 mm, all plans are virtually identical with pass rates of 100%. However, when switching to a most stringent criteria of 1%, 0 mm, the gamma index is anywhere from 73.2–54.0%. This predominantly high region of failure is occurring on the left side of the dose distribution in each case, and is caused by a relatively larger cedar gap in the phantom geometry (see Fig. 2b). Hence, in the lower density region the AAA calculation is overestimating the dose to the target, while the AXB algorithm compensates for photon attenuation of the target itself. Likewise, the greater overall discrepancies are generally occurring with the higher density MIP datasets.

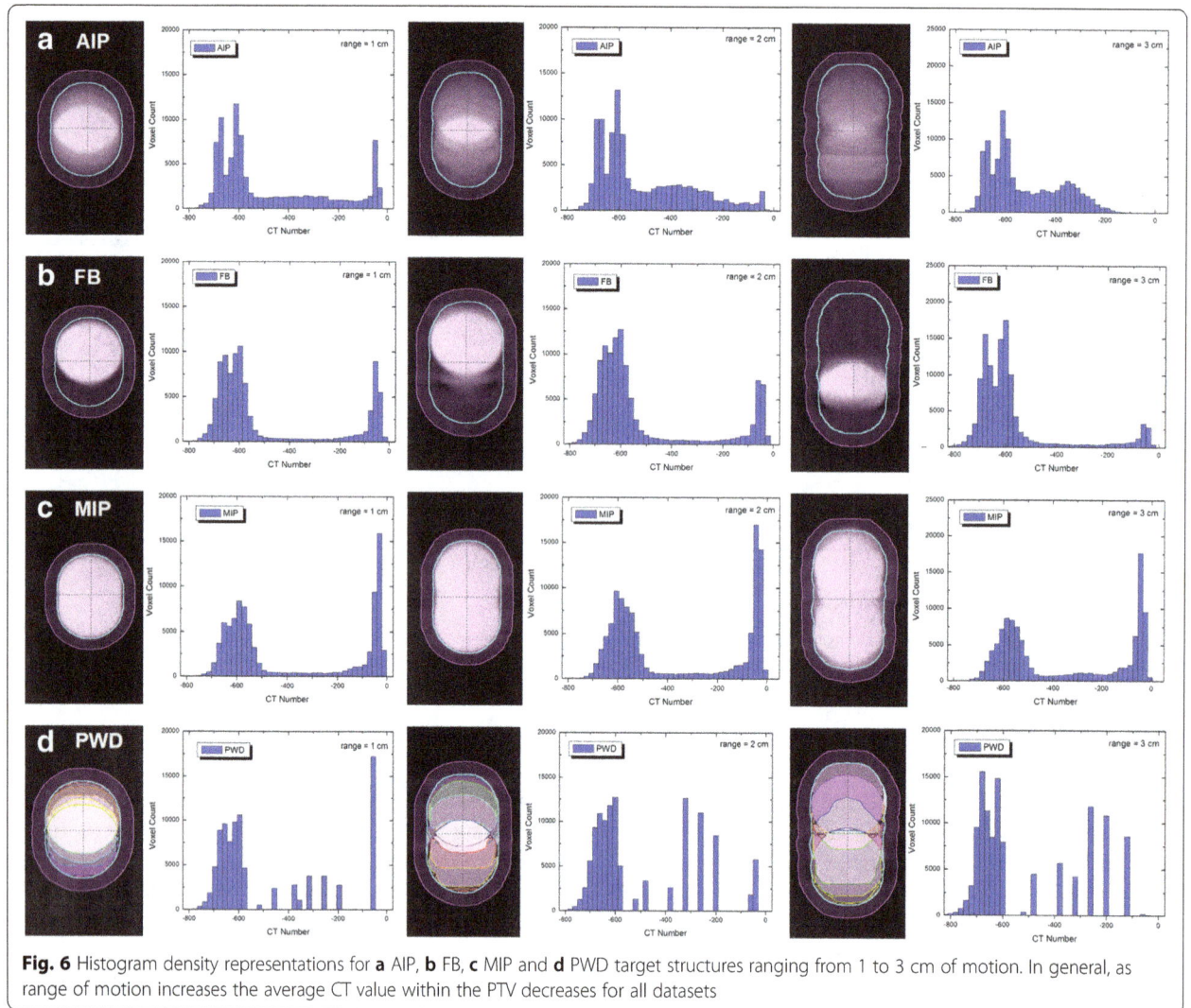

Fig. 6 Histogram density representations for **a** AIP, **b** FB, **c** MIP and **d** PWD target structures ranging from 1 to 3 cm of motion. In general, as range of motion increases the average CT value within the PTV decreases for all datasets

Table 2 The mean HU values per PTV and percentage difference for dosimetric parameters between AXB vs AAA calculations. For 1–3 cm superior-inferior target motion, the dose difference for FB, AIP, MIP and PWD datasets is given via $\Delta D = \left(\frac{D_{AXB} - D_{AAA}}{D_{AXB}}\right) x 100\%$

Target range	CT dataset	<HU> ±sd	ΔD_{max}	$\Delta D_{2\%}$	ΔD_{mean}	$\Delta D_{95\%}$	$\Delta D_{98\%}$
1 cm	AIP	-473 ± 223	−1.40	−1.40	0.06	−4.63	−4.80
	FB	−479 ± 246	−1.40	− 1.34	0.03	−4.39	− 5.22
	MIP	−370 ± 266	− 1.82	−2.17	− 0.09	−4.49	−4.79
	PWD	−472 ± 239	− 2.12	−2.52	− 0.33	−2.37	− 3.34
2 cm	AIP	− 503 ± 178	− 1.75	− 1.31	− 0.08	−5.07	− 5.43
	FB	−507 ± 227	− 0.91	− 0.50	0.23	− 4.92	− 6.73
	MIP	− 356 ± 259	− 1.91	− 2.15	−0.36	− 4.52	−4.32
	PWD	− 490 ± 207	−1.40	− 1.37	−0.06	− 4.26	− 5.43
3 cm	AIP	−524 ± 143	−1.54	− 1.16	− 0.23	−5.64	− 6.68
	FB	−569 ± 178	− 0.72	− 0.80	0.20	− 3.26	− 3.71
	MIP	− 352 ± 249	− 2.14	−2.10	−0.62	−5.42	− 6.91
	PWD	−507 ± 208	− 1.98	− 1.87	−0.37	−4.68	−5.28

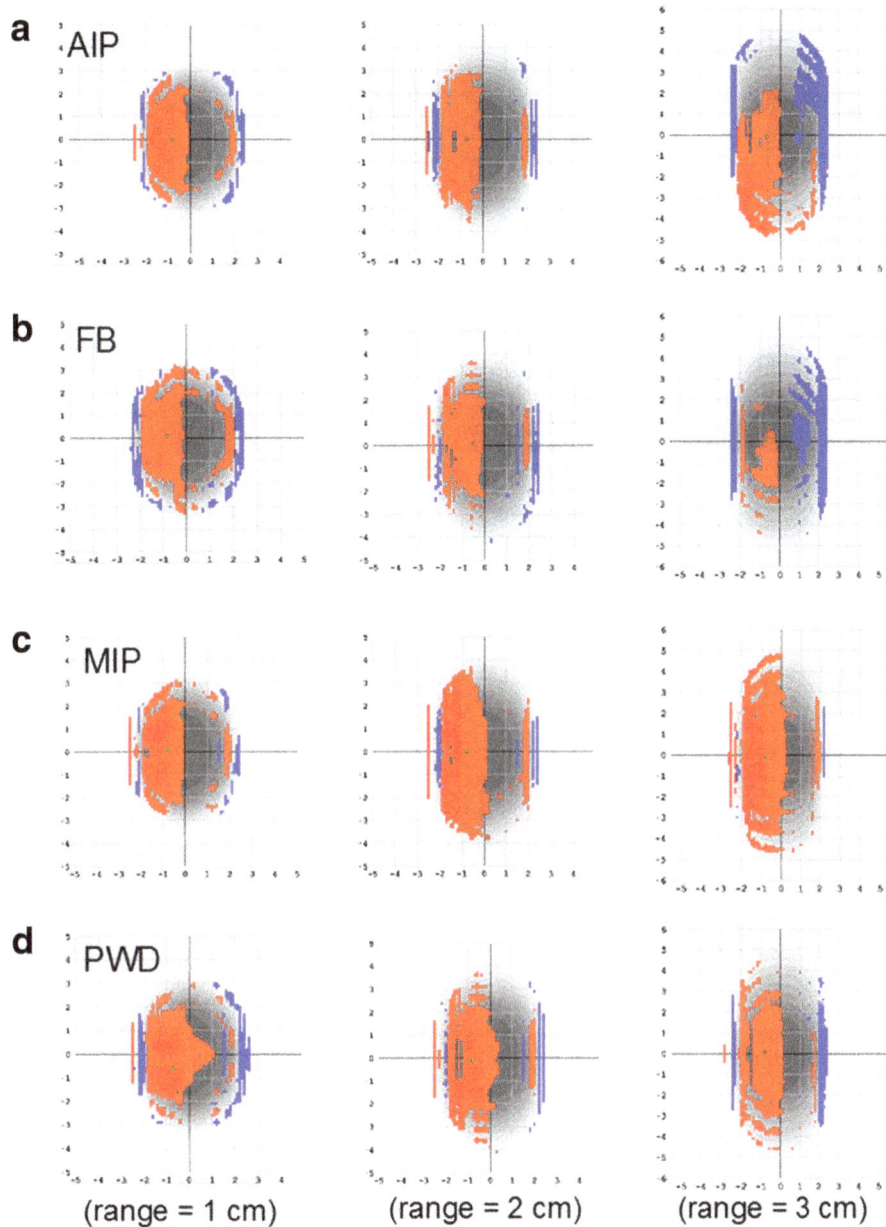

Fig. 7 A planner view of the dose distribution mismatch between AAA versus AXB computations. Plans were calculated for **a** AIP, **b** FB, **c** MIP, and **d** PWD data sets for target range of motion spanning from 1 to 3 cm (left to right). The analysis shown here is based on stringent gamma criteria (1%, 0 mm), where regions in red are indicating higher AAA dose calculation, versus blue for lower dose as with respect to AXB

Radiochromic film verification

All plans were measured using an identical lung insert phantom modified for PTW 0.125 cc ion chamber and were determined to be within < 2% agreement with the treatment planning system. However, these measurements yield only one data point at isocenter. Therefore, gafchromic film analysis was used for complete distribution comparisons for which the verification of the image registration and dose calibration process is shown in Fig. 8. Each static measurement was repeated three times in conjunction with our motion runs, for which the film was analyzed for the same plans calculated for AAA and AXB. These results demonstrate the accuracy and reproducibility for the systematic method of measurement used in this study when no motion was employed. Furthermore, they tend to rule out the inherent uncertainty that may be associated with the differences between both algorithms in question, and suggest the subsequent discrepancies have to do with

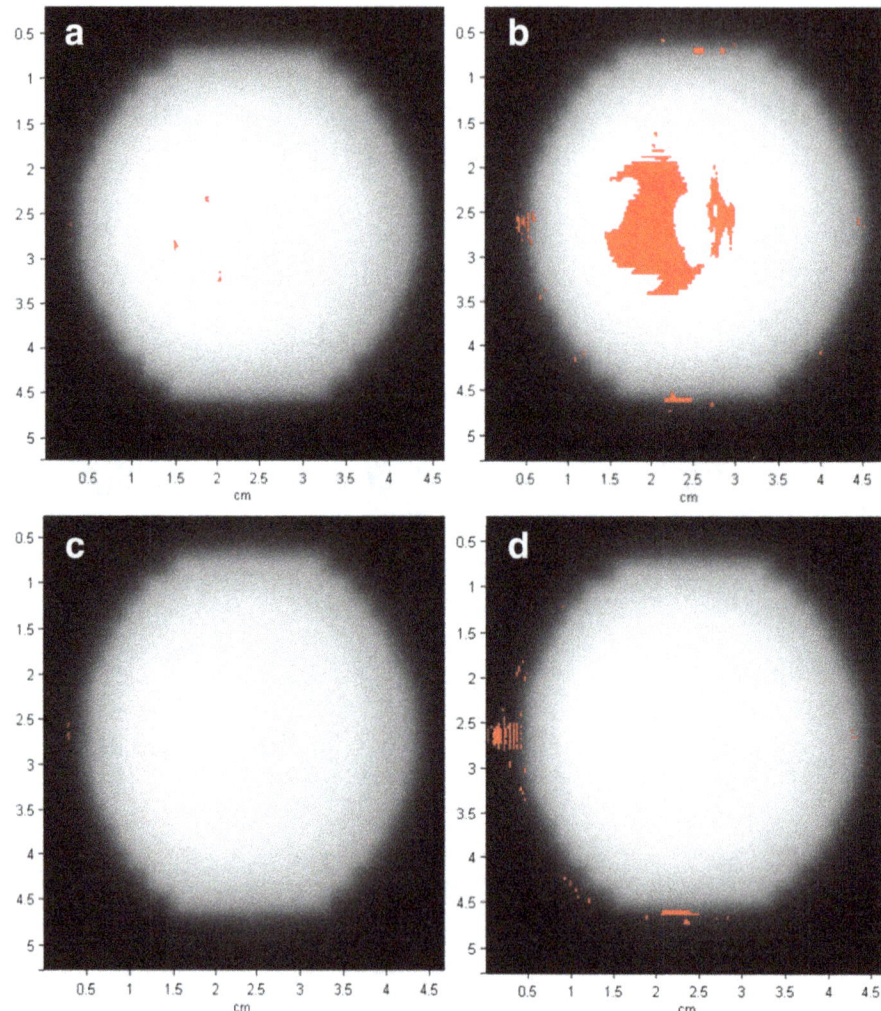

Fig. 8 Gafchromic film verification of image registration and dose calibration. Gamma pass rates for: **a** AAA (3%,3 mm) 99.0 ± 1.5%, **b** AAA (3%,1 mm) 91.1 ± 3.8%, **c** AXB (3%,3 mm) 99.7 ± 0.2%, and **d** AXB (3%,1 mm) 95.7 ± 3.6%. The red indicate failed pixels for which the gamma index is greater than 1 [28]

the density distributions that are represented by the CT datasets once the phantom was sent into motion.

Table 3 summarizes the film results for target motion amplitudes up to ±1.5 cm. Under conventional tolerances (gamma 3%, 3 mm), AIP and FB image sets generated plans with pass rates greater than 98% for both AAA and AXB based computations. When switching to SBRT tolerances (3%, 1 mm), MIP and PWD based AAA computations generally fell below 85% pass rates, and gradually degraded as range of motion increased. However, AXB pass rates for all image sets showed a substantial improvement in delivery accuracy when compared to AAA. Interestingly, the pass rates for the higher density MIP image set yielded comparable results (> 85%) to those of AIP and FB when calculated for AXB algorithm. Although PWD dataset did not perform well for large ranges of

motion when evaluated with AAA, PWD demonstrated a slightly better conformance over AIP and FB when using Acuros XB.

A comparison of the dose profiles for 3 cm of motion are shown in Fig. 9a–h. As seen in the left column, the TPS calculated dose for AAA is consistently overestimated with respect to that being measured, and more prominent with respect to MIP and PWD based computations. On the other hand, in the right column the AXB profiles show better conformance with TPS calculated versus measured dose, which give rise to higher pass rates.

Discussion

Motivation for this research was inspired by a related virtual slab phantom study performed by Aarup. He first reported a large discrepancy between MC and Pencil

Table 3 Summary of gamma pass rates (%) for gafchromic film measurements. All plans were measured on 3 separate instances where the error depicts the standard deviation

Range of motion (cm)	CT dataset	AAA		AXB	
		(3%, 3 mm)	(3%, 1 mm)	(3%, 3 mm)	(3%, 1 mm)
1 cm	AIP	99.4 ± 0.4	86.4 ± 5.2	99.8 ± 0.1	88.0 ± 4.1
	FB	98.7 ± 0.7	86.9 ± 5.0	99.8 ± 0.1	88.2 ± 3.6
	MIP	95.9 ± 3.6	80.5 ± 5.7	99.7 ± 0.2	89.8 ± 3.6
	PWD	97.1 ± 3.2	85.7 ± 3.5	99.7 ± 0.2	89.4 ± 5.7
2 cm	AIP	98.6 ± 0.7	85.0 ± 2.3	99.0 ± 0.4	86.8 ± 3.9
	FB	99.3 ± 1.2	87.1 ± 5.6	99.6 ± 0.8	86.8 ± 4.7
	MIP	98.2 ± 0.2	77.8 ± 4.5	99.5 ± 0.8	85.8 ± 4.0
	PWD	98.4 ± 2.5	83.2 ± 4.5	99.6 ± 0.3	89.1 ± 3.6
3 cm	AIP	98.1 ± 1.6	85.4 ± 4.5	99.1 ± 0.8	91.2 ± 1.7
	FB	98.4 ± 1.3	88.8 ± 3.5	99.1 ± 0.8	91.7 ± 4.6
	MIP	94.2 ± 3.8	69.4 ± 5.9	98.9 ± 0.8	88.1 ± 1.5
	PWD	94.1 ± 0.4	76.0 ± 5.2	99.3 ± 0.6	94.2 ± 4.2

Beam Convolution (PBC) based dose computations which systematically depended on the density of the surrounding lung tissue [30]. In other previous studies comparing alternative CT data sets, Huang et al. compared the dosimetric accuracy for AIP and MIP projection images for regular and irregular breathing motion [22], Han et al. compared geometric center differences for helical (FB) and AIP image sets [23], and Tian et al. reported on small but significant dosimetric differences between FB, MIP and AIP CT datasets [24]. In many respects, our study is more similar with Oechsner et al. who compared the same plans copied from AIP to FB, MIP and MidV datasets. These datasets were recalculated using the same monitor units to ensure the differences in dose were isolated to the density differences as defined by each dataset [25]. Although each of these previous studies used a single algorithm to compare the differences between datasets to one-another, Oechsner found that the greatest dose differences were between the MIP and FB with $D_{95\%} \leq 2.5\%$ when using AAA. Similarly, we observed our greatest dose difference was between MIP and FB datasets with $D_{98\%} \leq 2.9\%$ when using AXB. Nonetheless, we are general agreement with findings from another related study by Kroon et al. who compared volumetric modulated (VMAT) plans calculated for AXB and AAA. In Kroon's study, greater dose differences between algorithms occur with $D_{98\%}$ (– 3.2% average), with respect to smaller differences in D_{mean} (– 0.6% average) [31].

In other density related studies, Wiant et al. discovered plans which incorporated a density override region between the ITV and PTV margin [26]. These plans provided more accurate dose modeling and decreased

normal lung irradiation for lung SBRT. Interestingly, Liu et al. suggested the tolerance value of the CT number for lung material was ±20 HU in order to keep the associated dose uncertainty at 2–3% [29]. These results are in contrast with our current study where neither AAA nor AXB algorithms predicted a dose error at isocenter to be greater than 2% over a target density variation spanning a delta on the order of 200 HU. More recently, in a 20 patient study conducted by Zvolanek et al. treatment plans based on FB image sets were compared with AIP plans calculated for PBC, AAA, AXB and Voxel Monte Carlo (VMC) algorithms [27]. Even though their computations were done using multiple treatment planning systems, they found dose-differences to be small for Type C computations, so concluded FB and AIP image sets were essentially clinically equivalent. In retrospect, the number of studies directly concerning target density are relatively limited [26, 27, 29, 30]. Furthermore, these studies occasionally involve patient specific datasets where the dosimetric impact is fundamentally tied to the size of the delineation contour as defined by image set.

To the best of our knowledge, ours is the first systematic study to use a combination of 4DCT datasets and algorithms to best represent the temporal density dependence associated with lung tumor movement over an extended range of target motion in a representative heterogeneous phantom. Unlike previous virtual phantom studies, which are usually based on slab geometries to highlight worst case scenarios, this investigation concentrated on using a heterogeneous phantom to better replicate actual density variabilities in order to be more clinically applicable. We also introduced a phase weighted density technique, as an alternative to standard FB and AIP image sets most commonly used for lung dose calculations, and compared these datasets to treatment plans generated using MIP image set. In general, the dose error between AAA and AXB algorithms is small and more prominent when comparing plans generated using higher density MIP image sets. Nonetheless, when subject to stringent SBRT tolerances (gamma 3%, 1 mm), we found marginal discrepancies between datasets representing extreme degrees of tissue heterogeneity for plans calculated with the AXB algorithm. In all cases, however, a reduction in the calculated dose to the lung along with improved delivery accuracy was observed when using AXB over AAA as verified in previous studies [17, 31–33]. Since present organs at risk constraints (e.g. lung, etc.) have been determined using second generation computational algorithms, the "evidence based medicine" nature requires appropriate correction in the lung dose limits to be made before implementing Acuros XB.

Certain limitations of this study include irregular breathing cycles and target motion into the third

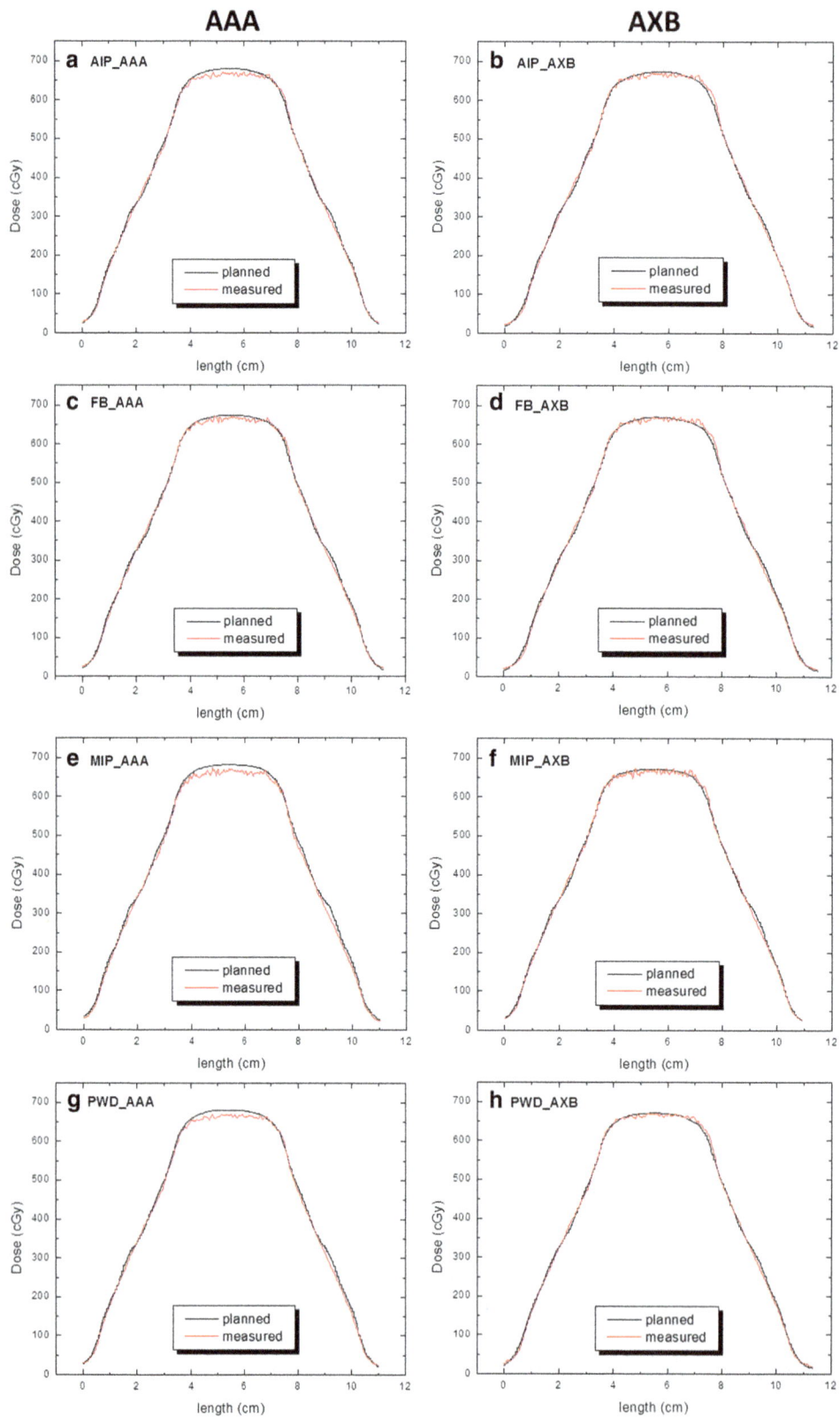

Fig. 9 a-h Dose profiles along the superior/inferior direction of travel as per dataset for AAA and AXB calculations (range of motion = 3 cm). The black curves represent the TPS dose as compared to measured dose indicated by the red curves

dimension which would affect target density distributions. In this investigation we minimized the trajectory variables in order to highlight the most clinically relevant scenarios while taking into consideration target densities associated with FB versus MIP datasets. These image sets represent the lowest versus highest density case scenarios, for which the inclusion of 3D motion and/or irregular breathing cycles would only yield a resulting density variation of somewhere in-between. Another limitation is only sparse sampling [10% phase increments] were used in this study. However, as per our experience, this is the normal sampling which is employed by our hospital, as well in a majority of worldwide clinics as it provides a best compromise of dose delivery accuracy along with acceptable work flow efficiency. Moreover, our motion has been very reproducible, and thus we felt 10% phase increments to be sufficient. At our site and at many others sites around the world, inconsistent breathing peaks are minimized by providing patients with audio/video feedback of their respiratory trace which seems to work very well. Excessive care should be taken when dealing with a sudden sneeze or cough which may result in involuntary breathing peaks compromising the quality of the entire 4DCT dataset.

Furthermore, we did not consider direct Monte Carlo dose computation in our comparison. However, in the retroactive study conducted by Zvolanek who evaluated 20 lung cancer patients, they found volumetric Monte Carlo (VMC) computation yielded similar results as AXB and concluded FB and AIP to be clinically equivalent for dose computation in the Monte Carlo era. With the results presented in this study, we have further corroborated the Zvolanek findings since our film analysis suggest the dosimetric discrepancies between FB, AIP, PWD and even MIP dataset indicate minimal favorability over the other when using Type C (MC and AXB) algorithms.

Arguably, although the PWD technique in its current development may be too time consuming to be implemented into clinical practice, it has been demonstrated to be a viable alternative, yielding a delivery accuracy comparable to that generated using the AIP and FB image sets. Additionally, it is noted many clinics have adopted the MIP image set as a way to define the ITV structure and have gone on to calculate dose using AIP of FB datasets. From the results presented in our study, dose computation using Type C algorithms show the dose discrepancies between MIP as compared to FB or AIP may be clinically acceptable. Furthermore, considering the photon attenuation dependence associated with Type C algorithms, an additional reduction of dose could be achieved when using the MIP image set for computation, although further investigation is needed.

Conclusions

In this heterogeneous phantom study, we evaluated lung target motion ranging up to 3 cm of motion using four distinct CT datasets and two dose algorithms. Despite the substantial density variations between computational datasets over an extensive range of target movement, the dose difference between CT datasets is small and could not be quantified with ion chamber. Radiochromatic film analysis suggests the optimal CT dataset is dependent on the dose algorithm used for evaluation. AIP and FB used with AAA resulted in the best conformance between "measured" verses "calculated" dose for target motion ranging up to 3 cm under both conventional and SBRT tolerance criteria. With AXB, pass rates improved for all datasets with the PWD technique demonstrating slightly better conformity over AIP and FB based computations (gamma 3%, 1 mm). As verified in previous studies, our results confirm a clear advantage in terms delivery accuracy and relative decrease in calculated lung dose when using Acuros XB over AAA. Great care has to be taken when adopting AXB in clinical practice as computed dose differences to various organs need to be correlated with the respective clinical results.

Abbreviations
4DCT: Four dimensional computed tomography; AAA: Analytical Anisotropic Algorithm; AIP: Average intensity projection; AXB: Acuros External Beam; FB: Free breathing; GTV: Gross tumor volume; ITV: Internal target volume; MC: Monte Carlo; MIP: Maximum intensity projection; PTV: Planned target volume; PWD: Phased weighted density; RTOG: Radiation Therapy Oncology Group; SBRT: Stereotactic body radiation therapy; TPS: Treatment planning system

Authors' contributions
Each author participated sufficiently in the work to take public responsibility for appropriate portions of the content. All authors read and approved the final manuscript.

Competing interests
The authors declare that they have no competing interests.

Author details
[1]Medical Physics Program, Jacobs School of Medicine and Biomedical Sciences, University at Buffalo, Buffalo, NY 14214-3005, USA. [2]Department of Radiation Medicine, Roswell Park Cancer Institute, Buffalo, NY 14293, USA. [3]Radiation Oncology, Cone Health Cancer Center, Greensboro, NC 27403, USA.

References

1. Wulf J, Haedinger U, Oppitz U, Thiele W, Mueller G, Flentje M. Stereotactic radiotherapy for primary lung cancer and pulmonary metastases: a noninvasive treatment approach in medically inoperable patients. Int J Radiat Oncol Biol Phys. 2004;60:186–96.

2. Benedict SH, Yenice KM, Followill D, et al. Stereotactic body radiation therapy: the report of AAPM task group 101. Med Phys. 2010;37:4078–101.

3. Bethesda, M. Tissue substitutes in radiation Dosimetry and measurement, Report 44 of the International Commission on Radiation Units and Measurements; 1989.

4. Keall PJ, Mageras GS, Balter JM, et al. The management of respiratory motion in radiation oncology report of AAPM Task Group 76a. Med Phys. 2006;33(10):3874–900.

5. Onishi H, Kuriyama K, Komiyama T, et al. CT evaluation of patient deep inspiration self-breath-holding: how precisely can patients reproduce the tumor position in the absence of respiratory monitoring devices? Med Phys. 2003;30(6):1183–7.

6. Mampuya WA, Nakamura M, Matsuo Y, et al. Interfraction variation in lung tumor position with abdominal compression during stereotactic body radiotherapy. Med Phys. 2013;40(9):091718.

7. Ling CC, Yorke E, Fuks Z. From IMRT to IGRT: frontierland or neverland? Radiother Oncol. 2006;78(2):119–22.

8. Gierga DP, Brewer J, Sharp GC, et al. The correlation between internal and external markers for abdominal tumors: implications for respiratory gating. Int J Radiat Oncol Biol Phys. 2005;61:1551–8.

9. Radiation Therapy Oncology Group. RTOG 0915: a randomized phase ii study comparing 2 stereotactic body radiation therapy (SBRT) schedules for medically inoperable patients with stage I peripheral non-small cell lung cancer. Philadelphia: RTOG; 2009.

10. Mexner V, Wolthaus JW, van Herk M, Damen EM, Sonke JJ. Effects of respiration-induced density variations on dose distributions in radiotherapy of lung cancer. Int J Radiat Oncol Biol Phys. 2009;74:1266–75.

11. Vanderstraeten B, Reynaert N, Paelinck L, et al. Accuracy of patient dose calculation for lung IMRT: a comparison of Monte Carlo, convolution/ superposition, and pencil beam computations. Med Phys. 2006;33:3149–58.

12. Ding GX, Duggan DM, Lu B, et al. Impact of inhomogeneity corrections on dose coverage in the treatment of lung cancer using stereotactic body radiation therapy. Med Phys. 2007;34:2985–94.

13. Miura H, Masai N, Oh RJ, Shiomi H, Yamada K, Sasaki J, Inoue T. Clinical introduction of Monte Carlo treatment planning for lung stereotactic body radiotherapy. J Appl Clin Medical Phys. 2014;15:38–46.

14. Chen WZ, Xiao Y, Li J. Impact of dose calculation algorithm on radiation therapy. World J Radiol. 2014;6:874.

15. Ojala JJ, Kapanen MK, Hyödynmaa SJ, Wigren TK, Pitkänen MA. Performance of dose calculation algorithms from three generations in lung SBRT: comparison with full Monte Carlo-based dose distributions. J Appl Clin Med Phys. 2014;15:4–18.

16. Van Esch A, Tillikainen L, Pyykkonen J, et al. Testing of the analytical anisotropic algorithm for photon dose calculation. Med Phys. 2006;33: 4130–48.

17. Bush K, Gagne IM, Zavgorodni S, Ansbacher W, Beckham W. Dosimetric validation of Acuros® XB with Monte Carlo methods for photon dose calculations. Med Phys. 2011;38:2208–21.

18. Sievinen J, Waldemar U, and Wolfgang K, "AAA photon dose calculation model in Eclipse™," 2005.

19. Failla GA, Wareing T, Archambault Y, Thompson S. Acuros XB advanced dose calculation for the eclipse treatment planning system. Palo Alto, CA: Varian Medical Systems; 2010.

20. Vedam SS, Kini VR, Keall PJ, Ramakrishnan V, Mostafavi H, Mohan R. Quantifying the predictability of diaphragm motion during respiration with a noninvasive external marker. Med Phys. 2003;30:505–13.

21. Rietzel E, Chen GT, Choi NC, Willet CG. Four-dimensional image-based treatment planning: target volume segmentation and dose calculation in the presence of respiratory motion. Int J Radiat Oncol Biol Phys. 2005;61: 1535–50.

22. Huang L, Park K, Boike T, et al. A study on the dosimetric accuracy of treatment planning for stereotactic body radiation therapy of lung cancer using average and maximum intensity projection images. Radiother Oncol. 2010;96:48–54.

23. Han K, Basran PS, Cheung P. Comparison of helical and average computed tomography for stereotactic body radiation treatment planning and normal tissue contouring in lung cancer. Clin Oncol. 2010;22:862–7.

24. Tian Y, Wang Z, Ge H, Zhang T, Cai J, Kelsey C, Yoo D, Yin FF. Dosimetric comparison of treatment plans based on free breathing, maximum, and average intensity projection CTs for lung cancer SBRT. Med Phys. 2012;39: 2754–60.

25. Oechsner M, Odersky L, Berndt J, Combs SE, Wilkens JJ, Duma MN. Dosimetric impact of different CT datasets for stereotactic treatment planning using 3D conformal radiotherapy or volumetric modulated arc therapy. Radiat Oncol. 2015;10(1):249.

26. Wiant D, Vanderstraeten C, Maurer J, Pursley J, Terrell J, Sintay BJ. On the validity of density overrides for VMAT lung SBRT planning. Med Phys. 2014; 41(8):081707.

27. Zvolanek K, Ma R, Zhou C, et al. Still equivalent for dose calculation in the Monte Carlo era? A comparison of free breathing and average intensity projection CT datasets for lung SBRT using three generations of dose calculation algorithms. Med Phys. 2017;44:1939–47.

28. Low DA, Harms WB, Mutic S, Purdy JA. A technique for the quantitative evaluation of dose distributions. Med Phys. 1998;25:656–61.

29. Liu Q, Liang J, Stanhope CW, Yan D. The effect of density variation on photon dose calculation and its impact on intensity modulated radiotherapy and stereotactic body radiotherapy. Med Phys. 2016;43:5717–29.

30. Aarup LR, Nahum AE, Zacharatou C, Juhler-Nøttrup T, Knöös T, Nyström H, Specht L, Wieslander E, Korreman SS. The effect of different lung densities on the accuracy of various radiotherapy dose calculation methods: implications for tumour coverage. Radiother Oncol. 2009;91:405–14.

31. Kroon PS, Hol S, Essers M. Dosimetric accuracy and clinical quality of Acuros XB and AAA dose calculation algorithm for stereotactic and conventional lung volumetric modulated arc therapy plans. Radiat Oncol. 2013;8(1):149.

32. Fogliata A, Nicolini G, Clivio A, Vanetti E, Cozzi L. Critical appraisal of Acuros XB and anisotropic analytic algorithm dose calculation in advanced non-small-cell lung cancer treatments. Int J of Radiat Oncol Biol Phys. 2012;83(5): 1587–95.

33. Huang B, Wu L, Lin P, Chen C. Dose calculation of Acuros XB and anisotropic analytical algorithm in lung stereotactic body radiotherapy treatment with flattening filter free beams and the potential role of calculation grid size. Radiat Oncol. 2015;10(1):53.

15

A novel model to correlate hydrogel spacer placement, perirectal space creation, and rectum dosimetry in prostate stereotactic body radiotherapy

Mark E Hwang[1], Paul J Black[1], Carl D Elliston[1], Brian A Wolthuis[1], Deborah R Smith[1], Cheng-Chia Wu[1], Sven Wenske[2] and Israel Deutsch[1*]

Abstract

Background: The SpaceOAR hydrogel is employed to limit rectal radiation dose during prostate radiotherapy. We identified a novel parameter – the product of angle θ and hydrogel volume – to quantify hydrogel placement. This parameter predicted rectum dosimetry and acute rectal toxicity in prostate cancer patients treated with stereotactic body radiotherapy to 36.25 Gy in 5 fractions.

Methods: Twenty men with low- and intermediate-risk prostate cancer underwent hydrogel placement from 2015 to 2017. Hydrogel symmetry was assessed on the CT simulation scan in 3 axial slices (midgland, 1 cm above midgland, 1 cm below midgland). Two novel parameters quantifying hydrogel placement – hydrogel volume and angle θ formed by the prostate, hydrogel, and rectum – were measured, and the normalized product of θ and hydrogel volume calculated. These were then correlated with perirectal distance, rectum maximum 1–3 cc point doses (rD_{max} 1–3 cc), and rectum volumes receiving 80–95% of the prescription dose (rV80–95%). Acute rectal toxicity was recorded per RTOG criteria.

Results: In 50% of patients, hydrogel placement was symmetric bilaterally to within 1 cm of midline in all three CT simulation scan axial slices. Lateral hydrogel asymmetry < 2 cm in any one axial slice did not affect rectum dosimetry, but absence of hydrogel in the inferior axial slice resulted in a mean increase of 171 cGy in the rD_{max} 1 cc ($p < 0.005$). The perirectal distance measured at prostate midgland, midline (mean 9.1 ± 4.3 mm) correlated strongly with rV95 (R^2 0.6, $p < 0.001$). The mean hydrogel volume and θ were 10.3 ± 4.5 cc and 70 ± 49°, respectively. Perirectal distance, rV95 and rD_{max} 1 cc correlated with hydrogel angle θ ($p < 0.01$), and yet more strongly with the novel metric θ*hydrogel volume ($p < 0.001$). With a median follow up of 14 months, no rectal toxicity >grade 2 was observed. Low grade rectal toxicity was observed in a third of men and resolved within 1 month of SBRT. Men who had these symptoms had higher rD_{max} 1 cc and smaller θ*hydrogel volume measurements.

Conclusions: Optimal hydrogel placement occurs at prostate midgland, midline. The novel parameter θ*hydrogel volume describes a large proportion of rectum dosimetric benefit derived from hydrogel placement, and can be used to assess the learning curve phenomenon for hydrogel placement.

Keywords: Prostate cancer, Stereotactic body radiotherapy, Rectal toxicity, SpaceOAR hydrogel, Dosimetry

* Correspondence: id2182@cumc.columbia.edu
[1]Department of Radiation Oncology, Columbia University Medical Center,
New York, New York 10032, USA
Full list of author information is available at the end of the article

Background

Hypofractionated prostate radiotherapy has gained popularity in prostate cancer treatment, with growing evidence that showed non-inferior tumor control and similar toxicity profile when compared against conventionally-fractionated, dose-escalated radiotherapy [1–3]. Stereotactic body radiotherapy (SBRT) for low risk prostate cancer was evaluated in RTOG 0938 and offered to eligible patients as a short course of radiotherapy lasting 2.5 weeks. Following per-protocol rectum dose constraints, under one quarter of prostate SBRT patients experienced 5-point changes in one-year Expanded Prostate Index Composite bowel scores after SBRT – well under the 35% considered acceptable for patients [4]. Ongoing efforts to minimize rectum toxicity in the context of a trend toward higher doses per fraction as seen in RTOG 0938 have thus remained a priority [5].

Research has shown that perirectal space enlargement with a temporary spacer material is one approach to reduce rectum dose. In one cadaveric study, a 20 cc hydrogel spacer generated a mean perirectal distance of 12.5 mm and a four-fold decrease in calculated rectum V70 Gy [6]. Multi-institutional evaluation of a different hydrogel spacer resulted in 7.5 mm of perirectal separation and a 10% reduction in rectum V40-70Gy when comparing pre- and post-spacer treatment plans [7]. More recently, the Augmenix SpaceOAR hydrogel, which received FDA approval following a 2014 phase III clinical trial, showed statistically significant reduction in grades 1 and 2 acute rectal toxicity in men receiving conventionally fractionated, dose escalated prostate radiotherapy [8]. Late grade 1 rectal toxicity at 3 years was also significantly lower in the SpaceOAR arm (42% v 17%, $p = 0.04$) [9]. This toxicity improvement is attributable to both reduced intrafraction motion, where the SpaceOAR hydrogel and daily rectal balloon usage are believed to be comparable immobilization tools [10], and improved rectal dosimetry based on posterior, rather than anterior, displacement of the anterior rectal wall with hydrogel instead of a rectal balloon [11]. A hydrogel spacer also has the additional benefit of allowing larger planning margins and higher target coverage due to improved rectal sparing [12, 13].

Recent publications have thus far correlated hydrogel distribution with rectum dosimetry in conventionally fractionated prostate radiotherapy, and demonstrated the dosimetric superiority of hydrogel over rectal balloon in prostate SBRT [11, 14]. Yet no study has correlated the *quality* of hydrogel placement with rectum dosimetry in prostate SBRT. Optimal hydrogel placement should have a greater impact on toxicity minimization in high-dose-per-fraction SBRT than in the conventionally fractionated setting. This need to examine hydrogel placement is important in the face of research that showed patients receiving prostate SBRT

doses up to 50 Gy in 10 Gy per fraction, but without use of a periprostatic spacer, suffered high grade rectal toxicity [5].

Identifying parameters that help optimize hydrogel placement will be clinically meaningful, especially in the context of rising hydrogel utilization and SBRT doses. In this study, we applied a previously published metric to analyze the symmetry of hydrogel placement in our SBRT patient cohort, developed a new metric to correlate the effect of hydrogel placement on rectum dosimetry, and report early toxicity outcomes.

Methods

Patients

We retrospectively reviewed all low- and intermediate-risk prostate cancer patients who were treated with linear-accelerator based SBRT to 36.25 Gy in 5 fractions. The twenty patients (Table 1) were extracted from our single-institution IRB approved databases from August 2015 to August 2017. Patients received pre- and post-hydrogel placement T2-weighted prostate MRI when possible. The post-hydrogel MRI was obtained at a median of 15 (range: 2–37) days after hydrogel placement. All patients underwent simultaneous periprostatic SpaceOAR hydrogel (Augmenix, Inc. Waltham, MA) and MRI-compatible Cybermark gold fiducial prostate

Table 1 Patient characteristics

Age ± stdev, y	69.7 ± 6.6
Range	55–82
PSA ± stdev, ng/mL	9 ± 5.3
Range	2.7–24.5
Gleason score 6 (%)	25
Gleason score 7 (%)	75
Primary GS 4 (%)	47
Cores involved ± stdev (#)	3.9 ± 2.4
Range	1–9
Cores involved ± stdev (%)	30 ± 19
Range	10–75
Clinical stage:	
cT1c	72
cT2a	17
cT2b	13
AUA score ± stdev[a]	9 ± 7
Range	0–20
SHIM score ± stdev[b]	14 ± 8.7
Range	0–26
Prostate volume ± stdev (cc)	40.1 ± 22.5
Range	13–108

[a]AUA = American Urological Association Symptom Score
[b]SHIM = Sexual Health Inventory for Men Score

marker (CIVCO Medical Instruments Co., Inc. Kalona, IA) placement 16–41 days (mean ± SD 29 ± 7.5 days) prior to starting radiotherapy. Only one SpaceOAR hydrogel kit was used per patient. All men underwent CT-based simulation, and the post-hydrogel MRI was fused to the CT simulation scan to facilitate hydrogel contouring. Normal tissue dose constraints, contours, and clinical target volume (CTV) to planning target volume (PTV) margin expansions were defined as per RTOG 0938. Prostate SBRT was planned on the Varian Eclipse treatment planning system and delivered with a Varian Truebeam Linear Accelerator (Varian Medical Systems, Palo Alto, Ca).

Quantifying SpaceOAR hydrogel placement

SpaceOAR hydrogel symmetry was first analyzed according to the rubric outlined by Fischer-Valuck et al. in patients receiving conventionally fractionated radiotherapy [14]. In their study, three axial slices on the CT simulation scan were selected for analysis (midgland, 1 cm above migland, and 1 cm below midgland). The presence or absence of hydrogel in each slice was recorded. Hydrogel placement was recorded as asymmetric if the hydrogel was present but deviated by greater than 1 cm from anatomic midline. Each patient received a composite hydrogel symmetry score that was compared with their final rectal dosimetry: Symmetry Score 1 (SYM1) = all 3 slices with symmetric distribution; Symmetry Score 2 (SYM2) = 1 of 3 slices with > 1 cm but < 2 cm asymmetry; Symmetry Scores 3–5 (SYM 3–5) were defined in their original publication as having progressively prominent asymmetry, but which were not needed in our study.

The SpaceOAR hydrogel, rectum, and CTV were identified and contoured on each patient's CT simulation scan. A post-hydrogel MRI T2-weighted sequence was fused with the CT simulation scan to facilitate hydrogel delineation. Volumes and center-of-mass coordinates were recorded for the prostate CTV, rectum, and hydrogel.

We quantified the hydrogel deviation from midline by measuring the angle, θ, formed by the posterior aspect of the CTV at CTV center (corresponding to prostate midgland, midline), hydrogel center of mass, and anterior wall of the rectum in 3-dimensional space (Fig. 1a, b).

Patient rectal toxicities were recorded per RTOG grading during treatment, 2–4 weeks after treatment, and every 3 months thereafter [15].

Quantifying the perirectal space

We measured the distances between the prostate and rectum at different locations to create a perirectal space map for each patient before and after hydrogel placement. Each perirectal distance was bounded anteriorly by the posterior aspect of the CTV, and posteriorly by the anterior portion of the rectum contour. We first measured the perirectal distance at the CTV center, which corresponded to the prostate midgland, at midline (Fig. 1a). Additional perirectal distances were then measured up to 2 cm superiorly, inferiorly, and bilaterally from the CTV center in 1 cm intervals. The perirectal space for each patient is thus mapped with 25 potential perirectal distance measurements that are spatially arranged in a 4 × 4 cm coronal grid (Fig. 1c). These measurements were performed on the CT simulation scan ($n = 20$), and repeated on each patient's pre- ($n = 13$) and post- ($n = 18$) hydrogel placement MRI T2-weighted scans. The *change* (Δ, n = 13) in perirectal space attributed to hydrogel placement was determined by subtracting the post- from pre-hydrogel perirectal distance measurements on MRI when both MRI scans were available. Perirectal distance measurements were then compared with the volume of rectum receiving 95, 90, and 80% of the prescription dose (rV95–80), as well as rectum maximum 1, 2, and 3 cc point doses (rD$_{max}$ 1–3 cc).

Statistical analysis

Statistical significance between SYM1 and all other symmetry groups was evaluated with student t test.

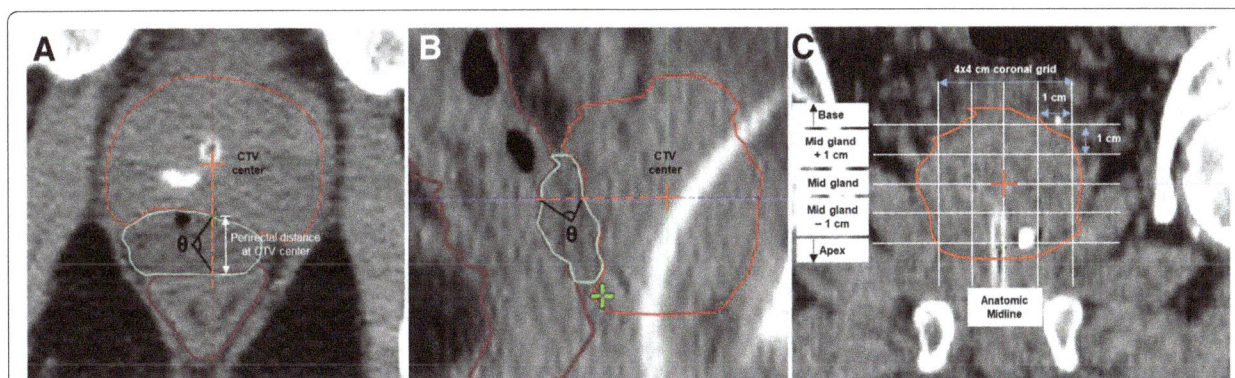

Fig. 1 Measurement of a perirectal distance at CTV center on axial CT image (**a**), and θ in 3-dimensional space on axial and sagittal CT images (**a**, **b**). The perirectal distance is measured at each vertex in a 4 × 4 cm coronal grid centered on the prostate midgland, at midline to generate a perirectal space map comprising up to 25 perirectal distance measurements for each patient (**c**)

Continuous variables were summarized with means and standard deviations and shown to approximate a normal distribution with a Shapiro-Wilk normality test. The relationships amongst continuous variables were quantified using Pearson correlation and multiple regression analysis. Analysis was performed in Office Suite Excel 2013 (Microsoft Corporation, Redmond, WA) and SPSS (IBM, Armonk, NY).

Results

SpaceOAR symmetry analysis

Hydrogel symmetry was analyzed on three axial slices from each patient's CT simulation scan, for a total of 60 analyzed axial slices from our cohort of 20 patients. SpaceOAR hydrogel was present in 51 axial slices and symmetric to within 1 cm of anatomic midline in 45 axial slices. Lateral hydrogel asymmetry was present in six slices but did not exceed 2 cm from midline. Hydrogel was completely absent in nine axial slices: four inferior to midgland, two at midgland, and three superior to midgland.

Thirteen patients (65%) had hydrogel present in all three axial slices. Ten patients (50%) had hydrogel present and symmetric bilaterally in all three axial slices, while three pateints (15%) had hydrogel present in all three axial slices but symmetric in only two of them (SYM 2). None of our patients met criteria for categorizing hydrogel placement into scores SYM3–5 (that denote asymmetry > 2 cm or asymmetry > 1 cm in more than one of three axial slices). SYM scores were not assigned to the remaining seven patients, five of whom had hydrogel in only two axial slices and two of whom had hydrogel in only one axial slice.

The rD_{max} 1 cc dose was not statistically different between groups SYM1 and SYM2 (Fig. 2). This is similar to results shown by Fischer-Valuck et al. [14]. However, rD_{max} 1 cc was on average 171 cGy higher in patients missing hydrogel in the inferior most axial slice versus patients with SYM1 scores (Fig. 2, $p < 0.005$).

Perirectal distance analysis on post-hydrogel simulation CT

Perirectal distance measurements from patient CT simulation scans are shown in Table 2. The mean perirectal distance measured at CTV center was 9.1 ± 4.3 mm. Perirectal distances were greatest at the superior-most axial slice, averaging 14.7 ± 10.3 mm, and smallest at the inferior-most slice, averaging 6.4 ± 4.5 mm. Averaging all perirectal distance measurements for each patient, the mean perirectal distance was 10.1 ± 7.4 mm, which closely approximated the single perirectal distance obtained at CTV center for each patient.

In none of our cohort was perirectal distance measurement possible in the inferior-most slice, 2 cm to the left

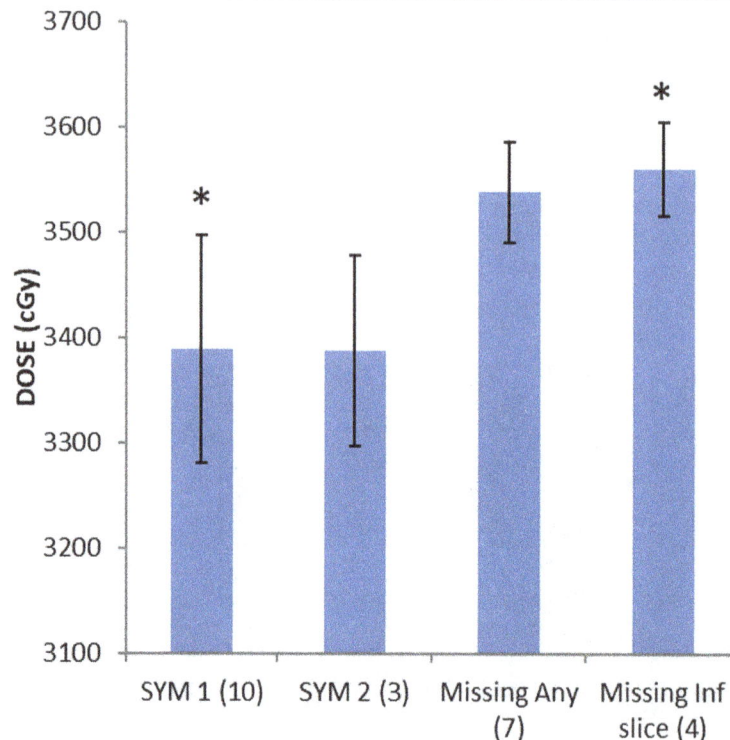

Fig. 2 Rectum maximum 1 cc point dose (rD_{max} 1 cc) by hydrogel symmetry (SYM) score. T-test comparison of means revealed a statistically significant difference between groups SYM1 and Missing Inf Slice, denoted by * = $p < 0.01$

Table 2 Mean perirectal distances (mm) measured on the CT simulation scan (*n* = 20). Standard deviation immediately beneath corresponding perirectal distance. The mean perirectal distance and standard deviation at each of 5 axial slices (right) and 5 sagittal slices (bottom) are also reported

		Left		Midline	Right		Mean	Stdev
		2 cm	1 cm	0	1 cm	2 cm		
Superior (base)	+ 2 cm	14.4	12.5	14.5	13.8	18.1	14.7	*10.3*
		6	*8.2*	*11.1*	*9.6*	*16.9*		
	+ 1 cm	19.1	11	9.9	11.3	13	12.9	*7.5*
		11.2	*7.5*	*5.8*	*5.9*	*10.7*		
Midgland	0	11.9	9	9.1	10.5	11.9	10.5	*5.3*
		4	*5.3*	*4.3*	*5.5*	*12.2*		
Inferior (apex)	− 1 cm	8.7	8.2	8.5	8.2	9.4	8.6	*5.6*
		2.6	*5.9*	*5.1*	*6.8*	*2.2*		
	− 2 cm		7.6	5.5	6.1		6.4	*4.5*
			4.3	*4.2*	*4.4*			
	Mean	13.5	9.7	9.5	10	13.1	10.1	*7.4*
	Stdev	*7.7*	*6.4*	*6.9*	*6.9*	*12.5*		

or right of midline, due to an absence of either CTV or rectum contour at this location.

Perirectal distance analysis on pre- and post-hydrogel MRI

Perirectal distances measured on the post-hydrogel MRI T2 sequence (Table 3B) were compared with those measured on post-hydrogel CT simulation scan. The perirectal distance at any given perirectal location was not statistically significantly different on t-test comparison of

Table 3 Mean perirectal distances (mm) on the T2-weighted MRI before (A, n = 13), and after SpaceOAR hydrogel (B, n = 18 patients). Mean change (**Δ**) in perirectal distances (C, *n* = 13)

			Left		Midline	Right	
			2 cm	1 cm	0	1 cm	2 cm
A	Superior (base)	+ 2 cm	12	9.1	11.7	10	14.3
		+ 1 cm	12.8	8.2	5.8	6.8	10.8
	Midgland	0	8.3	3	1	2.5	6.5
	Inferior (apex)	− 1 cm	6.5	1.8	0.6	2	7.6
		− 2 cm		3	1.5	5	
B	Superior (base)	+ 2 cm	15	13.6	14.6	12.2	16.2
		+ 1 cm	13.7	11.8	10.9	10.9	12
	Midgland	0	7.4	9.7	10.3	9.6	7
	Inferior (apex)	− 1 cm	7	8.7	10.3	9.2	10.6
		− 2 cm		8.1	7.3	6.8	
C	Superior (base)	+ 2 cm	0.5	3.5	4.8	4.6	2
		+ 1 cm	0	3.6	5.5	5.3	1
	Midgland	0	0	7.6	10	8.1	2.3
	Inferior (apex)	− 1 cm	0	7.9	9.8	8.8	1.3
		− 2 cm		5.2	5.9	4.5	

means between the post-hydrogel CT and MRI in the 18 men who had both scans (not shown, data available upon request). The greatest increase (Δ) in perirectal distance after hydrogel placement occurred at midline on the midgland axial slice (CTV center), and averaged 10 mm (Table 3C). The Δ perirectal space diminished at distances greater than 1 cm from CTV center.

Rectum dosimetry

RTOG 0938 rectum dose constraints were met in 18 of 20 patients. These constraints limited rD_{max} 1, 2 and 3 cc point doses, and rV95, rV90 and rV80. Two patients received rD_{max} 3 cc rectum doses of 3448 and 3460 cGy, which was slightly in excess of the 3440 cGy constraint.

Table 4 shows R^2 values from regressing different measures of rectum dosimetry against independent variables - perirectal distances, hydrogel volume, θ, and θ*hydrogel volume. The perirectal distance that explained the highest rectum dosimetry variance was that measured at CTV center (Table 4A, first row). Perirectal distance measurements that were inferior to this location, representing the perirectal space that is natively most closely approximated to the rectum, have slightly lower ability to explain rectum dosimetry variance (Table 4A, rows 2–3). Variance explanation strength decreased precipitously with perirectal distance measurements obtained further from the CTV center in all directions (results not shown).

Mean contoured hydrogel volume was 10.3 ± 4.5 cc, and mean θ was 70 ± 49°. Hydrogel volume and θ individually showed moderate power in explaining rectum dosimetry variance (Table 4B), with $R^2 < 0.43$ for any of rV80–95 and rD_{max} 1–3 cc. The product of θ, normalized to 180°, and hydrogel volume, normalized to the

Table 4 Coefficient of determination (R^2) values from simple linear regression models of rectum maximum 1, 2, and 3 cc point doses (rD_{max} 1, 2, 3 cc) and rectum volume receiving dose (rV95, 90, 80%) regressed against perirectal distance measurements obtained on CT (A) and hydrogel parameters (B)

		rD_{max}			rV		
		1 cc	2 cc	3 cc	95%	90%	80%
A	Perirectal Distance Measurement						
	CTV center	0.44	0.45	0.42	0.6	0.55	0.27
	1 cm inferomedial to CTV center	0.41	0.37	0.31	0.5	0.38	0.15
	2 cm inferomedial to CTV center	0.39	0.35	0.28	0.49	0.33	0.1
B	Hydrogel Parameters						
	Hydrogel volume (cc)	0.23	0.22	0.18	0.2	0.14	0.04
	θ	0.36	0.33	0.26	0.43	0.34	0.14
	Normalized θ*gel volume	0.64	0.62	0.55	0.60	0.52	0.25

volume of the single largest contoured hydrogel in this cohort, showed high power in explaining rectum dosimetry (R^2 for rV95 = 0.60, $p < 0.001$; rD_{max} 1 cc = 0.64, p < 0.001). CTV volume, with a mean and standard deviation of 40.1 ± 22.5 cc, had minimum ability to explain rectum dosimetry variance (not shown).

The parameter, θ*hydrogel volume, was as strongly correlated with, and explained the same proportion of variance in, rV95 as did the single perirectal distance measurement taken at CTV center (R^2 0.6, Table 4A, B; Fig. 3a, b). θ*hydrogel volume was even more strongly correlated with rD_{max} 1, 2 and 3 cc point doses than

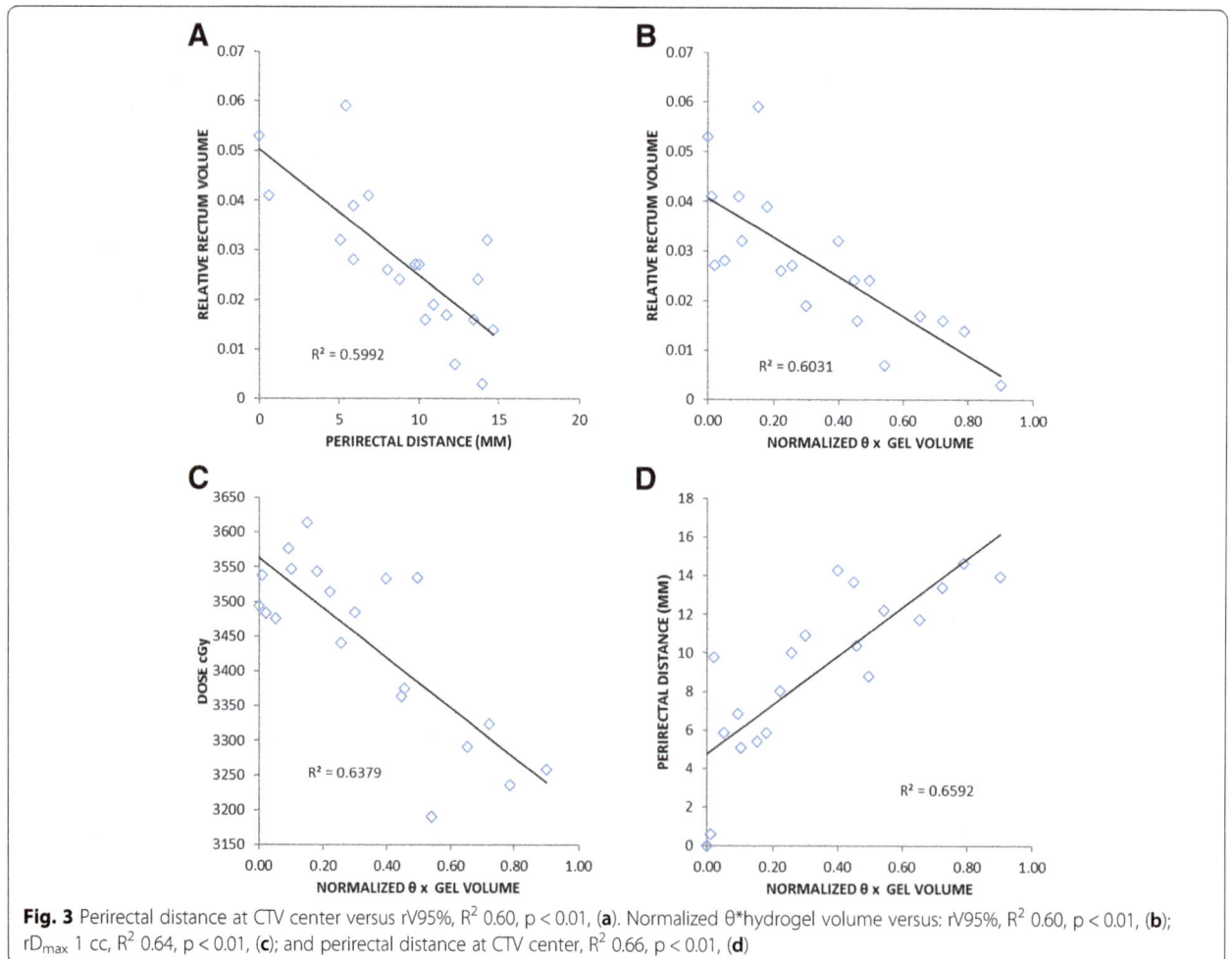

Fig. 3 Perirectal distance at CTV center versus rV95%, R^2 0.60, p < 0.01, (**a**). Normalized θ*hydrogel volume versus: rV95%, R^2 0.60, p < 0.01, (**b**); rD_{max} 1 cc, R^2 0.64, p < 0.01, (**c**); and perirectal distance at CTV center, R^2 0.66, p < 0.01, (**d**)

with any single perirectal distance measurement (Table 4A, B; Fig. 3c). This suggests that θ*hydrogel volume successfully describes the perirectal space creation effect of a given hydrogel (Fig. 3d).

Multiple linear regression was then used to identify predictive effects of independent variables θ, hydrogel volume, and θ*hydrogel volume on dependent variable rD_{max} 1 cc. Only the independent variable θ*hydrogel volume was a significant predictor of rD_{max} 1 cc, indicating a significant interaction component between θ and hydrogel volume in predicting rectum dosimetry (Standardized β = − 1.62; $t > − 3.05$; $R^2 = 0.694$; F = 12.08 (19,3)).

Acute rectal toxicity

With a median follow up of 18 months, 30% of men experienced Grade 1 ($n = 5$) or 2 ($n = 1$) acute rectal toxicity with soft stools during treatment. Symptoms completely resolved within two weeks in four men, and within four weeks in the remaining two men. No GI toxicity was reported on any subsequent follow up. Men with acute rectal toxicity tended to have higher rD_{max} 1 cc and lower θ*hydrogel volume scores (Fig. 4). No toxicity greater than Grade 2 was observed.

Discussion
Clinical relevance

Our institutional experience describes the early stages of SpaceOAR hydrogel implementation in high-dose per fraction SBRT setting, where the benefits of a well-placed spacer on rectum dosimetry quickly become clinically evident upon examination. Our objective was to develop a systematic method to quantify the perirectal space after hydrogel placement and identify a hydrogel placement metric to correlate perirectal space creation with rectum dosimetry. The findings showed increased perirectal space and optimal hydrogel placement have a positive impact on rectal dosimetry when we considered the θ*hydrogel volume metric. This metric was at least, if not more, predictive of rectum dosimetry than any perirectal space measurement. With longer follow up and greater sample size, this metric should have added utility of eventually tracking placement quality and operator experience.

Evidence of a learning curve in developing operative skillsets is well-established as seen in prostate brachytherapy implant quality that improves with experience up to a point [16, 17], after which proficiency is maintained with a minimum annual caseload [18]. The learning curve phenomenon for hydrogel placement was first reported by Pinkawa et al. in a study of 64 patients that showed improved lateral hydrogel symmetry, increased perirectal space, and better rectum dosimetry in the latter 32 patients compared with the first 32 patients [19]. Such a learning-curve effect is minimized in a well-established training environment with appropriate mentorship and operator feedback [20]. We expect that a well-designed hydrogel placement metric, such as we have described in this manuscript, would provide one such measure of feedback.

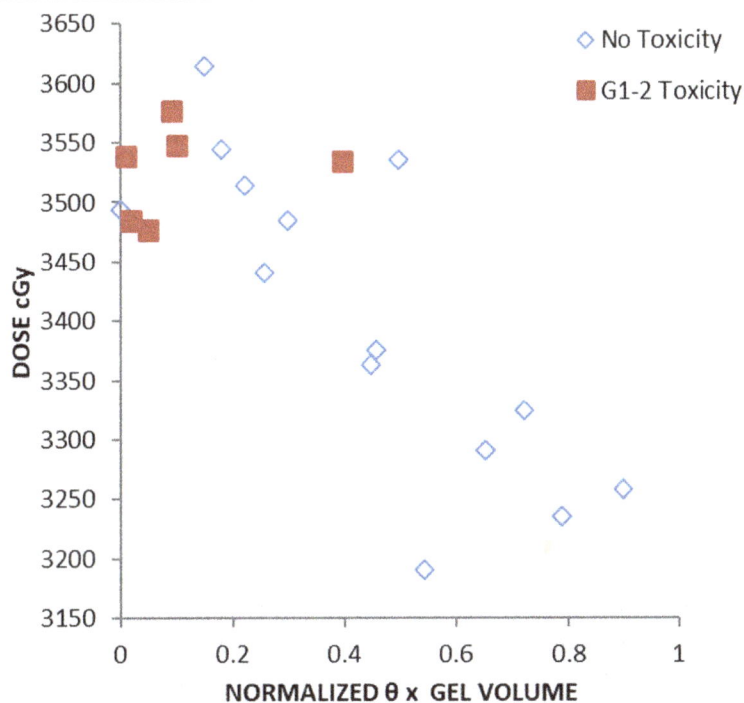

Fig. 4 Normalized θ*hydrogel volume versus rectum maximum 1 cc point dose (rD_{max} 1 cc), showing acute low grade rectal toxicity ($n = 6/20$)

Quantifying perirectal space

While results from this study are in agreement with the general expectation that a well-placed hydrogel is important for rectum dosimetry, to our knowledge this is the first time the post-hydrogel perirectal space has been rigorously mapped. We showed that precise perirectal space measurements can be obtained independently from either the post-hydrogel T2 weighted MRI or CT simulation scans (Tables 2 and 3). Prior to hydrogel placement, the prostate apex and midgland lie close to the rectum on the pre hydrogel placement MRI (Table 3A). Following hydrogel placement, almost all regions of the prostate have increased separation from the rectum, with the greatest mean increase seen at the prostate apex and midgland (Table 3C). Several publications have described a wide range of post-hydrogel perirectal separation ranging from 0.6 to over 2 cm, but to-date few have described in detail the optimal location to obtain this perirectal measurement, or Δ measurement, resulting from hydrogel placement [11, 14, 21–23].

From our perirectal space maps, we identified the perirectal distance measurement obtained posterior to the prostate at midgland, midline, or CTV center, as that which is most strongly correlated with rectum dosimetry (Table 4A). This is followed by the perirectal distance measurements 1 and 2 cm that are immediately inferior to it i.e. toward the prostate apex. As enlargement of the perirectal space at, or slightly inferior to, the prostate CTV center led to the greatest improvement in rectum dosimetry, this position represented the optimal location for hydrogel placement.

SpaceOAR characteristics and rectum dosimetry

Distribution of lateral hydrogel deviation in our patient cohort was nearly identical to that of earlier work by Fischer-Valuck et al. [14] Half ($n = 10$) of patients had symmetric gel placement (SYM1, lateral deviation < 1 cm) in all three axial slices, and 15% ($n = 3$) had hydrogel in all three axial slices but with lateral deviation < 2 cm in only one axial slice (SYM2). Consistent with their conclusions, the rV95% and rD$_{max}$ 1 cc were not significantly different between SYM1 and SYM2 hydrogels in our study (Fig. 2).

While the effect of lateral hydrogel deviation on rectum dosimetry is thus well-characterized, hydrogel distribution along the craniocaudal dimension has not been commented upon in existing literature. In our study minor hydrogel deviation along the craniocaudal axis had a more pronounced effect on rectum dosimetry than lateral deviation of a similar scale (~ 1 cm). The absence of hydrogel in the axial slice 1 cm inferior to midgland ($n = 4$) correlated to an increase in rD$_{max}$ 1 cc of 171 cGy ($p = 0.005$, Fig. 2).

This is unsurprising as the native perirectal space is most limited inferomedially, averaging 1–2 mm in our analysis. In the vast majority of patients, such close proximity between the prostate and rectum begins inferiorly at the prostate apex and extends superiorly at least as far as the prostate midgland. Whereas previous analysis emphasized the importance of lateral hydrogel symmetry, we conclude that hydrogel deviation must be accounted for in both the lateral and cranio-caudal dimensions to accurately predict rectum dosimetry.

As a result, we defined θ to quantify hydrogel deviation from the optimal CTV center location in three-dimensional space rather than along a single axis. θ alone correlated moderately with rD$_{max}$ 1 cc and rV95% and predicted only a minority of variance in these statistics ($R^2 = 0.36$ and 0.43, respectively; Table 4B) as it does not take into account the volume of hydrogel centered around the θ vertex.

Similarly, hydrogel volume alone was modestly correlated with rectum dosimetry (R^2 rD$_{max}$ 1 cc = 0.23; rV95%, 0.2). This is due to minimal enlargement of the perirectal space in the instance of suboptimal injection site (i.e. small θ). Indeed, hydrogel volume was not significant in two-variable regression of hydrogel volume and θ against rD$_{max}$ 1 cc (p$_{VOLUME}$ = 0.06, p$_\theta$ < 0.01, $n = 20$), but became significant only in the subset of patients with $\theta > 35°$ (p$_{VOLUME}$ = 0.04, p$_\theta$ < 0.01, $n = 16$).

We thus inferred that an interaction exists between hydrogel volume and θ such that the correlation of each θ and hydrogel volume influenced rectum dosimetry. Based on this examination of data, we tested the product θ*hydrogel volume which showed strong ability to explain rectum dosimetry (R^2 rD$_{max}$ 1 cc =0.64; rV95%, 0.6; Table 4B). A three-variable regression analysis of θ, hydrogel volume, and θ*hydrogel confirmed that θ*hydrogel was the only significant predictor of rV95 ($R^2 = 0.694$; F-value 12.08; $p = 0.008$). We thus conclude that the parameter θ*hydrogel volume quantifies perirectal space enlargement effect following hydrogel placement, and should be considered in evaluating hydrogel placement success.

Previous work has shown no statistically significant variation in rectum dose with CTV volume ranging up to 100 cc, and is consistent with our findings [21].

Acute rectal toxicity and θ*hydrogel volume

Hydrogel spacer use in prostate SBRT was documented as early as 2013 by Alongi et al. and continues to represent a growing proportion of SpaceOAR utilization [11, 24, 25]. Yet as of this study, the only published phase III randomized prostate hydrogel data were obtained in the conventionally fractionated setting [22]. In their control arm without hydrogel, acute rectal toxicity ≥grade 2 benefit was not statistically significant, but any late toxicity was improved 4.5-fold at 3 years.

We expected that relative toxicity benefits attributed to hydrogel use would be at least as prominent in the high-dose per fraction SBRT setting as it is in conventionally-fractionated treatment. In addition, projected cost-benefit decision analysis suggests that the use of hydrogel spacer will be cost-effective for toxicity management in the long term for all forms of prostate radiotherapy, but particularly so for prostate SBRT [26].

With the hydrogel spacer and prostate SBRT to a dose of 3625 cGy in five twice-weekly treatments, less than one third of patients developed grades 1–2 acute rectal toxicity either during or immediately after treatment, which resolved at the latest by the one-month post-treatment visit. It is noteworthy that these men had characteristics of rectum dosimetry, perirectal spacing, and θ*volume that we quantified as being in the less favorable half of our cohort (Fig. 4).

Likely as a result of small sample size, no statistically significant difference was observed in rD_{max} 1 cc, rV95%, perirectal distance at CTV center, and the metric θ*hydrogel volume, between men who developed acute rectal toxicity and men who did not. We suspect that the likelihood of statistically significant relationships between these parameters and symptomatic toxicity would emerge at the higher SBRT doses currently being evaluated in phase II clinical trials, with larger sample size, and longer follow-up.

We have nonetheless shown from our early hydrogel SBRT patient cohort a correlation between the metric θ*hydrogel volume and rectum dosimetry. We expect that the learning curve necessary to attain high-quality hydrogel placements will also become evident as measured by the θ*hydrogel volume metric as our experience with hydrogel placement increases.

The relatively wide range of hydrogel volumes as measured on post-hydrogel T2 weighted MRI bears further evaluation. Each SpaceOAR hydrogel is injected transperineally as a 10 cc suspension following dissection of Denonvillier's fascia with saline solution. Potential explanations for small hydrogel volumes include suboptimal placement, hydrogel dispersion prior to polymerization and incidental withdrawal of hydrogel along with the needle following the procedure. Explanations for large hydrogel volumes include contouring software volume overinterpolation and overcontouring of hydrogel. The latter may occur as saline solution used in the fascial dissection and SpaceOAR hydrogel is indistinguishable on the MRI T2 image obtained after hydrogel placement. In our cohort, the earliest post-hydrogel MRI was obtained two days after hydrogel placement.

Conclusions

After SpaceOAR hydrogel placement, the perirectal distance measurement at CTV center, which corresponds to the prostate midgland, midline, is shown to be highly correlated with rectum dosimetry. Hydrogel location can be quantified by θ as measured from the CTV center, with larger θ correlating with better placement. Hydrogel volume contributed more to perirectal space creation with increasing θ. The overall rectum dosimetric benefit from hydrogel placement strongly correlated with the novel metric θ*hydrogel volume, which can be used to track and minimize the learning curve phenomenon for hydrogel placement.

Abbreviations
CTV: clinical target volume; PTV: planning target volume; SBRT: stereotactic body radiotherapy; SYM: Symmetry Score

Acknowledgments
We thank Dr. Alvin Hwang, PhD, Director of AACSB Accreditation Management and Management Science at the Pace University Lubin School of Business for statistics support and analysis.

Authors' contributions
MEH analyzed organ-at-risk dosimetry, SpaceOAR hydrogel placement prior to radiotherapy, and patient toxicity following radiotherapy, and is the first author on this manuscript. PJB, CDE, BAW and DRS analyzed and correlated dosimetric data with SpaceOAR hydrogel placement. SW and ID provided clinical expertise in this project and were major contributors in writing the manuscript. All authors read and approved the final manuscript.

Competing interests
The authors declare that they have no competing interests.

Author details
[1]Department of Radiation Oncology, Columbia University Medical Center, New York, New York 10032, USA. [2]Department of Urology, Columbia University Medical Center, New York 10032, New York, USA.

References
1. Hegemann N-S, Guckenberger M, Belka C, Ganswindt U, Manapov F, Li M. Hypofractionated radiotherapy for prostate cancer. Radiat Oncol. 2014;9:275.
2. Katz AJ, Kang J. Stereotactic body radiotherapy as treatment for organ confined low- and intermediate-risk prostate carcinoma, a 7-year study. Front Oncol. 2014;4. https://doi.org/10.3389/fonc.2014.00240.
3. Katz AJ, Kang J. Quality of life and toxicity after SBRT for organ-confined prostate Cancer, a 7-year study. Front Oncol. 2014;4. https://doi.org/10.3389/fonc.2014.00301.
4. Lukka H, Stephanie P, Bruner D, Bahary JP, Lawton CAF, Efstathiou JA, et al. Patient-Reported Outcomes in NRG Oncology/RTOG 0938, a Randomized Phase 2 Study Evaluating 2 Ultrahypofractionated Regimens (UHRs) for Prostate Cancer. Int J Radiat Oncol. 2018;94:2.
5. Kim DWN, Cho LC, Straka C, Christie A, Lotan Y, Pistenmaa D, et al. Predictors of rectal tolerance observed in a dose-escalated phase 1-2 trial of stereotactic body radiation therapy for prostate Cancer. Int J Radiat Oncol. 2014;89:509–17.
6. Susil RC, McNutt TR, DeWeese TL, Song D. Effects of prostate-rectum separation on rectal dose from external beam radiotherapy. Int J Radiat Oncol. 2010;76:1251–8.
7. Song DY, Herfarth KK, Uhl M, Eble MJ, Pinkawa M, van Triest B, et al. A

multi-institutional clinical trial of rectal dose reduction via injected polyethylene-glycol hydrogel during intensity modulated radiation therapy for prostate Cancer: analysis of Dosimetric outcomes. Int J Radiat Oncol. 2013;87:81–7.

8. Hamstra DA, Mariados N, Sylvester J, Shah D, Karsh L, Hudes R, et al. Continued benefit to rectal separation for prostate radiation therapy: final results of a phase III trial. Int J Radiat Oncol. 2017;97:976–85.

9. Whalley D, Hruby G, Alfieri F, Kneebone A, Eade T. SpaceOAR hydrogel in dose-escalated prostate Cancer radiotherapy: rectal dosimetry and late toxicity. Clin Oncol. 2016;28:e148–54.

10. Hedrick SG, Fagundes M, Robison B, Blakey M, Renegar J, Artz M, et al. A comparison between hydrogel spacer and endorectal balloon: an analysis of intrafraction prostate motion during proton therapy. J Appl Clin Med Phys. 2017;18:106–12.

11. Jones RT, Hassan Rezaeian N, Desai NB, Lotan Y, Jia X, Hannan R, et al. Dosimetric comparison of rectal-sparing capabilities of rectal balloon vs injectable spacer gel in stereotactic body radiation therapy for prostate cancer: lessons learned from prospective trials. Med Dosim. 2017;42:341–7.

12. Müller A-C, Mischinger J, Klotz T, Gagel B, Habl G, Hatiboglu G, et al. Interdisciplinary consensus statement on indication and application of a hydrogel spacer for prostate radiotherapy based on experience in more than 250 patients. Radiol Oncol. 2016;50. https://doi.org/10.1515/raon-2016-0036.

13. Ruggieri R, Naccarato S, Stavrev P, Stavreva N, Fersino S, Giaj Levra N, et al. Volumetric-modulated arc stereotactic body radiotherapy for prostate cancer: dosimetric impact of an increased near-maximum target dose and of a rectal spacer. Br J Radiol. 2015;88:20140736.

14. Fischer-Valuck BW, Chundury A, Gay H, Bosch W, Michalski J. Hydrogel spacer distribution within the perirectal space in patients undergoing radiotherapy for prostate cancer: impact of spacer symmetry on rectal dose reduction and the clinical consequences of hydrogel infiltration into the rectal wall. Pract Radiat Oncol. 2017;7:195–202.

15. Cox JD, Stetz J, Pajak TF. Toxicity criteria of the radiation therapy oncology group (RTOG) and the European organization for research and treatment of cancer (EORTC). Int J Radiat Oncol Biol Phys. 1995;31:1341–6.

16. Lee WR, Bare RL, Marshall MG, McCullough DL. Postimplant analysis of transperineal interstitial permanent prostate brachytherapy: evidence for a learning curve in the first year at a single institution. Int J Radiat Oncol Biol Phys. 2000;46:83–8.

17. Zaorsky NG, Davis BJ, Nguyen PL, Showalter TN, Hoskin PJ, Yoshioka Y, et al. The evolution of brachytherapy for prostate cancer. Nat Rev Urol. 2017;14:415–39.

18. Thompson SR, Delaney GP, Gabriel GS, Izard MA, Hruby G, Jagavkar R, et al. Prostate brachytherapy in New South Wales: patterns of care study and impact of caseload on treatment quality. J Contemp Brachytherapy. 2014;4:344–9.

19. Pinkawa M, Klotz J, Djukic V, Schubert C, Escobar-Corral N, Caffaro M, et al. Learning curve in the application of a hydrogel spacer to protect the Rectal Wall during radiotherapy of localized prostate Cancer. Urology. 2013;82:963–8.

20. Acher P, Popert R, Nichol J, Potters L, Morris S, Beaney R. Permanent prostate brachytherapy: Dosimetric results and analysis of a learning curve with a dynamic dose-feedback technique. Int J Radiat Oncol. 2006;65:694–8.

21. Chao M, Ho H, Chan Y, Tan A, Pham T, Bolton D, et al. Prospective analysis of hydrogel spacer for patients with prostate cancer undergoing radiotherapy. BJU Int. 2018. https://doi.org/10.1111/bju.14192.

22. Karsh LI, Gross ET, Pieczonka CM, Aliotta PJ, Skomra CJ, Ponsky LE, et al. Absorbable hydrogel spacer use in prostate radiotherapy: a comprehensive review of phase 3 clinical trial published data. Urology. 2017. https://doi.org/10.1016/j.urology.2017.11.016.

23. Uhl M, Herfarth K, Eble MJ, Pinkawa M, van Triest B, Kalisvaart R, et al. Absorbable hydrogel spacer use in men undergoing prostate cancer radiotherapy: 12 month toxicity and proctoscopy results of a prospective multicenter phase II trial. Radiat Oncol. 2014;9:96.

24. Alongi F, Cozzi L, Arcangeli S, Iftode C, Comito T, Villa E, et al. Linac based SBRT for prostate cancer in 5 fractions with VMAT and flattening filter free beams: preliminary report of a phase II study. Radiat Oncol. 2013;8:171.

25. Wilton L, Richardson M, Keats S, Legge K, Hanlon M-C, Arumugam S, et al. Rectal protection in prostate stereotactic radiotherapy: a retrospective exploratory analysis of two rectal displacement devices. J Med Radiat Sci. 2017;64:266–73.

26. Hutchinson RC, Sundaram V, Folkert M, Lotan Y. Decision analysis model evaluating the cost of a temporary hydrogel rectal spacer before prostate radiation therapy to reduce the incidence of rectal complications. Urol Oncol Semin Orig Investig. 2016;34:291.e19–26.

16

Planning comparison of five automated treatment planning solutions for locally advanced head and neck cancer

J. Krayenbuehl[1*], M. Zamburlini[1], S. Ghandour[2], M. Pachoud[2], S. Tanadini-Lang[1], J. Tol[3], M. Guckenberger[1] and W. F. A. R. Verbakel[3]

Abstract

Background: Automated treatment planning and/or optimization systems (ATPS) are in the process of broad clinical implementation aiming at reducing inter-planner variability, reducing the planning time allocated for the optimization process and improving plan quality. Five different ATPS used clinically were evaluated for advanced head and neck cancer (HNC).

Methods: Three radiation oncology departments compared 5 different ATPS: 1) Automatic Interactive Optimizer (AIO) in combination with RapidArc (in-house developed and Varian Medical Systems); 2) Auto-Planning (AP) (Philips Radiation Oncology Systems); 3) RapidPlan version 13.6 (RP1) with HNC model from University Hospital A (Varian Medical Systems, Palo Alto, USA); 4) RapidPlan version 13.7 (RP2) combined with scripting for automated setup of fields with HNC model from University Hospital B; 5) Raystation multicriteria optimization algorithm version 5 (RS) (Laboratories AB, Stockholm, Sweden). Eight randomly selected HNC cases from institution A and 8 from institution B were used. PTV coverage, mean and maximum dose to the organs at risk and effective planning time were compared. Ranking was done based on 3 Gy increments for the parallel organs.

Results: All planning systems achieved the hard dose constraints for the PTVs and serial organs for all patients. Overall, AP achieved the best ranking for the parallel organs followed by RS, AIO, RP2 and RP1. The oral cavity mean dose was the lowest for RS (31.3 ± 17.6 Gy), followed by AP (33.8 ± 17.8 Gy), RP1 (34.1 ± 16.7 Gy), AIO (36.1 ± 16.8 Gy) and RP2 (36.3 ± 16.2 Gy). The submandibular glands mean dose was 33.6 ± 10.8 Gy (AP), 35.2 ± 8.4 Gy (AIO), 35.5 ± 9.3 Gy (RP2), 36.9 ± 7.6 Gy (RS) and 38.2 ± 7.0 Gy (RP1). The average effective planning working time was substantially different between the five ATPS (in minutes): < 2 ± 1 for AIO and RP2, 5 ± 1 for AP, 15 ± 2 for RP1 and 116 ± 11 for RS, respectively.

Conclusions: All ATPS were able to achieve all planning DVH constraints and the effective working time was kept bellow 20 min for each ATPS except for RS. For the parallel organs, AP performed the best, although the differences were small.

Keywords: Volumetric modulated arc therapy, Automated treatment planning, Head and neck carcinoma, Planning study, RapidPlan, Auto-planning, Raystation multicriteria optimization

* Correspondence: Jerome.krayenbuehl@usz.ch
[1]Department of Radiation Oncology, University Hospital Zurich, Rämistrasse 100, CH-8091 Zurich, Switzerland
Full list of author information is available at the end of the article

Background

In the past decade, intensity modulated radiotherapy (IMRT) and volumetric modulated radiotherapy (VMAT) became standard techniques for external beam radiotherapy treatments (EBRT) of many indications. The inverse optimization approach is an iterative process where optimization objectives are used in order to achieve the pre-defined clinical goals. Additionally, help structures are frequently defined to shape the dose distribution and further individualize and optimize the treatment plan. The complexity of the optimization increases with the number of organ at risks (OAR) and the number of target volumes. Head and neck carcinoma (HNC) is a typical complex case where a large number of OARs, typically 10–20, are surrounding the target volumes irradiated to different dose levels. This makes inverse planning optimization one of the most time consuming steps of the overall treatment planning process.

Additionally, plan quality may vary between planners and between clinical institutions. Plans produced by an experienced center may outperform those produced in a less experienced center [1] and the OAR sparing also depends on the planning target volume (PTV) dose homogeneity requirements [2]. Furthermore, evaluation of plan quality is often based on population-based dose volume histogram parameters (DVH), which neglect the nuances of an individual patients' geometry and therefore do not achieve the optimal solution based on a patient-individual level [3]. In order to overcome these issues, optimization modules were developed in order to automate part or the entire optimization [4–9] process. They all aim at reducing the inter-planner variability, reducing the planning time allocated for the optimization process and finally improving the overall plan quality [10, 11]. Nowadays, automated treatment planning and/or optimization systems (ATPS) are in the process of broad clinical implementation. However, since ATPS have to be customized in order to fulfill the specific constraints required by different medical centers, it could be that an ATPS implemented at one institution will not necessary work for patients from another institution. The goal of this study was to compare different ATPS for HNC planning in a multicenter setting.

Additionally, it was evaluated if a model for automated planning developed by one institution could be used for planning cases of another institution using similar but not the same structures and planning goals. This multi-institutional planning comparison of five ATPS solutions is, to the best of our knowledge, the first of its kind.

Methods

Study design

In this multi-institutional planning study, five automated treatment planning systems used in 3 different institutes were evaluated:

1) Automatic Interactive Optimizer (AIO) (in-house developed) in combination with RapidArc version 13.7 from Eclipse (Varian Medical Systems, Palo Alto, USA) from hospital B [4, 12];

2) Auto-Planning version 14.0 (AP) from Pinnacle (Philips Radiation Oncology Systems) from hospital A [6];

3) RapidPlan version 13.6 (RP1) from Eclipse (Varian Medical Systems, Palo Alto, USA) using HNC model from hospital A;

4) RapidPlan version 13.7 (RP2) combined with scripting for automated setup of fields with HNC model from hospital B [13];

5) Raystation multicriteria optimization algorithm version 5 (RS) (RaySearch Laboratories AB, Stockholm, Sweden), from hospital C.

Ten randomly selected locally advanced HNC cases were chosen from each of two different institutes (A and B). Two cases from each group were used to familiarize with the target volume, concepts, dose constraints and to generate an automated planning strategy. A single optimization using the same strategy was performed for the remaining cases. Only these eight cases for each institution, overall 16 cases, were included in the planning comparison.

Patients from institute A had three PTV dose levels, with doses of 70 Gy, 60 Gy and 54 Gy planned in 35 fractions using a simultaneous integrated boost (SIB), see Table 1 and Fig. 1. The dose was normalized to PTV 70Gy mean dose = 70 Gy.

Patients from institute B had two dose levels defined: 70 Gy and 54 Gy in 35 fractions using a SIB, see Table 1 and Fig. 1. The dose was normalized such that 95% of the PTV 70 Gy volume received 98% of the prescribed dose (70 Gy).

For both sets of patients, hard planning constraints were set for the PTVs and serial OAR, which had to be fulfilled by all planning system and patient cases, see Table 1. For the parallel OARs, the mean dose was asked to be kept as low as reasonably achievable. All plans were optimized with a 2 arc, 6 MV VMAT technique.

Plan evaluation

Dose-volume histogram (DVH) parameters were calculated for the PTVs and each of the OARs listed in Table 1. Maximum doses for the serial OAR were reported but the differences were not considered in this planning comparison. This allows the optimization algorithm to further reduce dose to the parallel organs. The dose bath was evaluated based on the volumes covered by the 50 Gy, 30 Gy and 5 Gy isodose surfaces.

Doses to parallel OARs were evaluated based on their mean dose. A ranking for each parallel OAR was performed per patient. A rank of 1 was given for the ATPS

Table 1 Targets, organs at risk and objectives used for plan optimization

Institution A	Institution B
Prescription	
70 Gy, 60 Gy and 54 Gy	70 Gy and 54 Gy
35 fractions with a simultaneous integrated boost	
Beam arrangement	
2 volumetric modulated arcs, 6MV photons	
PTVs	
PTV 70Gy Dmean = 70Gy	PTV 70Gy D95% = 98%
PTV 70Gy V95% > 95%	PTV 70Gy V107% < 5%
PTV 70Gy D2% > 75Gy	PTV 54Gy D95% > 98%
PTV 60Gy V95% > 95%	PTV 54Gy V107% < 5%
PTV 54Gy V95% > 95%	
Serial organs	
Brainstem Dmax < 54 Gy	Brainstem + 3 mm Dmax < 50 Gy
Brachial Plexus D0.5cm^3 < 60 Gy	
Mandible V70 Gy < 1 cm^3	Mandible Dmax < 70 Gy
Spinal cord < 45 Gy	Spinal cord + 3 mm Dmax < 54 Gy
Parallel organs	
	UAT Cricopharyngeal
Glottis	
	Larynx Lower
	Larynx Upper
Pharynx constrictor	
	Superior PCM
	Medial PCM
	Inferior PCM
Upper esophagus	Upper esophagus
	Upper Esophageal Sphincter
Thyroid	Thyroid
Trachea	Trachea
Oral cavity	Oral cavity
Parotids	Parotids
Submandibular glands	Submandibular glands

Abbreviation: *PCM* pharyngeal constrictor muscles, *UAT* upper aerodigestve tract

achieving the lowest mean dose for a given OAR. Each ATPS achieving a dose within 3 Gy to the lowest achieved dose was given a ranking of 1, assuming that a dose difference < 3 Gy was not clinically relevant in our case [14–16]. The ATPS achieving a dose within 3 Gy – 6 Gy to the lowest achieved dose had a rank of 2, within 6 Gy – 9 Gy, a rank of 3, etc. The mean ranking was calculated for the individual swallowing muscles plus trachea and thyroid gland resulting in a structure called upper aerodigestive tract (UAT).

Finally, an overall mean ranking was taken by averaging the mean rank for parotid glands, submandibular glands and oral cavity.

The time required to generate a plan was evaluated and divided into 2 parts:

1) The effective working time was defined as the time required by the planner to generate a plan. This included the time needed for the definition of auxiliary structures and definition of bolus structures if a PTV reached the skin surface. For RS, it also included the user navigation through the Pareto-optimal plan database. This time didn't include the time required for the optimization.

2) Optimization time, during which no interaction of the user was needed. For RS, it includes the automatic generation of Pareto-optimal plans and the final deliverable plan.

Automated treatment planning system
AIO
Using the application programming interface (API) of the Eclipse treatment planning system, several scripts were developed to; create the PTV structures used in the optimization; generate ring structures around the PTVs; position two RapidArc fields and the isocenter positioned in the center-of-mass of the total PTV. The scripts automatically positioned fixed optimization objectives for the PTVs, serial OARs, and ring structures, while for each parallel OAR, 10 optimization objectives are positioned evenly spread among the volume axis. After this, the user has to manually open the optimization window of the treatment planning system to start the automatic interactive optimization (AIO) process. AIO is a program that automatically adapts the optimization objectives of the parallel OAR during the optimization process, keeping them at a fixed distance from the DVH-line at all times [12, 17].

Auto-planning
Auto-Planning (AP), included in Pinnacle 14.0 (Philips Radiation Oncology Systems), is a fully integrated module in the TPS, similar to the "manual" inverse optimizer module and has been previously described [6, 18]. Briefly, Pinnacle AP is a template-knowledge based treatment planning system. During AP, a plan is automatically loaded and the isocenter placed at the center-of-mass of the total PTV. The optimizer is than automatically run multiple times with the individual optimization goals, constraints and weights automatically added and adjusts the priority of clinical goals based on their probability of being achieved.

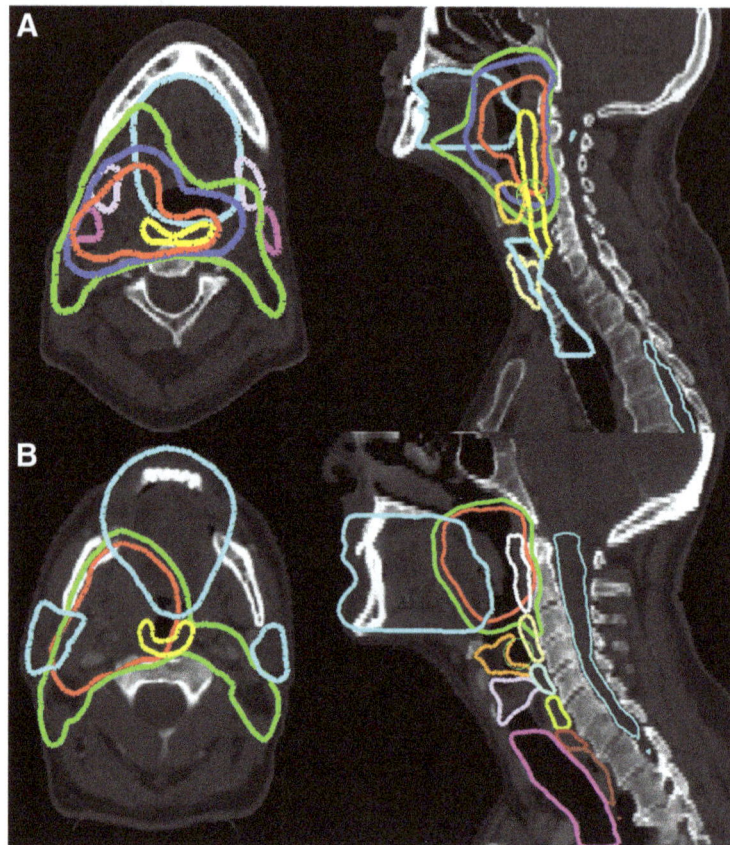

Fig. 1 Example of one head and neck case from institution A (**a**) and one from institution B (**b**). In red, blue and light green the PTVs 70 Gy, 60 Gy and 54 Gy respectively as well as the OARs

RapidPlan with a model from institute A (RP1)

Rapidplan (RP) is a knowledge-based automatic planning solution. A set of previously created plans representative of the internal hospital guidelines are fed into the program, which through a statistical modeling, creates a model. This model takes into account the geometrical and dosimetrical properties of the plans and is able to generate individualized constraints for the future plans taking into account their particular geometry, based on the library plans. Since RP is based on hospital-specific plans, the model is optimized to produce plans with a specific dose distribution and to accept OAR within a certain size and location. RP1 model was based on 83 clinically delivered HNC plans with SIB concept but variable dose levels created using 6MV photons and 2 full arcs. Since OAR definition from Institution A was different from Institution B, it was necessary to sum several OARs from Institution B before RP1 could be used.

RapidPlan with a model from institute B (RP2)

The same script as for AIO was used for the creation of the RapidPlan plans. However, instead of positioning all

optimization objectives as a preparation for AIO, a script was developed to call a RapidPlan model from institute B to predict achievable OAR doses and position optimization objectives for the various targets and OARs. This model was based on 177 clinical patient plans, which is an extension of a previously made model [13].

Raystation

The MultiCriteria optimization algorithm MCO is a convex optimization problem [19] based on the approximation of the Pareto surface-based technique [20] where a set of Pareto-optimal plans is automatically generated and stored in a database for each patient. The user can navigate through this "Pareto-optimal" plans database and assess in real-time the tradeoff between different objective functions assigned to each anatomical structure. The desired plan that meets the clinical goals is then selected by the planner and generated to be delivered to the patient [21]. In this study, the geometry of planning targets volumes PTVs were replaced with convex approximation geometry as a means to control the increased level of fluence modulation otherwise caused by a non-convex target shape. The DVH-based functions were used as hard constraints in order to respect the clinical constraints.

Statistical analysis

The mean dose to the parallel organs were reported as well as the standard deviation. The Wilcoxon signed rank test was used to compare the mean doses of the parallel organs of each planning system with those of the planning system that achieved the lowest mean dose. A $p \leq 0.05$ was considered significant.

Results

Dose distribution

The detailed results for the five ATPS are included in Tables 2 and 3. Each planning system were able to be modified successfully to achieve the hard constraints for the PTVs and serial organs for each patients listed in Table 1. Small variations in serial OAR doses were observed between the different ATPS but were judged as clinically irrelevant.

The dose bath $V_{50\ Gy}$ and $V_{30\ Gy}$ was lowest for RS, whereas AIO had the lowest $V_{5\ Gy}$, see Table 2. AP had on average the largest volume exposed to 50 Gy and 5 Gy. $V_{50\ Gy}$ and $V_{30\ Gy}$ were increased in comparison to RS by $1.9 \pm 10.6\%$ and $12.9 \pm 18.0\%$ (RP1), $6.1 \pm 10.4\%$ and $27.0 \pm 13.7\%$ (RP2), $8.7 \pm 12.4\%$ and $33.2 \pm 13.0\%$ (AIO), $18.5 \pm 17.6\%$ and $23.9 \pm 17.8\%$ (AP). $V_{5\ Gy}$ was increased in comparison to AIO by $2.4 \pm 3.7\%$ (RP2), $3.9 \pm 4.7\%$ (RS), $6.8 \pm 9.9\%$ (RP1) and $11.4 \pm 12.8\%$ (AP).

The mean dose results for the parallel organs are summarized in Table 3. Overall, AP had the best overall ranking for the parallel organs followed by RS ($p = 0.20$), AIO ($p = 0.03$), RP2 ($p = 0.01$), and RP1 ($p < 0.01$). When looking at each organ separately, the oral cavity mean dose was significantly lower with RS (31.3 ± 17.6 Gy) compared to AP (33.8 ± 17.8 Gy), RP1 (34.1 ± 16.7 Gy), AIO (36.1 ± 16.8 Gy) and RP2 (36.3 ± 16.2 Gy), $p < 0.05$. The lowest, respectively the highest, parotids mean dose was 21.2 ± 5.9 Gy (AP) and 22.8 ± 6.2 Gy (RP2) respectively. No significant differences were observed between the ATPS ($p > 0.2$). The submandibular glands mean dose was 33.6 ± 10.8 Gy (AP), 35.2 ± 8.4 Gy (AIO), 35.5 ± 9.3 Gy (RP2), 36.9 ± 7.6 Gy (RS) and 38.2 ± 7.0 Gy (RP1). Only RP1 and RS were significantly different to AP. In the subgroup of the UAT, large dose variations, up to 15 Gy, were observed for small structures such as the cricopharynx or the upper pharyngeal constrictor muscles between the ATPS. Averaging over all UAT structures reduced the differences. The lowest UAT mean dose was obtained with AIO (38.8 ± 9.3 Gy), AP (39.3 ± 9.4 Gy), RP2 (39.7 ± 8.9 Gy), RS (40.4 ± 8.4 Gy) and RP1 (43.4 ± 7.6 Gy). RP1 was the only ATPS having a significantly higher mean UAT dose compared to the ATPS achieving the lowest mean dose (AIO), $p < 0.01$.

Planning time

The effective working time required after volume definition by the clinicians to the end of the optimization process was evaluated for every planning system. This time was kept below 2 min for each plan optimized with AIO and RP 2, see Table 4. The mean effective working time was increased by 3 ± 1 for AP, 13 ± 2 by RP1 and 116 ± 11 min by RS, respectively.

Table 2 Detailed results for the PTVs, dose bath and serial organs

Structure			AIO		AP		RP1		RP2		RS	
			Mean	SD	Mean	SD	Mean	SD	Mean	SD	Mean	SD
Targets	PTV 70Gy	Dmean (Gy)	70.9	0.2	70.5	0.3	70.8	0.3	70.5	0.3	70.4	0.2
		V95% (%)	97.6	0.6	98.9	0.2	97.7	0.6	97.8	0.5	98.8	0.2
		D2% (Gy)	73.4	0.4	72.6	0.2	73.6	0.2	73.3	0.1	72.1	0.1
	PTV60Gy	V95% (%)	98.9	0.4	99.9	0.1	99.1	0.3	99.0	0.2	99.7	0.2
	PTV 54Gy	V95% (%)	98.2	0.4	98.7	0.6	98.3	0.4	98.8	0.3	98.0	0.6
Dose bath	Body	V50Gy (dm³)	1.02	0.34	1.12	0.34	0.96	0.30	1.00	0.32	0.94	0.32
		V30Gy (dm³)	2.50	0.62	2.32	0.66	2.12	0.56	2.38	0.61	1.88	0.43
		V5Gy (dm³)	6.39	1.28	7.12	1.40	6.83	1.35	6.54	1.40	6.64	1.36
Serial Organs	Brachial Plexus	D0.5 cm³ (Gy)	53.1	3.5	53.1	4.3	54.2	3.6	52.7	2.7	51.1	7.4
	Brainstem	Dmax (Gy)	30.2	15.5	27.4	13.6	26.2	14.7	30.6	12.8	23.7	13.4
	Mandible	Dmax (Gy)	67.8	4.6	66.6	5.5	68.0	7.9	67.1	12.0	67.0	3.2
	Spinal cord	Dmax (Gy)	40.7	0.8	41.5	2.2	41.3	2.1	40.8	1.3	36.0	2.9

Abbreviations: *AIO* automatic Interactive Optimizer, *AP* auto-planning, *RP* RapidPlan, *RS* Raystation, *V* $_{95\%}$ percentage volume receiving 95% of prescribed dose, *D* $_{2\%}$ dose corresponding to 2%, *D* $_{0.5\ cm^3}$ dose corresponding to 0.5 cm³, *V* $_{X\ Gy}$ volume receiving X Gy, *Dmax* maximal dose, *SD* standard deviation

Table 3 Detailed results for the parallel organs. Statistical significance was tested for each parallel organ group in comparison with the planning system that achieved lowest averaged mean dose (bold). Any $0.01 \leq p \leq 0.05$ is indicated with a *, and $p \leq 0.01$ is indicated with **

	AIO		AP		RP1		RP2		RS	
	Mean ± SD (Gy)	Rank± SD	Mean ± SD (Gy)	Rank ±SD	Mean ± SD (Gy)	Rank ±SD	Mean ± SD (Gy)	Rank ±SD	Mean ± SD (Gy)	Rank ±SD
OralCavity	36.1 ± 16.8 **	2.56 ± 1.21	33.8 ± 17.8*	1.63 ± 0.62	34.1 ± 16.7**	1.81 ± 0.75	36.3 ± 16.2**	2.75 ± 1.34	**31.3 ± 17.6**	1.06 0.25
Parotid	21.9 ± 6.3	1.31 ± 0.6	**21.2 ± 5.9**	1.19 ± 0.40	21.6 ± 6.3	1.25 ± 0.45	22.8 ± 6.2	1.50 ± 0.73	21.4 ± 6.2	1.19 ± 0.54
Submand. Glands	35.2 ± 8.4	1.94 ± 1.34	**33.6 ± 10.8**	1.44 ± 0.81	38.2 ± 7.0 **	2.88 ± 1.41	35.5 ± 9.3	1.88 ± 1.09	36.9 ± 7.6*	2.38 ± 1.15
UAT	**38.8 ± 9.3**	1.49 ± 0.37	39.3 ± 9.4	1.86 ± 0.64	43.4 ± 7.6**	2.99 ± 1.01	39.7 ± 8.9	1.89 ± 0.7	40.4 ± 8.4	2.00 ± 0.70
Average		1.83 ± 1.06*		**1.53 ± 0.67**		2.23 ± 1.20**		2.00 ± 1.08*		1.66 ± 0.91

Abbreviations: *AIO* automatic interactive optimizer, *AP* auto-planning, *RP* RapidPlan, *RS* Raystation, *SD* standard deviation, *UAT* upper aerodigestve tract

Discussion

This study presented a multi-institutional planning comparison study of five ATPS used in 3 different institutes, performed on 16 locally advanced head and neck cancer patients coming from two institutes. Although larger differences were observed for an individual patient, when looking at the mean results over all 16 patients, dosimetric differences between ATPS were generally small with Auto-Planning achieving the best ranking. Effective working time differed considerably more between ATPS, from 2 up till 116 minutes.

ATPS can be classified between automated optimization and automated planning, including optimization. The automated optimization can again be distinguished as optimization algorithm driven systems, such as AIO, AP and RS, were the objectives and/or priorities are automatically adjusted during the optimization and knowledge based planning systems based on plan libraries such as RP1 and RP2. The automated optimization algorithm driven systems can be easily modified to take into account possible changes in clinical protocols. This is not necessary the case for the knowledge based planning systems which rely on plans for a database of prior patients. Contrariwise, the use of a database allows a comparison between the predicted and achieved dose volume histogram [13].

The second classification can be performed based on automated planning where not only the optimization process is automated but also the field setup, gantry and collimator angles, the positioning of the isocenter and help structures such as bolus, rings structures or non-overlapping structures. This fully automated process was used by AIO, AP and RP2. RP1 and RS could also automate these planning process but it was not implemented.

After dose optimization, a single plan was generated by each ATPS except for RS where the user had to select a plan from a database of Pareto-optimal plans. This manual step will reduce the inter-planner standardization but will allow the user to choose the best dose trade-off between the targets and OARs.

Wu et al. [22] compared AP and RP, for oropharyngeal cancer patients and found that the plan quality from both systems was comparable. Differences between the two systems were in the range of 5%, which is in good agreement to the small differences observed in our study. To the best of our knowledge, no other ATPS comparisons are available.

The two sets of HNC were chosen to evaluate the flexibility of the different ATPS to take into account new structures, objectives and/or different dose levels. The model for AIO, AP and RS could be easily modified because they are based on a set of user pre-defined DVHs parameters, which were automatically adjusted during the optimization. However for the RS, the combination of objectives/constraints and the selection of their formulation had to be adjusted manually for each plan depending on the overlap between the PTV and OAR which affects directly the Pareto surface computation. This is not the case for RP models, which are based on previously generated site-specific plan libraries. In this

Table 4 Effective working time and optimization time

	AIO		AP		RP1		RP2		RS	
	Mean	StDev	Mean	StDev	Mean	StDev	Mean	StDev	Mean	StDev
Eff. working time (min)	< 2	< 1	5	1	15	2	< 1	< 1	116	11
Optimization time (min)	31	4	83	10	27	4	28	7	218	30

Abbreviations: *AIO* automatic interactive optimizer, *AP* auto-planning, *RP* RapidPlan, *RS* Raystation

case, the model had to be manually modified to take into account the structures not defined in the library. RP1 and RP2 were both used without considering whether a particular structure was an outlier. At later inspection, all OAR of the third case from group A were listed as "outside threshold values" for RP2 as the PTV_70Gy size of 585cm^3 was above the 90 percentile value of the model. This could have a negative effect on the predictions. RP2 parotid gland doses were 7 Gy higher than for AP for this case. Similarly, when applying RP1 to the patients in the group B, the Glottis was marked as outlier for each single patient, and the swallowing muscles received with RP1 in these patients the highest mean dose. This was also the organ in which the highest differences between RP1 and the other ATPs were observed, clearly showing that the model was not able to predict the correct objectives for this case. This could be overcome by deciding that patients with such warning signs by Rapid-Plan should not be subject to automated planning. In spite of this, we compared how RP1 and RP2 performed for each organ with the data from the own institution and the external patient data. We did not notice large dosimetric differences, demonstrating that rapidplan also works for patients with slightly different structure sets and prescriptions.

The time required to generate VMAT or IMRT plans has been reduced in the past years by improvement of the available tools in planning system as well as automation of steps in the optimization process time. Nowadays, planning templates, scripts and optimization automation are available in TPS. This allows a gain of time on one side and a standardization of the plan quality at a high level on the other side. The effective working time for ATPS planned with VMAT was reported to be less than 10 min with iCycle [23] and less than 4 min with AP [6], but the overall time was not recorded. The effective working time reported are in the same order as those from our study. By adding scripting to the automated optimization processes, effective planning time could be reduced to less than 2 min with RP and AIO. Similar scripting tools are also available in AP but were not implemented. This might have led to a similar reduction of the effective working time.

RS required substantially more time to generate VMAT plans as the other ATPS mainly for two reasons. The first reason is the technique employed in this study where each PTV geometry was approximated by a "more convex" or "less concave" geometry depending on the type of the nearest OAR (serial or parallel architecture). This additional planning step was introduced as earlier publications had shown that RS generated high quality plans in an efficient treatment planning time for convex target geometry [6, 17, 18]. Therefore, each PTV geometry was approximated by a "more convex" or "less concave" geometry depending on the type of the nearest OAR (serial or

parallel architecture). The second reason is that the HNC patients required a high-dimensional Pareto-surface approximation. Thus, the optimization time rises with the number of objective functions used during the optimization process. In our case, 20 objectives on average were used leading to a Pareto-surface approximation generated by 40 plans, as recommended by Craft et al. [20] for each patient. The optimization time was similar for RP for both institutions. AIO, which is running on the same system as RP, needed a few minutes longer to finish the optimization since the optimization is paused to automatically adjust the objectives. AP performs multitude steps of optimization and dose calculation where the objectives and help structures are automatically adjusted and created. This iterative process is time consuming and lasts typically between 1 h and 1.5 h. The optimization time is increased to three to 4 h with RS due to the reasons mentioned above. However, this approach allows the user to select the plan having the best balance between the targets and OARS dose. The optimization time mentioned above can be influenced by the number of users working in parallel on the server as well as its performances; therefore this parameter should be taken only as a rough estimation of the optimization time.

This study was focused on HNC treatment and whether similar results will be obtained for other sites still needs to be assessed.

Conclusion

The results obtained for the five ATPS evaluated on two different set of HNC patients show that all ATPS were able to fulfill the hard constraints. For the parallel organs, AP achieved the best results followed by RS, AIO, RP2 and RP1. Nevertheless, the differences were small. The effective working time was reduced to less than 20' for each ATPS, except RS, and could be reduced to less than 2' when using scripting, which was the case for AIO and RP2.

Abbreviations
AIO: Automatic interactive optimizer; AP: Auto-planning; ATPS: Automated treatment planning systems; D $_{0.5\ cm^3}$: Dose corresponding to 0.5 cm^3; D $_{2\%}$: Dose corresponding to 2%; Dmax: Maximal dose; DVH: Volume histogram parameters; EBRT: External beam radiotherapy treatments; HNC: Head and neck cancer; IMRT: Intensity modulated radiotherapy; OAR: Organ at risk; PCM: Pharyngeal constrictor muscles; PTV: Planning target volume; RP1: RapidPlan model from Hospital A; RP2: RapidPlan model from Hospital B; RS: Raystation; SD: Standard deviation; SIB: Simultaneous integrated boost; UAT: Upper aerodigestve tract; V $_{x\ Gy}$: Volume receiving X Gy; VMAT: Volumetric modulated radiotherapy

Authors' contributions
JK generated a model in AP, MZ generated a model for RP1, SG and MP generated a model for RS, JT and WFARV generated a model for RP2 and AIO. JK and MZ drafted the manuscript. JT, SL, MG and WFARV were

responsible for critical revision of the manuscript and provided senior input throughout the study. All authors read and approved the final manuscript.

Competing interests

The authors declare that they have no competing interests.

Author details

[1]Department of Radiation Oncology, University Hospital Zurich, Rämistrasse 100, CH-8091 Zurich, Switzerland. [2]Department of Radiation Oncology, Hôpital Riviera-Chablais, Avenue de la Prairie 3, CH-1800 Vevey, Switzerland. [3]Department of Radiotherapy, VU University Medical Center, De Boelelaan 1117, 1081, HV, Amsterdam, The Netherlands.

References

1. Chung H, Lee B, Park E, et al. Can all centers plan intensity-modulated radiotherapy (imrt) effectively? An external audit of dosimetric comparisons between three-dimensional conformal radiotherapy and imrt for adjuvant chemoradiation for gastric cancer. Oncol Biol Phys. 2008;71:1167–74.
2. Tol J, Dahele M, Doornaert P, et al. Different treatment planning protocols can lead to large differences in organ at risk sparing. Radiother Oncol. 2014; 113:267–71.
3. Wu B, Ricchetti F, Sanguineti G, et al. Patient geometry-driven information retrieval for imrt treatment plan quality control. Med Phys. 2009;36:5497–54505.
4. Tol J, Delaney A, Dahele M, et al. Evaluation of a knowledge-based planning solution for head and neck cancer. Int. J. Radiat. Oncol. Biol. Phys. 2015;91:612–20.
5. Appenzoller L, Michalski J, Thorstad W, et al. Predicting dose-volume histograms for organs-at-risk in imrt planning. Medical Phyics. 2012;39:7446–61.
6. Krayenbuehl J, Norton I, Studer G, Guckenberger M. Evaluation of an automated knowledge based treatment planning system for head and neck. Radiation Oncol (London, England). 2015;10:226. https://doi.org/10.1186/s13014-015-0533-2.
7. Fogliata A, Belosi F, Clivio A, et al. On the pre-clinical validation of a commercial model-based optimisation engine: application to volumetric modulated arc therapy for patients with lung or prostate cancer. Radiother Oncol. 2014;113: 385–91.
8. Breedveld S, Storchi P, Heijmen B. The equivalence of multi-criteria methods for radiotherapy plan optimization. Phys Med Biol. 2009;54:7199–209.
9. Ghandour S, Matzinger O, Pachoud M. Volumetric-modulated arc therapy planning using multicriteria optimization for localized prostate cancer. J Appl Clin Med Phys. 2015;16(3):258–69. https://doi.org/10.1120/jacmp.v16i3.5410.
10. Krayenbuehl J, Di M, Guckenberger M, et al. Improved plan quality with automated radiotherapy planning for whole brain with hippocampus sparing: a comparison to the rtog 0933 trial. Radiat Oncol. 2017;12
11. Winkel D, Bol G, van Asselen B, et al. Development and clinical introduction of automated radiotherapy treatment planning for prostate cancer. Phys Med Biol. 2016;61:8587–95.
12. Tol JP, Dahele M, Peltola J, Nord J, Slotman BJ, Verbakel WF. Automatic interactive optimization for volumetric modulated arc therapy planning. Radiat Oncol (London, England). 2015;10:75. https://doi.org/10.1186/s13014-015-0388-6.
13. Tol J, Dahele M, Delaney A, et al. Can knowledge-based dvh predictions be used for automated, individualized quality assurance of radiotherapy treatment plans? Radiat Oncol. 2015;10:1–14.
14. Bentzen S, Constine L, Deasy J, et al. Quantitative analyses of normal tissue effects in the clinic (quantec): an introduction to the scientific issues. Int. J. Radiat. Oncol. Biol. Phys. 2010;76:3–9.
15. Eisbruch A, Haken R, Kim H, et al. Dose, volume, and function relationships in parotid salivary glands following conformal and intensity-modulated irradiation of head and neck cancer. Int. J. Radiat. Oncol. Biol. Phys. 1999;45: 577–87.
16. Debelleix C, Pointreau Y, Lafond C, et al. Normal tissue tolerance to external beam radiation therapy: larynx and pharynx. Cancer Radiother. 2010;14:301–6.
17. Tol J, Dahele M, Doornaert P, et al. Toward optimal organ at risk sparing in complex volumetric modulated arc therapy: an exponential trade-off with target volume dose homogeneity. Medical Phyics. 2014;41:021722.
18. Hazell I, Bzdusek K, Kumar P, et al. Automatic planning of head and neck treatment plans. J Appl Clin Med Phys. 2016;17:272–82.
19. Bokrantz R. Multicriteria optimization for volumetric-modulated arc therapy by decomposition into a fluence-based relaxation and a segment weight-based restriction. Medical Phyics. 2012;39:6712–25.
20. Craft D, Halabi T, Shih H, et al. Approximating convex pareto surfaces in multiobjective radiotherapy planning. Medical Phyics. 2006;33:3399–33407.
21. Young MR, Craft DL, Colbert CM, Remillard K, Vanbenthuysen L, Wang Y. Volumetric-modulated arc therapy using multicriteria optimization for body and extremity sarcoma. J Appl Clin Med Physics. 2016;17(6):283–91.
22. Wu B, Kusters M, Kunze-busch M, et al. Cross-institutional knowledge-based planning (kbp) implementation and its performance comparison to auto-planning engine (ape). Radiother Oncol. 2017;123:57–62.
23. Della Gala G, Dirkx M, Hoekstra N, et al. Fully automated vmat treatment planning for advanced-stage nsclc patients. Strahlenther Onkol. 2017;193:402–9.

17

Image guidance and positioning accuracy in clinical practice: influence of positioning errors and imaging dose on the real dose distribution for head and neck cancer treatment

Katharina Bell[*], Norbert Licht, Christian Rübe and Yvonne Dzierma

Abstract

Background: Modern radiotherapy offers the possibility of highly accurate tumor treatment. To benefit from this precision at its best, regular positioning verification is necessary. By the use of image-guided radiotherapy and the application of safety margins the influence of positioning inaccuracies can be counteracted. In this study the effect of additional imaging dose by set-up verification is compared with the effect of dose smearing by positioning inaccuracies for a collective of head-and-neck cancer patients.

Methods: This study is based on treatment plans of 40 head-and-neck cancer patients. To evaluate the imaging dose several image guidance scenarios with different energies, techniques and frequencies were simulated and added to the original plan. The influence of the positioning inaccuracies was assessed by the use of real applied table shifts for positioning. The isocenters were shifted back appropriately to these values to simulate that no positioning correction had been performed. For the single fractions the shifted plans were summed considering three different scenarios: The summation of only shifted plans, the consideration of the original plan for the fractions with set-up verification, and the addition of the extra imaging dose to the latter. For both effects (additional imaging dose and dose smearing), plans were analyzed and compared considering target coverage, sparing of organs at risk (OAR) and normal tissue complication probability (NTCP).

Results: Daily verification of the patient positioning using 3D imaging with MV energies result in non-negligible high doses. kV imaging has only marginal influence on plan quality, primarily related to sparing of organs at risk, even with daily 3D imaging. For this collective, sparing of organs at risk and NTCP are worse due to potential positioning errors.

Conclusion: Regular set-up verification is essential for precise radiation treatment. Relating to the additional dose, the use of kV modalities is uncritical for any frequency and technique. Dose smearing due to positioning errors for this collective mainly resulted in a decrease of OAR sparing. Target coverage also suffered from the positioning inaccuracies, especially for individual patients. Taking into account both examined effects the relevance of an extensive IGRT is clearly present, even at the expense of additional imaging dose and time expenditure.

Keywords: IGRT, Positioning accuracy, NTCP modelling, Kilovoltage imaging, Megavoltage imaging, Treatment margins

* Correspondence: katharina.bell@uks.eu
Department of Radiotherapy and Radiation Oncology, Saarland University
Medical Centre, Kirrberger Str. Geb. 6.5/Saar, D-66421 Homburg, Germany

Introduction

Modern techniques in radiotherapy offer a more and more precise application of the dose to the target volume. This allows for an adequately sparing of the surrounding tissue while the tumor can be covered with dose as accurately as possible.

An exactly reproducible patient positioning is a prerequisite for the treatment to be successful, as any shift relative to the planned position can result in an underdosage of the target volume or an overdosage of the surrounding organs at risk (OAR). Beside the application of positioning and localization facilities like thermoplastic masks or laser marks, potential inter- and intrafractional shifts are already considered in the planning process by applying safety margins to expand the clinical target volume (CTV) to the planning target volume (PTV). Taking into account the systematic and random errors, there are several recipes to determine the width of these margins [1–3]. The more precisely patient positioning can be achieved the smaller can safety margins be chosen. At the same time OARs can be better spared using narrower margins, so exact positioning results in better sparing of OARs while offering the same target coverage.

To put this into effect, frequent positioning verification before treatment in the context of Image Guided Radiotherapy (IGRT) is the nowadays standard. Modern linear accelerators are equipped with different imaging modalities that can be applied in treatment position. However, as these modalities often use ionizing radiation, the accurate position verification implies a burden of an additional dose, which depends on the imaging energy, number of projections and frequency of the verifications. Ideally, the patients´ position should be controlled and corrected daily, however, the additional dose of the imaging cannot generally be neglected.

Hence there is a trade-off between two effects: By verifying the patients´ set-up regularly the positioning accuracy can be increased, undesirable dose smearing can be avoided and the CTV-PTV expansion margins can be decreased. However, the additional dose may also have a negative effect on the total dose.

The aim of this study is to examine these two effects. To analyze the effect of the additional imaging dose on the plan quality different realistic and representative imaging scenarios are simulated and the imaging dose is added to the original treatment plan, respectively. Within these scenarios we differentiate between imaging techniques (planar vs. 3D), different energies (kV vs. MV) and daily vs. non daily set-up verification. The effect of potential positioning uncertainties on the real dose distribution is also analyzed by simulating different scenarios with variable numbers of set-up corrections. So it can be investigated if the advantage of a higher precision with the possibility of steeper dose gradients and

smaller margins predominates over the disadvantage of the additional dose.

For both effects an evaluation of the dosimetrical plan quality is performed as well as modelling biological aspects in terms of normal tissue complication probabilities. These theoretical estimations are performed on an individual basis for a realistic collective of head and neck (H&N) cancer patients for best possible transferability into the clinical routine. H&N is one of the main indications for regular set-up verifications as the close vicinity of the OARs to the target volume and its complex shape requires steep dose gradients and an exact patient positioning [4, 5].

This is the first study to combine and balance both described aspects regarding IGRT. The current literature offers a number of studies either focusing on the additional imaging dose or the influence of positioning uncertainties on the dose distribution. Moreover, most studies regarding imaging dose primarily concentrate on the dose by itself [6–13], only few have the focus on the clinical consequences for plan quality [14–18]. There is one study to evaluate systematically the influence of different imaging scenarios on plan quality, however, this study deals with prostate treatment [19]. The effect of dose smearing is also sparsely examined by now, most studies on this topic rely on rather theoretical models of the average positioning errors and the resulting dose volume histogram [1, 3, 20–23]. So to our knowledge there is no such systematic investigation considering the clinical effect of imaging dose together with the effect of potential dose smearing, for both dosimetrically plan quality and biological aspects.

Material and methods

Collective and equipment

The analysis for this study was performed for a collective of 40 patients with head-and-neck cancer, treated at our institution in 2013. Several indications are included, the collective mostly consists of patients with pharyngeal cancer, cancer of the mouth- or base of the tongue, sporadically also tonsil, parotid and larynx.

The 40 patients were treated with a total of 1325 fractions, with 20–60 fractions per patient depending on indication and concept. Most patients received 30–35 treatment fractions. The prescribed dose to the PTV generally was 50 Gy (2 Gy daily) using a 7–13 beams IMRT with 6 MV photons. Partly, from a dose of 30 Gy, the single fraction dose had been changed from 2 Gy daily in one fraction to 1.4 Gy with two fractions per day following a hyperfractionated concept. With a similar number of beams the treatment plans of this collective include one or two boosts up to a total dose of 60–70 Gy. The CTV-PTV margin amounts to about 5–10 mm.

Planning was performed in the Pinnacle TPS V9.2 on the basis of planning CTs acquired with a Philips Brilliance Big Bore 120 kV.

At our department, three Siemens linacs, two Artistes and one Oncor, with different imaging modalities are available. All three machines can perform imaging using the 6 MV treatment beam line (TBL), the two Artistes are additionally equipped with a dedicated image beam line (IBL) with a nominal energy of 1 MV [24, 25]. A kV modality using an additional X-ray tube is installed at one of the two Artiste machines. Due to the different energies of the imaging modalities, the particular imaging dose differs, just as the image quality.

Imaging is individually performed as prescribed by the radiotherapist, also depending on the current workflow and schedule of the clinical routine. For immobilization, patients are positioned using thermoplastic masks, considering the room lasers to align with corresponding marks. The performed verification images are compared with the digitally reconstructed radiographs or the planning CT and positioning errors are corrected on-line with no action level.

Evaluation of the additional imaging dose

To analyze the effect of the additional imaging dose on the plan quality, the appropriate energies and beam properties of the imaging modalities need to be modelled and commissioned in the TPS. For our modalities this has already been realized in former studies [26, 27]. Additionally to the 6 MV treatment beam line, the IBL and kV imaging have been included in the TPS, so that the distribution of the imaging dose can be calculated and added to the original treatment plan for every patient.

As in our institution the kind and frequency of the executed set-up verifications depend on medical decisions and clinical workflow, patients receive different IGRT schemes. For H&N cancer patients imaging is generally not done daily, but about every third fraction.

To examine the influence of the imaging dose systematically for the different IGRT modalities, we simulated the following hypothetic scenarios (Table 1):

Scenario 1 represents the original treatment plan without imaging dose, as it was accepted for treatment. This serves as a reference for the comparison with the remaining scenarios.

Table 1 Imaging scenarios

Scenario 1	Original plan: without imaging dose
Scenario 2	Not daily: actual performed imaging
Scenario 3	Daily: kV CBCT 200°
Scenario 4	Daily: IBL CBCT 200°
Scenario 5	Daily: 1xTBL CBCT, 4× TBL planar images per week

For scenario 2 we consider the imaging dose every patient received in reality by their individual IGRT schedule. We obtained this data retrospectively from the Record and Verify (R&V) system. This scenario illustrates the non-daily but real imaging.

As it is desirable to verify the patients'position for every fraction, daily imaging is simulated in scenarios 3–5 for the different energies and techniques.

Scenario 3 contains the dose distribution for daily 3D imaging within the kV range. For this collective we consider CBCTs with a 200° rotation. For the kV modality an auto-exposure technique is available, so the mAs product is adapted individually to the patient by a "pre shot". For the calculation of the imaging beams the mean mAs value of the whole collective is used, which comes to a value of 112mAs per CBCT for this collective.

Analogue to this, scenario 4 implies daily 200° CBCTs for the IBL. For the calculation of the beams for this energy we use monitor units instead of the mAs product. The deposited IBL protocols apply about 6 MU for one H&N 200° CBCT.

Daily 3D imaging with the TBL entail a much too high additional dose, so for the 6 MV energy we choose a scenario (scenario 5) which considers one CBCT per week (200°, 7 MU) and planar images for the remaining days. Planar images are taken with gantry positions of 0° and 90° with 1 MU each.

Evaluation of the dose smearing

Positioning corrections are performed by shifting the table in the three spatial directions, anterior-posterior, left-right and superior-inferior. The values of these table shifts are also documented in the R&V system.

To analyze the influence of potential positioning errors, the isocenter was shifted back in the original treatment plan appropriately to the applied table shifts to simulate that no positioning correction had been done. The plans were recalculated for every single fraction and summed to a new plan, again considering different scenarios.

Firstly we consider an extreme scenario (extreme plan), in which only plans with shifted isocenters are summed and weighted equally. This simulates, that the patient's position would never be adapted and no verification imaging would be done. For example, for a patient with 10 verification images, 10 plans with isocenter shifts appropriate to the applied table shifts were recalculated, weighted with a factor of 0.1 respectively and summed up to a new plan. In a previous study we found that the applied table shifts are roughly Gaussian, so we can assume that these 10 fractions are representative for the remaining fractions without imaging [20].

Scenario two represents a more realistic case (realistic plan) where all fractions are considered. For those days on which positioning verification was performed, we can suppose that the patient's position was corrected and matches with the planning CT, so the original treatment plan is considered. Of course, this is an idealized assumption, minor positioning errors are expected even with image guidance. For all fractions without imaging we apply positioning errors observed on the other days and the previously calculated extreme plan is used. If a patient receives 30 fractions with 10 positioning verifications, the original plan is weighted with a third and the extreme plan with two thirds.

For scenario three (imaging plan) we combine the two examined effects to provide an inside into what would occur in reality. The additional imaging dose of each patient is added to the realistic plan calculated for scenario two. So for this scenario we consider the dose smearing caused by positioning errors as well as the actual imaging dose, individually for each patient.

For all scenarios the recalculation of the plans with shifted isocenters was carried out in the TPS, however, for the summation and further evaluation the single plans were exported in DICOM format and imported into the MATLAB- based Computational Environment for Radiotherapy Research (CERR) [28].

Assessment of plan quality

For both effects (additional imaging dose and dose smearing) plan quality was first analyzed visually by considering the dose distributions and dose-volume-histograms (DVH).

Sparing of OARs was assessed quantitatively on the base of clinically relevant DVH objectives (Table 2).

It is examined how many times these acceptance criteria failed with IGRT when passed by the original plan. Moreover, normal tissue complication probability was modelled regarding biological endpoints for particular toxicities (Table 3).

The different parameters could be entered into the TPS and CERR and the NTCP value could be calculated using the Lymann-Kutcher-Burrmann model (LKB) [31].

Table 2 Planning criteria (only valid, where the organ is not inside the PTV)

Parotid glands	Mean < 25Gy; V20Gy < 60%
Spinal chord	D2% < 42Gy
Larynx	D2% < 63Gy; Mean < 44Gy
Vocal chords	D2% < 25Gy

Table 3 Endpoints and paramters for the NTCP modelling [29, 30]]

Organ	Endpoint	m	n	Dose50 [Gy]
Parotid glands	Xerostomia	0.18	0.7	64.0
Spinal chord	Myelitis/Necrosis	0.175	0.05	66.5
Larynx	Edema	0.16	0.45	64.3

$$NTCP = \frac{1}{\sqrt{2\pi}} \int_{-\infty}^{u} \exp\left(\frac{-t2}{2}\right) dt$$

$$u = \frac{D - TD_{50}(V)}{m \cdot TD_{50}(V)}$$

with $TD_{50}(V) = TD_{50}(1)/V^n$

$TD_{50}(1)$ is the dose to the total organ which entails 50% complication risk, $TD_{50}(V)$ is the tolerance dose for a partial volume V, m is the slope of the sigmoidal curve, n describes the volume effect and D is the maximal dose to the organ.

For the effect of dose smearing, target coverage is also a point that needs to be checked by different measures of quality. The homogeneity index is calculated as

$$HI = \frac{D2\% - D98\%}{D50\%}$$

where Dx% is the dose received by x% of the volume of the PTV.

The amount of under- and overdosage can be assessed by the underdose- and overdose rate:

$$OR = \frac{TV_{PIV}}{PIV}$$

$$UR = \frac{TV_{PIV}}{TV}$$

where TV denotes the volume of the target, PIV is the volume receiving the prescribed dose, and TV_{PIV} is the volume of the target covered by the prescribed dose (95%). Paddick's conformity index [32] is given by

$$CI = OR \cdot UR$$

All these metrics are evaluated for the structure that receives the prescribed total dose (the boost in most cases) as this is most relevant for target coverage. The dose difference between the shifted plans and the original plans is also assessed for each scenario. With the constructed difference-plans it is possible to identify those points where dose deviations exceed a given level (e.g., 1%, 2%, 3%). In a way, this metric is similar to the gamma index pass rate, but disregarding the distance to agreement criteria (which would not make sense when evaluating the effect of spatial shifts).

For the statistical analysis all scenarios were pairwise compared using the Wilcoxon signed-rank test. The calculations were carried out in the Origin Pro 2015 software, taking a value of $p < 0.05$ as significant.

Results

Imaging dose

In Fig. 1 the dose distributions of all 5 imaging scenarios are illustrated for one patient. The tumor of this patient is located at the base of the tongue, the prescriped dose of 60 Gy is separated to a PTV of 50 Gy and a sequential boost of 10 Gy. The actual imaging scheme for this patient contains IBL CBCTs for 4 fractions, IBL planar images for 7 fractions and for one fraction planar images with 6 MV. The additional dose is reflected in small variations of the isodose lines, the 100% isodose spreads over the target volume according to the different scenarios. However, the visual inspection of the dose distribution shows only minor differences.

Figure 2 shows the dose distributions of only the imaging doses for the four scenarios without the treatment plan. It is conspicuous, that the course of the isodoses for the daily kV CBCTs differs from the others. As the

X-Ray tube is located opposite to the treatment head, it rotates below the back of the patients.

To analyze the influence of the additional imaging dose especially to the sparing of OAR, the DVHs of all scenarios for the same patient are presented in Fig. 3.

Scenario 2 and 3 reveal only small differences in comparison to the original plan, the curves almost run congruent. The 6 MV scenario shows a visible effect of the additional imaging dose. However, in comparison to a daily imaging with IBL CBCTs this effect is very slight, although daily MV imaging is used. Scenario 4 results in a marked shift of the curves to higher doses.

Figure 3 illustrates that the additional imaging dose causes an increase of the volume receiving a particular dose. For several patients this causes the DVH constraints for plan acceptability given in Table 2 to be exceeded. Table 4 lists the number of these exceedings for the different scenarios.

For scenario 2 only one DVH constraint is no longer satisfied in comparison with the original plan. With the kV scenario all criteria are still passed, so for these two scenarios plan acceptability is not markedly compromised by imaging. In contrast to that, scenario 4 results

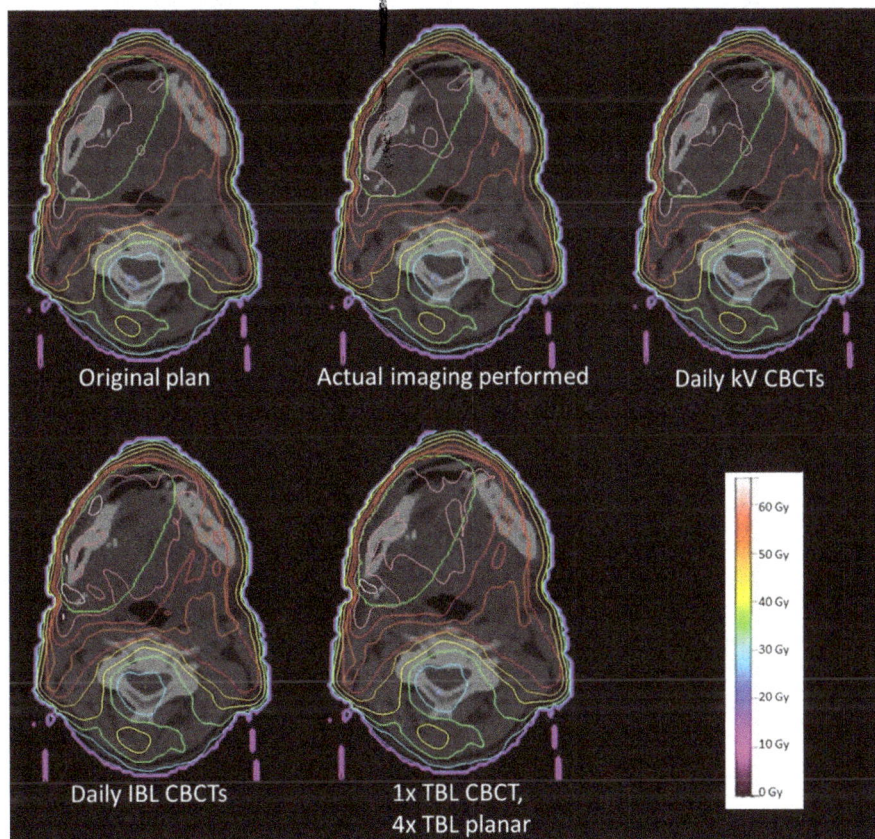

Fig. 1 Example Dose distributions of one patient for all scenarios

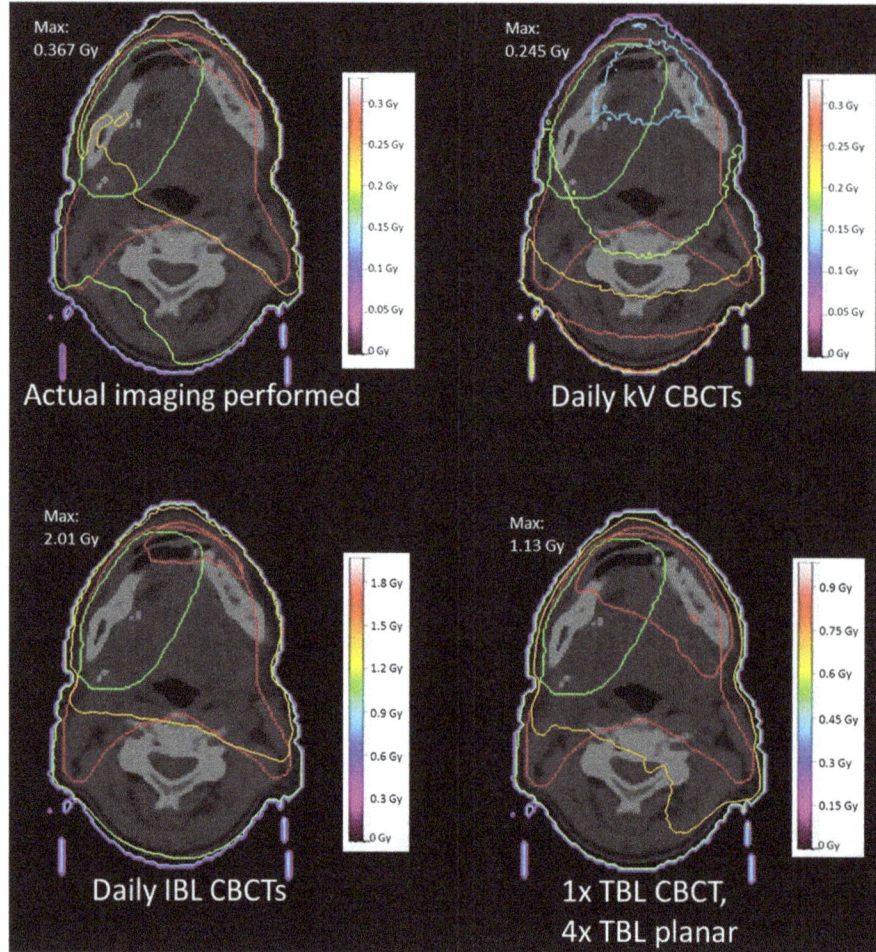

Fig. 2 Example Dose distributions of only the imaging doses without the treatment plan for the same patient as in Fig. 1

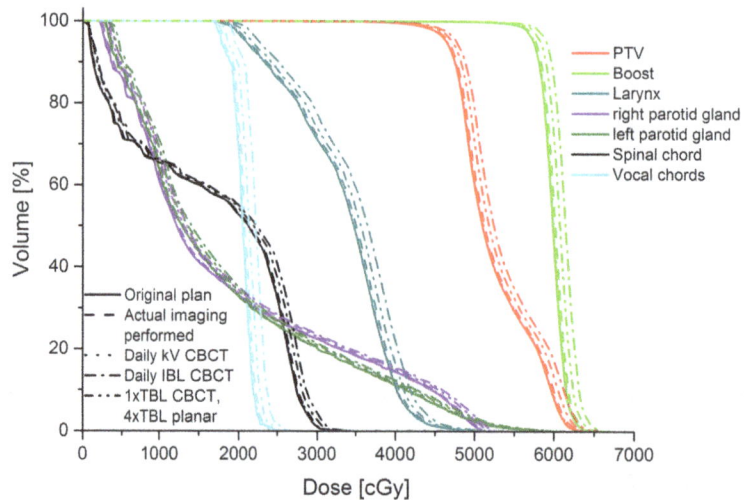

Fig. 3 Example DVH of the same patient as in Fig. 1 for all scenarios

Table 4 Number of exceedings of the considered planning criteria

Organ	Criteria	Original plan	Scenario 2	Scenario 3	Scenario 4	Scenario 5
Spinal chord	D2% < 42Gy	0	0	0	0	0
Parotid glands	Mean < 25Gy	4	5	4	12	8
	V20Gy < 60%	0	0	0	3	1
Larynx	D2% < 63Gy	2	2	2	4	4
	Mean < 44Gy	0	0	0	1	0
Vocal chords	D2% < 25Gy	2	2	2	8	4
Total		8	9	8	28	17

in a notable number of cases where the DVH constraints are no longer met, for the parotid glands the mean value exceeds the required 25 Gy for eight patients more than in the original plan. Nearly all DVH criteria are exceeded, some frequently, for this scenario leading to an entity of 20 cases, in which the given constraints are no longer satisfied. Obviously, fewer such cases can be found for the daily TBL scenario.

The mean values in Table 5 confirm these findings, scenario 2 and 3 showing only minor differences in comparison with the original plan. The daily kV imaging on average results in a smaller dose amount than the realistic scenario. Again, the table illustrates the marked influence of the IBL CBCTs on sparing of OARs, partly with an additional dose of up to a whole fraction dose. The values of scenario 5 range between those of scenario 2 and 3 and scenario 4. As expected, the statistical comparison results in clear significances (p-values < 0.001), in which the kV scenario results in a significant lower dose than the scenario considering the actual imaging for all parameters.

Table 5 also lists the mean values of the NTCP for the considered endpoints. The only relevant probability

Table 5 Mean values ±standard deviation and range of the DVH criteria and NTCP results for the different scenarios

Organ	Criteria/endpoint	Original plan	Scenario 2	Scenario 3	Scenario 4	Scenario 5
Spinal chord	D2% < 42 [Gy]	32.7 ± 3.8	32.9 ± 3.8	32.8 ± 3.8	34.0 ± 3.8	33.5 ± 3.8
		23.3–41-3	23.4–41.5	23.3–41.5	24.1–42.6	23.7–42.1
	Myelitis/Necrosis [%]	0.1 ± 0.4	0.1 ± 0.4	0.1 ± 0.4	0.1 ± 0.5	0.1 ± 0.5
		0–2	0–2	0–2	0–2	0–2
Right Parotid gland	Mean < 25 [Gy]	19.3 ± 4.6	19.5 ± 4.6	19.4 ± 4.6	20.6 ± 4.8	20.0 ± 4.7
		9.5–25.1	9.6–25.5	9.6–25.6	10.7–27.3	10.2–26.5
	V20Gy < 60 [%]	35.0 ± 14.8	35.5 ± 15.1	35.3 ± 15.0	38.2 ± 16.4	36.7 ± 15.6
		0.0–57.9	0.0–59.3	0.0–58.3	0.0–63.0	0.0–60.9
	Xerostomia [%]	0.5 ± 0.8	0.5 ± 0.8	0.5 ± 0.8	0.8 ± 1.2	0.7 ± 1.0
		0–3	0–3	0–3	0–5	0–4
Left Parotid gland	Mean < 25 [Gy]	20.7 ± 4.0	21.1 ± 4.0	20.9 ± 4.0	22.2 ± 4.2	21.6 ± 4.1
		12.6–25.6	12.8–25.7	12.7–25.6	13.6–27.3	13.2–26.5
	V20Gy < 60 [%]	41.0 ± 11.2	41.7 ± 11.5	41.3 ± 11.3	44.5 ± 12.5	43.1 ± 11.9
		17.8–56.8	18.0–57.4	17.9–57.0	18.9–61.3	18.4–59.1
	Xerostomia [%]	0.6 ± 0.9	0.6 ± 0.9	0.6 ± 0.9	1.1 ± 1.3	0.8 ± 1.0
		0–3	0–3	0–3	0–5	0–4
Larynx	D2% < 63 [Gy]	54.8 ± 5.2	55.2 ± 5.2	55.0 ± 5.2	56.5 ± 5.3	55.8 ± 5.2
		43.8–63.4	44.1–63.8	43.9–63.5	45.5–65.1	44.7–64.3
	Mean < 44 [Gy]	34.4 ± 4.7	34.8 ± 4.7	34.5 ± 4.8	36.1 ± 4.8	35.4 ± 4.8
		18.2–42.9	19.4–43.3	18.3–43.0	19.5–44.8	19.0–43.9
	Edema [%]	11.2 ± 8.2	11.8 ± 8.5	11.4 ± 8.3	15.5 ± 10.3	12.7 ± 9.4
		0–30	0–32	0–31	0–37	0–34
Vocal chords	D2% < 25 [Gy]	22.0 ± 2.2	22.3 ± 2.3	22.1 ± 2.2	23.7 ± 2.2	23.0 ± 2.2
		17.5–26.0	17.7–26.3	17.6–26.1	20.0–27.8	18.8–26.9

(values over 1%) refers to the occurrence of Larynx edema. Even for the original plan NTCP amounts over 10%, which increases to over 15% by the daily use of IBL CBCTs.

Positioning uncertainties

The visible inspection of the dose distributions and DVHs for all scenarios reveals only minor differences between the scenarios. Merely the combined scenario (imaging and positioning) leads to an expansion of the 100% isodose within the target volume (Fig. 4). Relating to OAR sparing, the right parotid gland and especially the vocal chords are best spared in the original plan, whereas the sparing of the left parotid gland is increased with the positioning uncertainties. However, for the whole collective the positioning errors result in a raised number of DVH constraints that are exceeded in comparison with the original plan (Table 6), especially for the parotid glands and the vocal chords.

In general, the same effects are observed for the realistic and the extreme plans, but in such a way that they are more pronounced for the extreme plan. This is not surprising, because the realistic plan is actually a weighted average of the extreme and the original plan, and should hence fall in between the two. It is also clear that due to the additional imaging dose the imaging plan contains more dose than the realistic scenario.

For the whole collective the mean values of the DVH constraints relating to sparing of OAR (Table 7) show a predominantly decreased sparing as a result of positioning errors, which is statistically significant for all cases besides the left parotid gland, with especial small p-values for the spinal chord and the vocal chords (< 0.001). Solely the left parotid gland is better spared with positioning inaccuracy (original plan:

19,82 Gy vs. extreme plan: 19,41 Gy). While the differences for the larynx are minor, the average values of the spinal chord and the right parotid gland differ about 1 Gy between original and extreme scenario, for the vocal chords even about 2 Gy (one whole fraction dose). As expected, the imaging scenario results for all cases in a significantly decreased sparing of OAR.

This is also reflected in the evaluation of NTCP. For all organs at risk NTCP values are lowest with the original scenario, especially for the larynx and the right parotid gland (Table 7). For these two organs pair-wise tests are significant (Larynx: original scenario vs. realistic scenario: $p = 0.021$, right parotid gland: original scenario vs. realistic scenario: $p = 0.031$).

For the examination of the influence of positioning errors on plan quality, measures of quality regarding PTV coverage are also considered (Table 7). The V95%, which is an important marker for the clinical routine, shows just minor deteriorations of target coverage as a result of positioning errors (differences of about 1% in comparison to the original plan). Homogeneity and conformity are also little affected by potential positioning errors for this collective. Although those measures of quality show just minor differences between the scenarios the statistical analysis results in significances for most cases (p-values< 0.03).

Figure 5 illustrates the dose deviations in terms of "hot spots" (red) and "cold spots" (blue) of the different scenarios in comparison to the original plan. Over- and underdosages are of the same magnitude, in general the positioning errors result in balanced shifts for all directions. The additional imaging dose leads to a marked expansion of the area with positive dose differences.

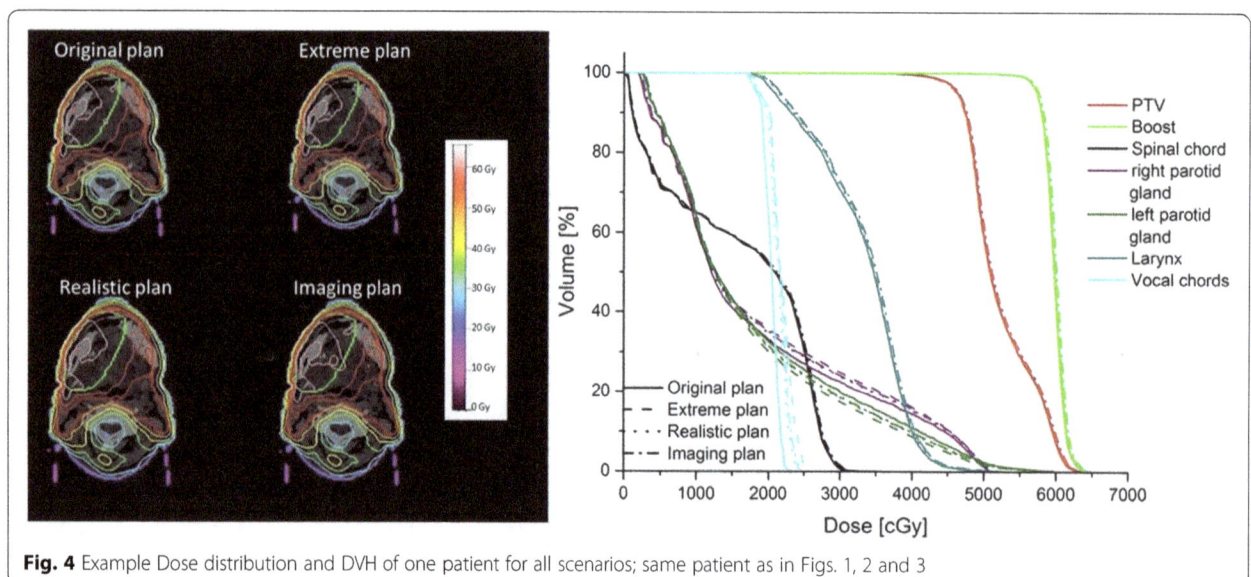

Fig. 4 Example Dose distribution and DVH of one patient for all scenarios; same patient as in Figs. 1, 2 and 3

Table 6 Number of exceedings of the considered planning criteria

Organ	Criteria	Original plan	Extreme plan	Realistic plan	Imaging plan
Spinal chord	D2% < 42Gy	0	1	0	0
Parotid glands	Mean < 25Gy	4	9	7	8
	V20Gy < 60%	0	2	1	2
Larynx	D2% < 63Gy	2	2	2	3
	Mean < 44Gy	0	0	0	0
Vocal chords	D2% < 25Gy	2	9	4	5
Total		8	23	14	18

For single cases even the realistic scenario shows dose differences of over 10 Gy (Table 8). The percentage of points with less than 2% and 3% dose differences yields values of over 90% for all scenarios. The 1% pass rates of the realistic and imaging scenarios are also still about 90% on average, whereas this is reduced for the extreme scenario to 83.8%. For all cases the large range shows that there are individual plans with extreme outliers.

Discussion

Interpretation

Currently there are numerous studies that deal with imaging dose in radiation therapy. However, in large parts they focus on the additional imaging dose itself, especially for the comparatively newer kV modalities [6–13]. Amer et al. [7] examined CBCT skin doses of an Elekta Synergy X-Ray System. They measured doses of about 1.6 mGy in the head-&-neck region. This can be confirmed by our findings of about 3–9 mGy for one head and neck CBCT [14]. In [14] we also give magnitudes for MV CBCTs, the IBL results in 34–62 mGy, while imaging using the treatment beam line provides about 80 mGy per CBCT in the head area. Further studies, in which imaging doses are explicitly calculated on the planning CT, also focus primarily on the kV modality. Alaei et al. [17] found an additional dose of about 30–40 mGy for 35 fractions head and neck treatment when using daily kV CBCT, which is comparatively less dose than our results for head and neck treatment show.

At our department the use of three energy-matched linacs with different imaging modalities leads to variations of set-up verifications regarding frequency and technique. While it is already shown in several previous tests, this study confirms that the actual performed imaging has little influence on plan quality. However, set-up verification is not done daily, so that uncorrected positioning errors could also affect plan quality. This trade-off between additional imaging dose and dose smearing was meant to be analyzed more accurately.

For daily imaging we can assume that no dose smearing comes into effect as positioning errors can be neglected. In a previous study we confirmed that for all imaging modalities set-up verifications can be performed with comparable precision [20].

Daily imaging using kV CBCTs just contributes a minor additional dose. This scenario is highly recommended for the clinical routine. Beside the low influence of the imaging dose on the plan quality, kV imaging yields the best image quality, so that image fusion is not restricted to bony structures. However, not every institution is equipped with a kV modality, so it should also be analyzed, if daily imaging is advisable for MV energies, too.

The Siemens specific IBL daily CBCT scenario leads to a very high dose amount of up to one additional fraction dose. Numerous DVH constraints are exceeded and NTCP is markedly increased, so that most of the plans are clinically not acceptable anymore. Caution is especially advised for the interpretation of the name of this modality. It is marketed as "kView", what pretends to be a kV-like modality. However, it should be kept in mind that the image beam line is a MV modality and the results show the negative effects of the additional dose although it is lower in comparison to the treatment beam line.

The use of daily CBCT with the TBL would result in inacceptable dose contributions. If the volumetric recordings are partly or completely replaced by planar images, this offers an acceptable alternative for daily 6 MV set-up verification. The dose can be even more reduced by the application of the IBL energy within this scenario.

If daily volumetric MV imaging is still required, it is also feasible to calculate the additional imaging dose already in the planning process. This leads to a realistic approximation and sparing of organs at risk and target coverage can be optimized in advance with the integration of the additional dose.

One point regarding frequency and technique of set-up verifications that should not be neglected is the treatment time. Imaging to control the patient's position is time consuming, which plays a central role for the schedule of the clinical routine. This point is also relevant for the patients. Long lay times should be avoided, especially for patients in pain but also to prevent from the opportunity of more patient-movements before the treatment starts. Generally,

Table 7 Mean values ±standard deviation and range of the quality metrics, DVH criteria and NTCP results for the different scenarios. HI: Homogeneity Index, CI: Conformity Index, UR: Underdose rate, OR: Overdose rate, GI: Gradient Index

Organ	Criteria/endpoint	Original plan	Extreme plan	Realistic plan	Imaging plan
V95%	≥95 [%]	90.95 ± 6.43	90.01 ± 6.21	90.58 ± 6.20	91.62 ± 5.96
		72.01–99.08	74.09–97.93	74.4–98.31	74.50–98.39
HI	the smaller the better	0.19 ± 0.14	0.19 ± 0.14	0.19 ± 0.14	0.19 ± 0.14
		0.07–0.89	0.07–0.89	0.07–0.89	0.07–0.89
CI	the closer to 1 the better	0.62 ± 0.15	0.63 ± 0.14	0.63 ± 0.14	0.62 ± 0.15
		0.20–0.87	0.23–0.87	0.22–0.87	0.20–0.87
UR	the closer to 1 the better	0.91 ± 0.06	0.90 ± 0.06	0.91 ± 0.06	0.92 ± 0.06
		0.72–0.99	0.74–0.98	0.74–0.98	0.75–0.98
OR	the closer to 1 the better	0.69 ± 0.18	0.70 ± 0.18	0.70 ± 0.18	0.69 ± 0.19
		0.21–0.96	0.24–0.97	0.23–0.97	0.20–0.96
Spinal chord	D2% < 42 [Gy]	32.6 ± 3.9	33.6 ± 3.9	33.1 ± 3.9	33.3 ± 3.8
		23.0–41.2	25.9–42.5	24.7–41.5	24.8–41.8
	Myelitis/Necrosis [%]	0.3 ± 0.7	0.3 ± 0.8	0.3 ± 0.7	0.3 ± 0.8
		0.0–4.0	0.0–4.6	0.0–4.3	0.0–4.5
Right Parotid gland	Mean < 25 [Gy]	19.0 ± 4.6	20.6 ± 4.8	19.9 ± 4.6	20.2 ± 4.6
		9.5–25.3	9.7–28.9	9.6–27.4	9.8–27.6
	V20Gy < 60 [%]	34.0 ± 14.6	39.8 ± 15.7	37.5 ± 14.8	38.1 ± 15.1
		0.0–57.8	0.0–64.9	0.0–60.8	0.0–62.2
	Xerostomia [%]	0.3 ± 0.4	0.7 ± 1.2	0.5 ± 0.9	0.6 ± 0.9
		0.0–1.8	0.0–5.0	0.0–3.5	0.0–3.6
Left Parotid gland	Mean < 25 [Gy]	19.8 ± 3.7	19.4 ± 4.3	19.6 ± 4.0	19.9 ± 4.1
		12.6–24.4	11.0–26.4	11.7–25.6	11.9–25.8
	V20Gy < 60 [%]	41.1 ± 10.9	40.7 ± 12.6	40.9 ± 11.6	41.7 ± 11.9
		17.4–54.8	11.6–59.1	14.9–57.5	15.1–58.3
	Xerostomia [%]	0.3 ± 0.4	0.4 ± 0.5	0.4 ± 0.5	0.4 ± 0.5
		0.0–1.3	0.0–2.3	0.0–1.9	0.0–2.0
Larynx	D2% < 63 [Gy]	54.4 ± 5.1	54.4 ± 5.2	54.4 ± 5.2	54.7 ± 5.2
		43.1–63.2	44.5–62.9	44.0–62.8	44.3–63.1
	Mean < 44 [Gy]	34.4 ± 4.7	34.8 ± 4.7	34.7 ± 4.7	35.0 ± 4.8
		18.3–42.6	19.0–43.6	18.8–43.3	18.9–43.7
	Edema [%]	10.7 ± 7.5	11.4 ± 7.9	11.1 ± 7.8	11.9 ± 8.1
		0.1–27.6	0.1–29.3	0.1–28.7	0.1–30.1
Vocal chords	D2% < 25 [Gy]	21.5 ± 2.2	23.6 ± 2.4	22.6 ± 2.2	23.0 ± 2.2
		17.7–26.9	19.7–27.4	19.3–26.9	19.5–27.5

daily set-up verifications for every single patient prove to be difficult. That is why the influence of potential positioning errors on plan quality should not be neglected.

We simulated an extreme case for the absence of verification images as well as a realistic case, where an exact positioning was supposed for those fractions with set-up verifications.

Sparing of OAR is markedly decreased due to positioning uncertainties, which is significant for the whole collective. This is also reflected in the NTCP modelled for clinical endpoints.

One last step was the creation of an imaging plan as an extension of the realistic case with the associated imaging dose. This serves as the actual case, where both effects are combined under real conditions. With the additional imaging dose, the decrease of OAR sparing due to positioning errors for this collective continues to deteriorate.

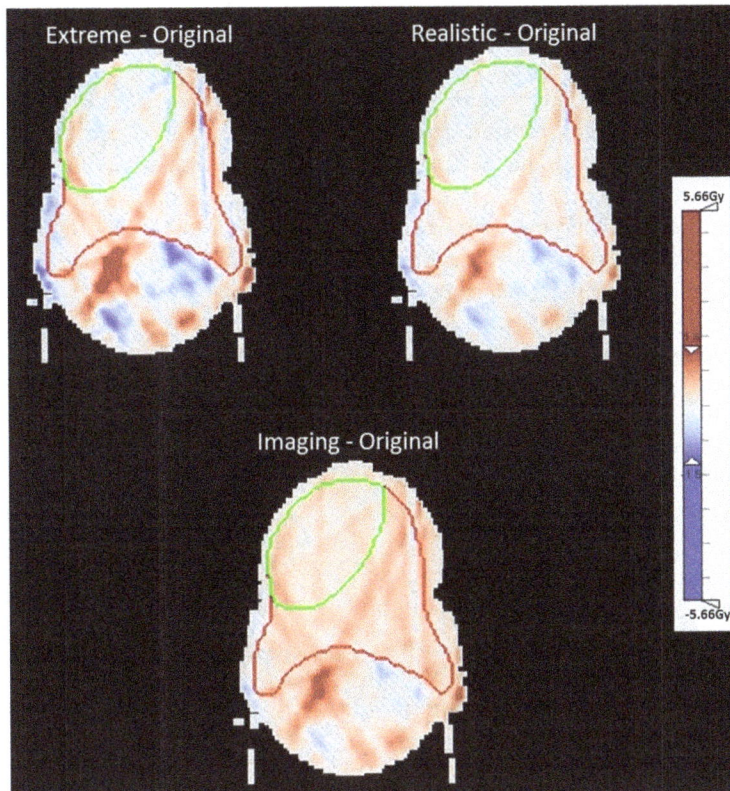

Fig. 5 Example dose differences (cold and hot spots) for the three scenarios in comparison with the original plan

This study shows that steady set-up verifications are reasonable and indispensable. The additional imaging dose can play a minor role, especially by the use of lower energy modalities. Daily imaging using kV energies was shown to have the least dosimetric impact. However, as the time schedule and technical circumstances do not always allow for applying this scenario, frequency and technique of the positioning verifications should be adapted to the relevant requirements. The thermoplastic masks for H&N treatments already offer a quite precise positioning. Generally, the IGRT concept should be a more individual decision. We saw large ranges in this study, an adaption on individual experiences for every patient after the first few fractions should be preferred compared to a fixed schedule.

Table 8 Mean values ± standard deviations and range of the dose differences and pass rates for the different scenarios in comparison with the original plan. "hot spot": points of overdosage in comparison to the original plan, "cold spot": points of underdosage in comparison to the original plan

Metric	Extreme	Realistic	Imaging
"cold spot" dose differences [Gy]	7.38 ± 3.53	4.61 ± 2.29	4.33 ± 2.30
	0.9–18.1	0.7–10.3	0.5–10.1
"hot spot" dose differences [Gy]	7.05 ± 3.85	4.37 ± 2.41	4.65 ± 2.41
	1.1–22.3	0.7–12.3	0.9–12.5
Pass rate for 3% local dose difference [%]	95.76 ± 3.94	98.09 ± 2.41	98.10 ± 2.37
	84.34–100	90.82–100	90.96–100
Pass rate for 2% local dose difference [%]	92.39 ± 5.79	96.08 ± 3.92	96.14 ± 3.90
	78.94–100	86.56–100	86.99–100
Pass rate for 1% local dose difference [%]	83.80 ± 8.50	89.82 ± 7.27	89.29 ± 7.20
	64.58–99.66	74.09–99.96	73.58–99.98

Limitations

All positioning uncertainties considered in this study result in an incorrect positioning of the patient. No anatomical deformations were included. This would be a more important point when considering prostate treatment, for example. However, in the head and neck area there is less proper motion of the organs relative to the bony structures to be accounted for. Moreover, considering only the patients'shifts does not yield any difficulties of changing OAR and PTV volumes, deformable registration and DVH dose accumulation. Besides, this approach allowed us to include set-up information from planar imaging rather than just CBCT in the analysis, which is clinically more relevant.

The usage of safety margins to avoid underdosage of the target volume due to positioning errors is standard nowadays. In our institution margins are adapted to potential positioning errors, but not necessarily in conjunction with an explicitly contouring of a CTV. The PTV is contoured directly with a safety margin of 5–10 mm to the tumor area. So in this study we returned the analysis only to the planning target volume, the influence of positioning errors on the clinical target volume could not be evaluated. In the framework of such an evaluation it would also be possible to determine the tumor control in terms of a TCP (Tumor Control Probability) analysis. However, in clinical reality it is the PTV that is normally considered for target coverage in many institutions – in our clinic, target coverage is considered acceptable as long as 95% of the PTV is covered by the 95% prescription isodose (However, this is not always feasible due to constraints on the OARs). Nonetheless, with an IGRT scenario featuring regular or even daily imaging the safety margins can be chosen considerably smaller. This leads automatically to a marked change in the initial dose distribution and indicate a clear benefit from using small meshed IGRT [33]. Beyond margin reduction, regular image-guidance can also allow for detecting pronounced anatomical changes and thus trigger a re-planning for the patient.

Conclusion

Plan quality is only marginally affected by the application of set-up verifications with kV energies. So this modality can be used for the clinical routine without reservation, even daily. If no kV modality is available, daily volumetric verification images should be avoided with MV energies without including the additional dose amount to the treatment plan beforehand. Within this energy a scenario with mostly planar imaging should be preferred.

Dose smearing due to positioning errors for this collective mainly resulted in a decrease of OAR sparing. Target coverage also suffered from the positioning

inaccuracies, especially for individual patients. The difference between the extreme scenario, in which the omission of any set-up verification is simulated, and the realistic scenario, in which those fractions with imaging are considered, shows the large benefit of regular positioning checks.

Taking into account both examined effects the relevance of an extensive IGRT is clearly present, even at the expense of additional imaging dose and time expenditure.

Abbreviations

CBCT: Cone Beam Computer Tomography; CERR: Computational Environment for Radiotherapy Research; CI: Conformity Index; CT: Computed Tomography; CTV: Clinical Target Volume; DICOM: Digital Imaging and Communication in Medicine; DVH: Dose Volume Histogram; H&N: Head and Neck; HI: Homogeneity Index; IBL: Imaging Beam Line; IGRT: Image Guided Radiation Therapy; LKB: Lymann Kutcher Burrmann; MU: Monitor Units; NTCP: Normal Tissue Complication Probability; OAR: Organ At Risk; OR: Overdose Ratio; PTV: Planning Target Volume; R&V: Record & Verify; TBL: Treatment Beam Line; TCP: Tumor Control Probability; TPS: Treatment Planning System; UR: Underdose Ratio

Acknowledgements

We thank the editor and two anonymous reviewers for their valuable comments on this manuscript.

Authors contributions

KB and YD designed the concept of the study. KB performed the analysis. All authors participated in the discussion of the results. KB drafted the manuscript. All authors read and approved the final manuscript.

Competing interests

The authors declare that they have no competing interests.

References

1. Suzuki M, Nishimura Y, Nakamatsu K, et al. Analysis of interfractional set-up errors and intrafractional organmotions during IMRT for head and neck tumors to define an appropriate planning target volume (PTV)- and planning organs at risk volume (PRV)-margins. Radiother Oncol. 2006;78:283–90.
2. Van Herk M. Errors and margins in radiotherapy. Semin Radiat Oncol 2004; 14:52–64.
3. Stroom JC, de Boer HC, Huizenga H, et al. Inclusion of geometrical uncertainties in radiotherapy treatment planning by means of coverage probability. Int J Radiat Oncol Biol Phys. 1999;43:905–19.
4. Graff P, Kirby N, Weinberg V, et al. The residual setup errors of different IGRT alignment procedures for head and neck IMRT and the resulting dosimetric impact. Int J Radiat Oncol Biol Phys. 2013;86(1):170–6.
5. Castelli J, Simon A, Acosta O, et al. The role of imaging in adaptive radiotherapy for head and neck cancer. IRBM. 2014;35:33–40.
6. Schneider U, Hälg R, Besserer J. Concept for quantifying the dose from image guided radiotherapy. Radiat Oncol. 2015;10:188.
7. Amer A, Marchant T. Sykes J, et al.. Imaging doses from the Elekta synergy X-ray cone beam CT system. Brit J Radiol. 2007;80:476–82.
8. Ding GX, Coffey CW. Radiation dose from kilovoltage cone-beam computed tomography in an image-guided radiotherapy procedure. Int J Radiat Oncol Biol Phys. 2009;73:610–7.
9. Gayou O, Parda DS, Johnson M, et al. Patient dose and image quality from mega-voltage cone beam computed tomography imaging. Med Phys. 2007; 34:499–506.
10. Islam MK, Purdie THG, Norrlinger BD, et al. Patient dose from kilovoltage cone beam computed tomography imaging in radiation therapy. Med Phys. 2006;33:1573–82.

Image guidance and positioning accuracy in clinical practice: influence of positioning errors...

163

11. Miften M, Gayou O, Reitz B, et al. IMRT planning and delivery incorporating daily dose from mega-voltage cone-beam computed tomography imaging. Med Phys. 2007;34:3760–7.

12. Morin O, Gillis A, Descovich M, et al. Patient dose considerations for routine megavoltage cone-beam CT imaging. Med Phys. 2007;34:1819–27.

13. Spezi E, Downes P, Jarvis R, et al. Patient-specific three-dimensional concomitant dose from cone beam computed tomography exposure in image-guided radiotherapy. Int J Radiat Oncol Biol Phys. 2012;83:419–26.

14. Dzierma Y, Ames E, Nuesken F, et al. Image quality and dose distributions of three linac-based imaging modalities. Strahlenther Onkol. 2015;191:365–74.

15. Alaei P, Spezi E. Commissioning kilovoltage cone-beam CT beams in a radiation therapy treatment planning system. J App Clin Med Phys. 2012;13:19–33.

16. Alaei P, Ding G, Guan H. Inclusion of the dose from kilovoltage cone beam CT in the radiation therapy treatment plans. Med Phys. 2012;37:244–8.

17. Alaei P, Spezi E, Reynolds M. Dose calculation and treatment plan optimization including imaging dose from kilovoltage cone beam computed tomography. Acta Oncol. 2014;53(6):839–44.

18. Alaei P, Spezi E. Imaging dose from cone beam computed tomography in radiation therapy. Phys Med. 2015;31(7):647–58.

19. Bell K, Heitfeld M, Licht N, et al. Influence of daily imaging on plan quality and normal tissue toxicity for prostate cancer radiotherapy. Radiat Oncol. 2017;12:7.

20. Dzierma Y, Beyhs M, Palm J, et al. Set-up errors and planning margins in planar and CBCT image-guided radiotherapy using three different imaging systems: a clinical study for prostate and head-and-neck cancer. Phys Med. 2015;31(8):1055–9.

21. Polat B, Wilbert J, Baier K, et al. Nonrigid patient setup errors in the head-and-neck region. Strahlenther Onkol. 2007;(9):506–11.

22. Wang J, Bai S, Chen N, et al. The clinical feasibility and effect of online cone beam computer tomography-guided intensity-modulated radiotherapy for nasopharyngeal cancer. Radiother Oncol. 2009;90:221–7.

23. Strbac B, Jokic VS. Evaluation of set-up errors in head and neck radiotherapy using electronic portal imaging. Phys Med. 2013;29:531–6.

24. Faddegon BA, Wu V, Pouliot J, et al. Low dose megavoltage cone beam computed tomography with an unflattened 4MV beam from a carbon target. Med Phys. 2008;35(12):5777–86.

25. Ostapiak OZ, O'Brien PF, Faddegon BA. Megavoltage imaging with low Z targets: implementation and characterization of an investigational system. Med Phys. 1998;25:1910–8.

26. Dzierma Y, Nuesken F, Licht NP, Ruebe C. Dosimetric properties and commissioning of cone-beam CT image beam line with a carbon target. Strahlenther Onkol. 2013;189:566–72.

27. Dzierma Y, Nuesken F, Otto W, et al. Dosimetry of an in-line kilovoltage imaging system and implementation in treatment planning. Int J Radiat Oncol Biol Phys. 2014;88(4):913–9.

28. Deasy JO, Aditya, A, Khullar D, et al. CERR: A computational environment for radiotherapy research. Version 3.0 beta 2007;4.

29. Luxton G, Keall P, King C. A new formula for normal tissue complication probability (NTCP) as a function of equivalent uniform dose (EUD). Phys Med Biol. 2008;53:23–36.

30. Rancati T, Schwarz M, Allen AM, et al. Radiation dose-volume effects in the larynx and pharynx. Int J Radiat Oncol Biol Phys. 2010;76(3):64–9.

31. Kutcher G, Burman C, Brewster L, et al. Histogram reduction method for calculating complication probabilities for three-dimensional treatment planning evaluations. Int J Radiat Oncol Biol Phys. 1991;21:137–46.

32. Paddick I. A simple scoring ratio to index the conformity of radiosurgical treatment plans. Technical note J Neurosurg. 2000;93(3):219–22.

33. Zeidan OA, Langen KM, Meeks SL, et al. Evaluation of image-guidance protocols in the treatment of head and neck cancers. Int J Radiat Oncol Biol Phys. 2007;67(3):670–7.

18

Assessing the impact of choosing different deformable registration algorithms on cone-beam CT enhancement by histogram matching

Halima Saadia Kidar[*] and Hacene Azizi

Abstract

Background: The aim of this work is to assess the impact of using different deformable registration (DR) algorithms on the quality of cone-beam CT (CBCT) correction with histogram matching (HM).

Methods and materials: Data sets containing planning CT (pCT) and CBCT images for ten patients with prostate cancer were used. Each pCT image was registered to its corresponding CBCT image using one rigid registration algorithm with mutual information similarity metric (RR-MI) and three DR algorithms with normalized correlation coefficient, mutual information and normalized mutual information (DR-NCC, DR-MI and DR-NMI, respectively). Then, the HM was performed between deformed pCT and CBCT in order to correct the distribution of the Hounsfield Units (HU) in CBCT images.

Results: The visual assessment showed that the absolute difference between corrected CBCT and deformed pCT was reduced after correction with HM except for soft tissue-air and soft-tissue-bone interfaces due to the improper registration. Furthermore, volumes comparison in terms of average HU error showed that using DR-NCC algorithm with HM yielded the lowest error values of about 55.95 ± 10.43 HU compared to DR-MI and DR-NMI for which the errors were 58.60 ± 10.35 and 56.58 ± 10.51 HU, respectively. Tissue class's comparison by the mean absolute error (MAE) plots confirmed the performance of DR-NCC algorithm to produce corrected CBCT images with lowest values of MAE even in regions where the misalignment is more pronounced. It was also found that the used method had successfully improved the spatial uniformity in the CBCT images by reducing the root mean squared difference (RMSD) between the pCT and CBCT in fat and muscle from 57 and 25 HU to 8HU, respectively.

Conclusion: The choice of an accurate DR algorithm before performing the HM leads to an accurate correction of CBCT images. The results suggest that applying DR process based on NCC similarity metric reduces significantly the uncertainties in CBCT images and generates images in good agreement with pCT.

Keywords: CBCT images, Deformable registration, Histogram matching, Adaptive radiation therapy

* Correspondence: kidar93@yahoo.fr
Department of Physics, Ferhat Abbas Setif University, El Bez Compus, 19000 Setif, Algeria

Background

In the past decade, on board cone-beam CT, integrated into linear accelerators was frequently used for image guidance of radiotherapy. It allowed the verification and the correction of patient's setup during the course of treatment in three dimensions with sufficient soft tissue contrast and low patient dose [1–4]. Therefore, it became a powerful tool for improving tumor targeting and reducing dose delivery to normal tissues [5].

Recently, the development of CBCT systems in terms of images acquisition, rapidity and improved image quality has underlined the question of using CBCT images for adaptive radiation therapy (ART). This technique aims to adapt the treatment planning with patient anatomy modification throughout the entire treatment; it is mainly based on three complex and consuming time processes: acquisition of daily CBCT images for making decision if the re-planning is necessary by comparing them to the CT images, the second process concerns the acquisition of new pCT images and the delineation of volumes of interest to provide a base for the last process which is the dose re-calculation [6]. However, repeated acquisition of CT images for each planning is unjustifiable, due to the accumulated dose. In addition, the preposition of using daily CBCT images directly for dose calculation is limited, owing to their reduced contrast compared to CT images, as shown in Fig. 1, and the large variation of Hounsfield Units caused by the increased amount of scattered radiation [7, 8].

Despite these drawbacks, several studies investigated the feasibility of CBCT images for dose calculation proposing three main "pCT-based" approaches to correct the HUs distribution and minimize as possible the density differences between CBCT and pCT to ensure an accurate dose calculation based on CBCT images. The first approach, known as HU mapping, consists of replacing the HUs values in CBCT by their equivalent points in pCT after the application of rigid or deformable registration. The accuracy of this approach is strongly dependent on region of body in which it is applied and it is available just for regions where the intra-scan motion and organs deformation are insignificant [9, 10]. The second approach is the Multilevel Threshold (MLT), it classifies all CBCT pixels with similar HUs into three or four different segments based on pCT. The use of such approach showed a high accuracy especially when combined with DR which minimizes the effect of organs deformation [11–14]. The last approach is the histogram matching (HM) which allows the adjustment of HUs values between CT and CBCT using cumulative histograms. This modification yielded a good agreement between CT and modified CBCT even for breast and prostate cancer where the intra-scan motion and organs deformation are significant [13, 15]. Other correction categories can be found in literature such as: "Scatter calibration" and "physics-based" techniques, which aim to directly use CBCT images without recourse to pCT-based strategies using empirical look-up-table (LUT) to calibrate CBCT images [16–18] and scatter measurement or simulation [19–23].

Focusing on pCT-based techniques, the previously cited works showed that the correction accuracy depends on the correspondence between the voxels of CBCT and pCT images. Therefore, the choice of DR algorithm must be validated.

The present paper aims to evaluate the impact of using different DR algorithms on the accuracy of CBCT enhancement by HM. A dataset containing CT and CBCT images for patients with prostate cancer was used to generate corrected CBCT, then, HUs values were compared for corrected CBCT and original CT using different metrics.

The remainder of this paper is organized as follows. In section "Methods and Materials", used data and each

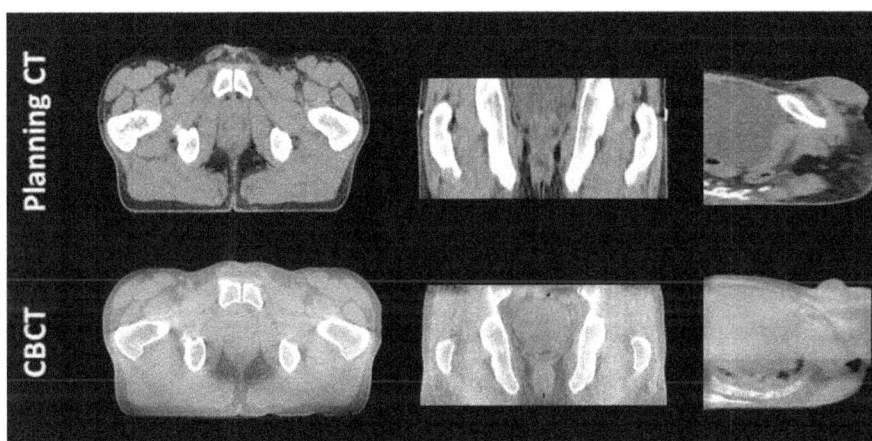

Fig. 1 pCT and CBCT for the same patient (axial, coronal and sagital views) displayed using the same window level

step to correct CBCT images are described. Numerical results based on ten prostate cancer patient data sets are presented in section "Results". In section "Discussion", we further discuss the performance and the effect of DR on the correction quality, and finally conclude the paper in section "Conclusion".

Methods and materials
Data description
This study was performed on data sets of 10 patients with prostate cancer containing pCT and CBCT images obtained by GE CT scan (General Electric Medical Systems) and on-board imager (OBI, Varian Medical Systems) mounted on the gantry of clinical iX21 linear accelerator, respectively. The settings of pCT and CBCT acquisition according to pre-defined protocols are recapitulated in Table 1. The slices number differed from a patient to another; it ranged from 123 to 159 slices in the pCT images and from 50 to 64 slices in the CBCT images giving sufficient information about the anatomical distribution and the motion artifact variations. For all these data CBCT images were acquired for the first day of treatment to minimize the error of patient's setup under the treatment machine. Since this technique is newly integrated in the clinical practice, the number of patients used in this study is limited.

Images pre-processing
Initially, collected CBCT and pCT contained not only the information describing the patient's body but also the couches of the CT scanner and the linear accelerator. For that reason, all images were pre-processed using the FIJI software [24] to select the region including the patient volume and remove the couches. Furthermore, to eliminate all unnecessary content, a fixed threshold was applied to assign all pixels outside the body surface (below − 700 HU for pCT and bellow -600HU for CBCT) to standard CT value for air (-1000HU) using the 3D Slicer software [25].

Corrected CBCT generation
In order to assess the impact of DR on the quality of CBCT enhancement, three intensity-based algorithms with different similarity metrics implemented in Elastix [26] were used. The workflow of corrected CBCT generation is described in Fig. 2.

Before starting the DR, the data sets for each patient were aligned using rigid 3D transformation with mutual

information similarity metric (step1 in Fig. 2). Moreover, to minimize the effect of difference in organ deformation between pCT and CBCT, a multi-resolution B-Spline transformation including 3 levels was performed (step2 in Fig. 2). It is mainly based on the displacement of control points around a control point grid that is put on fixed image, according to the considered similarity metric [26]. The B-Spline interpolator was used to estimate iteratively the deformation field in these points and at each iteration the control points displacement was optimized using the adaptive stochastic gradient descent (ASGD). In this DR process, three similarity metrics were considered: the Normalized Correlation Coefficient (NCC), the Mutual Information (MI), and the Normalized Mutual Information (NMI).

The Normalized Correlation Coefficient (NCC) is given by:

$$NCC(I_F, I_M) = \frac{\sum_{x_i \in \Omega_F}(I_F(x_i) - \overline{I_F})(I_M(T(x_i)) - \overline{I_M})}{\sqrt{\sum_{x_i \in \Omega_F}(I_F(x_i) - \overline{I_F})^2(I_M(T(x_i)) - \overline{I_M})^2}} \tag{1}$$

With I_F the fixed image, I_M the moving image using a given transformation T and $|\Omega_F|$ is the number of voxels of the fixed image. $\overline{I_F}$ and $\overline{I_M}$ are the average gray values for the fixed and the moving images respectively.

The Mutual Information (MI) is defined as:

$$MI(I_F, I_M) = H(I_F) + H(I_M) - H(I_F, I_M) \tag{2}$$

Where: $H(I_F) = - \int p_{I_F}(a) \log p_{I_F}(a) da$ and $H(I_M) = - \int p_{I_M}(b) \log p_{I_M}(b) db$.

With: H(I_F) and H(I_M) the entropies of I_F and I_M respectively. $p_{I_F}(a)$ and $p_{I_M}(b)$ are the pixel's probabilities with values a and b in I_F and I_M respectively. $H(I_F, I_M)$ is the joint entropy of I_F and I_M.

The NMI is given by:

$$NMI(I_F, I_M) = 1 + \frac{MI(I_F, I_M)}{H(I_F, I_M)} = \frac{H(I_F) + H(I_M)}{H(I_F, I_M)} \tag{3}$$

After DR, the 3D slicer software [25] was used to match the histograms of the CBCT images against the corresponding deformed pCT (step3 in Fig. 2). This processing method aims to adjust the HU values between pCT and CBCT images using their cumulative

Table 1 Acquisition settings

Protocol	Tube current (mA)	Exposure time (ms)	Tube voltage (kVp)	Axial image size (pixels)	Voxel size (mm³)
CT	360	500	100	512×512	0.8496 × 0.8496 × 3
CBCT	80	8632	125	512×512	0.8789 × 0.8789 × 2.5

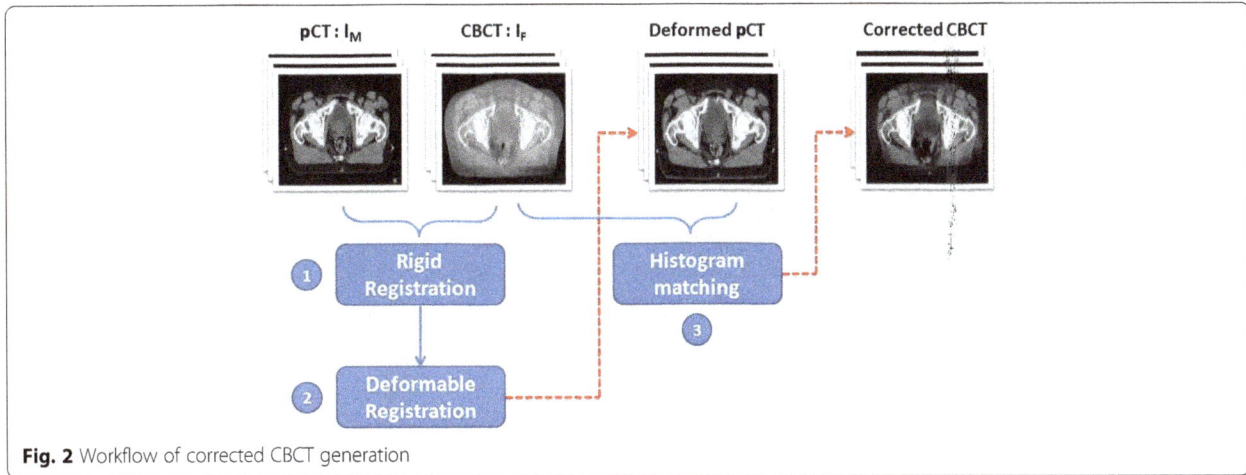

Fig. 2 Workflow of corrected CBCT generation

histograms. Each pixel value in the CBCT images is replaced by the HU having the same cumulative value in the pCT images according to the following formula:

$$CBCT(H_1) = pCT(H_2) \qquad (4)$$

Where $CBCT(H_1)$ represents the HU values for CBCT and $pCT(H_2)$ represents the HU values for pCT [13, 15].

Data analysis

To evaluate the quality of corrected CBCT, deformed pCT images were considered as a reference for each patient. A visual assessment was performed by the calculation of absolute difference between pCT and CBCT images before and after HM to assess the discrepancies between them.

Furthermore, to evaluate quantitatively the agreement between corrected CBCT and pCT, three methods were used. The first one consists of the average HU error estimation over the entire volume [27] given by:

$$V_{err} = \sqrt{mean\left(\left[HU_{pCT}(x,y,z) - HU_{CBCT}(x,y,z)\right]^2\right)} \qquad (5)$$

The second method is the Mean Absolute Error (MAE) plots creation which allows comparing the different tissue classes. It is based on the calculation of the MAE between pCT and corrected CBCT in equidistant bins across the HU scale. For this comparison a size of 20 HU was taken for each bin and the formula describing the MAE is given by:

$$MAE = \frac{1}{N}\sum_{0}^{N}|HU_{pCT} - HU_{CBCT}| \qquad (6)$$

Where N is the number of pixels having intensities in [HU-10, HU + 10] in the pCT [28].

The third one is the image quality evaluation in terms of spatial uniformity. For this method, the mean pixel value among five regions of interest (ROIs) having 10 by 10 pixels and positioned in regions of the same soft tissue area is measured [29]. Then, the RMSD between the mean pixel values in the pCT and the CBCT images before and after correction are calculated.

Results
Visual assessment

Figure 3 shows the absolute difference between deformed pCT and CBCT images for one patient before and after HM using three DR algorithms (DR-NCC, DR-MI and DR-NMI). Obtained results for a RR algorithm are also included to confirm the effect of morphologic deformation between pCT and CBCT on the quality of correction. The effect of applying HM is clearly visualized; it reduced the amount of artefacts in CBCT and yielded corrected images in good agreement with deformed pCT. However, high differences in bony regions and soft tissue-air interfaces are present due to the misalignment between CBCT and pCT.

Volumes comparison

Results of volumes comparison for each patient in terms of HU average error between deformed pCT and CBCT before and after correction are shown in Table 2. The mean and the standard deviation are also presented.

The largest magnitude of V_{err} is observed for unprocessed CBCT images especially when using RR process where the mean HU error value was about 206.47 ± 52.21 HU. For the DR process, a significant decrease was obtained with error values ranging from 64.15 ± 9.50 to 68.20 ± 10.12 HU which confirms the performance of DR algorithms. Whereas, after the correction of CBCT images reduced values of HU of about 55.95 ± 10.43 HU, 56.58 ± 10.51 HU and 58.60 ± 10.35 HU were obtained for DR-NCC, DR-NMI and DR-MI,

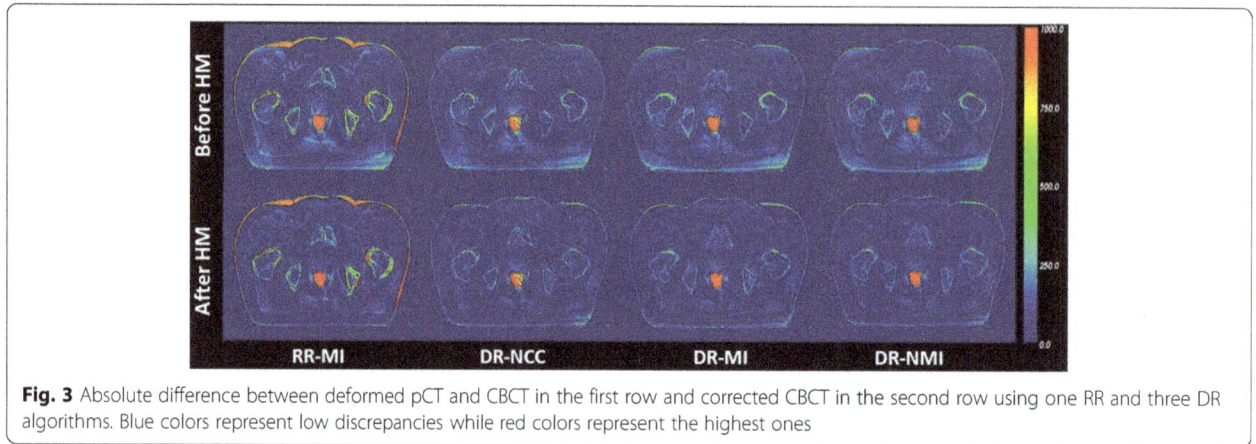

Fig. 3 Absolute difference between deformed pCT and CBCT in the first row and corrected CBCT in the second row using one RR and three DR algorithms. Blue colors represent low discrepancies while red colors represent the highest ones

respectively, indicating that the HM after using DR-NCC yielded corrected CBCT images in good agreement with pCT images compared to unprocessed CBCT images.

Tissue class's comparison

Since volumes comparison may not give information about the presence of large errors and their location, the MAE plots for each algorithm over the HU scale are illustrated in Fig. 4. Similarly to [13], HU scale for pCT images was divided according to the tissue type on different classes. All the values lower than – 400 HU was considered as air. The HU values between – 400 and 250 HU were associated to soft tissues, while those between 250 and 600 HU presented the soft bone. The remaining values (higher than 600 HU) were considered as bone.

Figure 4a compares MAE results using RR algorithm before HM with those obtained after HM. It shows

obviously that the use of HM with RR increases the uncertainties in CBCT images, due to the misalignment between pCT and CBCT images. However, in (Fig. 4b, c, d) the MAE becomes lower and the combination of DR with HM contributes significantly to reduce the errors after correction, especially for pixels with CT number higher than 200 HU. For the values below – 200 HU a mismatch is observed and the MAE values after correction are higher than before. This is due to the low number of pixels in corrected CBCT containing the same HU values as pCT in the interfaces soft tissue-air, which is in agreement with the visual assessment where high errors were noticeable in those regions owing to the improper registration.

The DR performance comparison is depicted in Fig. 5. Plotting together the MAE values before and after correction against each other (Fig. 5a and b respectively) shows that the use of DR based on NCC metric was

Table 2 HU average error values between deformed pCT and CBCT before and after HM for each patient with the mean and the standard deviation

V_{err} [HU]								
Patient's number	RR-MI		DR-NCC		DR-MI		DR-NMI	
	Before HM	After HM	Before HM	After HM	Before HM	After HM	Before HM	After HM
1	138.50	141.33	71.03	64.70	75.94	68.07	73.53	65.67
2	140.00	143.01	57.89	49.10	60.77	51.76	59.90	49.87
3	260.62	288.10	73.58	65.17	76.33	66.71	75.09	64.84
4	257.67	274.16	65.76	55.10	71.23	57.05	68.51	54.03
5	239.04	267.54	67.48	55.73	73.34	59.89	71.44	58.02
6	258.85	269.82	82.09	77.88	87.37	80.24	86.24	79.04
7	171.96	195.80	57.74	47.26	60.12	48.18	58.90	46.26
8	193.20	194.09	54.89	45.74	58.68	47.75	57.23	46.03
9	153.75	173.61	51.82	45.90	56.13	51.47	54.33	49.09
10	251.15	269.41	59.29	52.92	62.16	54.96	60.62	53.01
Mean	206.47	**221.68**	64.15	**55.95**	68.20	**58.60**	66.57	**56.58**
SD	52.21	**57.97**	9.50	**10.43**	10.12	**10.35**	10.06	**10.51**

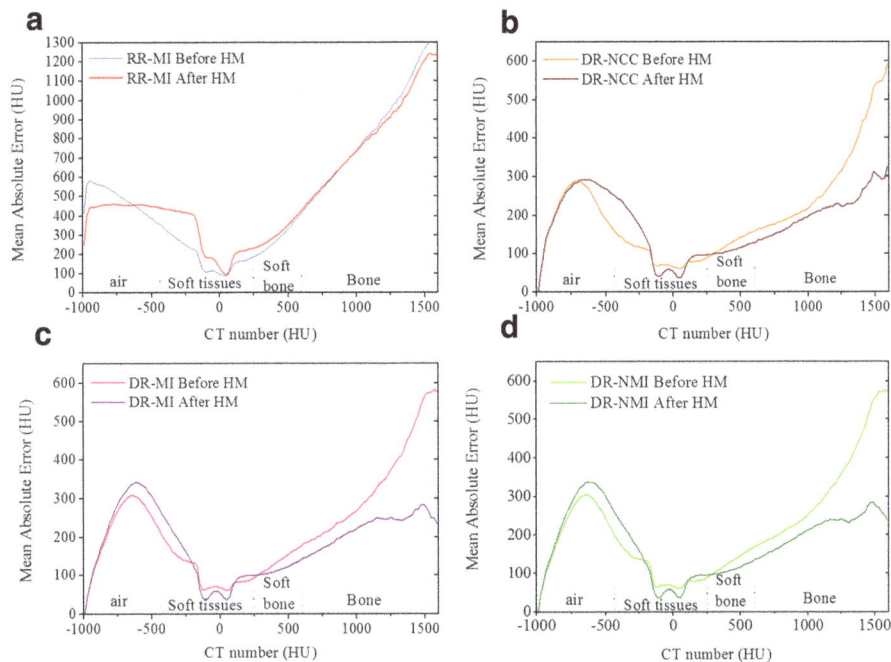

Fig. 4 MAE values of CBCT images before and after correction using **a**) RR-MI, **b**) DR-NCC, **c**) DR-MI and **d**) DR-NMI

better than MI and NMI especially in soft tissue-air interfaces. Moreover, using the NCC metric in combination with HM produced more accurate CBCT images.

Concerning the uniformity of resulted CBCT images, the RMSD of the mean pixel values of ROIs between CBCT, corrected CBCT and pCT images are summarized in Table 3. The obtained results showed that the use of HM reduced the RMSD in fat and muscle (soft tissues) from about 57 and 25 HU to 8 HU, respectively, indicating that the CBCT image quality was brought closer to the pCT image quality through this correction technique.

Discussion

In this work, the impact of choosing different registration algorithms on the quality of CBCT correction by HM was studied. One RR algorithm based on MI similarity metric and three DR algorithms including NCC, MI and NMI similarity metrics were validated.

Several studies investigated the accuracy of dose calculation based on corrected CBCT using HM with DR based on MI [13, 15] but our strategy differs from those studies because it aims to initially choose the appropriate DR algorithm, and then generate corrected CBCT images.

All the results confirmed that the performance of DR of each algorithm is strongly dependent on the region in which the transformation was applied. It was shown that all DR algorithms provided a good alignment between anatomical structures in pCT and CBCT compared to RR registration but their reduced ability to align some regions as soft tissue-air and soft tissue-bone interfaces

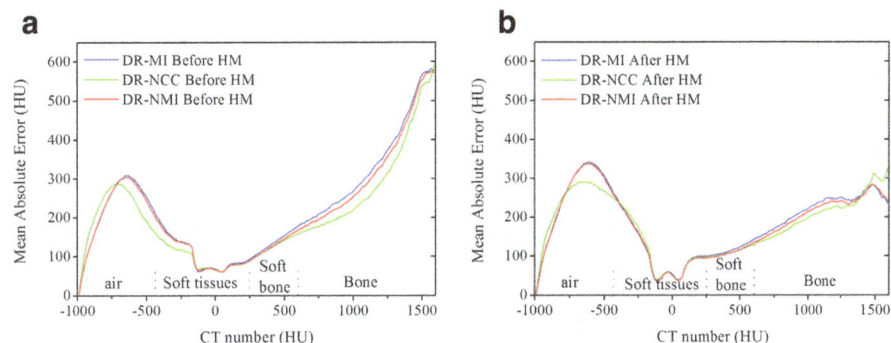

Fig. 5 MAE values of CBCT images for each algorithm before HM (**a**) and after HM (**b**)

Table 3 Comparison of the mean pixel values in fat and muscle between the pCT, CBCT and corrected CBCT images with the three different DR algorithms

Mean pixel values [HU]

Patient's number	Fat				
	pCT	CBCT	CBCT$_{DR-NCC}$	CBCT$_{DR-MI}$	CBCT$_{DR-NMI}$
1	−108.16	−144.37	−90.73	−92.50	−92.06
2	−87.68	−163.92	−84.98	−88.25	−85.77
3	−104.83	−139.75	−90.03	−91.48	−91.16
4	−103.80	−151.60	−104.64	−105.23	−105.19
5	−103.43	−170.34	−102.28	−103.16	−102.89
6	−109.43	−130.55	−98.50	−99.30	−99.09
7	−97.70	−148.56	−97.08	−98.47	−97.97
8	−108.62	−213.92	−108.76	−108.53	−108.04
9	−110.23	−160.35	−105.87	−106.76	−106.82
10	−99.50	−123.33	−100.24	−101.55	−101.40
RMSD		56.83	8.19	7.38	7.57
	Muscle				
1	49.45	−1.37	31.76	30.62	30.68
2	51.61	25.39	42.09	41.12	41.68
3	47.59	59.00	53.25	54.53	53.25
4	42.17	45.81	50.65	51.61	50.93
5	48.87	11.70	47.66	47.66	47.65
6	49.68	40.03	50.09	50.78	50.25
7	49.73	28.39	45.44	46.12	46.01
8	46.46	13.39	36.65	39.04	39.34
9	48.85	56.30	52.18	51.95	51.86
10	49.44	51.98	45.97	47.25	46.40
RMSD		25.49	7.72	8.28	8.02

was clearly visualised. In addition, the sensitivity of HM process to the quality of registration has been proved. It has been found that the better the alignment the more significant is the HM contribution to correct the HU distribution in CBCT images. For that reason, the best compromise for this correction method seems to be the use of DR with NCC similarity metric for which the MAE values after correction were found to be the lowest as indicated in Fig. 5. Also, this choice can be justified by Table 2 where reduced HU errors in corrected CBCT were obtained for the DR-NCC algorithm.

Despite the influence of DR accuracy on the HM process, the use of DR-NCC before HM yielded acceptable HU errors values compared to other studies investigating pCT-based approaches and direct approaches without recourse to pCT [29, 30]. In [29], Kida et al. applied a deep convolutional neural network (DCNN) method to improve the quality of CBCT images acquired for 20 prostate cancer patients. They reported that the RMSD of the mean pixel values for corrected

CBCT images was about 11 and 14 HU in fat and muscle, respectively, while in our study the same evaluation showed that the RMSD was about 8 HU. This suggests that our proposed workflow had successfully improved the spatial uniformity in the CBCT images. Besides, Poludniowski et al. [30] studied for 12 patients (6 brain, 3 prostate and 3 bladder cancer patients) four correction methods based on "scatter calibration" and "scatter measurement" using CBCT images acquired by other linear accelerator (Elekta Linac). They reported that for prostate cancer the average HU error for each method, called also Root Mean Squared Difference, were about 95.5, 91.5, 73.1 and 67.7 HU. Whereas, in our study the HM considered as pCT-based approach resulted in average HU error of about 55.95 ± 10.43 HU when using DR-NCC indicating that although our CBCT images differs from theirs; our results are better than their findings.

To improve the correctness of the proposed workflow, the minimization of its limitations as the existence of non-comparable regions in the pCT and CBCT images, e.g. regions of gas in the rectum, is a priority. Thus, further investigations taking into account the correction of these regions before performing DR and HM are required. In addition, dosimetric evaluation is needed to validate the efficiency of using corrected CBCT for dose calculation in the context of adaptive radiation therapy. Also, we are looking forward to applying this workflow on large number of patients and translate it to other body regions.

Conclusion
In this study, the impact of using different DR algorithms on the HM process to correct CBCT images was evaluated. The results showed that the quality of correction is strongly dependent to the accuracy of DR process and revealed that performing HM after DR with the NCC similarity metric contributed significantly to reduce the uncertainties in CBCT images. On the basis of this study, a combination of the present workflow with automatic segmentation algorithms could be a promising way towards online adaptive radiation therapy.

Abbreviations
ART: Adaptive Radiation Therapy; ASGD: Adaptive Stochastic Gradient Descent; CBCT: Cone Beam Computed Tomography; DCNN: Deep Convolutional Neural Network; DR: Deformable Registration; DR-MI: Deformable Registration based on Mutual Information similarity metric; DR-NCC: Deformable Registration based on Normalized Correlation Coefficient similarity metric; DR-NMI: Deformable Registration based on Normalized Mutual Information similarity metric; HM: Histogram Matching; HU: Hounsfield Unit; LUT: Look Up Table; MAE: Mean Absolute Error; MLT: Multilevel Threshold; OBI: On-Board Imager; pCT: Planning Computed Tomography; RMSD: Root Mean Squared Difference; ROIs: Regions of Interest; RR-MI: Rigid Registration based on Mutual Information similarity metric; V$_{err}$: Average HU error over the entire volume

Acknowledgements
Not applicable.

Funding
Not applicable.

Authors' contribution
HS K designed and executed the experiment process, analyzed and interpreted the results and was major contributor in writing the manuscript. HA supervised the whole study. Both authors read and approved the final manuscript.

Competing of interests
The authors declare that they have no competing interests.

References
1. Letourneau D, Martinez AA, Lockman D, et al. Assessment of residual error for online cone-beam CT-guided treatment of prostate cancer patients. Int J Radiat Oncol Biol Phys. 2005;62:1239–46.
2. Oldham M, et al. Cone-beam CT guided radiation therapy: a model for on-line application. Radiother Oncol. 2005;75:271.e1–271.e8.
3. Gukenberger M, Meyer J, Vordermark D, Baier K, et al. Magnitude and clinical relevence of translational and rotational patient setup errors: a cone-beam CT study. Int J Radiat Oncol Biol Phy. 2006;65:934–42.
4. Streink MF, Bezak E. Technological approaches to in-room CBCT imaging. Phys Eng Sci Med Australas. 2008;31:167–79.
5. Jaffray DA, Siewerdsen JH, Wong JW, Martinez AA. Flat-panel cone-beam computed-tomography for image-guided radiation therapy. Int J Radiat Oncol Biol Phys. 2002;53:1337–49.
6. Lafond C, Simon A, Henry O, Prichon N. Radiothérapie adaptative en routine? Etat de l'art: point de vue du physicien médical. Cancer Radiothérapie. 2015; In press.
7. Kim S, Yoo S, Yin FF. Kilovoltage cone-beam CT: comparative dose and image quality evaluation in partial and full-angle scan protocols. Med Phys. 2010;37:3648–459.
8. Stock S, Pasler M, Birkfellner W. Image quality and stability of image-guided radiotherapy (IGRT) devices: a comparatives study. Radiother Oncol. 2009;93:1–7.
9. Zijtveld MV, Dirkx M, Heijmen B. Correction of cone beam CT values using a planning CT for derivation of the dose of the day. Radiother Oncol. 2007;85:195–200.
10. Yang Y, Schreibmann E, Li T, Wang C, Xing L. Evaluation of on-board kv cone beam CT (CBCT)-based dose calculation. Phys Med Biol. 2007;52:685–705.
11. Boggula R, Lorenz F, Abo-Madyan Y, Lohr F, Wolff D, Boda-Heggemann J, et al. A new strategy for online adaptive prostate radiotherapy on cone-beam CT. Med Phys. 2009;19:264–76.
12. Fotina I, Hopfgartner J, Stock M, Steininger T, Ltegendorf-Cancig C, George D. Feasibility of CBCT-based dose calculation: comparative analysis of HU adjustment techniques. Radiother Oncol. 2012;104:249–56.
13. Onozato Y, Kadoy N, Fujita Y, Arai K, Dobashi S, Tekeda K, et al. Evaluation of on board kv cone-beam computed tomography-based dose calculation with deformable image registration using housnfeild unit modification. Int J Radiot Oncol Biol Phys. 2014;89:416–23.
14. Almatani T, Hugtenburg RP, Lewis RD, Barley SE, Edwards MA. Automated algorithm for CBCT- based dose calculations of prostate radiotherpay with bilateral hip protheses. Br J Radiol. 2016;89:20160443.
15. Amit G, Purdie TG. Automated planning of breast radiotherapy using cone beam CT imaging. Med Phys. 2015;42:770–9.
16. Yoo S, Yin FF. Dosimetric feasibility of cone-beam CT-based treatment planning compared to CT-based treatment planning. Int J Radiat Oncol Biol Phys. 2006;66(5):1553–61.
17. Letourneau D, Wong R, Moseley D, et al. Online planning and delivery technique for radiotherapy of spinal metastases using cone-beam CT: image-quality and system performance. Int J Radiat Oncol Biol Phys. 2007;67(4):1229–37.
18. Ritcher A, Hu Q, Steglich D, et al. Investigation of the usability of cone beam CT data sets for dose calculation. Radiat Oncol. 2008;3:42.
19. Jarry G, Graham SA, Moseley DJ, et al. Characterization of scattered radiation in kV CBCT images using Monte Carlo simulations. Med Phys. 2006;33(11):4320–9.
20. Zhu L, Xie Y, Wang J, et al. Scatter correction for cone-beam CT in radiation therapy. Med Phys. 2009;36(6):2258–68.
21. Sun M, Star-lack JM. Improved scatter correction using adaptive scatter kernel superposition. Phys Med Biol. 2010;55(22):6695–720.
22. Poludniowski G, Evans PM, Hansen VN, et al. An efficient Monte Carlo-based algorithm for scatter correction in keV cone-beam CT. Phys Med Biol. 2009;56(12):3847–64.
23. Poludniowski G, Evans PM, Kavanagh A, et al. Removal and effects of scatter-glare in cone-beam CT with an amorphous-silicon flat-panal detector. Phys Med Biol. 2011;56(6):1837–51.
24. Schindelin J, Arganda-Carreras I, Frise E, et al. Fiji: an open-source platform for biological-image analysis. Nat Methods. 2012;9(7):676–82.
25. Fedorov A, Beichel R, Kalpathy-Cramer J, Finet J, et al. 3D slicer as an image computing platform for the quantitative imaging network. Magn Reas Imaging. 2012;30:1323–41.
26. Klein S, Staring M, Murphy K, Viergever MA, Pluim JPW. Elastix: a toolbox for intensity based medical image registration. IEEE Trans Med Imaging. 2010;29(1):196–205.
27. Thing RS, Bernchou U, Mainegra-Hing E, et al. Hounsfield unit recovery in clinical coen beam CT images of the thorax acquired for image guided radiation therapy. Phys Med Biol. 2016;61:5781–802.
28. Boydev C, et al. Zero echo time MRI-only treatment planning for radiation therapy of brain tumors after resection. Phys Med. 2017; In press.
29. Kida S, Nakano M, et al. Cone beam computed tomography image improvement using a deep convolutional neural network. Cureus. 2018;10(4):e2548.
30. Poludniowski G, Evans PM, Webb S. Cone beam computed tomography number errors and consequences for radiotherapy planning: an investigation of correction methods. Int J Radiat Oncol Biol Phys. 2012;84(1).e109–14.

19

Decreases in TGF-β1 and PDGF levels are associated with echocardiographic changes during adjuvant radiotherapy for breast cancer

Hanna Aula[1,2]* [iD], Tanja Skyttä[1,2], Suvi Tuohinen[1,3,4], Tiina Luukkaala[5,6], Mari Hämäläinen[7], Vesa Virtanen[1,3], Pekka Raatikainen[4], Eeva Moilanen[7] and Pirkko-Liisa Kellokumpu-Lehtinen[1,2]

Abstract

Background: Radiation-induced heart disease is mainly caused by activation of the fibrotic process. Transforming growth factor-beta 1 (TGF-β1) and platelet-derived growth factor (PDGF) are pro-fibrotic mediators. The aim of our study was to evaluate the behavior of TGF-β1 and PDGF during adjuvant radiotherapy (RT) for breast cancer and the association of these cytokines with echocardiographic changes.

Methods: Our study included 73 women with early-stage breast cancer or ductal carcinoma in situ (DCIS) receiving post-operative RT but not chemotherapy. TGF-β1 and PDGF levels in serum samples taken before and on the last day of RT were measured by an enzyme-linked immunosorbent assay. Echocardiography was also performed at same time points. Patients were grouped according to a ≥ 15% worsening in tricuspid annular plane systolic excursion (TAPSE) and pericardium calibrated integrated backscatter (cIBS).

Results: In all patients, the median TGF-β1 decreased from 25.0 (IQR 21.1–30.3) ng/ml to 23.6 (IQR 19.6–26.8) ng/ml ($p = 0.003$), and the median PDGF decreased from 18.0 (IQR 13.7–22.7) ng/ml to 15.6 (IQR 12.7–19.5) ng/ml ($p < 0.001$). The baseline TGF-β1, 30.7 (IQR 26.0–35.9) ng/l vs. 23.4 (IQR 20.1–27.3) ng/l ($p < 0.001$), and PDGF, 21.5. (IQR 15.7–31.2) ng/l vs. 16.9. (IQR 13.0–21.2) ng/ml, were higher in patients with a ≥ 15% decrease in TAPSE than in patients with a < 15% decrease. In patients with a ≥ 15% decrease in TAPSE, the median TGF-β1 decreased to 24.7 (IQR 20.0–29.8) ng/ml ($p < 0.001$), and the median PDGF decreased to 16.7 (IQR 12.9–20.9) ng/ml ($p < 0.001$). The patients with a < 15% decrease had stable TGF-β1 ($p = 0.104$), but PDGF decreased to 15.1 (IQR 12.5–18.6), $p = 0.005$. The patients with a ≥ 15% increase in cIBS exhibited a decrease in TGF-β1 from 26.0 (IQR 21.7–29.7) to 22.5 (IQR 16.6.-26.7) ng/ml, $p < 0.001$, and a decrease in PDGF from 19.8 (IQR 14.6–25.9) to 15.7 (IQR 12.8–20.2) ng/ml, $p < 0.001$. In patients with a < 15% increase, TGF-β1 and PDGF did not change significantly, $p = 0.149$ and $p = 0.053$, respectively.

Conclusion: We observed a decrease in TGF-β1 and PDGF levels during adjuvant RT for breast cancer. Echocardiographic changes, namely, in TAPSE and cIBS, were associated with a greater decrease in TGF-β1 and PDGF levels. Longer follow-up times will show whether these changes observed during RT translate into increased cardiovascular morbidity.

Keywords: Cardiotoxicity, Breast cancer, Radiotherapy, Transforming growth factor beta-1, Platelet-derived growth factor, Echocardiography

* Correspondence: hanna.aula@uta.fi
[1]Faculty of Medicine and Life Sciences, University of Tampere, PO Box 100, 33014 Tampere, Finland
[2]Department of Oncology, Tampere University Hospital, PO Box 2000, 33521 Tampere, Finland
Full list of author information is available at the end of the article

Decreases in TGF-β1 and PDGF levels are associated with echocardiographic changes during...

173

Background

Late adverse effects of radiotherapy (RT), including radiation-induced heart disease, are mostly caused by fibrotic processes and take years to manifest [1]. Although the relationship between fibrosis and early inflammatory responses to microvascular damage caused by radiation is still unclear, it has been shown that pro-fibrotic mediators, including the fibroblast activating cytokines transforming growth factor-beta 1 (TGF-β1) and platelet derived growth factor (PDGF), are released by inflammatory, endothelial and epithelial cells [2]. Increased expression of TGF-β1 and PDGF in response to irradiation has been reported in animal and in vitro studies [3], but evidence describing the behavior of circulating TGF-β1 and PDGF in humans is varying [4–6].

High plasma or serum levels of TGF-β1 before RT have been associated with fibrosis of the breast [4, 5]. Regardless of whether patients received intra-operative RT or not, TGF-β1 concentrations in wound fluid were similar 24 h after surgery [7]. The relationship between TGF-β1 and RT has been most extensively studied in lung cancer patients. A meta-analysis concluded that the risk of radiation pneumonitis was increased in lung cancer patients receiving RT with a post-RT/pre-RT TGF-β1 ratio ≥ 1 [6]. TGF-β1 expression is also induced after a myocardial infarction (MI), but the exact role of TGF-β1 in MI remains elusive [3].

Increased PDGF levels are linked to the development of fibrosis, and PDGF also acts as a pro-angiogenic mediator [8]. In one study, serum PDGF levels declined after RT of non-Hodgkin lymphoma with varying target sites [9], and in another study, serum PDGF levels did not change after chemotherapy and mediastinal RT for Hodgkin's lymphoma [10]. In animal studies, inhibition of PDGF or both TGF-β1 and PDGF during RT attenuated the development of pulmonary fibrosis [11, 12]. To our knowledge, PDGF has not been previously studied in relation to breast cancer RT.

The aim of our study was to evaluate the behavior of serum TGF-β1 and PDGF during adjuvant RT for early breast cancer and to find associations with changes in echocardiographic parameters.

Materials and methods

Patients

This observational, prospective, single-center study included 73 women with early stage breast cancer or ductal carcinoma in situ (DCIS). All patients received postoperative RT after breast conserving surgery (n = 72) or mastectomy (n = 1), but did not receive chemotherapy. The patient characteristics of the study population are shown in Table 1. The inclusion and exclusion criteria have been previously described [13]. The Tampere University hospital ethics committee approved the

Table 1 Patient characteristics (n = 73)

Age, Md (IQR; range)	64	(58–66; 49–79)
BMI, Md (IQR; range)	26.3	(24.2–29.9; 20–41), n = 69
Left-sided BC, n (%)	50	(68.5)
AI use, n (%)	26	(35.6)
Tamoxifen use, n (%)	6	(8.2)
ACE or ARB use, n (%)	22	(30.1)
ASA use, n (%)	8	(11.0)
Beta-blocker use, n (%)	12	(16.4)
Statin use, n (%)	15	(20.5)
CAD, n (%)	3	(4.1)
Diabetes, n (%)	6	(8.2), n = 69
Hypertension, n (%)	30	(41.1)
Hypothyroidism, n (%)	12	(16.4)
Smoking, n (%)	8	(11)

Md median, *IQR* interquartile range, *BMI* body mass index, *BC* breast cancer, *AI* aromatase inhibitor, *ACE* angiotensin converting enzyme inhibitor, *ARB* angiotensin II receptor blocker, *ASA* low dose acetylsalicylic acid, *CAD* coronary artery disease, *Diabetes* use of diabetes medication

study (R10160), and informed consent was obtained from all participants.

Radiotherapy

The RT protocol has been previously described in detail [14]. Patients received either 50 Gy in 2 Gy fractions or 42.56 Gy in 2.66 Gy fractions. The planning target volume (PTV) was the remaining breast with margins for patients with breast conserving surgery and the chest wall with margins for the post-mastectomy patient. Two patients had positive axillary nodes, and the PTV included axillary and supraclavicular areas.

Serum biomarker analysis

Serum samples were drawn before RT and on the last day of RT, and they were stored at − 80 °C until analysis. TGF-β1 and PDGF-AB concentrations were determined with an enzyme-linked immunosorbent assay using the reagents from R&D Systems Europe Ltd. (Abingdon, UK). The detection limit and the inter-assay coefficient of variation were 7.8 pg/ml and 5.4% for TGF-b1 and 3.9 pg/ml and 4.6% for PDGF-AB, respectively.

Echocardiographic examination

Echocardiographic examinations were performed by a single cardiologist (ST) before and at the end of RT. A commercially available ultrasound machine (Philips iE33 ultrasound system; Philips, Bothell, WA, USA) and a 1–5 MHz matrix-array X5–1 transducer were used to perform the examination, as previously described [13], in a standardized manner following current guidelines [15–18]. The patients were divided into two groups, one with a ≥ 15% decline and the other with a < 15% decline in tricuspid annular plane systolic excursion (TAPSE), as we earlier reported marked changes in these two parameters [13, 19]. The decline was chosen to represent an approximately 4-mm decrease in TAPSE, which can be considered a clinically meaningful change as in patients with pulmonary hypertension with every 1-mm decrease in TAPSE, risk of death was increased by 17% [20]. Also, in our earlier study the significant average reduction of TAPSE was 2.1 ± 3.2 mm and TAPSE decreased by 4 mm in 39% of patients [19]. Similarly, a ≥ 15% increase and a < 15% increase in the pericardium calibrated integrated backscatter (cIBS) were used to categorize patients into two groups. As the magnitude of a clinically meaningful change is not known for cIBS, a 15% cutoff was used to keep the change similar to the change in TAPSE.

Statistical analysis

As the distribution of all continuous variables was skewed, medians and interquartile ranges were calculated. The Wilcoxon signed-rank test was utilized to test for changes in the biomarkers and the echocardiographic parameters from before to after RT. To test the linear relationships among the biomarkers, Spearman's correlation was used. The patients were divided into two groups for further analysis according to a 15% change in TAPSE or cIBS as described above. To test for differences in patient characteristics, biomarker levels and radiation doses between the described groups, Fisher's exact test for categorical variables, and the Mann–Whitney U-test for continuous variables were used. Multivariable logistic regression was used to test the change in TGF-β1 or PDGF and the change in TAPSE and cIBS using age, use of hypertension medication and mean heart dose as predictors. IBM SPSS statistics for Windows (version 23, IBM Corp., Armonk, NY, USA) was used for all statistical analysis. P-values less than 0.05 were considered statistically significant.

Results

TGF-β1 and PDGF

The TGF-β1 and PDGF levels of all 73 patients were measured before and after RT. In these patients, the median (Interquartile Range; IQR) TGF-β1 levels decreased from 25.0 (IQR 21.1–30.3) ng/ml before RT to 23.6 (IQR 19.6–26.8) ng/ml after RT, $p = 0.003$ (Fig. 1). Similarly, the median PDGF levels decreased from 18.0 (IQR 13.7–22.7) ng/ml before RT to 15.6 (IQR 12.7–19.5) ng/ml after RT, $p < 0.001$ (Fig. 1). TGF-β1 and PDGF exhibited a strong correlation before RT (Spearman's rho = 0.802) and after RT (rho = 0.817). The change in TGF-β1 also correlated with the change in PDGF (rho = 0.817) (Fig. 2). There was no significant correlation between change in TGF-β1 or PDGF and the time from surgery to RT (Additional file 1: Table S1) or radiation doses to the heart (Additional file 2: Table S2). Median time from surgery to start of RT was 56.0 (IQR 49.0–64.5) days.

Transforming growth factor-beta 1, platelet-derived growth factor and cardiac function

TGF-β1 and PDGF levels and changes in TAPSE

Sixty-six of the 73 (90%) patients had echocardiography completed before and after RT. TAPSE declined by ≥15% in 20 patients and by < 15% in 46 patients. In the 20 patients with a ≥ 15% TAPSE decline, TAPSE was 25.0 (IQR 23.3–30.0) mm before RT and 20.5 (IQR 18.0–23.0) mm after RT, $p < 0.001$. However, in the 46 patients with a < 15% decline, the median TAPSE was stable with 22.5 (IQR 20.0–26.0) mm and 22.0 (IQR 19.0–25.3) mm ($p = 0.298$) before and after RT, respectively. The baseline TAPSE was significantly higher in the group with a ≥ 15% TAPSE decline than in the group with a < 15% decline, $p = 0.021$. The groups were similar in body mass index (BMI), age, smoking status, proportion of left-sided breast cancer, coronary artery disease, hypertension, and use of aromatase inhibitors (AI), tamoxifen, acetylsalicylic acid (ASA), statins, levothyroxine, diabetes medication, angiotensin converting enzyme

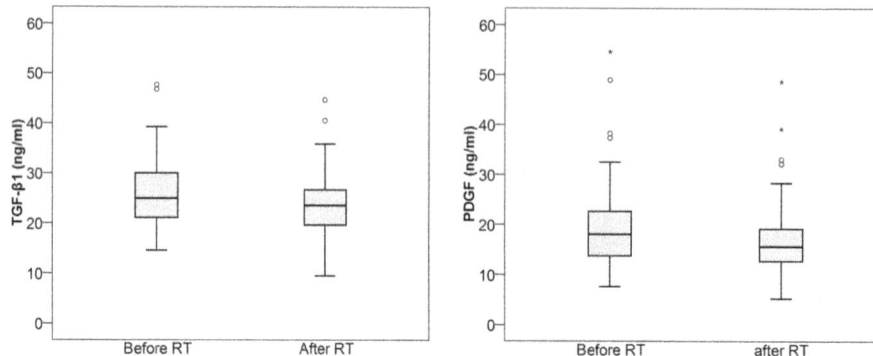

Fig. 1 TGF-β1 and PDGF levels decreased significantly during RT, $p = 0.003$ and $p < 0.001$, respectively

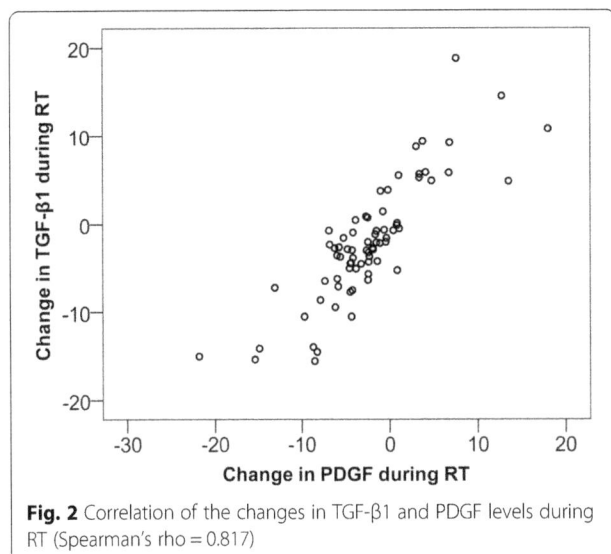

Fig. 2 Correlation of the changes in TGF-β1 and PDGF levels during RT (Spearman's rho = 0.817)

(ACE) inhibitors or angiotensin reseptor blockers (ARB) and β-blockers (Additional file 3: Table S3).

In the patients with a ≥ 15% decline in TAPSE, the median TGF-β1 level decreased from 30.7 (IQR 26.0–35.9) ng/ml before RT to 24.7 (IQR 20.0–29.8) ng/ml after RT, $p < 0.001$ (Fig. 3). TGF-β1 remained stable in patients with a < 15% decline in TAPSE, with a median TGF-β1 of 23.4 (IQR 20.1–27.3) ng/ml before RT and 22.6 (IQR 19.0–25.6) ng/ml after RT, $p = 0.104$. The baseline TGF-β1 level was also significantly higher, $p < 0.001$, in those with a ≥ 15% TAPSE decline than in those without. There was no correlation between change in TGF-β1 and the change in TAPSE (Additional file 4: Table S4). In a multivariable logistic regression analysis the change in TGF-β1 remained significant, OR 0.85 (95% CI 0.75–0.96) when age, hypertension and mean heart dose were included in the model to test variables associated with ≥15% and < 15% decline in TAPSE (Additional file 5: Table S5).

PDGF levels decreased significantly in both groups. In patients with a ≥ 15% decline in TAPSE, PDGF levels decreased from a median of 21.5 (IQR 15.7–31.2) ng/ml before RT to a median of 16.7 (IQR 12.9–20.9) ng/ml after RT, $p < 0.001$. In patients with a < 15% decline, PDGF levels decreased from a median of 16.9 (IQR 13.0–21.2) ng/ml before RT to a median of 15.1 (IQR 12.5–18.6) ng/ml after RT, $p = 0.005$ (Fig. 3). In addition, the baseline PDGF level was significantly higher, $p = 0.020$, in patients with a ≥ 15% decline than in those with a < 15% decline. The change in PDGF did not correlate with the change in TAPSE (Additional file 4: Table S4). In a multivariable logistic regression analysis the change in PDGF remained significant, OR 0.85 (95% CI 0.75–0.97) when age, hypertension and mean heart dose were included in the model (Additional file 6: Table S6).There was no difference in radiation doses to the heart between the groups with ≥15% or < 15% decline in TAPSE (Table 2).

Fifty patients had left-sided breast cancer. TGF-β1 and PDGF behavior was similar in the left-sided patients as described above for the whole group. During RT, TGF-β1 levels decreased from 24.1 (IQR 20.9–29.8) ng/ml to 23.4 (IQR 19.4–26.9) ng/ml, $p = 0.025$, and PDGF levels decreased from 17.6 (IQR 13.4–22.8) ng/ml to 15.3 (IQR 12.7–19.8) ng/ml, $p = 0.001$. When the patients with left-sided breast cancer were grouped according to the ≥15% or < 15% decline in TAPSE, the mean radiation dose to the heart was higher in the group with a ≥ 15% decline than in those with a < 15% decline, with 3.9 (IQR 3.2–4.3) Gy and 2.2 (IQR 1.6–3.7) Gy received, respectively, $p = 0.024$. Similarly, the mean doses to the left descending coronary artery (LAD), 1.1 (IQR 0.4–1.5) Gy vs. 0.7 (IQR 0.4–0.9) Gy ($p = 0.006$), and the left ventricle, 7.0 (IQR 4.2–8.0) Gy vs. 3.8 (IQR 2.1–5.6) Gy ($p = 0.005$), were significantly higher in the ≥15% group compared to the < 15% group.

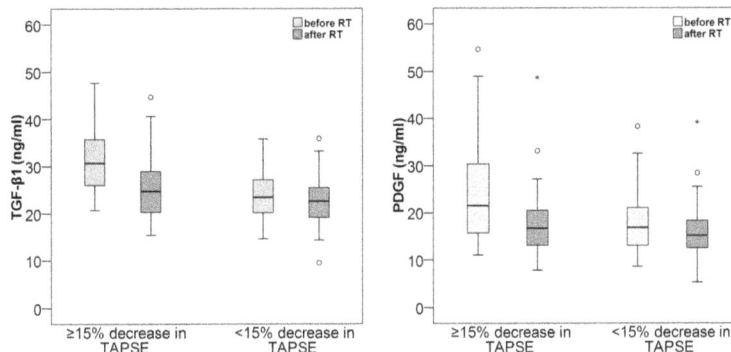

Fig. 3 Baseline TGF-β1 and PDGF levels were higher, $p < 0.001$ and $p = 0.020$, respectively, and both decreased significantly, $p < 0.001$, in patients with a ≥ 15% decrease in TAPSE compared with patients with a < 15% decrease in TAPSE. TGF-β1 levels were stable, but PDGF levels decreased significantly, $p = 0.005$, in patients with a < 15% decrease in TAPSE

Table 2 Radiation doses according to TAPSE decline

	≥15% decrease in TAPSE (n = 20) Md (IQR)	< 15% decrease in TAPSE (n = 46) Md (IQR)	p
Heart			
Dmean (Gy)	3.39 (0.8–4.2)	1.8 (0.8–3.5)	0.343
Dmax (Gy)	46.1 (5.3–49.0)	45.9 (11.8–47.5)	0.676
V45 (%)	0.2 (0–1.3)	0.1 (0–0.7)	0.630
V20 (%)	4.3 (0–5.2)	1.4 (0–4.8)	0.330
LAD			
Dmean (Gy)	23.7 (0.3–28.5)	10.3 (2.3–23.5)	0.414
Dmax (Gy)	44.1(0.7–48.1)	40.8 (5.0–46.1)	0.460
V45 (%)	0(0–5.2)	0(0–7.3)	0.663
V20 (%)	43.6 (0–67.6)	19.7(0–54.9)	0.193
Left ventricle			
Dmean (Gy)	4.6 (0.2–7.2)	2.7 (1.2–5.5)	0.273
Dmax (Gy)	44.6 (0.8–47.6)	44.1 (5.0–46.7)	0.691
V45 (%)	0.1 (0–2.0)	0 (0–0.4)	0.360
V20 (%)	6.0 (0–11.7)	1.7 (0–7.8)	0.192
V10 (%)	8.8 (0–15.1)	3.4 (0–11.0)	0.150
Right ventricle			
Dmean (Gy)	2.0 (0.8–7.2)	1.6 (0.9–2.9)	0.692
Dmax (Gy)	27.6 (3.1–43.4)	21.3 (3.3–42.8)	0.988
V45 (%)	0 (0–0)	0 (0–0)	0.925
V20 (%)	0.1 (0–1.3)	0 (0–1.3)	0.848
V10 (%)	0.7 (0–3.6)	0.1 (0–3.8)	0.714
Ipsilateral lung			
Dmean (Gy)	8.1 (6.4–9.1)	7.7 (6.2–9.0)	0.484
Dmax (Gy)	49.2 (46.2–52.7)	48.5 (47.1–51.6)	0.994

Md median, *IQR* interquartile range, *Dmean* mean radiation dose to the structure, *Dmax* maximum radiation dose within the structure, *V45* percentage of the structure volume receiving 45 Gy of radiation, *V20* percentage of the structure volume receiving 20 Gy of radiation, *V10* percentage of the structure volume receiving 10 Gy of radiation, *LAD* left anterior descending coronary artery

TGF-β1, PDGF and change in cIBS

Sixty-four of the 73 (88%) patients had cIBS measured by echocardiography. Twenty-nine patients had a ≥ 15% increase in cIBS, from a median of – 19.8 (IQR -22.6- -16.6) dB before RT to a median of – 13.3 (IQR -15.3- -9.5) dB after RT, p < 0.001. The group of 35 patients with a < 15% increase in cIBS had a significant decrease in cIBS from – 17.1 (IQR -21.5- -14.6) dB before RT to – 18.3 (IQR -24.0- -16.7) dB after RT, p = 0.033. The baseline cIBS values between the groups did not differ significantly, p = 0.257. Furthermore, the groups had similar baseline characteristics (Additional file 7: Table S7). There was a tendency for patients with a ≥ 15% increase to be older than those with a < 15% increase, 65 (IQR 59.5–69) years old and 62 (IQR 58–66) years old, respectively (p = 0.079). Additionally, smokers tended to more likely have a < 15% increase in cIBS (p = 0.063).

In patients with a ≥ 15% increase in cIBS, the median TGF-β1 level decreased significantly from 26.0 (IQR 21.7–29.7) ng/ml before RT to 22.5 (16.6–26.7) ng/ml after RT (p < 0.001) (Fig. 4). TGF-β1 remained stable in patients with a < 15% increase in cIBS, with a median TGF-β1 level of 24.0 (IQR 20.7–31.4) ng/ml and 24.1 (IQR 21.1–22.5) ng/ml before and after RT, respectively (p = 0.149). The baseline TGF-β1 levels were similar in both groups, p = 0.518. There was no correlation between the change in TGF-β1and the change in cIBS (Additional file 4: Table S4). In a multivariable logistic regression analysis the change in TGF-β1 remained borderline significant, OR 0.91 (95% CI 0.82–1.00) when age, hypertension and mean heart dose were included in the model (Additional file 5: Table S5).

In addition to declining TGFβ-1 levels, a significant decrease in PDGF levels was observed from 19.8 (IQR 14.6–25.9) ng/ml before RT to 15.7 (IQR 12.8–20.2) ng/

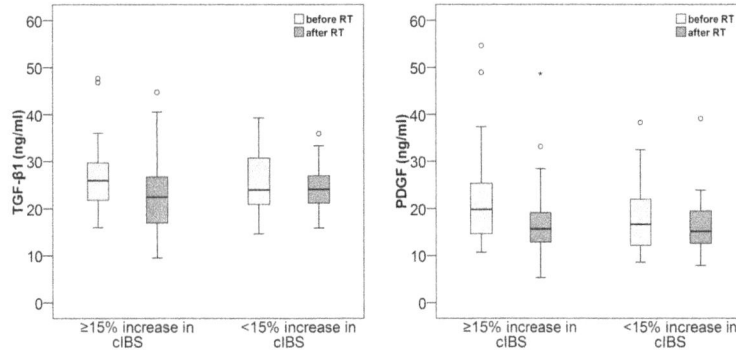

Fig. 4 TGFβ-1 and PDGF levels decreased significantly in patients with a ≥ 15% increase in cIBS, $p < 0.001$ for both, but remain stable in patients with a < 15% increase in cIBS

ml after RT, $p < 0.001$, in patients with a ≥ 15% increase in cIBS. There was no significant change in PDGF levels in patients with a < 15% increase in cIBS, with a median PDGF of 16.6 (IQR 11.7–22.6) before RT and 15.2 (IQR 12.6–19.8) after RT, $p = 0.053$. The baseline PDGF level tended to be higher in those with a ≥ 15% increase than in those with a < 15% increase in cIBS, $p = 0.050$. The change in PDGF did not correlate with the change in cIBS (Additional file 4: Table S4). In a multivariable logistic regression analysis change in PDGF remained significant, OR 0.88 (95% CI 0.78–0.99), when age, hypertension and mean heart dose were included in the model (Additional file 6: Table S6).

The radiation doses, especially those to the left side of the heart and to the ipsilateral lung, were higher in those with a ≥ 15% increase in cIBS than those with a < 15% increase in cIBS. Table 3 presents a detailed depiction of the radiation doses.

Discussion

In this study, we demonstrated the behavior of serum TGF-β1 and PDGF during adjuvant RT for breast cancer. A small decline was observed in all patients, but the decline was most pronounced in patients with worsening cardiac function and structural changes observed in echocardiography. We also found a strong correlation between baseline TGF-β1 and PDGF levels and the change in TGF-β1 and PDGF levels during RT. This correlation is probably explained by the same origin of both cytokines, which are produced by macrophages, although TGF-β1 is additionally produced by endothelial and mesenchymal cells [1, 2]. This result suggests that the behavior of both cytokines depict the same phenomenon during adjuvant RT for breast cancer. The time from surgery to RT did not affect TGF-β1 and PDGF levels and change in these levels. This is probably because the wound was healed by the time RT started and the half-life of TGF-β1 and PDGF in serum is short [21].

Transforming growth factor-beta 1 and cardiac function

It is generally accepted that TGF-β1 is a pro-fibrotic cytokine that initiates fibrosis in response to RT [1, 2]. Additionally, it plays a role in cardiac remodeling after myocardial infarction [3]. Earlier studies have shown that an increase in TGF-β1 during RT for non-small cell lung cancer is likely to be predictive for the development of radiation pneumonitis [6]. However, some studies do not confirm this finding, and in patients who do not develop radiation pneumonitis, a decrease in TGF-β1 levels is seen [22, 23]. In lung cancer, this decline is thought to represent a decrease in production of TGF-β1 by tumor cells. However, this explanation probably does not explain the decline in TGF-β1 in our study since our patients underwent breast conserving surgery or mastectomy and the likelihood of macroscopic tumor residual is extremely small.

The dynamics of TGF-β1 during adjuvant RT for breast cancer have not been previously reported; however, two studies found that an increased TGF-β1 level before RT was predictive of fibrosis of the breast [4, 5]. Neither of these studies reported the behavior of TGF-β1 during RT. In our patients with a 15% decline in TAPSE, the baseline TGF-β1 level was higher than that in patients without the decline, indicating an association between high TGF-β1 levels and right ventricular dysfunction induced by RT.

TGF-β1 also seems to be a marker of radiosensitivity. A decrease in TGF-β1 levels during RT is associated with a positive response to RT [24]. Additionally, in vitro experiments suggest that blockade of TGF-β1 during RT for non-small cell lung cancer and breast cancer increases radiosensitivity [25, 26]. Therefore, increased TGF-β1 levels seem to be a marker for both radioresistance and radiosensitivity, depending on the tissue in question. As the association of TGF-β1 and echocardiographic has not been studied during RT, we present a novel finding. Levels of TGF-β1 decreased significantly in patients with a decline in TAPSE and an increase in cIBS. TAPSE is in wide

Table 3 Radiation doses according to the change in cIBS

Structure	≥15% increase in cIBS (n = 29)	< 15% increase in cIBS (n = 35)	
	Md (IQR)	Md (IQR)	p
Heart			
Dmean (Gy)	3.4 (1.1–4.2)	1.6 (0.8–2.7)	**0.011**
Dmax (Gy)	47.2 (15.0–48.8)	44.5 (6.4–47.1)	0.068
V45 (%)	0.5 (0–1.7)	0 (0–0.4)	**0.025**
V20 (%)	4.4 (0–6.2)	1.1 (0–2.4)	**0.005**
LAD			
Dmean (Gy)	22.9 (2.3–27.3)	7.3 (0.4–18.0)	**0.042**
Dmax (Gy)	45.9 (5.3–46.8)	36.3 (0.6–45.3)	**0.040**
V45 (%)	0.4 (0–13.9)	0 (0–0.3)	**0.008**
V20 (%)	42.7 (0–68.7)	8.9 (0–38.4)	**0.041**
Left ventricle			
Dmean (Gy)	4.9 (1.2–7.0)	2.3 (0.2–3.8)	**0.023**
Dmax (Gy)	45.8 (9.0–47.8)	41.7 (0.7–45.9)	0.080
V45 (%)	0.1 (0–2.9)	0 (0–0.2)	0.006
V20 (%)	6.7 (0–10.4)	1.3 (0–4.7)	**0.021**
V10 (%)	9.0 (0–15.0)	3.0 (0–6.5)	**0.006**
Right ventricle (n = 49)			
Dmean (Gy)	2.4 (1.1–3.1)	1.5 (0.9–2.3)	0.074
Dmax (Gy)	29.6 (3.6–44.0)	8.1 (3.0–39.3)	0.189
V45 (%)	0 (0–0)	0 (0–0)	0.150
V20 (%)	0.1 (0–2.7)	0 (0–0.4)	0.053
V10 (%)	0.9 (0–6.5)	0 (0–1.4)	**0.019**
Lung			
Dmean (Gy)	8.2 (7.6–9.6)	6.8 (5.5–8.2)	**0.001**
Dmax (Gy)	50.1 (47.9–56.7)	47.5 (46.4–49.7)	**0.009**

Md median, *IQR* interquartile range, *Dmean* mean radiation dose to the structure, *Dmax* maximum radiation dose within the structure, *V45* percentage of the structure volume receiving 45 Gy of radiation, *V20* percentage of the structure volume receiving 20 Gy of radiation, *V10* percentage of the structure volume receiving 10 Gy of radiation, *LAD* left anterior descending coronary artery

clinical use as a reliable measurement of the right ventricular function, and a decline in TAPSE correlates with poor cardiac prognosis in many patient groups [17, 20]. Myocardial reflectivity can be determined with off-line analysis of the echocardiography acquisition (cIBS). Even though the exact basis for the changes in cIBS are not completely understood, an increase in cIBS presents changes in three-dimensional myocardial structure due to factors such as tissue edema or interstitial fibrosis [27].

In studies of cardiac function after an experimental myocardial infarction in mice, blockade of TGF-β1 by an antibody increased mortality and left ventricular dilatation [28]. Another study concluded that early inhibition of TGFβ-1 was detrimental and that later inhibition was beneficial to the cardiac function of mice after an MI, which indicates that the role of TGFβ-1 may be different in various phases of the healing process [29]. In obese, hypertensive patients, an abundance of circulating TGF-β1 is associated with left ventricular filling abnormalities [30]. As concluded by a review conducted by Bujak, the role of TGF-β1 after an MI remains elusive [3].

Platelet-derived growth factor and cardiac function
PDGF consists of two linked chains, designated A, B, C or D. It can be assembled as a hetero- or homodimer [8]. We measured the heterodimer PDGF-AB and found that RT induced a decrease in PDGF that was associated with a decrease in TAPSE and an increase in cIBS. The role of PDGF in long-term adverse effects of RT is not as extensively studied as is the role of TGFβ-1. During RT, PDGF levels were decreased in non-Hodgkin lymphoma patients with varying RT sites, some with preceding chemotherapy and some without [9]. In patients receiving chemotherapy and RT, PDGF and TGF-β1 levels remained unchanged [10]. Because the sites of RT varied, some patients had intact tumors and some patients had

chemotherapy that also may influence cytokine levels, indicating that the studies were quite different from our study.

The effect of PDGF has also been studied through inhibition of the PDGF receptor. In mice, treatment with a PDGF receptor tyrosine kinase inhibitor, imatinib, attenuated the development of lung and skin fibrosis [11, 31]. The function of PDGF in cardiac tissue remains elusive, as blockade of PDGF receptor improved cardiac function [32], but injection of exogenous PDGF-AB or PDGF-BB improved heart function after an MI [33–35].

Echocardiographic changes associate with radiation doses

In our earlier study, we reported changes in TAPSE during RT of left-sided breast cancer patients but found no association with radiation doses [19]. In this study, only patients with available serum samples were included. We found that patients with left-sided breast cancer that had a ≥ 15% decline in TAPSE had higher radiation doses to the whole heart, the left ventricle and the LAD than those with a < 15% decline in TAPSE. There were even more differences in the radiation doses to the whole heart or parts of the heart when patients were grouped according to ≥15% and < 15% increases in cIBS. An increase in cIBS represents an increase in the reflectivity of the cardiac tissue, probably due to structural changes caused by RT-induced inflammation. TAPSE is a parameter depicting longitudinal function of the right ventricle. Its decrease may portray inflammatory changes because the thinness of the right ventricle makes it more sensitive to RT-induced changes [19].

Study limitations

The limitations to our study are that the population is rather small and the follow-up time is very short, as we only studied the changes that occurred during adjuvant RT. At this stage, we do not know if the echocardiographic changes are permanent or if they are associated with the development of fibrosis, which is thought to be responsible for the increased risk of cardiac morbidity after irradiation of the heart [36]. Thus, longer follow-up times are needed to determine whether the behavior of TGF-β1 and PDGF during adjuvant RT depict permanent damage to the heart.

Conclusion

In this study, we demonstrated that RT induces a decrease in TGF-β1 and PDGF levels in accordance with worsening cardiac function and structural changes, namely, a decrease in TAPSE and an increase in cIBS. Additionally, higher baseline TGF-β1 and PDGF levels were associated with a decrease in TAPSE, possibly indicating a higher susceptibility to RT-induced cardiac changes. Decreases in TGF-β1 and PDGF levels and the

association of these cytokines with echocardiographic changes could depict increased sensitivity of the heart to the effects of radiation. These novel findings are preliminary and need to be confirmed by more studies and longer follow-up, as serum biomarkers are an attractive, minimally invasive and easily available option to identify RT patients in need of closer cardiological follow-up.

Additional files

Additional file 1: Table S1. Spearman's correlation coefficients. RT radiotherapy, TFGβ transforming growth factor, PDGF platelet derived growth factor

Additional file 2: Table S2. Spearman's correlation coefficient between changes in TFG-β1 and PDGF and radiation doses. *Dmean*, mean radiation dose to the structure; *Dmax*, maximum radiation dose within the structure; *V45* percentage of the structure volume receiving 45 Gy of radiation; *V20*, percentage of the structure volume receiving 20 Gy of radiation; *V10*, percentage of the structure volume receiving 10 Gy of radiation; *LAD*, left anterior descending coronary artery.

Additional file 3: Table S3. Baseline characteristic according to change in TAPSE. *TAPSE*, tricuspid annular plane systolic excursion; *BMI*, body mass index; *bc*, breast cancer; *Hypertension*, use of hypertension medication; *ASA*, low dose acetylsalicylic acid; *Diabetes*, use of diabetes medication; *ACE* angiotensin converting enzyme inhibitor; *ARB*, angiotensin II receptor blocker; *AI* aromatase inhibitor use.

Additional file 4: Table S4. Spearman's correlation coefficient between changes in TFG-β1, PDGF, TAPSE and cIBS. *TFG-β1*, transforming growth factor beta 1; *PDGF*, platelet derived growth factor; *TAPSE*, tricuspid annular plane systolic excursion; *cIBS*, pericardium calibrated integrated backscatter.

Additional file 5: Table S5. Multivariable logistic regression analysis with change < 15% or ≥ 15% in TAPSE and cIBS. *TAPSE*, tricuspid annular plane systolic excursion; *cIBS*, pericardium calibrated integrated backscatter; *TFG-β1*, transforming growth factor beta 1

Additional file 6: Table S6. Multivariable logistic regression analysis with change < 15% or ≥ 15% in TAPSE and cIBS. *TAPSE*, tricuspid annular plane systolic excursion; *cIBS*, pericardium calibrated integrated backscatter; *PDGF*, platelet derived growth factor.

Additional file 7: Table S7. Baseline characteristic according to change in cIBS. *cIBS*, pericardium calibrated integrated backscatter; *BMI*, body mass index; *bc*, breast cancer; *Hypertension*, use of hypertension medication; *ASA*, low dose acetylsalicylic acid; *Diabetes*, use of diabetes medication; *ACE* angiotensin converting enzyme inhibitor; *ARB*, angiotensin II receptor blocker; *AI* aromatase inhibitor use.

Abbreviations

AI: Aromatase inhibitor; ASA: Acetylsalicylic acid; BMI: Body mass index; cIBS: Pericardium calibrated integrated backscatter; DCIS: Ductal carcinoma in situ; IQR: Interquartile range; LAD: Left descending coronary artery; MI: Myocardial infarction; PDGF: Platelet derived growth factor; PTV: Planning target volume; RT: Radiotherapy; TAPSE: Tricuspid annular plane systolic excursion; TGF-β1: Transforming growth factor beta 1

Acknowledgements
Ms. Terhi Salonen is warmly acknowledged for excellent technical assistance.

Funding
Financial support was provided by the Seppo Nieminen fund (150620 and 150636), the competitive state financing of the expert responsibility area of the Tampere University Hospital and the Paulo Foundation.

Authors' contributions

HA prepared the draft of the manuscript and all other authors provided critical revisions of the content. HA, TS, ST, MH, VV, PR, EM and PK contributed to the conception or design of the study. MH and EM were responsible for the analysis of the samples. HA and TL performed and interpreted statistical analyses. All authors read and approved the final manuscript.

Competing interests

The authors declare that they have no competing interests.

Author details

[1]Faculty of Medicine and Life Sciences, University of Tampere, PO Box 100, 33014 Tampere, Finland. [2]Department of Oncology, Tampere University Hospital, PO Box 2000, 33521 Tampere, Finland. [3]Heart Hospital, Tampere University Hospital, PO Box 2000, 33521 Tampere, Finland. [4]Department of Cardiology, Heart and Lung Center, Helsinki University Hospital, PO Box 340, Tampere 00029, Finland. [5]Research, Development and Innovation Center, Pirkanmaa Hospital District, PO Box 2000, 33521 Tampere, Finland. [6]Health Sciences, Faculty of Social Sciences, University of Tampere, PO Box 100, 33014 Tampere, Finland. [7]The Immunopharmacology Research Group, Faculty of Medicine and Life Sciences, University of Tampere and Tampere University Hospital, PO Box 100, 33014 Tampere, Finland.

References

1. Westbury CB, Yarnold JR. Radiation fibrosis - current clinical and therapeutic perspectives. Clin Oncol. 2012;24:657–72.
2. Yarnold J, Vozenin Brotons M-C. Pathogenetic mechanisms in radiation fibrosis. Radiother Oncol. 2010;97:149–61. https://doi.org/10.1016/j.radonc.2010.09.002.
3. Bujak M, Frangogiannis N. The role of TGF-β signaling in myocardial infarction and cardiac remodeling. Cardiovasc Res. 2007;74:184–95. https://doi.org/10.1016/j.cardiores.2006.10.002.
4. Li C, Wilson PB, Levine E, Barber J, Stewart AL, Kumar S. TGF-beta1 levels in pre-treatment plasma identify breast cancer patients at risk of developing post-radiotherapy fibrosis. Int J Cancer. 1999;84:155–9.
5. Boothe DL, Coplowitz S, Greenwood E, Barney CL, Christos PJ, Parashar B, et al. Transforming growth factor β-1 (TGF-β1) is a serum biomarker of radiation induced fibrosis in patients treated with Intracavitary accelerated partial breast irradiation: preliminary results of a prospective study. Int J Radiat Oncol Biol Phys. 2013;87:1030–6. https://doi.org/10.1016/j.ijrobp.2013.08.045.
6. Zhang X-J, Sun J-G, Sun J, Ming H, Wang X-X, Wu L, et al. Prediction of radiation pneumonitis in lung cancer patients: a systematic review. J Cancer Res Clin Oncol. 2012;138:2103–16. https://doi.org/10.1007/s00432-012-1284-1.
7. Scherer SD, Bauer J, Schmaus A, Neumaier C, Herskind C, Veldwijk MR, et al. TGF-β1 is present at high levels in wound fluid from breast Cancer patients immediately post-surgery, and is not increased by intraoperative radiation therapy (IORT). PLoS One. 2016;11:e0162221. https://doi.org/10.1371/journal.pone.0162221.
8. Li M, Jendrossek V, Belka C. The role of PDGF in radiation oncology. Radiat Oncol. 2007;2:5. https://doi.org/10.1186/1748-717X-2-5.
9. Ria R, Cirulli T, Giannini T, Bambace S, Serio G, Portaluri M, et al. Serum levels of angiogenic cytokines decrease after radiotherapy in non-Hodgkin lymphomas. Clin Exp Med. 2008;8:141–5. https://doi.org/10.1007/s10238-008-0170-2.
10. Villani F, Busia A, Villani M, Vismara C, Viviani S, Bonfante V. Serum cytokine in response to chemo-radiotherapy for Hodgkin's disease. Tumori. 2008;94:803–8. https://doi.org/10.1700/396.4659.
11. Abdollahi A, Li M, Ping G, Plathow C, Domhan S, Kiessling F, et al. Inhibition of platelet-derived growth factor signaling attenuates pulmonary fibrosis. J Exp Med. 2005;201:925–35. https://doi.org/10.1084/jem.20041393.
12. Dadrich M, Nicolay NH, Flechsig P, Bickelhaupt S, Hoeltgen L, Roeder F, et al. Combined inhibition of TGFβ and PDGF signaling attenuates radiation-induced pulmonary fibrosis. Oncoimmunology. 2016;5:e1123366. https://doi.org/10.1080/2162402X.2015.1123366.
13. Tuohinen SS, Skytta T, Virtanen V, Virtanen M, Luukkaala T, Kellokumpu-Lehtinen P-L, et al. Detection of radiotherapy-induced myocardial changes by ultrasound tissue characterisation in patients with breast cancer. Int J Cardiovasc Imaging. 2016;32:767–76.
14. Skytta T, Tuohinen S, Boman E, Virtanen V, Raatikainen P, Kellokumpu-Lehtinen P-L. Troponin T-release associates with cardiac radiation doses during adjuvant left-sided breast cancer radiotherapy. Radiat Oncol. 2015;10:141.
15. Lang RM, Badano LP, Mor-Avi V, Afilalo J, Armstrong A, Ernande L, et al. Recommendations for cardiac chamber quantification by echocardiography in adults: an update from the American Society of Echocardiography and the European Association of Cardiovascular Imaging. Eur Heart J Cardiovasc Imaging. 2015;16:233–70.
16. Galderisi M, Henein MY, D'hooge J, Sicari R, Badano LP, Zamorano JL, et al. Recommendations of the European Association of Echocardiography: how to use echo-Doppler in clinical trials: different modalities for different purposes. Eur J Echocardiogr. 2011;12:339–53.
17. Rudski LG, Lai WW, Afilalo J, Hua L, Handschumacher MD, Chandrasekaran K, et al. Guidelines for the echocardiographic assessment of the right heart in adults: a report from the American Society of Echocardiography endorsed by the European Association of Echocardiography, a registered branch of the European Society of Cardiology, and t. J Am Soc Echocardiogr. 2010;23:685–8.
18. Nagueh SF, Appleton CP, Gillebert TC, Marino PN, Oh JK, Smiseth OA, et al. Recommendations for the evaluation of left ventricular diastolic function by echocardiography. Eur J Echocardiogr. 2009;10:165–93.
19. Tuohinen SS, Skytta T, Virtanen V, Luukkaala T, Kellokumpu-Lehtinen P-L, Raatikainen P. Early effects of adjuvant breast cancer radiotherapy on right ventricular systolic and diastolic function. Anticancer Res. 2015;35:2141–7.
20. Forfia PR, Fisher MR, Mathai SC, Housten-Harris T, Hemnes AR, Borlaug BA, et al. Tricuspid annular displacement predicts survival in pulmonary hypertension. Am J Respir Crit Care Med. 2006;174:1034–41. https://doi.org/10.1164/rccm.200604-547OC.
21. Coffey RJ, Kost LJ, Lyons RM, Moses HL, LaRusso NF. Hepatic processing of transforming growth factor beta in the rat. Uptake, metabolism, and biliary excretion. J Clin Invest. 1987;80:750–7. https://doi.org/10.1172/JCI113130.
22. De Jaeger K, Seppenwoolde Y, Kampinga HH, Boersma LJ, Belderbos JSA, Lebesque JV. Significance of plasma transforming growth factor-beta levels in radiotherapy for non-small-cell lung cancer. Int J Radiat Oncol Biol Phys. 2004;58:1378–87. https://doi.org/10.1016/j.ijrobp.2003.09.078.
23. Novakova-Jiresova A, Van Gameren MM, Coppes RP, Kampinga HH, Groen HJM. Transforming growth factor-beta plasma dynamics and post-irradiation lung injury in lung cancer patients. Radiother Oncol. 2004;71:183–9. https://doi.org/10.1016/j.radonc.2004.01.019.
24. Fu Z-Z, Gu T, Fu B-H, Hua H-X, Yang S, Zhang Y-Q, et al. Relationship of serum levels of VEGF and TGF-β1 with radiosensitivity of elderly patients with unresectable non-small cell lung cancer. Tumor Biol. 2014;35:4785–9. https://doi.org/10.1007/s13277-014-1628-3.
25. Bouquet F, Pal A, Pilones KA, Demaria S, Hann B, Akhurst RJ, et al. TGF 1 inhibition increases the Radiosensitivity of breast Cancer cells in vitro and promotes tumor control by radiation in vivo. Clin Cancer Res. 2011;17:6754–65. https://doi.org/10.1158/1078-0432.CCR-11-0544.
26. Du S, Bouquet S, Lo C-H, Pellicciotta I, Bolourchi S, Parry R, et al. Attenuation of the DNA damage response by transforming growth factor-Beta inhibitors enhances radiation sensitivity of non–small-cell lung Cancer cells in vitro and in vivo. Int J Radiat Oncol. 2015;91:91–9. https://doi.org/10.1016/j.ijrobp.2014.09.026.
27. Mor-Avi V, Lang RM, Badano LP, Belohlavek M, Cardim NM, Derumeaux G, et al. Current and evolving echocardiographic techniques for the quantitative evaluation of cardiac mechanics: ASE/EAE consensus statement on methodology and indications endorsed by the Japanese Society of Echocardiography. Eur J Echocardiogr. 2011;12:167–205. https://doi.org/10.1093/ejechocard/jer021.
28. Frantz S, Hu K, Adamek A, Wolf J, Sallam A, KG Maier S, et al. Transforming growth factor beta inhibition increases mortality and left ventricular dilatation after myocardial infarction. Basic Res Cardiol. 2008;103:485–92. https://doi.org/10.1007/s00395-008-0739-7.
29. Ikeuchi M, Tsutsui H, Shiomi T, Matsusaka H, Matsushima S, Wen J, et al. Inhibition of TGF-beta signaling exacerbates early cardiac dysfunction but prevents late remodeling after infarction. Cardiovasc Res. 2004;64:526–35. https://doi.org/10.1016/j.cardiores.2004.07.017.
30. Parrinello G, Licata A, Colomba D, Di Chiara T, Argano C, Bologna P, et al. Left ventricular filling abnormalities and obesity-associated hypertension:

relationship with overproduction of circulating transforming growth factor β1. J Hum Hypertens. 2005;19:543–50. https://doi.org/10.1038/sj.jhh.1001864.

31. Horton JA, Chung EJ, Hudak KE, Sowers A, Thetford A, White AO, et al. Inhibition of radiation-induced skin fibrosis with imatinib. Int J Radiat Biol. 2013;89:162–70. https://doi.org/10.3109/09553002.2013.741281.

32. Liu C, Zhao W, Meng W, Zhao T, Chen Y, Ahokas RA, et al. Platelet-derived growth factor blockade on cardiac remodeling following infarction. Mol Cell Biochem. 2014;397:295–304. https://doi.org/10.1007/s11010-014-2197-x.

33. Zheng J, Shin JH, Xaymardan M, Chin A, Duignan I, Hong MK, et al. Platelet-derived growth factor improves cardiac function in a rodent myocardial infarction model. Coron Artery Dis. 2004;15:59–64.

34. Hsieh PCH, MacGillivray C, Gannon J, Cruz FU, Lee RT. Local controlled Intramyocardial delivery of platelet-derived growth factor improves Postinfarction ventricular function without pulmonary toxicity. Circulation. 2006;114:637–44. https://doi.org/10.1161/CIRCULATIONAHA.106.639831.

35. Chin A, Zheng J, Duignan I, Edelberg JM. PDGF-AB-based functional cardioprotection of the aging rat heart. Exp Gerontol. 2006;41:63–8. https://doi.org/10.1016/j.exger.2005.10.012.

36. Sardaro A, Petruzzelli MF, D'Errico MP, Grimaldi L, Pili G, Portaluri M. Radiation-induced cardiac damage in early left breast cancer patients: risk factors, biological mechanisms, radiobiology, and dosimetric constraints. Radiother Oncol. 2012;103:133–42. https://doi.org/10.1016/j.radonc.2012.02.008.

20

Comorbidity indexing for prediction of the clinical outcome after stereotactic body radiation therapy in non-small cell lung cancer

Julia Dreyer, Michael Bremer and Christoph Henkenberens[*] (iD)

Abstract

Purpose: To determine the prognostic impact of comorbidity and age in medically inoperable early-stage non-small cell lung cancer (NSCLC) treated with stereotactic body radiotherapy (SBRT) using the age-adjusted Charlson Comorbidity Index (aCCI).

Patients and methods: Between November 2008 and January 2015, 196 consecutive patients with medically inoperable NSCLC were treated with SBRT at a single institution. The prescribed isocenter dose was either 60.0 Gray (Gy) in six fractions for central lung cancer or 56.25 Gy in three fractions for peripheral lung cancer. Baseline comorbidities were retrospectively retrieved according to available outclinic medical records as well as the hospital information system. The aCCI was scored for each patient and subjected according to outcome and toxicity as well as all of the single items of the aCCI and other clinical parameters using univariate and multivariate analysis.

Results: Thirty-one point 6 % (62/196) of patients were deceased, of whom 17.3% (34/196) died due to lung cancer and 14.3% (28/196) due to comorbidities. The median overall survival (OS) was 15.0 months (95% CI [11.9–18.1]), whereas the median cancer-specific survival (CSS) was not reached. An aCCI $\geq$7 compared with an aCCI $\leq$6 was significantly associated with an increased risk of death (HR 1.79, 95% CI [1.02–2.80], $p = 0.04$) and cancer-specific death (HR 9.26, 95% CI [4.83–24.39], $p < 0.001$), respectively. Neither OS nor CCS were significantly associated with age, sex, side (left vs. right), lobe, localization (central vs. peripheral), packyears, TNM, or any item of the aCCI. Considering the 14.3% (28/196) of deceased patients who died due to comorbidities, aCCI $\geq$9 was significantly associated with non-cancer-related death (HR 3.12, 95% CI [1.22–8.33], $p = 0.02$). The observed cumulative rate of radiation pneumonitis (RP) $\geq$2 was 12.7% (25/196). The aCCI had no statistical association with RP.

Conclusion: Advanced age and numerous comorbidities characterizing this patient population were successfully assessed using the aCCI in terms of survival. Therefore, we recommend that age and comorbidity be indexed using the aCCI as a simple scoring system for all patients treated with SBRT for lung cancer.

Introduction

Lobectomy remains the standard of care for early-stage non-small cell lung cancer (NSCLC) in medically fit patients [1], but approximately 20% of patients are medically inoperable due to comorbidities, old age, or both [2].

Among the strategies to improve control rates, stereotactic body radiotherapy (SBRT) is the most favored. Numerous reports have indicated extremely good local control after SBRT with an excellent toxicity profile [3–5].

However, the reported overall survival rates after SBRT for early-stage NSCLC tend to be worse than local control. This has frequently been attributed to competing comorbidities because patients are treated with SBRT instead of surgery due to their comorbidities [6–9]. The choice against surgery and in favor SBRT has been found to depend on local practice [6] and patient-specific

* Correspondence: henkenberens.christoph@mh-hannover.de
First author: Julia Dreyer
Co-Author: Michael Bremer
Last/Senior author: Christoph Henkenberens
Department of Radiotherapy and Special Oncology, Medical School
Hannover, Carl-Neuberg-Str. 1, 30625 Hannover, Germany

factors [7–9]. Baseline comorbidities and their prognostic impacts on the clinical outcome have not been assessed using a simple and objective comorbidity score. With this study, we aimed to make another step towards this goal. The objective of this retrospective study cohort was therefore to use the age-adjusted Charlson Comorbidity Index (aCCI) [10], as it is tempting to use given its simplicity, to investigate the impact of comorbidities on the outcome of NSCLC treated with SBRT.

Patients and methods

Patients

Between November 2008 and January 2015, 196 patients with medically inoperable NSCLC were treated with SBRT at a single institution. Patient were collected by reviewing the available outclinic medical records and the medical records of the hospital information system. Comorbidities were encoded using the aCCI (Table 1). The selection criteria were medically unfit for surgery or declination of surgery and staging of tumor and distant metastasis based on positron emission tomography (PET) computed tomography (CT) and biopsy of the tumor if the medical condition allowed bronchoscopy or CT guided biopsy.

Table 1 Age-adjusted Charlson Comorbidity Index (aCCI) [10]

Score	Comorbid condition
1	Myocardial infarction
	Congestive heart failure
	Cerebral vascular disease
	Peripheral vascular disease
	Dementia
	COPD
	Connective tissue disease
	Peptic ulcer disease
	Mild liver disease
	Age[a]
2	Diabetes
	Hemiplegia
	Moderate(Severe renal disease
	Diabetes with end-organ damage
	Solid tumor
	Leukemia
	Lymphoma
3	Moderate/severe liver disease
6	Metastatic solid tumor
	Acquired immunodeficiency syndomre

[a]1pint is added to aged 41–50 years, 2 points for those aged 51–60 years, 3 points for those 61–70 years, and 4 points for those 71 years or older

Radiotherapy

Patients were fixed in a stereotactic body frame system with a customized vacuum pillow (Elekta, Stockholm, Sweden) using abdominal compression and free breathing. The gross tumor volume was defined based on CT findings in lung and soft tissue windows including all small spiculae. Slow scan cone beam computed tomography was performed to determine the internal target volume (ITV) until October 2014, and 4-dimensional CT was used after that. We added a margin of 4 mm in all directions to the ITV to define the planning target volume (PTV). SBRT treatment planning was conducted with Oncentra Masterplan (Elekta, Stockholm, Sweden). Irradiation was performed as multifield irradiation using a linac accelerator every second day. The prescribed isocenter dose for peripheral located tumors was 18.75 Gy (PTV border covered by the 67% isodose), and the total dose was 56.25 in three fractions. Centrally located tumors usually received an isocenter dose of 7.5 Gy (PTV boarder covered by the 80% isodose), and the total dose was 60.0 Gy. Dosimetric calculation was conducted using a pencil beam algorithm with heterogeneity correction. The constraints for RT planning are described elsewhere [5, 11]. In some patients, the dose was individually adjusted to the dose exposure of organs at risk. The detailed patient characteristics are summarized in Table 2.

Follow-up

Follow-up visits were performed every 3 months and included CT of the chest and abdomen. ^{18}F-fluorodeoxyglucose positron emission tomography (FDG-PET) was performed when CT was suspicious for relapse. The date of relapse was determined as the date when FDG-PET was assessed as positive for local and/or distant relapse by experienced nuclear physicians or when biopsy proved relapse in medically fit patients. Overall survival (OS) was defined as the period from the last day of SBRT to the date of death from any cause. Lung cancer death was defined as death resulting from the progression of lung cancer (local and/or distant), and non-lung cancer death was defined as death of any other cause due to comorbidities. Locoregional relapse was defined as any relapse within the lung or mediastinum, and distant metastases were defined as lung cancer lesions outside the lung and mediastinum.

Toxicity

Toxicity was assessed weekly during SBRT by anamnesis and physical examination. Acute toxicity was defined from the start of SBRT up to 90 days after the last day of irradiation and was graded according to the Common Toxicity for Criteria Adverse Events (CTCAE V 4.0) [12]. Late toxicity was defined as symptoms > 90 days

Table 2 Patient characteristics

	n = 196 (%); median	range
Sex		
female	73 (37.1)	
male	123 (62.9)	
Medically inoperable	182 (92.8)	
Medically operable	14 (7.2)	
Localization		
-central	83 (42.3)	
-peripheral	113 (57.7)	
Side		
-left	86 (43.9)	
-right	110 (56.1)	
Grading (G)		
G1	7 (3.6)	
G2	74 (37.8)	
G3	42 (21.4)	
Stage according to UICC (7th edition)		
-I	113 (57.7)	
-II	68 (34.6)	
-IIIa	15 (7.7)	
Histology		
-Adenocarcinoma	49 (39.9)	
-Squamous cell carcinoma	71 (57.7)	
-Large cell carcinoma	3 (2.4)	
-No biopsy due to comorbidities	73 (37.2)	
Age	67	29–86
0–50	6 (3.1)	
50–65	63 (32.1)	
66–80	101 (51.5)	
> 80	26 (13.3)	
aCCI	7	3–16
0–3	4 (2.0)	
4–6	63 (32.1)	
7–9	62 (31.6)	
10–12	44 (22.4)	
> 12	23 (11.9)	
Hypertension	119 (60.7)	
Diabetes with or without end-organ damage	52 (26.6)	
Moderate/severe renal damage	63 (32.1)	
COPD	167 (85.2)	
-Gold 1 + 2	51 (26.0)	
-Gold 3	61 (31.1)	
-Gold 4	55 (28.1)	
Peripheral vascular disease	49 (25)	

Table 2 Patient characteristics (Continued)

	n = 196 (%); median	range
Myocardial infarction	31 (15.8)	
Congestive heart failure	71 (36.2)	
Cerebral vascular disease	13 (6.6)	
Mild liver disease	9 (4.5)	
Isocenter Dose		
-peripheral tumor	18.75	18–20
-central tumor	7.5	7–9
Packyears	40	0–120

after the last fraction of SBRT and was classified according to the Late Effects on Normal Tissue-Subjective, Objective, Management scales (LENT-SOMA) [13].

Statistics

The outcomes were statistically assessed using Kaplan Meier analysis with log-rank test and Cox regression analysis.

Toxicity was statistically assessed with univariate analyses using the Chi-squared-test for non-parametric parameters and Student's t-test for parametric parameters. Multivariate logistic regression analysis included all significant parameter from the univariate analysis using backwards elimination to determine the parameters that contributed the most to toxicity. The factors evaluated were age, sex, histology, grading, side, localization, TNM stage, packyears, aCCI and all single items of the aCCI. Statistical analysis was performed with a commercially available software package (SPSS V.24, IBM, Armonk, NY, USA).

Results
Outcome

The median overall survival was 15.0 (3.0–64.0) months for all patients and the median follow-up was 24.0 months (6–64.0) for patients who were alive (66.8% [131/196]. Concerning all patients, 31.6% (62/196) were deceased and 1.6% (3/196) were lost to follow-up. Seventeen point 3 % (34/196) of patients died due to lung cancer, 6.1% (12/196) due to locoregional failure and 11.2% (22/196) due to distant extrapulmonary metastases. Furthermore, 14.3% (28/196) of patients died due to comorbidities. The detailed results are shown in Table 3.

The median OS was 15.0 months (95% CI [11.9–18.1], Fig. 1a), whereas the median cancer-specific survival (CSS) was not reached (Fig. 1b). In addition, 45.2% (28/62) of the deceased patients died from competing comorbidities and 54.8% (34/62) from lung cancer. Neither OS (Fig. 2a) nor CCS (Fig. 2b) was significantly worse for central tumors compared with peripheral tumors (HR 1.05, 95% CI [0.64–1.70], p = 0.85; HR 1.40, 95% CI [0.73–2.70],

Table 3 Descriptive outcome analysis

Status	n	%
Alive	131	66.8
Deceased	62	31.6
Unknown	3	1.6
Death from lung cancer	34	17.3
Locoregional failure	12	6.2
Distant progression	22	11.2
Death from comorbidities	28	14.3
cardiovascular	8	4.1
lung	6	3.1
infection	4	2.0
stroke	3	1.5
other	7	3.6

$p = 0.31$). Considering the survival of the presented patient cohort divided by the median aCCI of 7, aCCI ≥ 7 compared with a aCCI of ≤ 6 was found to be significantly associated with an increased hazard for death (HR 1.79, 95%CI [1.02–2.80], $p = 0.04$) and cancer-specific death (HR 9.26, 95% CI [4.83–24.39], $p < 0.001$), respectively. The corresponding Kaplan Meier curves of the OS and CCS are shown in Fig. 3. Neither OS nor CCS was significantly associated with age, sex, side (left vs. right), lobe, localization (central vs. peripheral), packyears, TNM, or any item of the aCCI. Considering the 14.3% (28/196) of deceased patients who died due to comorbidities, aCCI ≥ 9 was significantly associated with non-cancer-related death (HR 3.12, 95% CI [1.22–8.33], $p = 0.02$).

Toxicity

Due to the low number of events, the frequencies of acute and late toxicity were assessed cumulatively. We observed no fatal toxicity related to SBRT.

Radiation pneumonitis (RP) of grade 1 occurred in 34.7% (68/196), of grade 2 in 11.2% (22/196), of grade 3 in 1.0% (2/196), of grade 4 in 0.5% (1/196) and of grade 5 in 0% (0/196) of patients, respectively. This resulted in a cumulative RP ≥ 2 rate of 12.7% (25/196). Univariate analysis revealed that tumors located on the right lung side ($p = 0.01$) were associated with clinically relevant RP $\geq$ grade 2. Age, sex, lobe, localization (central vs. peripheral), packyears, TNM, aCCI nor any item of the aCCI were statistically associated with RP $\geq$ grade 2.

In total, 7.7% (15/196) of patients developed a radiation esophagitis (RE) grade ≥ 2. No patients (0/113) with peripheral tumors developed an RE grade ≥ 2, whereas 16.9% (14/83) of the patients with central tumors developed acute RE grade 2, and 1.2% (1/83) acute RE grade 3, respectively. No late RE $\geq$ grade 1 was observed. Univariate statistical analysis revealed no significant parameters associated with RE. Furthermore, in 2.1% (4/196), a mild chest wall toxicity (CWT) grade 1 with no need for narcotics was observed. No CWT $\geq$ grade 2 was observed. In addition, none of the assessed toxicities (RP, RE, CWT) were associated with items of the aCCI.

Discussion

To our best knowledge, the presented study represents the largest early-stage lung cancer population treated with SBRT to quantify the impact of baseline co-morbidities on the clinical outcome.

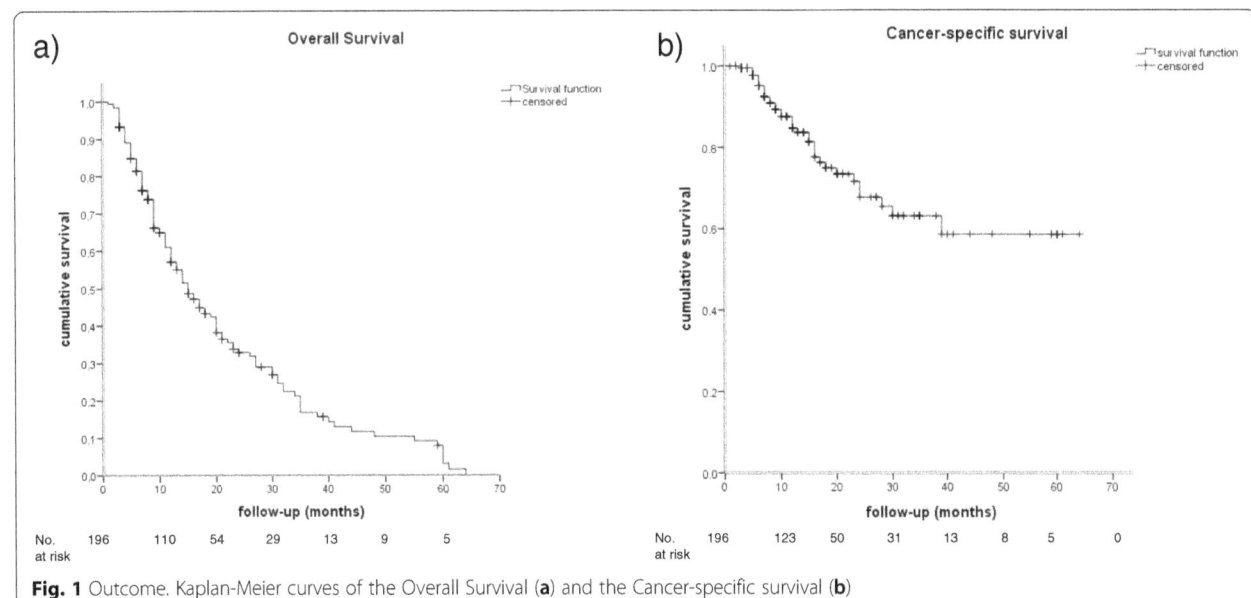

Fig. 1 Outcome. Kaplan-Meier curves of the Overall Survival (**a**) and the Cancer-specific survival (**b**)

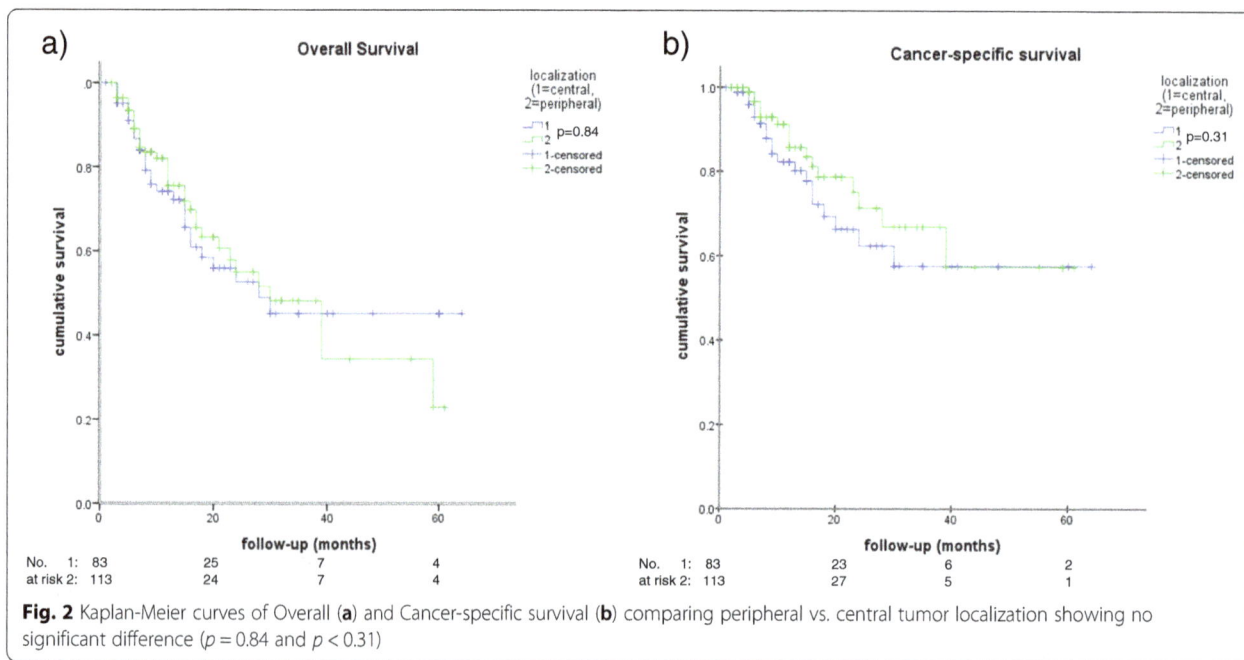

Fig. 2 Kaplan-Meier curves of Overall (**a**) and Cancer-specific survival (**b**) comparing peripheral vs. central tumor localization showing no significant difference ($p = 0.84$ and $p < 0.31$)

The observed median overall survival of 15.0 months was low, although this rate is consistent with other studies [14–16]. Convincing data suggest that poor survival–despite high local control rates–is attributed to advanced age and competing comorbidities because subgroup analysis revealed that medically operable patients treated with SBRT had a much higher survival than medically inoperable patients treated with SBRT [17–20], which was recently confirmed in a prospective single-arm phase 2 study conducted by the NRG Oncology Radiation Therapy Oncology Group [21]. Although a large randomized trial comparing surgery with SBRT for medically operable early stage NSCLC does not exist; SBRT is a good alternative to surgery [17–21] with lower direct medical costs and better quality-adjusted life expectancies [22]. Furthermore, Eguchi et al. showed in a competing risks analysis of curative-intent resection of stage I lung cancer that high age was a significant parameter for worse short-term outcome and 1-point increase of the CCI (not age-adjusted) decreased the overall survival by 14% [23].

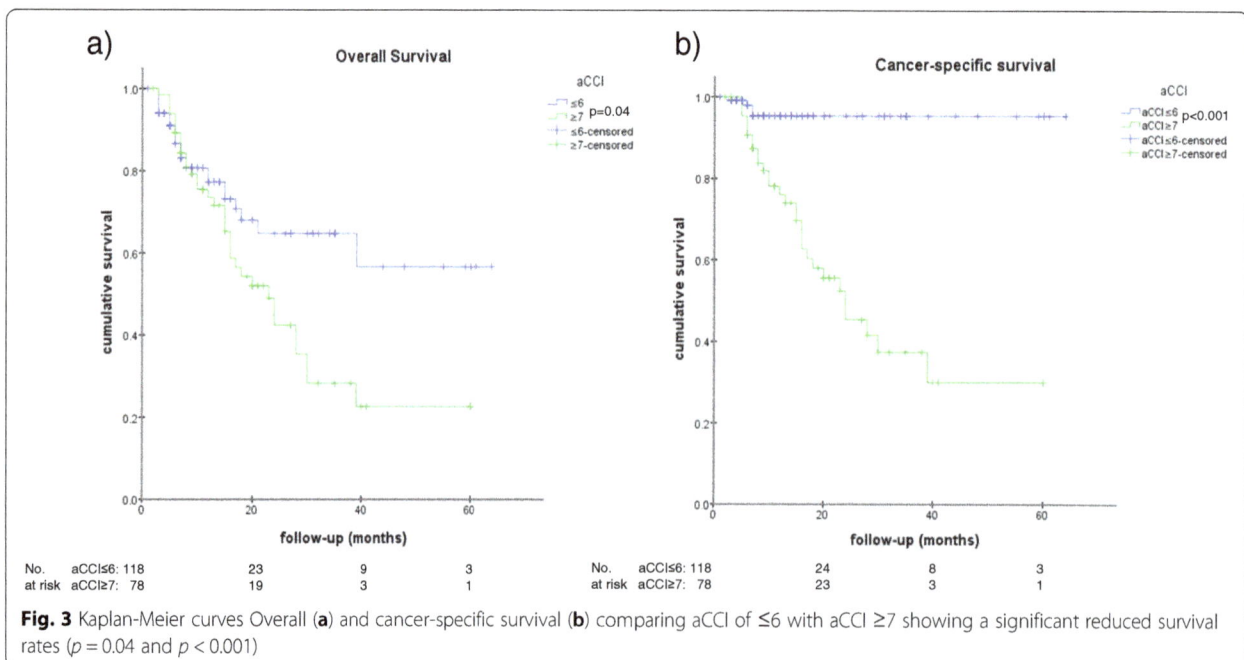

Fig. 3 Kaplan-Meier curves Overall (**a**) and cancer-specific survival (**b**) comparing aCCI of ≤6 with aCCI ≥7 showing a significant reduced survival rates ($p = 0.04$ and $p < 0.001$)

Therefore, it is lucid to assume that reported data from lung cancer patients treated with SBRT are biased by not precisely recorded high age, number and severity of comorbidities and not by the technique of SBRT itself, which may compromise survival. Therefore, the age-adjusted Charlson Comorbidity Index (aCCI) was used in this study to assess the prognostic significance of age and co-morbidity. The improved survival of early-stage NSCLC –particularly in medically unfit patients- is related to the widespread adoption of SBRT to the clinical routine [24–27]. A direct comparison of the survival between lobectomy and SBRT is limited by the inherent unmeasured biases of databases warranting dedicated prospective trials [24, 25].

The results of our analysis provide some reassurance that it is indeed advanced age coupled with competing baseline comorbidity rather than overlooked treatment-related mortality that is largely responsible for the low observed OS and CSS rates post-SBRT. Patients with aCCI ≥7 had a significantly increased hazard for death and cancer-specific death compared with patients with an aCCI ≤6. The median aCCI was 7, suggesting usually three other competing comorbidities for a patient cohort with a median age of 70. This is considerably higher than in other reports [14, 28, 29], although some studies do not use the age-adjusted CCI [14, 29]. Nevertheless, in our analysis neither age nor any of the single comorbidities of the aCCI were significantly associated with outcome suggesting that an age-adjusted comorbidity index, such as the aCCI, should be used instead of an index that does not adjust for age because age is generally associated with poor survival after SBRT for lung cancer [30]. The CCI in general does not graduate severity of comorbidities in a precise way, and Extermann et al. were cautious about the CCI due to its tendency to underrate the functional status of older cancer patients [31]. In the particular case of SBRT, lung cancer patients are often not eligible for surgery due to chronic obstructive pulmonary disease (COPD) Gold III or Gold IV, which is the major reason for allocating to SBRT. The aCCI distinguishes chronic pulmonary disease as yes or no but does not take into account that patients with severe COPD Gold III or IV have a substantially reduced life expectancy, even without lung cancer [32, 33]. The severity of COPD classified according to the Gold criteria was not assessed, although that might have been a confounder that influenced survival analysis using aCCI. An alternative score is the Cumulative Illness Rating Scale for Geriatrics (CIRS-G), which allows a subjective grading of severity of comorbidities in elderly patients [34, 35], but the CIRS-G has never been used in a large patient cohort with mainly medically inoperable lung cancer patients treated with SBRT [20]. The CIRS-G is much more complex, more labor-intensive and less user-friendly than the aCCI because the user of the CIRS-G needs complex multidisciplinary knowledge, and sometimes the CIRS-G even requires further medical consultation [20, 34, 35]. Therefore, the aCCI is a more applicable and faster scoring system than the CIRS-G.

RP is considered to be the most important toxicity with rates of RP ≥2 ranging from 9 to 28% [36]. We observed no abnormally increased rate of clinically relevant RP ≥2 of 12.7% in the presented patient collective with mainly multimorbid patients. Several risk factors, such as age, sex, severity of COPD, baseline lung function and smoking status, have been reported with controversial results [22, 37–39]. Statistical analyses showed that tumor location on the right lung was associated with RP ≥2, which was also observed by Chaudari et al. [37]. Basically, it can be assumed that the small patient cohorts and the low incidence of RP have introduced bias into the statistical results, and thus, the results of statistical analyses have to be interpreted with caution. Therefore, we cannot rule out that the statistical association with RP ≥2 and tumor on the right lung side might be a random result.

Some limitations of this study should be acknowledged. First, its retrospective character has inherent limitations and might have introduced a selection bias. Second, this study included a selected cohort with mainly medically inoperable patients. Therefore, caution should be applied when transferring the observed results to medically fit and operable patients. Third, the aCCI certainly does not include all outcome relevant comorbidities and does not grade comorbidities according to their severity in a precise way. Additionally, the aCCI was not developed specifically for carcinoma patients, but is a more general tool to estimate the prognosis of patients. Fourth, this study is based on clinical parameters, although dosimetric parameters also have impact on outcome and side effects [5, 22, 40, 41]. Fifth, the follow-up period of 24 months for patients who were alive and the number of deceased patients (cancer related and non-cancer related death) might be insufficient to make definitive statements about long-term cancer survival and survival of comorbidities. Therefore we cannot predict long-term outcome and claim that we successfully assessed age and numerous comorbidities in general. Ideally, there would be a validation cohort for this purpose.

Nevertheless, the observed results are robust and the aCCI was a simple tool for estimation of prognosis in medically unfit patients.

Conclusion

The results of the present study indicate that SBRT for early stage lung cancer is a well-tolerated treatment modality that offers long-term tumor control. The advanced age and numerous comorbidities characterizing this patient population were successfully assessed with the aCCI in terms of survival. Therefore, we recommend that age and comorbidity should be indexed using the aCCI as a simple score for all patients treated with SBRT for lung cancer.

Abbreviations

aCCI: Age-adjusted Charlson Comorbidity Index; CIRS-G: Cumulative Illness Rating Scale for Geriatrics; COPD: Chronic obstructive pulmonary disease; CSS: Cancer-specific survival; CT: Computed tomography; CTCAE: Common Toxicity for Criteria Adverse Events; CWT: Chest wall toxicity; FDG: ^{18}F-fluorodeoxyglucose; G: Grading; Gy: Gray; ITV: Internal target volume; LENT-SOMA: Late Effects on Normal Tissue-subjective, objective, management scales; NSCLC: Non-small cell lung cancer; OS: Overall survival; PET: Positron emission tomography; PTV: Planning target volume; RE: Radiation esophagitis; RP: Radiation pneumonitis; SBRT: Stereotactic body radiotherapy

Acknowledgements

We thank Mr. Bernhard Vaske for his statistical support.

Funding

Not applicable.

Authors' contributions

DJ and HC performed the data acquisition, statistical analyses and wrote the manuscript. BM revised the manuscript. All authors read and approved the final manuscript.

Competing interest

The authors declare that they have no competing interests.

References

1. Crino L, Weder W, van Meerbeck J, Felip E. ESMO guidelines working group. Early stage and locally advanced (non-metastatic) non-small-cell lung cancer: ESMO clinical practice Guidleines for diagnosis, treatment and follow-up. Ann Oncol. 2010;21(Suppl 5):v103–15.
2. Raz DJ, Zell Ja OSH, Gandara SR, Anton-Culver H, Jablons DM. Natural history of stage I non-small cell lung cancer: implications for early detection. Chest. 2007;132:193–9.
3. Timmerman RD, Park C, Kavanagh BD. The north American experience with stereotactic body radiation therapy in non-small cell lung cancer. J Thorac Oncol. 2007;2:101–12.
4. Chang JY, Senan S, Paul MA, Mehran RJ, Louie AV, Balter P, et al. Stereotactic ablative radiotherapy versus lobectomy for operable stage I non-small-cell lung cancer: a pooled analysis of two randomized trials. Lancet Oncol. 2015;16:630–7.
5. Guckenberger M, Andratschke N, Alheit H, Holy R, Nestle U, Sauer O. Definition of stereotactic body radiotherapy: principles and practice for the treatment of stage I non-small cell lung cancer. Strahlenther Onkol. 2014; 190:26–33.
6. Khakwani A, Al R, Powell HA, Tata LJ, Stanley RA, Baldwin DR, et al. Lung cancer survival in England: trends in non-small-cell lung cancer survival over the duration of the National Lung Cancer Audit. Br J Cancer. 2013;109:2058–65.
7. Crabtree TD, Denlinger CE, Meyers BF, El Naqa I, Zoole J, Krupnick AS, et al. Stereotactic body radiation therapy versus surgical resection for stage I non-small cell lung cancer. J Thorac Cardiovasc Surg. 2010;140:377–86.
8. Palma D, Senan S. Improving outcomes for high-risk patients with early-stage non-small-cell lung cancer. Insight from population-based data and the role of stereotactic ablative radiotherapy. Clin Lung Cancer. 2013;14:1–5.
9. Palma DA, Visser O, Lagerwaard FJ, Belderbos J, Slotman B, Senan S. Treatment of stage I NSCLC in elderly patients: a population-based matched-pair comparison of stereotactic radiotherapy versus surgery. Radiother Oncol. 2011;101:240–4.
10. Charlson ME, Szwatrowski TP, Peterson J, Gold J. Validation of a combined index. J Clin Epidemiol. 1994;47:1245–51.
11. Benedict SH, Yenice KM, Followill D, Galvin JM, Hinson W, Kavangh B, et al. Stereotactic body radiation therapy: the report of AAPM task group 101. Med Phys. 2010;37:4078–101.
12. National Cancer Institute. Common Terminology Criteria for Adverse Events v4.0 https://evs.nci.nih.gov/ftp1/CTCAE/CTCAE_4.03/Archive/CTCAE_4.0_2009-05-29_QuickReference_8.5x11.pdf. Accessed 22 Apr 2018.
13. LENT SOMA scales for all anatomic sites. Int J Radiat Oncol Biol Phys. 1995; 31:1049–92.
14. Mohkles S, Nuyttens JJ, Maat AP, Birim Ö, Aerts JG, Bogers AJ, et al. Survival and treatment of non-small cell lung cancer stage I-II treated surgically or with stereotactic body radiotherapy: patient and tumor-specific factors affect the prognosis. Ann Surg Oncol. 2015;22:316–23.
15. Nyman J, Johansson KA, Hulten U. Stereotactic hypofractionated radiotherapy for stage I non-small cell lung cancer – mature results for medically inoperable patients. Lung Cancer. 2006;51:97–103.
16. Wulf J, Haedinger U, Oppitz U, Thiele W, Mueller G, Flentje M. Stereotactic radiotherapy for primary lung cancer and pulmonary metastases: a noninvasive treatment approach in medically inoperable patients. Int J Radiat Oncol Biol Phys. 2004;60:186–96.
17. Onishi H, Shirato H, Nagata Y, Hiraoka M, Fujino M, Gomi K, et al. Hypofractionated stereotactic radiotherapy (HypoFXSRT) for stage I non-small cell lung cancer: updated results of 257 patients in a Japanese multi-institutional study. J Thorac Oncol. 2007;2:94–100.
18. Uematsu M, Shioda A, Suda A, Fukui T, Ozeki Y, Hama Y, et al. Computed tomography-guided frameless stereotactic radiotherapy for stage I non-small cell lung cancer: a 5-year experience. Int J Radiat Oncol Biol Phys. 2001;51:666–70.
19. Onishi H, Kuriyama K, Komiyama T, Tanaka S, Sano N, Marino K, et al. Clinical outcomes of stereotactic radiotherapy for stage I non-small cell lung cancer using a novel irradiation technique: patient self-controlled breath-hold and beam switching using a combination of linear accelerator and CT scanner. Lung Cancer. 2004;45:45–55.
20. Firat S, Bousamra M, Gore E, Byhardt RW. Comorbidity and KPS are independent prognostic factors in stage I non-small-cell lung cancer. Int J Radiat Oncol Biol Phys. 2002;52:1047–57.
21. Timmermann RD, Paulus R, Pass HI, Gore EM, Edelman MJ, Galvin J, et al. Stereotactic body radiation therapy for operable early-stage lung Cancer: findings from the NRG oncology RTOG 0618 trial. Jama Oncol. 2018;4:1263–6.
22. Paix A, Noel G, Falcoz PE, Levy P. Cost-effectiveness analysis of stereotactic body radiotherapy and surgery for medically operable early stage non small cell lung cancer. Radiother Oncol. 2018;128:534–40.
23. Eguchi T, Bains S, Lee MC, Tan KS, Hristov B, Buitrago D, et al. Impact of increasing age on cause-specific mortality and morbidity in patients with stage I non-small-cell lung Cancer: a competing risks analysis. J Clin Oncol. 2017;35:281–90.
24. Boyer MJ, Williams CD, Harpole DH, Onaitis MW, Kelley MJ, Salama JK. Improved survival of stage I non-small cell lung Cancer: a VA central registry analysis. J Thorac Oncol. 2017;12:1814–23.
25. Bryant AK, Mundt RC, Sandhu AP, Urbanic JJ, Sharabi AB, Gupta S, et al. Stereotactic body radiation therapy versus surgery for early lung Cancer among US veterans. Ann Thorac Surg. 2018;105:425–31.
26. Hague W, Verma V, Polamraju P, Farach A, Butler EB, The BS. Stereotactic body radiation therapy versus conventionally fractionated radiation therapy for early stage non-small cell lung cancer. Radiother Oncol. 2018; [Epub ahead of print].
27. Von Reibnitz SF, Wu AJ, Trehame GC, Dick-Godfrey R, Foster A, et al. Stereotactic body radiation therapy (SBRT) improves local control and overall survival compared to conventionally fractionated radiation for stage I non-small cell lung cancer (NSCLC). Actac Oncol. 2018; [Epub ahead of print].
28. Kopek N, Paludan M, Petersen J, Hansen A, Grau C, Hoyer M. Co-morbidity index predicts for mortality after stereotactic body radiotherapy for medically inoperable early-stage non-small cell lung cancer. Radiother Oncol. 2009;93:402–7.
29. Baker R, Han G, Sarangkasiri S, DeMarco M, Turke C, Stevens CW, et al. Clinical and Dosimetric predictors of radiation pneumonitis in a large series of patients treated with stereotactic body radiation therapy to the lung. Int J Radiat Oncol Biol Phys. 2013;85:190–5.
30. Zheng X, Schipper M, Kidwell K, Lin J, Reddy R, Ren Y, et al. Survival outcome after stereotactic body radiation therapy and surgery for stage I non-small cell lung cancer: a meta-analysis. Int J Radiat Oncol Biol Phys. 2014;90:603–11.
31. Extermann M, Overcash J, Lyman GH, Parr J, Balducci L. Comorbidity and functional status are independent in older cancer patients. J Clin Oncol. 1998;16:1582–7.

32. Shavelle RM, Paculdo DR, Kush SJ, Dm M, Strauss DJ. Life expectancy and years of life lost in chronic obstructive pulmonary disease: findings from the NHANES III follow-up study. Int J Chron Obstruct Pul Dis. 2009;4:137–48.

33. Suissa S, Dell'Aniello S, Ernst P. Long-term natural history of chronic obstructive pulmonary disease: severe exacerbations and mortality. Thorax. 2012;67:957–63.

34. Kirkhus L, Jordhøy M, Šaltytė Benth J, Rostoft S, Selbaek G, Jensen Hjermstad M, et al. Comparing comorbidity scales: attending physician score versus the cumulative illness rating scale for geriatrics. J Geriatric Oncol. 2016;7:90–8.

35. Grønberg BH, Sundstrøm S, Kaasa S, Bremnes RM, Flotten O, Amundsen T, et al. Influence of comorbidity on survival, toxicity and health-related quality of life in patients with advanced non-small-cell lung cancer receiving platinum-doublet chemotherapy. Eur J Cancer. 2010;46:2225–34.

36. Yamashita H, Takahashi W, Haga A, Nakagawa K. Radiation pneumonitis after stereotactic radiation therapy for lung cancer. World J Radiol. 2014;6:708–15.

37. Chaudhuri AA, Binkley MS, Rigdon J, Carter JN, Aggarwal S, Dudley SA. (2016) pre-treatment non-target lung FDG-PET uptake predicts symptomatic radiation pneumonitis following stereotactic ablative radiotherapy (SABR). Radiother Oncol. 2016;119:454–60.

38. Wang J, Cao J, Ji W, Arenberg D, Dai J, Stanton P, et al. Poor baseline pulmonary function may not increase the risk of radiation-induced lung toxicity. Int J Radiat Oncol Biol Phys. 2013;85:798–804.

39. Takeda A, Kunieda E, Ohashi T, Aoki Y, Oku Y, Enomoto T, et al. Severe COPD is correlated with mild radiation pneumonitis following stereotactic body radiotherapy. Chest. 2012;141:858–66.

40. Schanne DH, Nestle U, Allgäuer M, Andratschke N, Appold S, Dieckmann U, et al. Stereotactic body radiotherapy for centrally located stage I NSCLC: a multicenter analysis. Strahlenther Onkol. 2015;191:125–32.

41. Moustakis C, Blanck O, Ebrahimi Tazehmahalleh F, Ka Heng Chan M, Ernst I, Krieger T, et al. planning benchmark study for SBRT of early stage NSCLC : results of the DEGRO working group stereotactic radiotherapy. Strahlenther Onkol. 2017;193:780–90.

21

Bone density and pain response following intensity-modulated radiotherapy versus three-dimensional conformal radiotherapy for vertebral metastases - secondary results of a randomized trial

Tanja Sprave[1,3], Vivek Verma[2], Robert Förster[1,3,4], Ingmar Schlampp[1,3], Katharina Hees[2,5], Thomas Bruckner[2,5], Tilman Bostel[1], Rami Ateyah El Shafie[1,3], Thomas Welzel[1], Nils Henrik Nicolay[1,3,6], Jürgen Debus[1,3] and Harald Rief[1,3*] [iD]

Abstract

Background: This was a prespecified secondary analysis of a randomized trial that analyzed bone density and pain response following fractionated intensity-modulated radiotherapy (IMRT) versus three-dimensional conformal radiotherapy (3DCRT) for palliative management of spinal metastases.

Methods/materials: Sixty patients were enrolled in the single-institutional randomized exploratory trial, randomly assigned to receive IMRT or 3DCRT (30 Gy in 10 fractions). Along with pain response (measured by the Visual Analog Scale (VAS) and Chow criteria), quantitative bone density was evaluated at baseline, 3, and 6 months in both irradiated and unirradiated spinal bodies, along with rates of pathologic fractures and vertebral compression fractures.

Results: Relative to baseline, bone density increased at 3 and 6 months following IMRT by a median of 24.8% and 33.8%, respectively ($p < 0.01$ and $p = 0.048$). These figures in the 3DCRT cohort were 18.5% and 48.4%, respectively ($p < 0.01$ for both). There were no statistical differences in bone density between IMRT and 3DCRT at 3 ($p = 0.723$) or 6 months ($p = 0.341$). Subgroup analysis of osteolytic and osteoblastic metastases showed no differences between groups; however, mixed metastases showed an increase in bone density over baseline in the IMRT (but not 3DCRT) arm. The 3-month rate of the pathological fractures was 15.0% in the IMRT arm vs. 10.5% in the 3DCRT arm. There were no differences in pathological fractures at 3 ($p = 0.676$) and 6 ($p = 1.000$) months. The IMRT arm showed improved VAS scores at 3 ($p = 0.037$) but not 6 months ($p = 0.430$). Using Chow criteria, pain response was similar at both 3 ($p = 0.395$) and 6 ($p = 0.732$) months.

Conclusions: This the first prospective investigation evaluating the impact of IMRT vs. 3DCRT on bone density. Along with pain response and pathologic fracture rates, significant rises in bone density after 3 and 6 months were similar in both cohorts. Future randomized investigations with larger sample sizes are recommended.

Trial registration: NCT, NCT02832830. Registered 14 July 2016

Keywords: Bone metastases, Spine, Intensity-modulated radiation therapy, Bone density, Palliative radiotherapy

* Correspondence: harald.rief@gmx.at
[1]University Hospital of Heidelberg, Department of Radiation Oncology, Im Neuenheimer Feld 400, 69120 Heidelberg, Germany
[3]Heidelberg Institute of Radiation Oncology (HIRO), Im Neuenheimer Feld 280, 69120 Heidelberg, Germany
Full list of author information is available at the end of the article

Introduction

Spinal metastases, which occur in up to 40% of advanced-stage cancer patients, can be a major source of symptomatic burden and quality of life detriment [1]. These include not only pain and immobility, but also neurological deficits and risk of pathological fractures. Historically, conventionally fractionated three-dimensional conformal radiotherapy (3DCRT) has been the technique of choice to palliate these cases [2, 3]. However, the advancement of technologies such as intensity-modulated radiation therapy (IMRT) allows for safer dose-escalation by means of higher conformality, image guidance, and decreased doses to nearby organs-at-risk (OARs).

Because much of current research on spinal metastases involves stereotactic radiotherapy (achieved in 5 or fewer fractions), fractionated IMRT has remained an understudied option for these cases. Although stereotactic radiotherapy may be accomplished by inverse-planned IMRT, volumetric modulated arc therapy (VMAT), or TomoTherapy techniques, fractionated IMRT (most commonly 30 Gy in 10 fractions as in this study), which can also be performed with any of the aforementioned techniques, has largely been overshadowed to date and thus deserves further study.

There are known serious adverse events associated with spinal irradiation, such as decreases in bone density potentially resulting in vertebral compression fractures (VCFs). There are no randomized data evaluating these parameters in IMRT versus 3DCRT to date. This was a prespecified secondary analysis of a randomized trial, which evaluated bone density and pain response following IMRT versus conventional 3DCRT as part of palliative management of painful spinal metastases.

Materials and methods

Trial design and participants

The randomized trial, registered on clinicaltrials.gov (NCT02832830), was approved by the Heidelberg University Independent Ethics Committee (Nr. S-238/2016). Details of the study design have been published previously [4]. The primary endpoint of this randomized, single-institutional, pilot trial was 3-month RT-induced toxicity following delivery of 30 Gy in 10 fractions of image-guided IMRT versus conventional 3DCRT in patients with previously untreated spinal metastases. All patients had an established indication for RT, including pain and/or neurological deficits. The present study was a prespecified secondary analysis of bone density, as well as pain response and rates of pathologic fracture and VCF.

A block randomization approach (block size of 6) was used to ensure that the two groups were balanced. In addition to the above, inclusion criteria were ages 18–85, a Karnofsky performance score ≥ 50, and ability to provide written informed consent. Exclusion criteria were subjects with significant neurological or psychiatric disorders precluding informed consent, previous RT to the given irradiation site, or multiple myeloma or lymphoma histology. Number or location of metastases were not specific criteria for inclusion or exclusion, nor was the presence of spinal cord compression.

Assessment of endpoints

Per protocol, bone density in irradiated and non-irradiated vertebral bodies, other pathologic vertebral fractures, and VCFs were assessed at baseline and at 3 and 6 months after RT. Bone density was assessed with the Syngo Osteo CT workstation in manually selected regions of interest. Hounsfield units (HU) were used for bone density measurements. The Siemens Somatom Sensation Open (Siemens, Erlangen, Germany) scanner was used for all CT examinations. Measurements were carried out at the appropriate site by a single physician in light of interobserver bias. During the observation period, because most participants received anti-osteoresoptive treatment, changes in bone density in unaffected vertebrae were also measured.

Pathologic fractures were diagnosed by experienced radiologists by means of CT and/or MRI imaging by comparing to baseline imaging tests. New fractures were, by definition, not present on initial imaging, whereas progressive fractures referred to visibly increasing size and/or number of fracture gaps, dislocation of fracture fragments, or increasing sintering of the VCF. A VCF was defined as the reduction of the vertebral body height by more than 20%. Each of these was grouped under the term of "pathologic fractures".

In addition to evaluating neuropathic pain, overall pain response to RT was quantified by the visual analog scale (VAS), measured at the irradiated region prior to, immediately following, and at 3 and 6 months after RT. Pain response was designated as complete response (CR), partial response (PR), pain progression (PP), and intermediate pain (IP) according to the International Bone Consensus response categories by Chow et al. [5]. Complete response (CR) was defined as no pain (VAS = 0) after 3 months and partial response (PR) as an improvement by at least two points after 3 and 6 months. CR referred to VAS = 0 with no concurrent increase in analgesic intake (stable or reducing analgesics in daily oral morphine equivalents). PR was pain reduction of 2 or more without increase in analgesics, or analgesic reduction of at least 25% from baseline without an increase in pain. PP was defined as increase in pain score of ≥2 above baseline with stable oral morphine equivalents, or an increase of 25% or more in the latter with the pain score stable or 1 point above baseline. Any response not covered by the CR, PR or PP definitions was

Table 1 Baseline characteristics of randomly assigned participants

	IMRT group n = 30		3D group n = 30		p-value
	n	%	n	%	
Age (years)					0.219
Mean (SD)	66,1 (10,5)		62,5 (11,8)		
Karnofsky-Perfomance Status					0.283
Mean (SD)	64,9 (9,32)		61,3 (9,7)		
Gender					0.795
Male	17	56,7	16	53,3	
Female	13	43,3	14	46,7	
Weight (kg, SD)	75,8 (14,9)		76,2 (19,4)		0.929
Height (cm, SD)	171,6 (8,8)		172,2 (8,6)		0.790
Body mass index (BMI)					0.960
Mean (SD)	25,7 (4,4)		25,6 (5,7)		
Primary site					
Lung cancer	11	36,7	16	53,3	
ABreast cancer	7	23,3	6	20	
Prostata cancer	6	20	1	3,3	
Other	6	20	7	23,3	
Volume of metastases at baseline					
Mean size (mm^3)	30	1166,6	30		0.191
Localization metastases					0.261
Cervical	4	13,3	5	16,7	
Thoracic	15	50	15	50	
Lumbar	11	36,7	7	23,3	
Sacrum	0	0	3	10	
Number metastases					0.140
1 metastase	17	56,7	10	33,3	
2 metastases	4	13,3	9	30	
3 metastases	9	30	11	36,7	
Distant metastases at baseline					
Viszeral	14	46,7	10	33,3	0.292
Lung	7	23,3	6	20	0.754
Brain	4	13,3	5	16,7	0.718
Tissue	5	16,7	5	16,7	1.000
Hormontherapy	12	40	6	20	0.091
Immuntherapy	4	13,3	5	16,7	0.718
Chemotherapy	14	46,7	20	66,7	0.118
Surgery	18	60	13	43,3	0.196
Neurological deficit at baseline	4	13,3	3	10	0.688
Bisphosphonate at baseline	13	43,3	7	23,3	0.100
Orthopedic corset at baseline	9	30	10	33,3	0.781
Medication at baseline					
Sleeping medication	5	16,7	2	6,7	0.228
Psychiatric medication	9	30	6	20	0.371
Opiate	20	66,7	17	56,7	0.426

Table 1 Baseline characteristics of randomly assigned participants *(Continued)*

	IMRT group *n* = 30		3D group *n* = 30		*p*-value
	n	%	*n*	%	
NSAID	23	76,7	19	63,3	0.260

Explanation: Others: carcinoma of unknown primary (CUP), gastrointestinal stromal tumor (GIST), melanoma, mesothelioma, pancreatic cancer, renal cancer.
Abbreviations: *NSAID* nonsteroidal inflammatory drug

called "stable pain". Responders were defined as having CR or PR, and non-responders as having PP or IP.

Exploratory analysis of overall survival (OS) was performed and defined as the time from initial diagnosis until death or censored at last contact.

Radiotherapy

CT simulation was performed with custom immobilization using Aquaplast® (Aquaplast Corporation, Wyckoff, NJ, USA) head masks for cervical spine cases and Wingstep/Prostep® (Elekta, Stockholm, Sweden) devices for thoracolumbar cases. In addition to OARs (dose constraints for which were per QUANTEC recommendations), the clinical target volume (CTV) was delineated on the planning CT and encompassed the affected vertebral body [6]. The planning target volume (PTV) was an isotropic 1 cm expansion of the CTV and was to be covered by the 90% isodose line. The prescription dose for both cohorts was 30 Gy in 10 fractions.

The IMRT group received image-guided (mega- or kilovoltage cone beam computed tomography) RT by means of step-and-shoot IMRT, VMAT (Elekta Versa HD accelerator), or helical TomoTherapy (Accuray Inc., Madison, WI). The 3DCRT cohort was most commonly delivered

with two or three anteroposterior 6 MV individually-formed beams. Position verification was applied by weekly kilo-voltage CT and before each fraction by comparing orthogonal portal images with digitally reconstructed radiographs from the planning CT.

Statistical analysis

Complete details regarding statistical analysis are presented elsewhere [4]. Owing to the exploratory nature of this study, a complete power calculation was not possible; however, with 30 patients in each group, it was possible to detect a standardized mean-value effect of 0.8 with 80% power at a significance level of 0.05.

All variables were analyzed descriptively by tabulation of the measures of the empirical distributions. According to the scale level of the variables, means (Hodges-Lehmann estimates) and standard deviations or absolute and relative frequencies, respectively, were reported. Additionally, for variables with longitudinal measurements, the time courses of individual patients and summarized by treatment groups. Descriptive *p*-values of the corresponding statistical tests comparing the treatment groups were given. Analysis of covariance (ANOVA) with repeated measurements, with treatment group as a

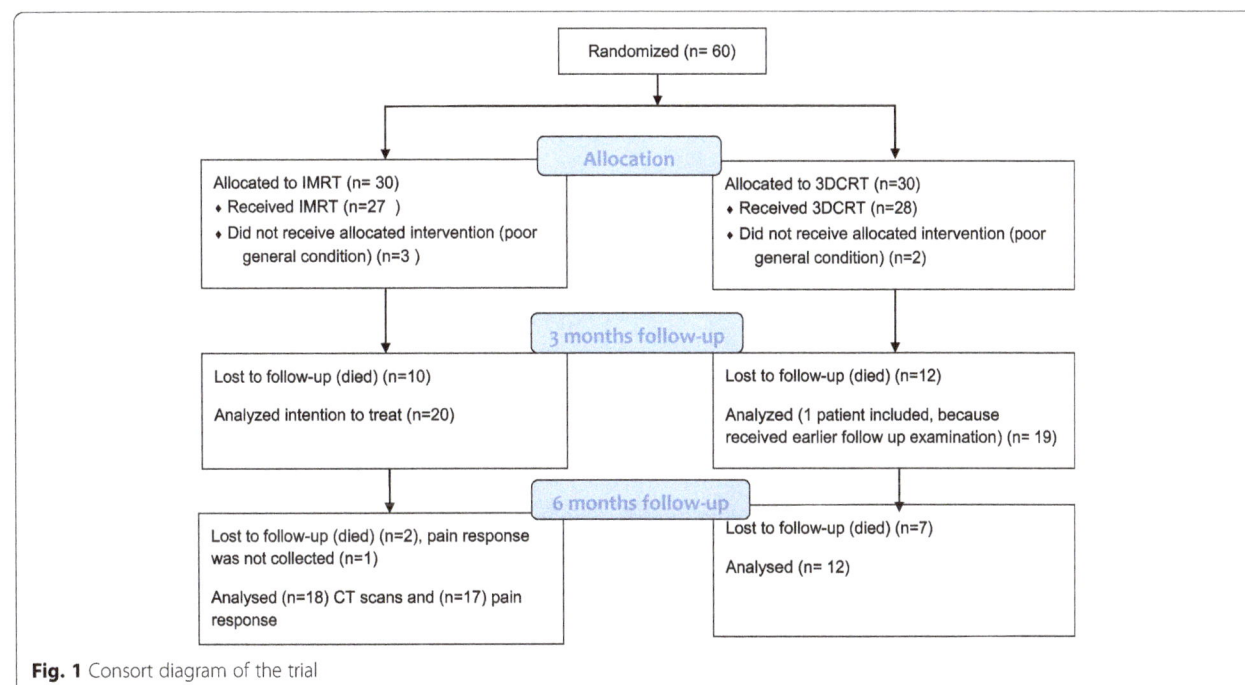

Fig. 1 Consort diagram of the trial

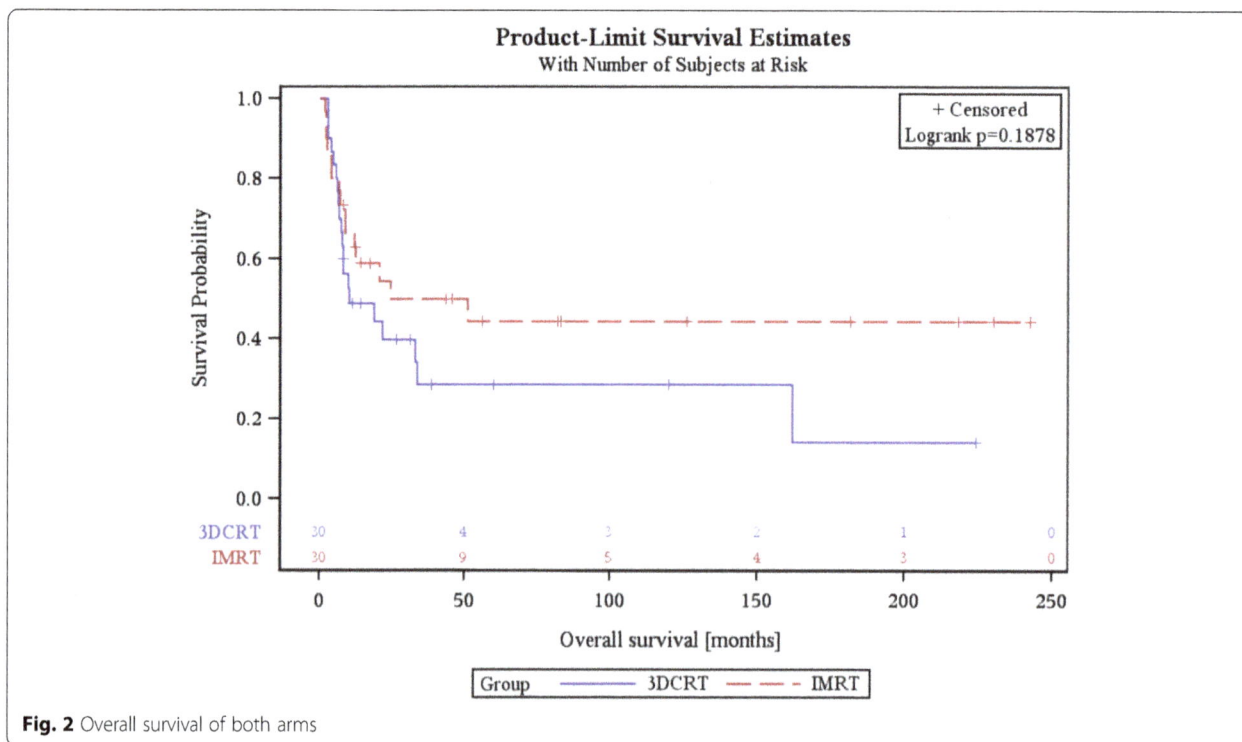

Fig. 2 Overall survival of both arms

factor, and pain medication as covariates, were done. The Wilcoxon rank-sum test was used to detect possible differences between groups after 3 and 6 months. All statistical analyses were done using SAS software Version 9.4 or higher (SAS Institute, Cary, NC, USA).

Funding source

The sponsors of the study had no role in study design, data analysis, data interpretation and wording of the report. The corresponding author (HR) had full access to the entire data of the study and had final responsibility regarding the decision to submit for publication.

Results

From November 2016 to May 2017, 60 patients were randomized. No patients were excluded post randomization. Baseline characteristics were balanced between the two treatment arms (Table 1, as previously reported) [7].

Although all surviving patients completed all assessments, not all patients survived by the three and six month time periods. Within the first 3 months, 10 patients

Table 2 Bone density of both groups in metastatic bone before RT (baseline), as well as 3 and 6 months after RT

	IMRT group			Within group	3DCRT group			Within group	Differences between groups		
	n	Median	SD	p-value	n	Median	SD	p-value	HL	95% CI	p-value
All metastases											
HU Baseline	30	258.5	183.3		30	195.0	125.4		62	5.0–126.0	0.037
HU T2	20	419.3	232.7		19	300.0	165.7		−59.5	−194.0-59.0	0.232
HU T3	18	416.8	277.7		12	454.0	185.4		61.5	− 146.0-229	0.641
3 months											
HU T0-T2	20	90.5	134.2	< 0.01	19	35.0	87.1	< 0.01	−25.0	− 86.0-42.0	0.407
HU T0-T2 (%)	20	24.8	51.0	< 0.01	19	18.5	38.7	< 0.01	−4.5	−25.5-21.9	0.723
6 months											
HU T0-T3	18	124.0	166.0	0.023	12	132.0	157.7	< 0.01	59.0	−73.0-193.0	0.330
HU T0-T3 (%)	18	33.8	61.6	0.048	12	48.4	70.7	< 0.01	34.0	−20.3-91.1	0.341

The results were presented by absolute and relative values (%) of HU within and between groups as median (Hodges–Lehmann estimate) and IQR

Table 3 The subgroup analysis of the bone density (HU = Hounsfield units) in metastatic bone before RT (baseline), as well as 3 and 6 months after RT

	IMRT group			3DCRT group			Differences between groups		
	n	Median	SD	n	Median	SD	HL	95% CI	p-value
Mixed									
HU Baseline	17	242.0	100.1	10	230.5	77.3	−41.5	− 128.0-40.0	0.238
HU T2	11	360.0	153.1	5	418.0	89.4	58.0	− 114-204.0	0.450
HU T3	9	355.0	174.1	4	559.5	132.0	190.5	−61.0-416.0	0.190
3 months									
HU T0-T2	11	102.0	92.2	5	164.0	68.4	59.0	−43.0-174.0	0.213
HU T0-T2 (%)	11	38.8	41.2	5	60.8	48.5	25.7	−32.5-89.5	0.256
6 months									
HU T0-T3	9	176.0	123.1	4	301.0	89.4	161.5	73.0–341.0	0.025
HU T0-T3 (%)	9	55.0	61.1	4	145.9	42.2	80.7	8.7–155.1	0.037
Osteolytic									
HU Baseline	6	178.5	74.3	14	156.5	60.9	20.0	−60.0 − 82.0	0.536
HU T2	4	269.5	198.4	8	181.5	70.8	84.0	-82.0-387.0	0.270
HU T3	4	153.0	127.7	3	295.0	82.8	126.5	− 184.0-277.0	0.377
3 months									
HU T0-T2	4	35.5	171.2	8	16.0	38.0	19.5	−53.0-364.0	0.489
HU T0-T2 (%)	4	20.3	83.11	8	9.3	21.2	12.2	−27.5-178.4	0.489
6 months									
HU T0-T3	4	10.0	95.3	3	64.0	89.1	110.0	−60.0-315.0	0.212
HU T0-T3 (%)	4	−0.8	55.4	3	27.7	55.0	46.9	−61.2-174.2	0.377
Osteoblastic									
HU Baseline	7	419.0	247.6	6	426.0	159.8	−94.5	− 415.0-172.0	0.520
HU T2	5	574.0	327.0	6	481.5	174.4	145.5	− 284.0-604.0	0.411
HU T3	5	700.0	374.8	5	475.0	196.4	255.0	− 367.0-711.0	0.296
3 months									
HU T0-T2	5	52.0	188.3	6	13.0	103.3	45.0	− 311.0-155.0	0.647
HU T0-T2 (%)	5	15.4	35.8	6	3.1	27.5	3.0	−57.0-30.8	1.000
6 months									
HU T0-T3	5	130.0	241.7	5	57.0	102.9	42.0	− 408.0-224.0	0.676
HU T0-T3 (%)	5	15.4	47.2	5	13.6	27.3	1.7	−77.9-53.4	1.000

The results were presented by absolute and relative values (%) of HU within and between groups as median (Hodges–Lehmann estimate) and IQR. Abbreviations: HU Hounsfield units, IQR interquartile range, T0 baseline, T2 3 months, T3 6 months, T0–T2 difference in baseline minus 3 months, T0-T3 difference in baseline minus 6 months

Table 4 Results of pathological fractures of both groups

	IMRT group			3DCRT group			Differences between groups
	n	n/(%)		n	n/(%)		p-value
		No	Yes		No	Yes	
Baseline	30	29 (96.7%)	1 (3.3%)	30	26 (86.7%)	4 (13.3%)	0.161
3 months	20	17 (85.0%)	3 (15%)	19	17 (89.5%)	2 (10.5%)	0.676
6 months	18	15 (83.3%)	3 (16.7%)	12	10 (83.3%)	2 (16.7%)	1.000

Abbreviations: n = alive participants; n/% = total number of pathological fractures in absolute and percentage terms

Table 5 Response according to Brief Pain Inventory score at 3 and 6 months in the per-protocol cohort

	IMRT group n = 20		3DCRT group n = 19		
After 3 months	n	%	n	%	p-value
CR	10	50	5	26,3	0.395
PR	4	20	4	20,1	
PP	1	5	3	15,8	
IP	5	25	7	36,8	
Responders	14	70	9	47,4	0.151
Non-responders	6	30	10	52,6	
	IMRT group n = 17		3DCRT group n = 12		
After 6 months					
CR	7	41,2	3	25	0.732
PR	5	29,4	4	33,3	
PP	2	11,8	3	25	
IP	3	17,7	2	16,7	
Responders	12	70,8	7	58,3	0.494
Non-responders	5	29,4	5	41,7	

Abbreviations: *CR* complete response, *PR* partial response, *PP* pain progression, *IP* intermediate pain

(33.3%) in the IMRT group had died, along with 11 patients (36.7%) in the 3DCRT arm. Between 3 and 6 months, another 2 patients (10%) died from tumor progression in the IMRT cohort, along with a further 7 patients (36.8%) in the 3DCRT arm (Fig. 1). OS did not differ between groups ($p = 0.187$) (Fig. 2). The mean follow-up was 6.3 months (IQR 2.5–9.3) for both groups.

As compared to baseline, bone density became significantly higher at 3 and 6 months following IMRT by a median percentage of 24.8% and 33.8% ($p < 0.01$ for 3 months and $p = 0.048$ for 6 months), respectively (Table 2). These figures in the 3DCRT cohort were 18.5% and 48.4% (p < 0.01 for both), respectively. There were no statistical differences in bone density between IMRT and 3DCRT at 3 ($p = 0.723$) or 6 months ($p = 0.341$).

Subgroup evaluation of solely osteolytic lesions at 3 and 6 months showed no significant differences between groups ($p = 0.489$ and $p = 0.377$ respectively) (Table 3). There were no differences between bone density changes in osteoblastic metastases in the IMRT and 3DCRT groups at 3 or 6 months ($p = 1.000$ for both) (Table 3). Subgroup evaluation of mixed lesions showed a significant difference ($p = 0.037$) at 6 months but not at 3 months ($p = 0.256$) (Table 3).

Bone density in unaffected vertebrae did not show substantial changes within groups at 3 and 6 months following RT (IMRT: $p = 0.623$ and $p = 0.167$, 3DCRT: $p = 0.934$ and $p = 0.147$). There were also no significant differences between the IMRT and 3DCRT arms at 3 ($p = 0.574$) or 6 months ($p = 0.949$).

Preexisting pathological fractures existed in 3.3% patients in the IMRT arm vs. 13.3% in the 3DCRT group ($p = 0.161$) (Table 4). By 3 and 6 months, these numbers rose to 15.0% vs. 10.5% ($p = 0.676$) and 16.7% vs. 16.7% (p = 1.000), respectively. No pathological fractures in either group required salvage surgical intervention.

Pain assessment, using VAS scoring, was similar between cohorts at baseline ($p = 0.882$) and immediately following RT ($p = 0.075$). Although the IMRT arm showed improved pain response at 3 months (p = 0.037), this was not observed at 6 months ($p = 0.430$). There were also no differences in neuropathic pain at 3 ($p = 0.946$) or 6 ($p = 0.661$) months. Using Chow criteria, pain response was statistically similar at both 3 ($p = 0.395$) and 6 ($p = 0.732$) months (Table 5). At 3 months, 70.0% of patients that underwent IMRT were categorized as responders, as compared to 47.4% in the 3DCRT arm ($p = 0.151$); these numbers at 6 months were 70.8% and 58.3%, respectively ($p = 0.494$).

There were no differences in the pattern of recorded OMED consumption between groups at both 3 and 6 months after RT (Fig. 3).

Discussion

This prespecified secondary evaluation of a prospective randomized trial is the first to investigate the impact of image-guided IMRT on bone density as compared to 3DCRT. No differential effects on bone density or other secondary endpoints were expected between IMRT and 3DCRT techniques at the time of study creation. The significant rises in bone density after 3 and 6 months, along with pathologic fracture rates and pain response, were similar in both cohorts.

Despite rightful concerns regarding its cost-effectiveness for palliative vertebral irradiation, IMRT is an attractive option in part owing to the ability to perform simultaneous integrated boosting (SIB). This refers to allowing multiple target volumes to receive different doses per fraction, while maintaining the same total number of fractions. Although no patient in this trial received SIB, this topic will be better understood following maturation of the IRON-2 trial, which consists of four arms: 20 Gy in 5 fractions (with or without SIB to 30 Gy in 5 fractions) and 30 Gy in 10 fractions (with or without SIB to 40 Gy in 10 fractions) [8]. Evaluating bone density in such instances will be essential to evaluate whether higher fractional doses are safe from the bone density standpoint as well.

From these data, it was noteworthy that baseline bone density was higher in the IMRT arm ($p = 0.037$). Although numerically higher at 3 months as well (median 419 versus 300), this did not reach statistical significance ($p = 0.232$), likely owing to the lower sample sizes available at 3 months. Nevertheless, 6 month values were numerically comparable. Moreover, the relative magnitude of bone density change at 3 and 6 months was also

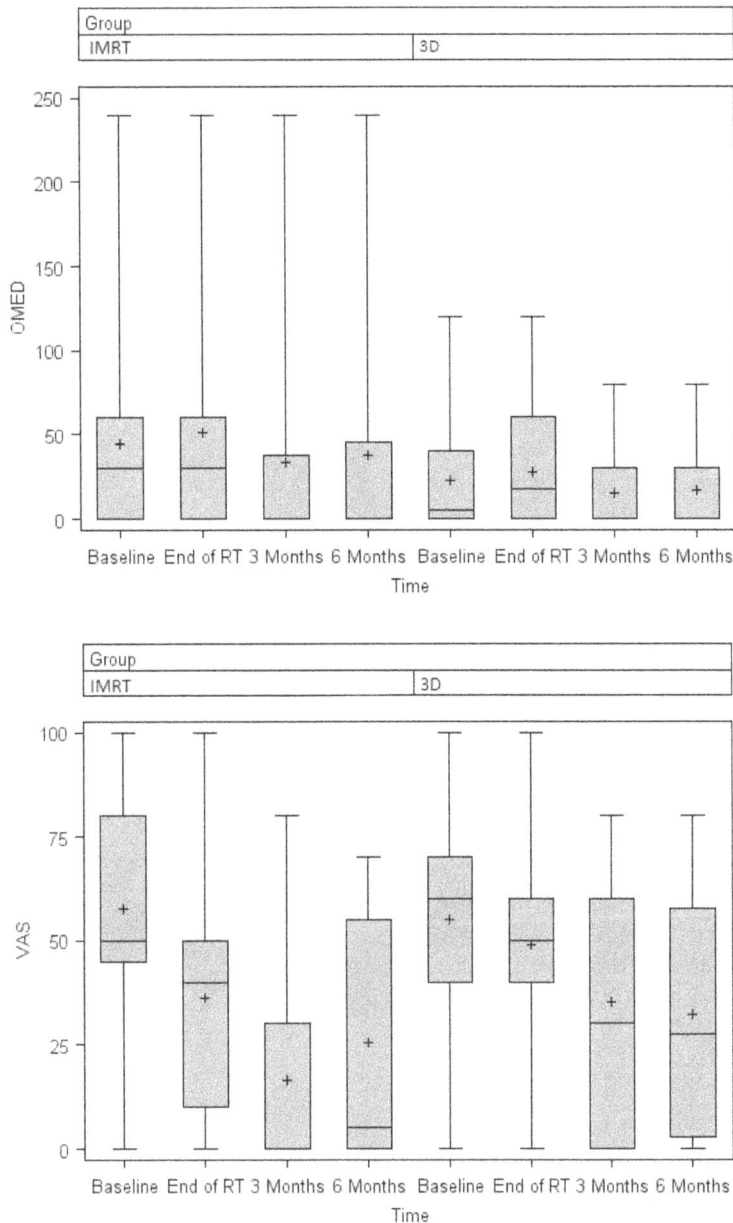

Fig. 3 OMED and VAS of both groups at measured points

numerically and statistically comparable between both groups. This implies that components of bone density changes specifically related to RT are likely similar between both cohorts.

What is less clear are the findings related to mixed osteolytic-osteoblastic lesions at 6 months. The three-month values were not significantly different between cohorts, nor were those for purely osteolytic or osteoblastic metastases. As such, these analyses with clearly small sample sizes may not provide robust conclusions in this subgroup of patients. Additionally, only a few previous studies included mixed or osteoblastic metastases. In

contrast to our results, Eggermont et al. did not observe any bone density changes in mixed proximal femur lesions after 4 and 10 weeks [9]. This could possibly result from an earlier date of collection and lower doses (prescription up to 20 or 24 Gy). In line with these results, less remineralization in the extremities was reported by Rieden and coauthors [10].

Wachenfeld et al. reported an increase in CT density in osteolytic metastases to approximately 150% of the initial value at 3 months after multi-fraction irradiation [11]. Koswig and Budach showed improvement of bone density in osteolytic metastases by 173% at 6 months after multi-fraction irradiation [12]. In this trial, however, the differences were 20.3% and 9.3% in the IMRT and 3DCRT arms, respectively, at 3 months; 6-month values were – 0.8% and 27.7%, respectively. There are several causes of these discrepancies, including the specific patient population, histology, size of metastases and several other factors.

The improved pain response based on VAS in the IMRT group ($p = 0.037$) at 3 months could have been from a greater use of hormonal therapy in metastatic prostate carcinoma. That being said, potential imbalances in anti-osteoresorptive therapies are an unlikely cause of the findings herein, as densities of unaffected vertebrae yielded no differences between groups. Rief et al. studied the impact of resistance training concomitantly with conventional multi-fraction 3DCRT on bone density in a randomized controlled study and found no significant differences in the uninvolved spine [13]. Therefore, it has been suggested that bisphosphonates may not exert decisive effects in this circumstance.

Despite the randomized design and standardized evaluation of bone density and recording of all pathological structures, several limitations must be noted. In addition to the lower sample size and shorter follow-up, robust conclusions based on statistical comparisons cannot be made, as partially discussed above. Second, a possible methodological weakness in our study was the lack of a control group. Third, many patients did not receive concurrent radiotherapy and chemotherapy, so the relationship of systemic therapy on bone density changes cannot be entirely excluded [14–18]. Fourth, some participants received immunotherapy and prior or subsequent radiotherapy to other distant metastases. The abscopal effect in this setting has been sporadically described but not sufficiently clarified [19, 20], but our study did not investigate this causality. Fifth, few studies can entirely account for other factors influencing bone density such as diet, particular medications, or vitamin supplementation. There may also be heterogeneity in this population given the specific location of vertebral metastases (e.g. vertebral body versus lamina/pedicle) as well as degree of soft tissue extension. Although these may limit applicability to other studies, larger randomized data are recommended to validate these results.

Conclusions

This prespecified secondary evaluation of a prospective randomized trial is the first to investigate the impact of image-guided IMRT on bone density as compared to 3DCRT. The significant rises in bone density after 3 and 6 months, along with pain response and pathologic fracture rates, were similar in both cohorts. Future randomized investigations with larger sample sizes are recommended.

Abbreviations
CR: Complete response; CT: Computed tomography; CTV: Clinical target volume; 3DCRT: conventional 3D conformal radiotherapy; EBRT: external body radiotherapy; Gy: Gray; HU: Hounsfield unit; IMRT: Intensity-modulated radiotherapy; kV: kilo-voltage; MV: Megavoltage; SIB: simultaneous integrated boost; OAR: Organ at risk; OMED: oral equivalent morphine dose; OS: Overall survival; PP: Progression pain; PR: Partial response; PTV: Planning target volume; QoL: Quality of life; RT: Radiotherapy; SBRT: Stereotactic body radiation therapy; IP: Intermediate pain; SRS: Stereotactic radiosurgery; VAS: Visual analog scale; VCF: Vertebral compression fracture; VMAT: Volumetric modulated arc therapy

Acknowledgements
We thank the German Bone Cancer Research Group Members for their great effort.

Funding
Not applicable.

Authors' contributions
HR and JD developed and planned this trial. TB was responsible for statistical considerations. TS, VV, RF, IS, NHN, TB, RES and HR performed the examinations and RT supervisions. TW (radiologist) planned the diagnostic examination of computed tomography. HR and TS made the data collection. All authors read and approved the final manuscript.

Competing interests
The authors declare that they have no competing interests.

Author details
[1]University Hospital of Heidelberg, Department of Radiation Oncology, Im Neuenheimer Feld 400, 69120 Heidelberg, Germany. [2]Department of Radiation Oncology, Allegheny General Hospital, Pittsburgh, PA, USA. [3]Heidelberg Institute of Radiation Oncology (HIRO), Im Neuenheimer Feld 280, 69120 Heidelberg, Germany. [4]University Hospital Zurich, Department of Radiation Oncology, Raemistrasse 100, 8091 Zurich, Switzerland. [5]University Hospital of Heidelberg, Department of Medical Biometry, Im Neuenheimer Feld 305, 69120 Heidelberg, Germany. [6]University Hospital of Freiburg, Department of Radiation Oncology, Robert-Koch-Strasse 3, 79106 Freiburg, Germany.

References
1. Wong DA, Fornasier VL, MacNab I. Spinal metastases: the obvious, the occult, and the impostors. Spine. 1990;15(1):1–4.
2. Sze WM, Shelley M, Held I, Mason M. Palliation of metastatic bone pain: single fraction versus multifraction radiotherapy - a systematic review of the randomised trials. Cochrane Database Syst Rev. 2004;2:CD004721.
3. McQuay HJ, Collins SL, Carroll D, Moore RA. Radiotherapy for the palliation of painful bone metastases. Cochrane Database Syst Rev. 2000;2:Cd001793.
4. Meyerhof E, Sprave T, Welte SE, Nicolay NH, Forster R, Bostel T, Bruckner T, Schlampp I, Debus J, Rief H. Radiation-induced toxicity after image-guided and intensity-modulated radiotherapy versus external beam radiotherapy for patients with spinal bone metastases (IRON-1): a study protocol for a randomized controlled pilot trial. Trials. 2017;18(1):98.
5. Chow E, Wu JS, Hoskin P, Coia LR, Bentzen SM, Blitzer PH. International consensus on palliative radiotherapy endpoints for future clinical trials in bone metastases. Radiother Oncol. 2002;64(3):275–80.
6. Marks LB, Yorke ED, Jackson A, Ten Haken RK, Constine LS, Eisbruch A, Bentzen SM, Nam J, Deasy JO. Use of normal tissue complication probability models in the clinic. Int J Radiat Oncol Biol Phys. 2010;76(3 Suppl):S10–9.
7. Sprave T, Verma V, Forster R, Schlampp I, Bruckner T, Bostel T, Welte SE,

Tonndorf-Martini E, El Shafie R, Nicolay NH, et al. Radiation-induced acute toxicities after image-guided intensity-modulated radiotherapy versus three-dimensional conformal radiotherapy for patients with spinal metastases (IRON-1 trial) : First results of a randomized controlled trial. Strahlentherapie und Onkologie. 2018. https://doi.org/10.1007/s00066-018-1333-z Epub ahead of print.

8. Sprave T, Welte SE, Bruckner T, Forster R, Bostel T, Schlampp I, Nicolay NH, Debus J, Rief H. Intensity-modulated radiotherapy with integrated-boost in patients with bone metastasis of the spine: study protocol for a randomized controlled trial. Trials. 2018;19(1):59.

9. Eggermont F, Derikx LC, Verdonschot N, Hannink G, Kaatee R, Tanck E, van der Linden YM. Limited short-term effect of palliative radiation therapy on quantitative computed tomography-derived bone mineral density in femora with metastases. Advances in radiation oncology. 2017;2(1):53–61.

10. Rieden K, Adolph J, Lellig U, Zum Winkel K. The radiotherapeutic effect on bone metastases in relation to the frequency of metastases, sites of metastases and histology of the primary tumor. Strahlentherapie und Onkologie. 1989;165(5):380–5.

11. Wachenfeld I, Sanner G, Bottcher HD, Kollath J. The remineralization of the vertebral metastases of breast carcinoma after radiotherapy. Strahlentherapie und Onkologie. 1996;172(6):332–41.

12. Koswig S, Budach V. Remineralization and pain relief in bone metastases after after different radiotherapy fractions (10 times 3 Gy vs. 1 time 8 Gy). A prospective study. Strahlenther Onkol. 1999;175(10):500–8.

13. Rief H, Omlor G, Akbar M, Welzel T, Bruckner T, Rieken S, Haefner MF, Schlampp I, Gioules A, Habermehl D, et al. Feasibility of isometric spinal muscle training in patients with bone metastases under radiation therapy - first results of a randomized pilot trial. BMC Cancer. 2014;14:67.

14. Strang P, Bergqvist J. Does palliative chemotherapy provide a palliative effect on symptoms in late palliative stages? An interview study with oncologists. Acta oncologica. 2017;56(10):1258–64.

15. Daimon T, Kosaka T, Oya M. A metastatic castration resistant prostate cancer patient with multiple bone metastases has durable biochemical and radiological response to docetaxel chemotherapy. American journal of clinical and experimental urology. 2016;4(2):28–31.

16. Nieder C, Haukland E, Mannsaker B, Norum J. Impact of intense systemic therapy and improved survival on the use of palliative radiotherapy in patients with bone metastases from prostate cancer. Oncol Lett. 2016; 12(4):2930–5.

17. Steinauer K, Huang DJ, Eppenberger-Castori S, Amann E, Guth U. Bone metastases in breast cancer: frequency, metastatic pattern and non-systemic locoregional therapy. Journal of bone oncology. 2014;3(2):54–60.

18. Groenen KH, Pouw MH, Hannink G, Hosman AJ, van der Linden YM, Verdonschot N, Tanck E. The effect of radiotherapy, and radiotherapy combined with bisphosphonates or RANK ligand inhibitors on bone quality in bone metastases. A systematic review. Radiother Oncol. 2016; 119(2):194–201.

19. Leung HW, Wang SY, Jin-Jhih H, Chan AL. Abscopal effect of radiation on bone metastases of breast cancer: a case report. Cancer Biol. Ther. 2018; 19(1):20–4.

20. Brix N, Tiefenthaller A, Anders H, Belka C, Lauber K. Abscopal, immunological effects of radiotherapy: narrowing the gap between clinical and preclinical experiences. Immunol Rev. 2017;280(1):249–79.

22

Urinary function and quality of life after radiotherapy for prostate cancer in patients with prior history of surgical treatment for benign prostatic hyperplasia

Mélanie Guilhen, Christophe Hennequin, Idir Ouzaid, Ingrid Fumagalli, Valentine Martin, Sophie Guillerm, Pierre Mongiat-Artus, Vincent Ravery, François Desgrandchamps and Laurent Quéro*ⓘ

Abstract

Background: To evaluate long-term IPSS score and urinary quality of life after radiotherapy for prostate cancer, in patients with prior history of surgical treatment for benign prostatic hyperplasia (BPH).

Methods: In this retrospective study, we reviewed medical records of patients treated in our department, between 2007 and 2013 with surgery for BPH followed by radiotherapy for localized prostate cancer. Patients were contacted to fill in IPSS questionnaire and they were also asked for urinary quality of life. Predictive factors known to be associated with bad urinary function were also analysed.

Results: Fifty-nine patients were included in our study. Median age was 70 years. Median follow-up was 4.6 years. Median radiotherapy dose was 78 Gy (5×2 Gy/week). Thirty patients (48.5%) received hormone therapy in combination with RT. Main surgery indications were urinary symptoms (65%) and urinary retention (20%). Five-year biochemical-disease free survival was 75% and 5-year clinical relapse free survival was 84%. At the time of the study, the IPSS after radiotherapy was as follows: 0–7: 77.6%; 8–19:20.7%; 20–35: 1.7%. Urinary quality of life was satisfactory for 74.2% of patients. After multivariate analysis, a high dose of RT and a medical history of hypertension were associated with a poorer quality of urinary life ($p = 0.04$).

Conclusion: External radiotherapy remains an appropriate treatment option without a major risk for deterioration in urinary function in patient with antecedent surgery for BPH. High dose of RT and a medical history of hypertension were associated with a poorer quality of urinary life.

Keywords: Radiotherapy, TURP, Prostate, Cancer, IPSS, Toxicity, Quality of life, Hypertension, Dose

Background

External beam radiotherapy (RT) is a well-established treatment for clinically localized prostate cancer. Benign prostatic hyperplasia (BPH) is a very common urological problem in elderly patients, and transurethral resection of the prostate (TURP) is the most common type of surgery for the treatment of BPH. Thus, many patients may have a personal medical history of TURP or significant urinary symptoms at the time of radiotherapy for prostate cancer treatment.

Currently, TURP still represents the gold standard in the operative management of BPH. The major two late complications of TURP are urethral strictures (2.2–9.8%) and bladder neck contractures (0.3–9.2%) [1]. However, it has been reported up to 29% of urethral stricture in patients who had radiotherapy after TURP [2]. Mechanical perturbations of the mucosa leading to scarring remain the most commonly reported causative factor, and fibroblast proliferation suggests that a history of multiple TURPs would be a significant risk factor for higher urinary toxicity after RT.

TURP after radiotherapy is commonly associated with poor urinary function outcome. Liu et al. reported

* Correspondence: laurent.quero@aphp.fr
Radiation Oncology Department, Saint Louis Hospital, 1, avenue Claude Vellefaux, 75010 Paris, France

patients treated by TURP after RT, may have 5 times more long-term urinary incontinence [3]. Several studies observed an increase urinary morbidity incidence in case of previous medical history of TURP before RT but authors did not conclude to a major risk [4, 5].

Urinary quality of life evaluation is not usually reported in studies combining TURP and radiotherapy. In the present study, we report on International prostate symptom score (IPSS) and long-term urinary quality of life of patients treated with high dose 3D RT with prior medical history of TURP.

Methods

Study setting

We retrospectively identified from our medical database patients treated with radiotherapy between November 2008 and February 2013, for non-metastatic prostate cancer. To be included, patients had to have biopsy proven prostate cancer and a prior medical history of TURP or adenectomy within 4 years before the diagnosis of prostate cancer. Patients treated with androgen deprivation therapy (ADT) before RT start could be included but patients with previous history of prostatectomy or prostate brachytherapy were excluded from the study.

Treatment and assessment

The primary endpoint of our study was late urinary function evaluation (> 2 years after RT) using IPSS. The IPSS is based on the answers to 7 questions concerning urinary symptoms (score 0 to 35) Urinary symptoms of patients can be classified as follows: mildly symptomatic (IPSS score = 0–7) moderately symptomatic (IPSS score = 8–19) or severely symptomatic (IPSS score = 20–35). We evaluated the urinary quality of life question using the eighth question of the IPSS (QOL IPSS). QOL IPSS is rated from 0 (Delighted) to 6 (Terrible). Long-term urinary toxicity (urinary tract pain, macroscopic hematuria, urinary incontinence and urinary retention), using Common Terminology Criteria for Adverse Events (CTCAE) version 4.0 grading system [6] was also evaluated. In our study, we analyzed factors correlated with poor late urinary function defined by both an IPSS $\geq$7 and QOL IPSS $\geq$3. Following factors were analyzed: initial prostate volume, volume of the prostate removed by TURP, time interval between surgical procedure and radiotherapy, radiotherapy dose to the prostate, volume of the clinical target volume (CTV) (in cubic centimeter), volume of the bladder receiving 70 Gy (B70Gy), and comorbidities (Diabetes mellitus and arterial hypertension).

All patients underwent a planning computed tomography scan before RT and were treated by 3D RT to a median dose of 78.5 Gy (range, 70 to 80 Gy), prescribed

to the planning target volume (PTV), according to ICRU 50 and 62 reports. Patients received initial treatment to the prostate and seminal vesicles alone (40–46 Gy) followed by a prostatic boost. A PTV expansion was typically 1 cm in all directions around the clinical target volume, except 0.5 cm posteriorly. Patients who had a high risk for regional lymphatic involvement (ie $\geq$15%) according to Roach formula [7], also received 44–46 Gy to the pelvic lymph-nodes. RT treatment was delivered with six individually shaped coplanar fields, with 18 MV X-rays in daily fractions of 2 Gy, 5 days per week. To minimize toxicity, dose–volume histograms were used to evaluate the dose to the rectum, the bladder, the femoral heads and the bowel. Prostate localization during RT treatment was done once weekly by portal imaging or Cone beam computerized tomography (CBCT) depending on the time period during which the patients were treated. Acute urinary toxicity was scored according to Common Terminology Criteria for Adverse Events (CTCAE) version 4.0.

The use of androgen deprivation therapy (ADT) was at the discretion of the physician.

Statistical analysis

Statistical analyses were performed using the Stata software version 14.1 (stataCorp, TX, USA). Univariate analysis was performed using Student t-test for the quantitative variables and the Chi-2 test for the qualitative variables.

Bravais-Pearson correlation coefficient was used to confirmation a correlation between variables (correlation coefficient (r)). Statistical significance was set at a p-value less than 0.05.

Results

During the study period, 422 patients treated by radiotherapy in our department for non-metastatic prostate cancer were identified. Sixty-two patients who had a prior history of prostate surgery for BPH (TURP or adenectomy) were included for analysis. The indication for prostate surgery was urinary disorders in 38 patients, acute urinary retention in 11 patients, a large prostate in 4 patients and unknown reason in 11 patients. Median follow-up of the study was 4.6 years after the end of RT (range 2.2–6.9 years). Median time interval between surgery and RT was 10.6 months (range 2.2–51.6). The characteristics of patients are listed in Table 1. Thirty-three patients had arterial hypertension and 19 were treated by antihypertensive drugs. Among patients treated for hypertension, 12, 6, 9 and 5 patients were treated by angiotensin receptor blockers, beta-blockers, calcium channel blockers and diuretics respectively. Only one patient was treated by alpha blockers. Some patients received combination of

Table 1 Patient characteristics

Median age (years)	69,9 [58.6–78.3]
D'Amico risk stratification	
Low risk	13 (21%)
Intermediate risk	23 (37%)
High risk	26 (42%)
Median pre-treatment PSA level	13.7 ng/mL [1.5–94]
Gleason score	
6	22 (35.5%)
7 (3 + 4)	18 (29%)
7 (4 + 3)	9 (14.5%)
≥ 8	13 (21%)
T Stage	
T1a/b	5 (8%)
T1c	27 (43.5%)
T2	20 (32.5%)
T3a	5 (8%)
T3b	5 (8%)
N Stage	
N0	60 (96.7%)
N1	2 (3.3%)
Prostate surgery	
TURP	52 (84%)
Vaporization	2 (3%)
Adenectomy	8 (13%)
Androgen deprivation therapy	30 (48.5%)
Diabete mellitus (n = 61)	11 (18%)
Arterial hypertension (n = 61)	33 (54%)
Medical treatment[a]	7 (11.3%)
Prostatic volume before surgery (n = 59)	59.5 cc [3–150]
Prostatic volume after surgery (n = 54)	26.8 cc [3–100]
Median RT dose	78.5 Gy [70–80]
70 Gy	3 (4.9%)
76 Gy	15 (24.2%)
80 Gy	44 (70.9%)
Whole-pelvis RT	6 (9.6%)
Bladder volume receiving 70 Gy (n = 57)	34.7 cc [1–86]

RT Radiotherapy, TURP (Trans-urethral resection of prostate)
[a] alpha blocker or anticholinergic (solifenacin succinate)

multiple classes of antihypertensive drugs. Five-year biochemical disease-free survival was 75% and 5-year clinical relapse free survival was 84%. During the follow-up, 10 patients had biochemical recurrence, 7 patients had loco-regional progression, 3 patients had metastatic progression and 3 patients died: one from cardio-vascular cause and two from unknown causes unrelated to cancer. Patients who have died during the

follow-up were excluded from the functional analysis (Fig. 1). The incidence of acute urinary toxicity was 45% (26/58), 45% (26/58), 8.5% (5/58), 1.5% (1/58) for grade 0, 1, 2 and 3 respectively. There was no acute grade 4 urinary toxicity.

Fifty-nine living patients were evaluable for QoL IPSS and long-term urinary toxicity. Among those patients, ten had biochemical relapse. One patient could not answer to the IPSS questionnaire because he had a urinary sheath. Median time interval between the end of radiotherapy and the urinary function evaluation by questionnaire was 4.5 years +/– 1.1. The median IPSS was 5.5 (range 0–25): 45 patients had mild urinary symptoms 45/58 (77.6%), 12 had moderate urinary symptoms (12/58 (20.7%)) and 1 had severe urinary symptoms (1/58 (1.7%)) (Fig. 2). Quality of urinary life according to the eighth question of the IPSS was as follows: Forty-three patients reported to have a good urinary quality of life (QOL IPSS < 3) (3/58 (74.1%)) but 15 patients reported to have a poor urinary quality of life (QOL IPSS ≥3) ((15/58) (25.9%)) (Fig. 3). A statistically significant correlation was observed between the IPSS score and the QOL IPSS ($r = 0,56$; $p = 0.00001$). Fifty-five patients (55/59 (93.2%)) had grade < 2 long-term urinary toxicity according to the CTCAE scale and only 4 patients ((4/59 (6.8%)) had grade ≥ 2 long-term urinary toxicity (Fig. 4). One patient and three patients had grade 2 and grade 3 urinary retention respectively and one patient had grade 2 urinary incontinence. No patient had grade 4 long-term urinary toxicity.

A significant correlation was observed between RT dose and the QOL IPSS ($r = 0.3$; $p = 0.02$) (Fig. 5) but not between RT dose and the IPSS.

A significant correlation was also observed between the arterial hypertension (HTA) and the QOL IPSS ($p = 0.04$) (Table 2) but not between the acute urinary toxicity and the QOL IPSS ($p = 0.064$). There was no correlation observed between diuretic intake and QOL IPSS ($p = 0.167$). Three patients with HTA were excluded from the analysis because they have died during the follow-up. We also found a correlation between HTA and IPSS> 7 but this correlation was not statistically significant ($p = 0.5$) (Table 2). It is important to note that the nine patients who had medical history of HTA and a QOL IPSS≥3 did not take diuretics at the time of RT.

A non-significant trend was found between an IPSS < 7 and a small prostate volume (p = 0.06). We found no significant correlation between a poor lower urinary function and the prostate volume after surgery for BPH, the B70Gy, the prostate CTV, the time interval between surgery and RT, diabetes mellitus and androgen deprivation therapy.

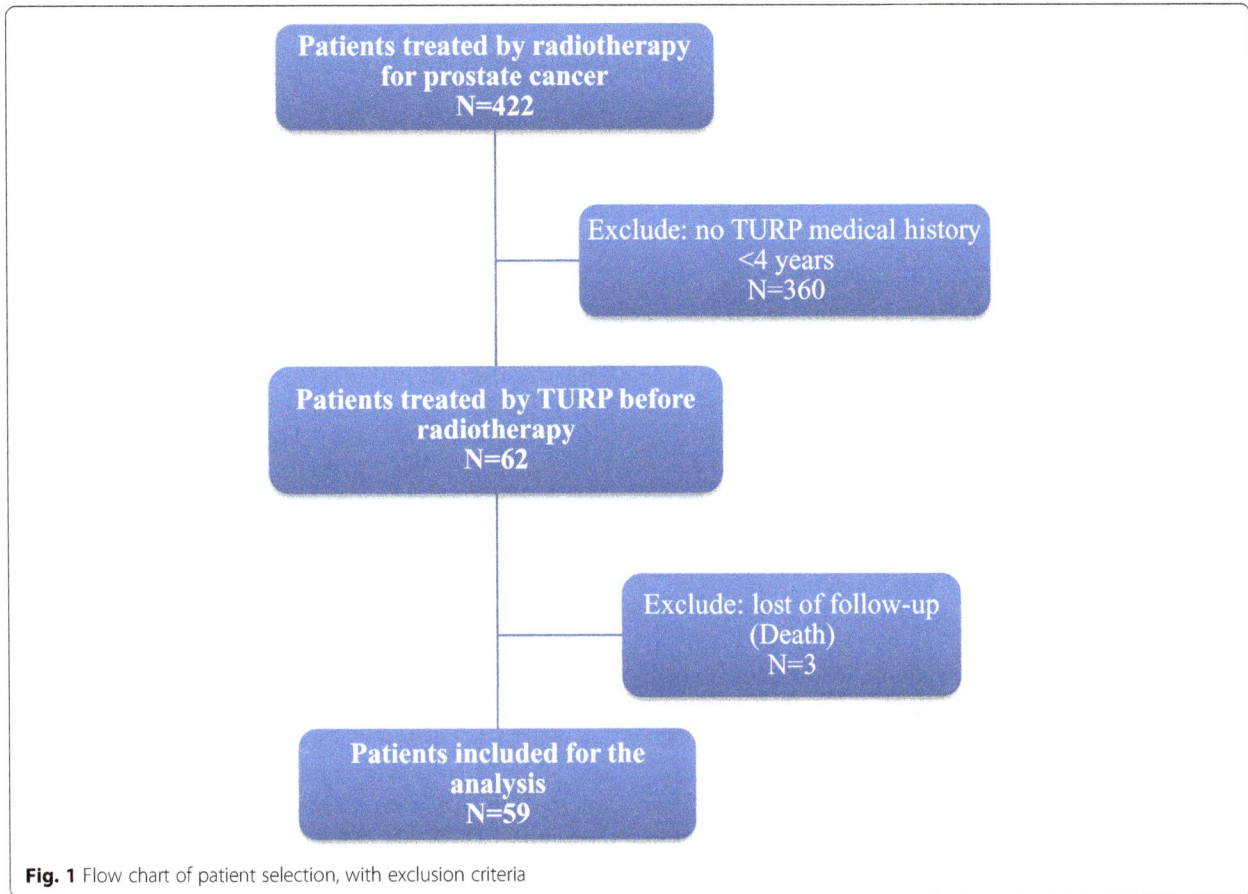

Fig. 1 Flow chart of patient selection, with exclusion criteria

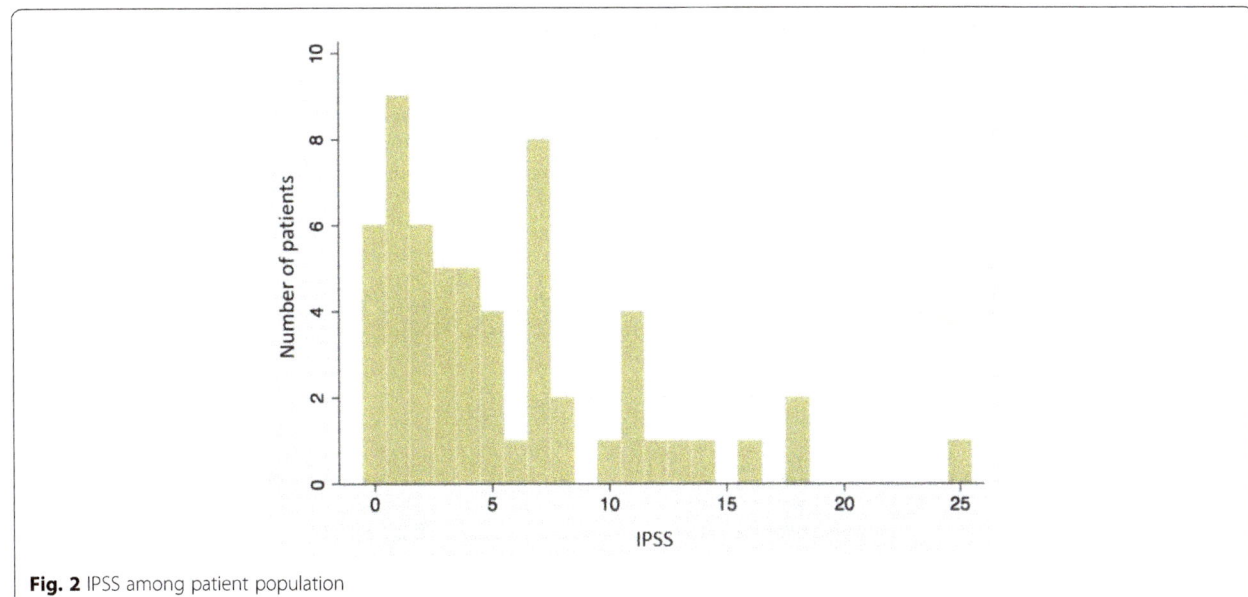

Fig. 2 IPSS among patient population

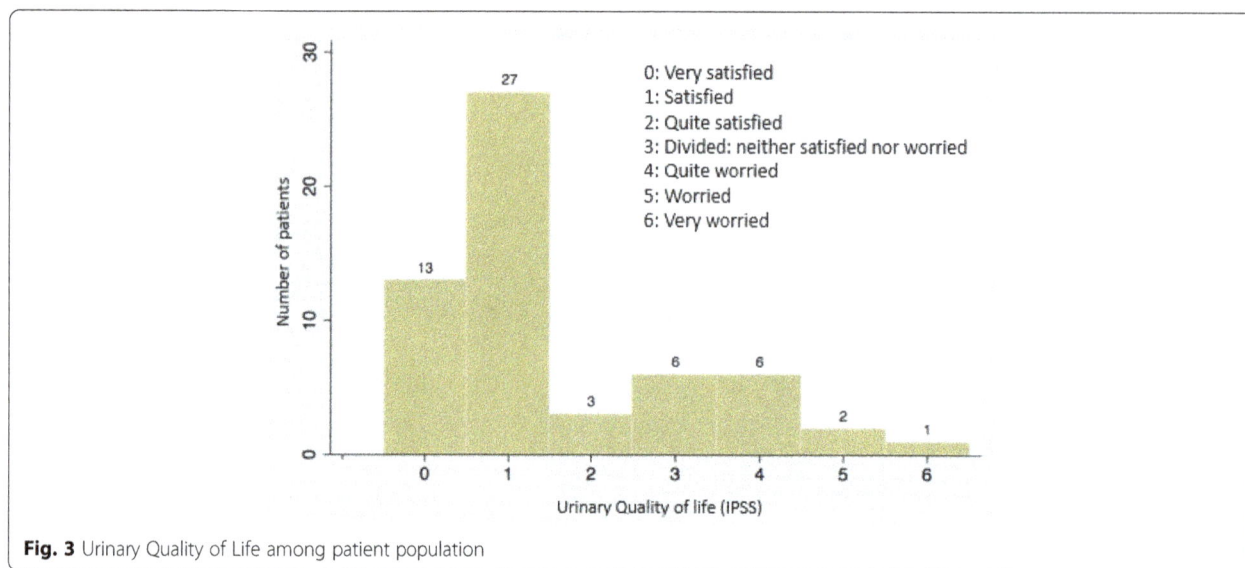

Fig. 3 Urinary Quality of Life among patient population

Discussion

In our study, we reported that almost 75% of patients had a good urinary quality of life after RT (QOL IPSS < 3), despite a previous medical history (PMH) of surgery for BPH.

In the literature, the results of the studies about toxicity after RT in patients previously treated by TURP are debated: the late urinary incontinence rate varies from 0 to 13.3% (Table 3).

Lee et al. reported on a late urinary incontinence rate of 2% vs 0.2% after RT in patients with or without a PMH of TURP respectively. Despite a lower incidence of late urinary incontinence rate, the difference was significant [5]. In two independent studies, Perez et al. reported on a non-significant increase in the incontinence rate: 13% vs 4% in the first study and 2% vs 0% in the second study [8, 9]. It is important to note that all

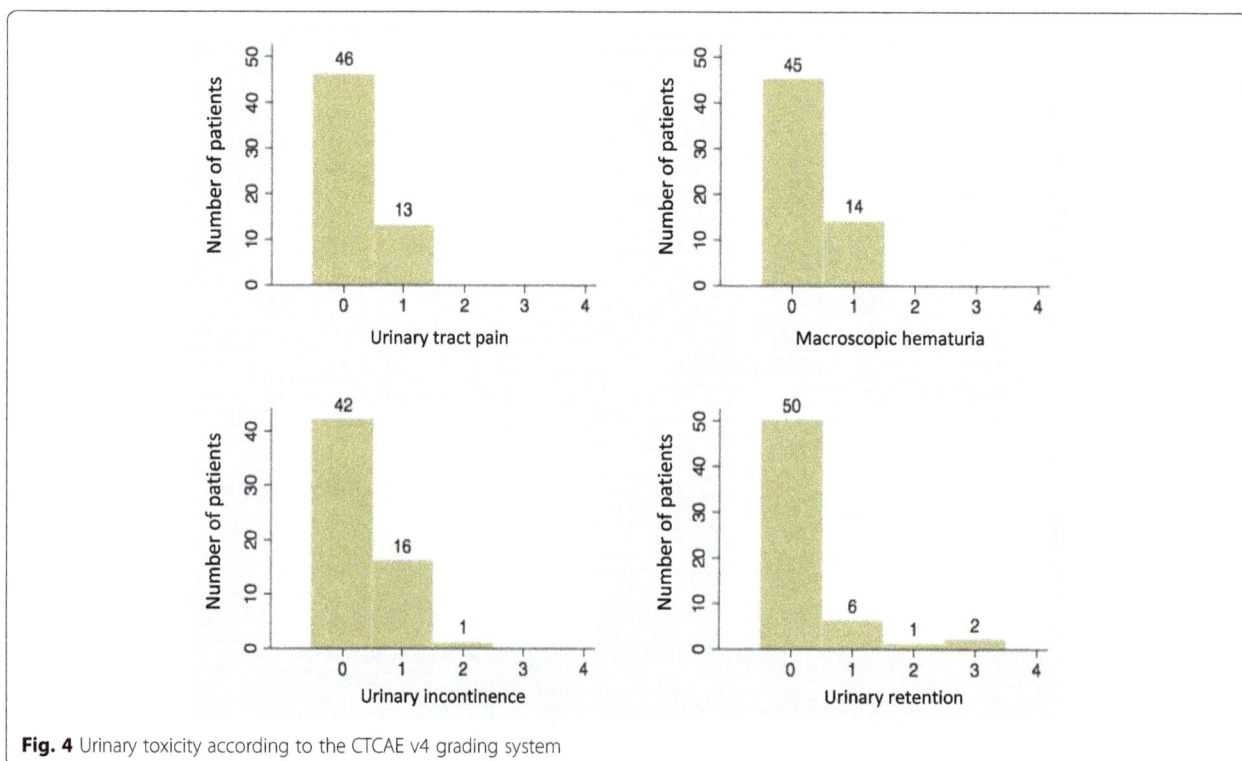

Fig. 4 Urinary toxicity according to the CTCAE v4 grading system

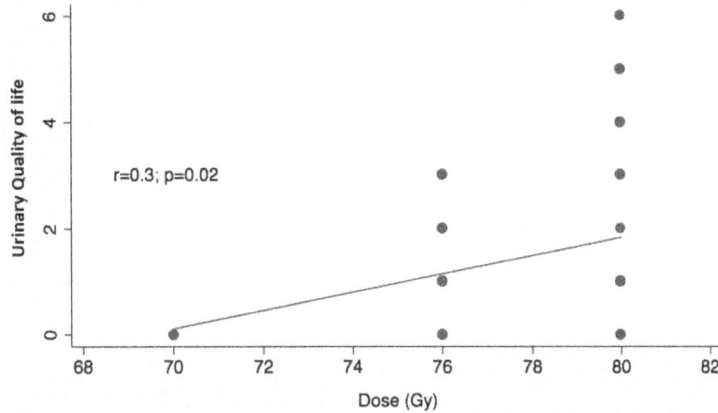

Fig. 5 Urinary Quality of life and radiotherapy dose

patients in these studies were treated with old 2DRT technics. In a study on 1192 patients, published in 2004, Liu et al. evaluated urinary incontinence in patients treated by 2DRT or 3DRT for prostate cancer. Two hundred and forty-six patients had a previous medical history of TURP. Grade ≥ 1 incontinence rate at 5 years was greater in patients with a PMH of TURP in comparison with those without PMH of TURP (10% vs 6%, p = 0.03) [3]. N. et al. evaluated 285 patients treated with 3DRT at a dose of 79.2Gy, of whom, of whom 13% had a TURP beforehand [10]. Grade 2–3 urinary toxicity at

5 years was greater for patients with PMH of TURP (25.7% vs 6.1%, p = 0.0002).

S. et al., did not find any difference regarding grade ≥ 2 long-term overall urinary toxicity in patients treated by 3DRT or IMRT with or without a PMH of TURP (10 vs 9%) [11].

In a systematic review of the literature, 13 studies among 14, reported a higher incontinence rate in patients with PMH of TURP compared with patients without PMH of TURP. Among these studies, four demonstrated a statistically significant increase of

Table 2 Risk factors associated with long term urinary toxicity (Univariate analysis)

	IPSS ≤7	IPSS > 7	p	QOL < 3	QOL ≥3	p	CTCAE Grade < 2	CTCAE Grade ≥ 2	p
Initial prostate volume (g)	56	71	0.06	58	64	0.24	60	36	0.08
Resected prostate Volume (g)	28	24	0.3	26	30	0.2	27	16	0.1
CTV prostate (cc)	45	61	0.07	50	59	0.1	53	37	0.08
V70Gy (cc)	34	37	0.2	35	36	0.4	34	40	0.2
TURP-RT time interval (days)	312	398	0.2	312	382	0.2	306	614	0.05
Total dose of radiotherapy (Gy)	78.3	78.7	0,3	78	79.4	0.04	78.4	79	0.3
Hypertension									
No	24	3	0.5	21	6	0.04	27	0	0.05
Yes	20	10		21	9		27	4	
TURP indication									
Unknown	5	0	0.1	4	1	0.1	5	0	0.8
Urinary symptoms	28	10		26	12		36	3	
Urinary retention	10	1		11	0		10	1	
High prostate volume	2	2		2	2		4	0	
Androgen deprivation therapy									
No	23	9	0.2	25	6	0.2	29	3	0.3
Yes	22	4		18	9		26	1	

IPSS International prostate symptom score, *QOL* urinary quality of life, *CTCAE* (Common Terminology Criteria for Adverse Events) version 4 grading system, *TURP* transurethral resection of the prostate

Table 3 Studies on toxicity after radiotherapy in patients previously treated by TURP

Authors	Years	n	Dose RT	Late urinary incontinence rate
Gibbons et al. [24]	1979	71	66.8 Gy (Mean)	0%
Perez et al. [9]	1980	60	60–70 Gy	13.3%
Pilepich et al. [25]	1981	88	65–70 Gy	2.3%
Green et al. [26]	1990	130	65 Gy	5.5%
Amdur et al. [27]	1990	114	65–70 Gy	3%
Perez et al. [8]	1994	242	62–72%	2%
Lee et al. [5]	1996	132	68–79 Gy	2%
Sandhu et al. [11]	2000	120	64.8–81 Gy	10%
Liu et al. [3]	2005	246	66 Gy (median)	10%
Devissety et al. [2]	2010	71	70 Gy (Median)	3%
Current study	2018	59	78 Gy (Median)	2%

incontinence [4]. Acute grade ≥ 2 urinary toxicity, longer follow-up time, and stage $\geq$T3 were reported as risk factors for incontinence in this group. In our study, high RT dose to the prostate was associated with a long-term poor urinary QOL. Indeed, in our study, patients with an IPSS> 7 received a higher average dose to the prostate and the 3 patients who received only 70 Gy to the prostate had a QOL IPSS = 0. Despite a relatively high median dose delivered to the prostate (78.6 Gy) with 70.9% of patients receiving 80 Gy and 24.2% 76 Gy, most of the patients were overall satisfied with their urinary QOL.

D. et al. reported on a study of 609 patients, treated by RT for prostate cancer, a non-significant increase risk of urinary toxicity in patients with a PMH of TURP or a RT dose greater than 74 Gy [2]. In several studies it was shown that the RT dose is associated with a higher urinary toxicity. Z. et al. reported on a higher urinary toxicity grade ≥ 2 rate for patients treated with a dose > 75.6 Gy delivered by 3DRT (14% vs 5%, $p < 0.001$) [12, 13].

However, modern irradiation technics such as Intensity Modulated Radiotherapy (IMRT)/ Volumetric Modulated Arc Therapy (VMAT)/ Image Guided Radiotherapy (IGRT) could decrease late urinary toxicity rate in patients treated with high-dose radiotherapy. Zapatero et al. reported that compared with 3DCRT, high-dose IMRT/IGRT was associated with a lower rate of late urinary complications (6.4% vs 10.8%, $p = 0.056$) in spite of higher radiation dose (80.7 Gy vs 78.7 Gy, p < 0.001) [14]. In patients treated with high dose IMRT (86.4 Gy) + IGRT, Z. et al. have reported a lower rate of 3-year likelihood of grade 2+ urinary toxicity in comparison with patients treated without IGRT (10.4% vs 20.0%, $p = 0.02$) [15].

Few studies have both evaluated urinary function and quality of life using the IPSS questionnaire after definitive RT for prostate cancer. In our study, we also evaluated QOL IPSS, to take into account the patient's point of view about their urinary toxicity. In our study, 45/58 (77.6%) of patients had a mild, 12/58 (20.1%) a moderate and 1/58 (1.7%) a severe IPSS. For the urinary QOL IPSS, 43/58 (74%) were satisfied, 6/58 (11%) were neither satisfied nor worried and 9/58 (15%) were quite worried to very worried.

Despite the PMH of TURP, only one patient had a severe IPSS, the vast majority of our patients had a mild IPSS and a good urinary quality of life. Our results are comparable with those published by L. et al., who reported IPSS in 154 patients treated by 3DRT or 2DRT without TURP: 79% of patients had a mild IPSS score, 14% had a moderate IPSS score and 6% had a severe IPSS score. For the urinary QOL IPSS, 87% of the patients were satisfied, 10% were shared and 3% were annoyed [16]. In a study of 60 patients treated by 3DRT without TURP for prostate cancer, Pastorello et al. reported at 48 months after RT, a median IPSS = 11. The median IPSS of their patients was higher compared with the median IPPS of our patients treated by TURP and RT (11 vs 5.5) [17].

We also found in our study, a correlation between a worse QOL IPSS and a PMH of hypertension. Our results are in accordance with Cozzarini et al., who observed in a study of 742 patients more grade 2–3 late urinary toxicity in patients with hypertension and treated with postoperative RT [18]. Hypertension has also been found to be associated with an increased risk of urethral stricture after prostate brachytherapy [19].

It has been observed that circulating catecholamine levels are high in patients with arterial hypertension [20, 21]. Increase catecholamine levels may influence the lumbosacral cord and therefore increase urinary frequency [22].

No other statistically significant risk factors for long-term urinary toxicity were found.

Due to the retrospective nature of our study, baseline IPSS before RT was not available, therefore we did not evaluate the relationship between baseline IPSS and post RT IPSS or QOL IPSS.

Chevli et al. who evaluated 368 patients treated with RT, did not show an association between the volume of the prostate gland (VP) before treatment and urinary toxicity at 1 year [23]. VP does not appear to be a good indicator of radiotherapy toxicity in patients with or without TURP.

The absence of correlation between surgery-RT delay and long-term urinary function observed in our study could be explained by our local procedure, which recommends a minimum delay between the TURP and the start of radiotherapy of 10 or more weeks, to allow sufficient time for the tissues to heal.

Our study has a number of limitations, including its retrospective nature, a small sample and the fact that it was conducted at a single institution. Patients have been questioned on their urinary function at different interval after RT.

Conclusion

RT in patients previously treated by surgery for BPH is feasible, well tolerated and is associated with low IPSS score, a satisfactory quality of life and a low incidence of severe long-term urinary toxicities, similar to those without surgery for BPH, reported in the literature. External radiotherapy remains an appropriate treatment option without a major risk for deterioration in urinary function in patient with antecedent surgery for BPH and with prior medical history of arterial hypertension. In practice, for patients with poor urinary function, surgery may be a good option to alleviate urinary symptoms, albeit requiring a waiting time to heal before RT.

Abbreviations

ADT: Androgen deprivation therapy; BPH: Benign prostatic hyperplasia; CBCT: Cone beam computerized tomography; CTCAE: Common terminology criteria for adverse events; CTV: Clinical target volume; ICRU: International commission on radiation units and measurements; IPSS: International prostate symptom score; PMH: Previous medical history; PTV: Planning target volume; RT: External beam radiotherapy; TURP: TransUrethral Resection of the Prostate

Funding
This research did not receive any specific grant from any funding agency in the public, commercial or not-for-profit sector.

Authors' contributions
Data acquisition: MG, CH. Conception and design: MG, CH, LQ. Data analysis: MG, CH, LQ. Patient treatment and manuscript review: MG, CH, IO, IF, VM, SG, PMA, VR, FD, LQ. All authors read and approved the final manuscript.

Competing interests
The authors declare that they have no competing interests.

References

1. Rassweiler J, Teber D, Kuntz R, Hofmann R. Complications of transurethral resection of the prostate (TURP)--incidence, management, and prevention. Eur Urol. 2006;50:969–79 discussion 980.
2. Devisetty K, Zorn KC, Katz MH, Jani AB, Liauw SL. External beam radiation therapy after transurethral resection of the prostate: a report on acute and late genitourinary toxicity. Int J Radiat Oncol Biol Phys. 2010;77:1060–5.
3. Liu M, Pickles T, Berthelet E, et al. Urinary incontinence in prostate cancer patients treated with external beam radiotherapy. Radiother Oncol. 2005;74:197–201.
4. Ishiyama H, Hirayama T, Jhaveri P, et al. Is there an increase in genitourinary toxicity in patients treated with transurethral resection of the prostate and radiotherapy? A systematic review. Am J Clin Oncol. 2014;37:297–304.
5. Lee WR, Schultheiss TE, Hanlon AL, Hanks GE. Urinary incontinence following external-beam radiotherapy for clinically localized prostate cancer. Urology. 1996;48:95–9.
6. Services, UDoHaH. National Cancer Institute. Common Terminology Criteria for Adverse Events (CTCAE) version 4.03: National Institutes of Health; 2010.
7. Roach M 3rd, Marquez C, Yuo HS, et al. Predicting the risk of lymph node involvement using the pre-treatment prostate specific antigen and Gleason score in men with clinically localized prostate cancer. Int J Radiat Oncol Biol Phys. 1994;28:33–7.
8. Perez CA, Lee HK, Georgiou A, Lockett MA. Technical factors affecting morbidity in definitive irradiation for localized carcinoma of the prostate. Int J Radiat Oncol Biol Phys. 1994;28:811–9.
9. Perez CA, Walz BJ, Zivnuska FR, Pilepich M, Prasad K, Bauer W. Irradiation of carcinoma of the prostate localized to the pelvis: analysis of tumor response and prognosis. Int J Radiat Oncol Biol Phys. 1980;6:555–63.
10. Nakamura RA, Monti CR, Castilho LN, Trevisan FA, Valim AC, Reinato JA. Prognostic factors for late urinary toxicity grade 2-3 after conformal radiation therapy on patients with prostate cancer. Int Braz J Urol. 2007;33:652–9 discussion 660-651.
11. Sandhu AS, Zelefsky MJ, Lee HJ, Lombardi D, Fuks Z, Leibel SA. Long-term urinary toxicity after 3-dimensional conformal radiotherapy for prostate cancer in patients with prior history of transurethral resection. Int J Radiat Oncol Biol Phys. 2000;48:643–7.
12. Zelefsky MJ, Fuks Z, Hunt M, et al. High dose radiation delivered by intensity modulated conformal radiotherapy improves the outcome of localized prostate cancer. J Urol. 2001;166:876–81.
13. Zelefsky MJ, Leibel SA, Gaudin PB, et al. Dose escalation with three-dimensional conformal radiation therapy affects the outcome in prostate cancer. Int J Radiat Oncol Biol Phys. 1998;41:491–500.
14. Zapatero A, Roch M, Buchser D, et al. Reduced late urinary toxicity with high-dose intensity-modulated radiotherapy using intra-prostate fiducial markers for localized prostate cancer. Clin Transl Oncol. 2017;19:1161–7.
15. Zelefsky MJ, Kollmeier M, Cox B, et al. Improved clinical outcomes with high-dose image guided radiotherapy compared with non-IGRT for the treatment of clinically localized prostate cancer. Int J Radiat Oncol Biol Phys. 2012;84:125–9.
16. Lilleby W, Fossa SD, Waehre HR, Olsen DR. Long-term morbidity and quality of life in patients with localized prostate cancer undergoing definitive radiotherapy or radical prostatectomy. Int J Radiat Oncol Biol Phys. 1999;43:735–43.
17. Pastorello M, Romano M, Porcaro A, et al. Urodynamic patterns after prostate radiotherapy. Evaluation at 2, 18, 48 and 60 months. Neurourol Urodyn. 2017;36:472.
18. Cozzarini C, Fiorino C, Da Pozzo LF, et al. Clinical factors predicting late severe urinary toxicity after postoperative radiotherapy for prostate carcinoma: a single-institute analysis of 742 patients. Int J Radiat Oncol Biol Phys. 2012;82:191–9.
19. Sullivan L, Williams SG, Tai KH, Foroudi F, Cleeve L, Duchesne GM. Urethral stricture following high dose rate brachytherapy for prostate cancer. Radiother Oncol. 2009;91:232–6.
20. Binggeli C, Corti R, Sudano I, Luscher TF, Noll G. Effects of chronic calcium channel blockade on sympathetic nerve activity in hypertension. Hypertension. 2002;39:892–6.

21. Esler M, Rumantir M, Kaye D, et al. Sympathetic nerve biology in essential hypertension. Clin Exp Pharmacol Physiol. 2001;28:986–9.

22. Sugaya K, Kadekawa K, Ikehara A, et al. Influence of hypertension on lower urinary tract symptoms in benign prostatic hyperplasia. Int J Urol. 2003;10: 569–74 discussion 575.

23. Chevli C, Narayanan R, Rambarran L, Kubicek G, Chevli KK, Duff M. Effect of pretreatment prostate volume on urinary quality of life following intensity-modulated radiation therapy for localized prostate cancer. Res Rep Urol. 2013;5:29–37.

24. Gibbons RP, Mason JT, Correa RJ Jr, et al. Carcinoma of the prostate: local control with external beam radiation therapy. J Urol. 1979;121:310–2.

25. Pilepich MV, Perez CA, Walz BJ, Zivnuska FR. Complications of definitive radiotherapy for carcinoma of the prostate. Int J Radiat Oncol Biol Phys. 1981;7:1341–8.

26. Green N, Treible D, Wallack H. Prostate cancer: post-irradiation incontinence. J Urol. 1990;144:307–9.

27. Amdur RJ, Parsons JT, Fitzgerald LT, Million RR. Adenocarcinoma of the prostate treated with external-beam radiation therapy: 5-year minimum follow-up. Radiother Oncol. 1990;18:235–46.

23

Delineation of lung cancer with FDG PET/CT during radiation therapy

J. Ganem[1,2], S. Thureau[1,2,3*], I. Gardin[1,2,3], R. Modzelewski[1,2], S. Hapdey[1,2] and P. Vera[1,2]

Abstract

Objectives: To propose an easily applicable segmentation method (perPET-RT) for delineation of tumour volume during radiotherapy on interim fluorine 18 fluorodeoxyglucose (FDG) positron emission tomography/computed tomography (PET/CT) in patients with non-small cell lung cancer (NSCLC).

Material and methods: Sixty-seven patients (51 primary tumours, 60 lymph nodes), from 4 prospective studies, underwent an FDG PET/CT scan during the fifth week of radiation therapy, using different generations of PET/CT. Per-therapeutic PET/CT scans were delineated in consensus by two experienced physicians leading to the gold standard threshold to be applied. The mathematical expression of Th_{opt}, the optimal threshold to be applied as a function of the maximum standard uptake value (SUV_{max}), was determined. The performance of this method (perPET-RT) was assessed by computing the DICE similarity coefficient (DSC) and was compared with 8 fixed threshold values and 3 adaptive thresholding methods.

Results: Th_{opt} verified the following expression: $Th_{opt} = A.\ln(1/SUV_{max}) + B$ where A and B were 2 constants. A and B were independent from the generation of PET/CT, but depended on the type of lesions (primary lung tumours vs. lymph nodes). PerPET-RT showed good to very good agreement in comparison to the gold standard. The mean and standard deviation of DSC value was 0.81 ± 0.13 for lung lesions and 0.78 ± 0.15 for lymph nodes. PerPET-RT showed a significant better agreement than the other segmentation methods ($p < 0.001$), except for one of the adaptive thresholding method ADT ($p = 0.11$).

Conclusion: On the database used, perPET-RT has proven its reliability and accuracy for tumour delineation on per-therapeutic FDG PET/CT using only SUV_{max} measurement. This method may be used to delincate tumour volume for dose-escalation planning.

Trial registration: NCT01261598, NCT01261585, NCT01576796.

Keywords: Delineation, Radiation therapy, PET/CT, Lung cancer, perPET-RT

Introduction

Non-Small Cell Lung Cancer (NSCLC) represents a leading cause of death by cancer in the world, especially in Europe and North America. Treatment modalities should be personalized according to the patient's clinical condition, tumor staging, histological/molecular profile, whether disease is resectable, locally advanced or

* Correspondence: Sebastien.thureau@chb.unicancer.fr;
sebastien.thureau@chb.unicancer.fr
[1]Nuclear Medicine Department, Henri Becquerel Cancer Centre and Rouen University Hospital, Rouen, France
[2]QuantIF-LITIS (EA [Equipe d'Accueil] 4108-FR CNRS [Fédération de Recherche-Centre National pour la Recherche Scientifique] 3638), Faculty of Medicine, University of Rouen, Rouen, France
Full list of author information is available at the end of the article

advanced and may comprise surgery, radiation therapy and chemotherapy [1–3].

FDG PET/CT (^{18}F-fluorodeoxyglucose positron emission tomography/computed tomography) has proven utility to accurately to delineate the tumour volume for external radiation therapy [4, 5]. In the case of NSCLC, pre-therapeutic FDG PET/CT allows the delineation of the metabolic tumour volume (MTV), the exclusion of non-tumoral abnormalities (such as atelectasis) and also improves inter and intra observers reproducibility [6, 7], which are one of the main limitations when delineating on CT modality alone.

Several radiation therapy strategies have been considered so far Bradley et al. showed that high dose conformational radiation therapy was not better than standard-dose radiation therapy and even potentially harmful, due to increased toxicity [8].

Current radiotherapy techniques make it possible to deliver a heterogeneous dose by IMRT. FDG PET/CT can help define patients or volumes at risk of recurrence. However, Aerts et al. [9] and Calais et al. [10] showed that high FDG uptake areas on pre-therapeutic FDG PET/CT scans were highly correlated to the sites of local relapse or persistent abnormalities on post-therapeutic scans. These findings lead to consider the idea of dose-escalation on a smaller volume, allowing a better local control of the disease and minimising in parallel early and late toxicity.

The FDG PET/CT fixing per-treatment can also be a volume of interest. Per-radiotherapy FDG PET/CT can be performed without artefacts (lung inflammation) and the persistence of 42Gy fixation is very pejorative [11, 12]. As a result, we proposed a French multicenter study with dose increase on per-radiotherapy FDG volume (RTEP7, NCT02473133). Another study is also underway in the USA by the RTOG (RTOG 1106) and encouragingpreliminary results have been published by Kongs et al. in a phase 2 [13].

The definition of BTV (Biologic Target Volume) is a crucial step of treatment planning in radiation therapy. Many methods of pre-treatment segmentation have been defined but there is no segmentation method in the process of radiotherapy. For Until now, manual delineation of FDG PET positive tissues is the gold standard, despite poor reproducibility [14].

For pre-radiotherapy, many methods have been proposed in the literature. The first methods are a fixed standard uptake value (SUV), for example 2.5 [15, 16] or a threshold value around 40% of the maximum standard uptake value (SUV$_{max}$) within the lesion [16, 17]. The last recommendations, published by the European Association of Nuclear Medicine (EANM), suggested a delineation of the MTV by applying 3D isocontours at 41% or 50% of SUV$_{max}$ [5, 18, 19].

However, these methods are not optimal for low contrast or small volumes [20]. which can be the case on per-therapeutic PET/CT images. Thus, several complex methods have been developed [18–29]. None of them has proven its superiority yet [30]. This absence of consensus can be a problem in multicentre trials, where acquisition reproducibility is poor and devices correspond to different PET/CT models, possibly from different generation technologies. Another limitation comes from the availability of delineation softwares, especially in case of sophisticated approaches.

The aim of this article is to propose a reliable, reproducible and easy delineation method applicable in clinical routine and suitable for multicentre studies, in the specific context of per-therapeutic FDG PET/CT with potentially small volume and low contrast. This step was a prerequisite for the RTEP7 study.

Material and methods

Patient population and treatment

Data were extracted from 4 prospective studies corresponding to a total of 67 patients, respectively S1, S2, S3 and S4, where S1–3 correspond to monocentric clinical trials (Centre Henri Becquerel, Rouen, France) [11, 12, 31] (NCT01261598, NCT01261585) and S4 (NCT01576796) an ongoing multicentre clinical trial study [31], in which patients had given written and informed consent. All patients were treated with radiation therapy alone or concomitant chemoradiotherapy for inoperable stage II or III NSCLC. Patients were treated by conformational radiation therapy. The dose prescription corresponded to 66 Gy in 33 fractions, with 2 Gy per fraction given daily, 5 days a week. The mean age was 59 years. There were 13 women and 54 men presenting stage II (10%) or stage III (90%) NSCLC. Clinical data are summarized in Table 1.

PET/CT imaging

For patients treated at the Centre Henri Becquerel, the per-therapeutic PET/CT was performed on a Biograph Sensation 16 Hi-Rez device (Siemens Medical Solutions, Erlangen, Germany), without time of flight system or image reconstruction algorithm incorporating point-spread function. Forty-six patients underwent their PET/CT on this device. They were unrolled in S1–3 monocentric clinical trials (39 patients), and in S4 (7 patients). As the PET/CT device

Table 1 Clinical, pathological and therapeutic data

Number of patients	67
Age (years)	Mean: 59 (min 38; max 80)
Sex (number of patients)	Women: 13; Men: 54
Tumoral stage:	
- II A	2
- II B	5
- III A	25
- III B	35
Histology:	
- Adenocarcinoma	24 (5 poorly differentiated)
- Squamous cell carcinoma	37
- Undifferentiated carcinoma	6
Type of treatment:	
- Radiation therapy	21
- Concomitant radiochemotherapy	46
Dose received before per-therapeutic PET/CT	Mean: 43 Gy (min: 32 Gy; max: 52 Gy)

corresponded to an old generation model, these patients were grouped into a database called S_{old}.

Patients who underwent their FDG PET/CT on a new generation of positron-emission tomograph came from S4 study. All the image reconstruction algorithms incorporated a point-spread function, while some of them used a time of flight system (ToF). They were grouped into a database called S_{New} (21 patients). The PET/CT models and their characteristics are listed in Appendix.

All 67 patients underwent a FDG PET/CT during the fifth week of radiation therapy. Protocols of acquisition and reconstruction followed EANM procedure guidelines [5], but they were inherent to each nuclear medicine department. On the other hand, they were the same for a given device.

PET/CT analysis

First, per-therapeutic PET/CT scans were delineated in consensus using a Planet Onco workstation (PlanetOnco, v.2.0; DOSISoft) at the Centre Henri Becquerel (Rouen, France) by two experienced physicians of the same center: one nuclear medicine physician and one radiation oncologist with clinical practice in lung cancer. The delineation was performed using different thresholds until the volume corresponded with the one obtained by manual delineation, leading to Th_{GStd}, the gold standard threshold. SUV_{max} of the lesion was also extracted leading to (Th_{GStd}, SUV_{max}) pairs of values.

Then, primary lung tumours (pr) were isolated from lymph nodes (no), leading to 4 classes of lesions: $S_{Old}(pr)$, $S_{New}(pr)$, $S_{Old}(no)$ and $S_{New}(no)$ lesions.

PerPET-RT segmentation method

The graphical representation of y (Th_{GStd}) as a function of x (SUVmax) showed that the shape of the curve could be approximated as the natural logarithm of the reciprocal of x.

The method proposed to easily segment the MTV on a per-therapeutic PET/CT during the fifth week of treatment of NSCLC, called perPET-RT, is based on an adaptive thresholding method according to the following expression:

$Th_{opt} = A . \ln(1/SUV_{max}) + B$ *Eq. 1.*

where Th_{opt}(%) is the optimal threshold to be applied, SUV_{max} the maximum of the SUV in the tumour (primary or node) to be segmented, and A and B, two constants depending on the kind of lesion (primary or node) leading respectively to (A_{pr}, B_{pr}) and (A_{no}, B_{no}).

One can note that Eq. 1 corresponds to a linear relationship between Th_{opt} and X = $\ln(1/SUV_{max})$, where A is the slope of the line and B the intercept, leading to the following expression:

$Th_{opt} = A . X + B$ *Eq. 2.*

Segmentation methods for performance comparison

The performance of perPET-RT was compared to several segmentation methods, based on thresholding, applied by a third experienced physician, independently from the consensual delineation used for the gold standard:

- Fixed SUV-values: 2; 2.5; 3; 3.5;
- Fixed threshold corresponding to a percentile of the maximum SUV (% of SUV_{max}): 40, 50, 60, 70%;
- An adaptive thresholding method, called AOV, where the threshold to be applied corresponds to 1.5 times the mean SUV measured in an aorta volume of 1 cc [21];
- Two adaptive thresholding methods: COA and ADT [20, 22]. The two methods were calibrated according to the recommendations respectively from Schaefer et al. [20] and Vauclin et al. [23] for Biograph Sensation 16 Hi-Rez device.

Data analysis
Regression function of perPET-RT

For primary tumours and nodes, the couples of values (Th_{opt}, SUV_{max}) were defined, as well as the associated couple of constants (i. e. (A_{pr}, B_{pr}) and (A_{no}, B_{no})) of the linear regression (*Eq. 2*). The fits were obtained by minimizing the residuals by computing their coefficient of determination (R^2).

The robustness of the adaptive threshold calibration procedure was evaluated by testing whether the slopes and the intercepts of the two datasets issued from the two PET models (old vs. new) were significantly different [33].

First, slopes were compared. If this first *p*-value was less than 0.05, it could be concluded that the lines were significantly different. In that case, there was no point in comparing the intercepts. Otherwise, intercepts were compared. If this second p-value was high, there was no compelling evidence that the lines were different. The software used was GraphPad Prism 5 (Version 5.0 SAS Institute Inc., CA, USA).

Agreement of segmented volumes

The performance of perPET-RT method was evaluated using the Dice similarity coefficient (DSC) according to the following expression:

$$DSC = \frac{2(X \cap Y)}{(X \cup Y)}$$ *Eq. 3.*

Where X corresponds to the gold standard volume and Y the volume segmented by perPET-RT.

The agreement between the segmented volumes using other segmentation methods was also performed using DSC.

As two adaptive thresholding methods (ADT and COA) were calibrated only on the Biograph Sensation

16 Hi-Rez device, the segmentation was only done on S_{old} data for these 2 methods.

At, first a descriptive analysis of DSC was performed for each segmentation method by computing median (DSC_{med}), minimum (DSC_{min}) and maximum (DSC_{max}) of DSC. For this analysis, first/third quartiles and first/ninth deciles of DSC-values were also extracted leading to the estimation of the inter-quartile range (difference between third and first quartiles, i.e. including 50% of the data) and the inter-decile range (difference between ninth and first deciles, i.e. including 80% of the data. Box and Whiskers plots were established. In order to compare the segmentation methods, a non-parametric analysis of DSC was performed. A *p*-value less than 0.05 was considered to be statistically significant. A Bonferonni *post-hoc* test was used.

The following criteria for the Cohen κ test were chosen to qualify the agreement of the segmentation methods: 0–0.2, poor agreement; 0.21–0.40, fair agreement; 0.41–0.60,

moderate agreement; 0.61–0.80, good agreement; and 0.81–1.00, very good agreement (21).

Results
Per-therapeutic PET results
Patients underwent per-therapeutic PET/CT after a mean dose of 43 Gy (see Table 1). Sixty-one of the 67 patients (91%) had persistent hypermetabolic lesions on these scans, but MTV and SUV_{max} were lower on PET/CT during the treatment if compared to those of pre-therapeutic PET/CT. An example is given in Fig. 1.

A total of 111 lesions were identified: 51 lung tumours and 60 mediastinal nodes. Their main characteristics such as metabolic volume, SUV_{max} and threshold applied by the experts for delineation are reported in Table 2.

Regression function
In Fig. 2, are given the pairs of points (Th_{GStd},Ln (1/SUV_{max})) for both primary tumours and nodes. This Fig.

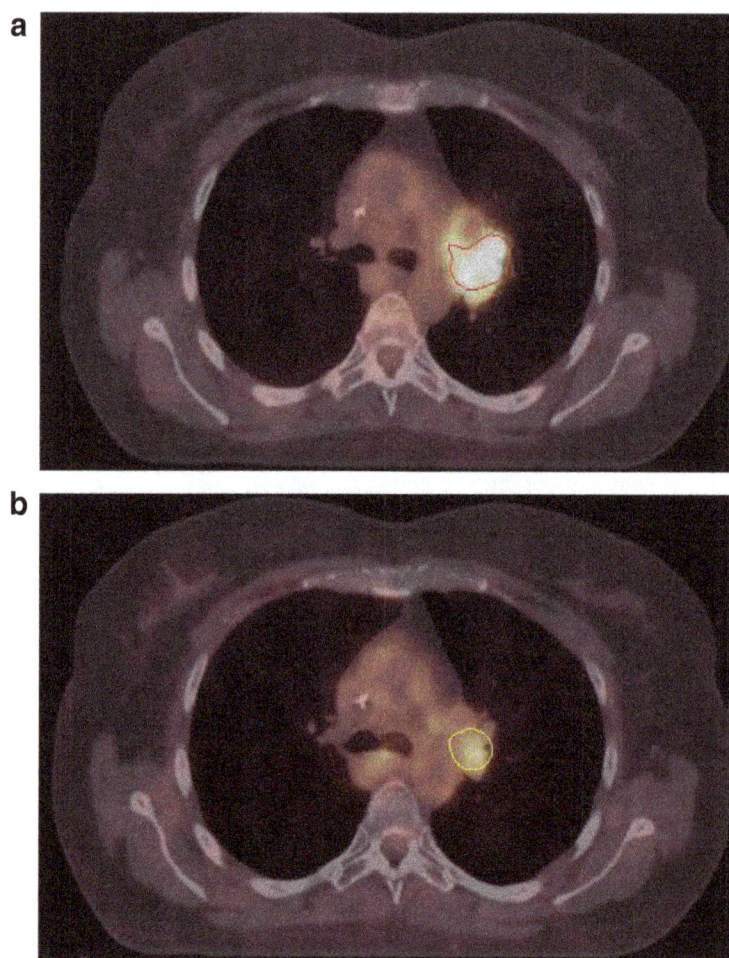

Fig. 1 Patient with stage IIIA left lung adenocarcinoma. FDG PET/CT performed before (**a.**) and during (**b**) radiation therapy. Pre therapeutic scan (**a**) show left para-hilar hypermetabolism with SUV_{max} = 9.6 and MTV = 15.4 cc defined with a threshold value of 41% SUV_{max}. Per-therapeutic data (**b**) reveals a decrease in FDG uptake (SUV_{max} = 4.2) and MTV = 4.8 cc. defined by the experts with a threshold value of 55% of SUV_{max}

Table 2 Metabolic characteristics of primary tumours (pr) and involved lymph nodes (no), FDG uptake, threshold used by the experts for metabolic tumour volume delineation and corresponding volume. New and Old refer to the generation of PET device

	SUV_{max} range	SUV_{max} Mean/*Median*	Thresholds range (%SUV_{max})	Thresholds Mean/ *Median* (%SUV_{max})	Volumes range (cc)	Volumes Mean/ *Median* (cc)
S_{Old}(pr) ($n=32$)	2.5–14.1	6.2/*5.8*	34–66	50/*50*	0.26–65	12/*17*
S_{Old}(no) ($n=38$)	2.4–8.4	4.6/*4.6*	46–73	60/*59*	0.26–13	3/*2*
S_{New}(pr) ($n=19$)	2.5–36.5	10.5/*8.0*	16–65	43/*44*	0.47–140	20/*10*
S_{New}(no) ($n=22$)	2.6–9.3	5.4/*4.6*	44–71	57/*59*	0.57–25	4.5/*1.5*

2 shows also the plots corresponding to the two linear regressions (primary vs. nodes). There was no statistical difference between slopes. However, a significant difference existed between their intercepts ($p < 0.01$). On the other hand, for a given type of lesion, no significant difference was found between the lines obtained with the old and the new generation PET/CT devices.

Agreement of segmented volumes

In Fig. 3a are given the descriptive statistics of perPET-RT and the other segmentation methods (AOV, fixed threshold methods) using all the lesions. The segmentation with perPET-RT showed a good to a very good agreement with respect to the experts since the mean value and standard deviation of DSC were 0.78 ± 0.15 for mediastinal lymph nodes and 0.81 ± 0.13 for lung tumours. In Fig. 3b are also given the descriptive statistics of perPET-RT and ADT and COA, but only on the 70 lesions observed on the Biograph Hi-Rez device.

PerPET-RT showed a significant better agreement compared to the other segmentation methods ($p < 0.001$), except for ADT ($p = 0.11$) which showed a DSC mean value and standard deviation of 0.75 ± 0.17.

Discussion

With this study, we propose a perPET-RT segmentation method easy to use and adapted to multicentre studies. There are no reference methods for segmentation during radiotherapy, but standard techniques may overestimate target volumes (low fixation during the treatment). The method proposed in the present study, with data extracted from 4 prospective studies, is satisfying, with good to very good agreement when compared to manual delineation during radiation therapy.

This study has several limitations. We have a limited number of patients because all patients had to have a per-radiotherapy PET/CT with persistent 42Gy fixation. If you want to increase the dose to a low volume, it is important to define it precisely and the use of 4D PET could be interesting in this context. All patients were included in studies in which 4D PET was not requested. However, the large volumes or node volumes in the case of radiochemotherapy are not very mobile.

With this method, only one dose level is possible but dose painting techniques could be interesting with heterogeneous doses depending on the FDG fixation. The dose painting could take into account the dose in relation to the FDG fixation but also the dose to be

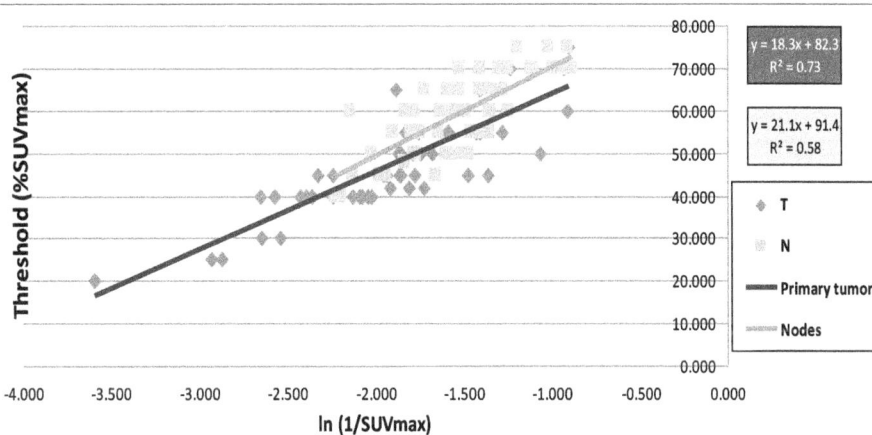

Fig. 2 Each lesion is represented as a diamond for lung lesions and a square for involved lymph nodes. Th_{opt}, the optimal threshold to be applied for delineation is expressed as a linear regression such as $Th_{opt} = A.[\ln (1/SUV_{max})] + B$ of the maximum standard uptake value (SUV_{max}). The expression of Th_{opt} for lung lesions and lymph nodes are presented with their respective coefficient of determination R^2

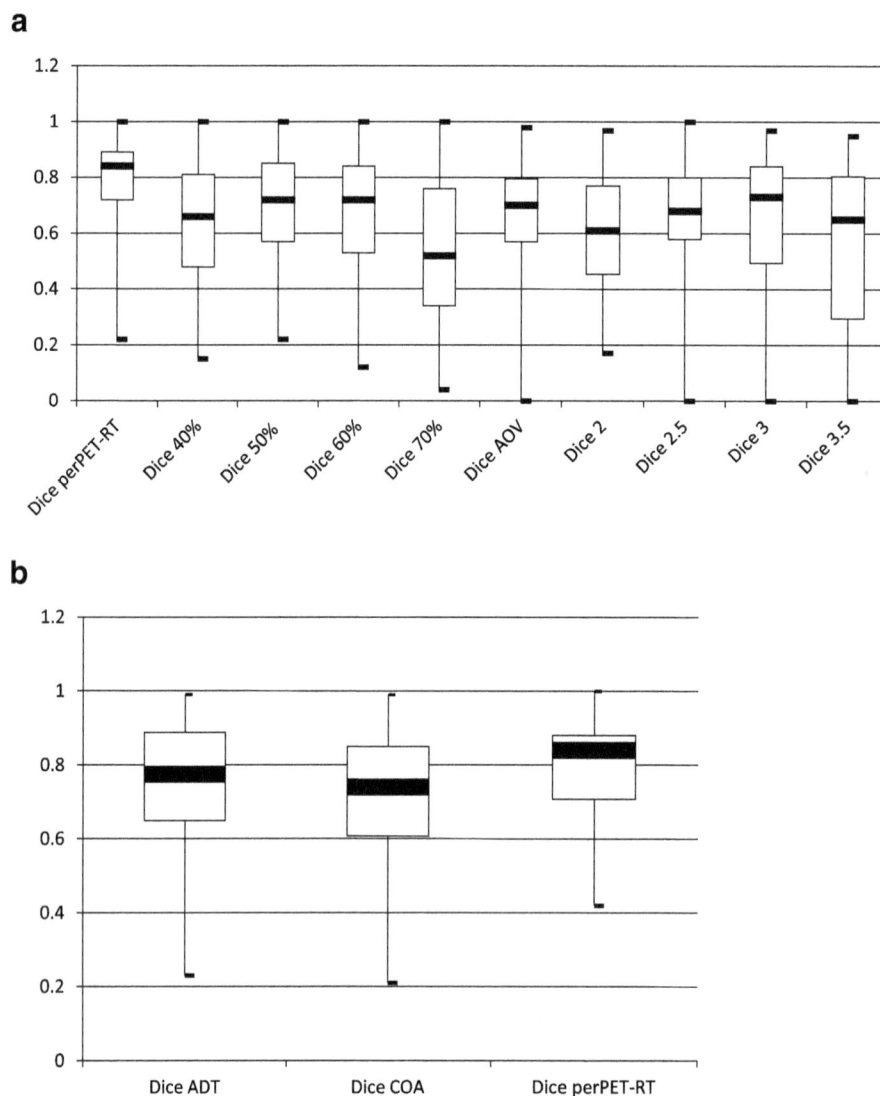

Fig. 3 Descriptive statistics of DSC for each segmentation methods represented as Box-and-whisker plots for perPET-RT, AOV and fixed thresholding methods for the 111 lesions (**a**) and for perPET-RT, ADT and COA for the 70 lesions observed on the Biograph Hi-Rez (**b**)

delivered to organs at risk, particularly for lymph node fixation.

Despite combination of chemotherapy and radiation therapy, survival rates remain poor for stage III NSCLC [34, 35]. Patients with locally advanced NSCLC have a very high risk of relapse and/or progression leading to death within the year if they express high metabolic profiles on a per-therapeutic PET/CT scans performed during the fifth week of radiation therapy [12]. The dose-escalation on a smaller volume delineated on the per-therapeutic PET/CT is aiming for a better local control of the disease and to avoid exacerbated early and late toxicity. Nevertheless, this concept is altered the lack of available FDG PET segmentation methods in clinical routine adapted to per-therapeutic FDG PET/CT

(around 43 Gy). A randomized phase II dose-escalation trial demonstrated the feasibility of significant dose-escalation on the primary tumour or the high FDG uptake subvolume of the primary tumour without violating the dose constraints for the organs at risk [36]. Dose-escalation planning based on interim FDG PET/CT scans (around 50 Gy of radiation therapy) is feasible, but none of the semi-automatic segmenting tools (including threshold of 2.5, 40% of SUV_{max} or AOV method) seemed reliable to define volumes correctly [37]. All the methods developed have essentially been developed for tumors more than for lymph node fixation and for tumors before treatment. Radiation therapy modifies the tumor to background ratio. In our study, there was a good agreement between the different methods, but the perPET-RT method had the best agreement with the experts. The ADT method was not significantly different from our method, this is probably due to the fact that it was developed specifically for lung cancers as in our case.

In addition, ongoing clinical trials are evaluating the impact of dose escalation on progression-free survival and overall survival. One of them [32] proposes to increase the dose to hypoxic tumoral areas. Another current clinical trial, lead by the RTOG group, seeks to determine if the dose to the tumour can be increased when a personalized radiation treatment is planned with a PET/CT scan acquired at 40–46 Gy of radiotherapy in patients with inoperable or unresectable stage III NSCLC. The method used for tumoral volume delineation corresponds to the AOV method [38].

PerPET-RT is one of the thresholding-based approaches which are the most widely available techniques in clinical routine. It requires knowing the type of lesion (primary or node) and the measurement of SUV_{max}, which is, in practice, easier and more reproducible than thresholding methods based on contrast (COA and ADT) or a mean SUV measurement (AOV). Another advantage of perPET-RT is that there is no need to calibrate the method on PET/CT models, unlike many adaptive thresholding methods. In our database, the method was not sensitive to the generation of PET models. This result has to be confirmed on other databases. Nevertheless, the concept of using such an approach in clinical routine or in mono or multicentre clinical trials is possible and easy to implement. As gold standard, a consensus threshold value was used. Palie et al. showed that there was an excellent reproducibility in delineation of MTVs by the physicians [39]. In addition, a recently published study demonstrated the added value of consensus methods in delineation [23]. PerPET-RT was compared with other thresholding methods (fixed or adaptive) due to the ease of use of these techniques. On the other hand, more sophisticated algorithms were not used due to the lack of availability in the context of multicenter clinical trials.

The clinical impact of dose-escalation on the volumes defined by this method is yet to be evaluated by a recently started multicentre clinical trial [40].

Conclusion

PerPET-RT, a thresholding-based approach, was proposed and validated on 4 prospective studies. We have showed that this method is reliable, easy to use and accurate for tumoral delineation on per-therapeutic FDG PET/CT. This method may be used to delineate tumoral volumes for dose-escalation planning. A clinical trial evaluating the impact of dose-escalation radiation therapy in NSCLC has already started in France (PHRC 2014, IFCT 1402-RTEP7).

Appendix

Table 3 New generation PET/CT devices with their respective system characteristics and the number of patients per device

Type of PET/CT device	Constructor	Number of patients and lesions (tumor, node)	Reconstruction algorithm with point-spread function	ToF system
Gemini TF	Philips	3 (2, 4)	Yes	Yes
GE 690	General Electrics	8 (8, 12)	Yes	Yes
Biograph mCT 40	Siemens	4 (3, 2)	Yes	Yes
Biograph 6	Siemens	4 (4, 1)	Yes	No
Biograph mCT	Siemens	2 (2, 3)	Yes	Yes

Abbreviations
FDG: fluorine 18 fluorodeoxyglucose; MTV: metabolic tumour volume; NSCLC: non-small cell lung cancer; PET/CT: positron emission tomography/computed tomography; SUV_{max} : the maximum standard uptake value

Acknowledgements
Not applicable.

Funding
Not applicable.

Disclosure
No potential conflict of interest relevant for this article was reported.

Authors' contributions
JG, IG, and ST wrote the article. RM collected the data. ST, JG and PV have been working on data. SH has been working on PET data quality. All authors read and approved the final manuscript.

Competing interests
The authors declare that they have no competing interests.

Author details
[1]Nuclear Medicine Department, Henri Becquerel Cancer Centre and Rouen University Hospital, Rouen, France. [2]QuantIF-LITIS (EA [Equipe d'Accueil] 4108-FR CNRS [Fédération de Recherche-Centre National pour la Recherche Scientifique] 3638), Faculty of Medicine, University of Rouen, Rouen, France. [3]Department of Radiotherapy and Medical Physics, Henri Becquerel Cancer Centre and Rouen University Hospital, Rouen, France.

References
1. PDQ Adult Treatment Editorial Board. Non-small cell lung Cancer treatment (PDQ®): health professional version. In: PDQ Cancer information summaries. Bethesda: National Cancer Institute (US); 2002. http://www.ncbi.nlm.nih.gov/books/NBK65865/.

2. Albain KS, Swann RS, Rusch VW, Turrisi AT, Shepherd FA, Smith C, et al. Radiotherapy plus chemotherapy with or without surgical resection for stage III non-small-cell lung cancer: a phase III randomised controlled trial. Lancet Lond Engl. 2009;374(9687):379–86.

3. Goldstraw P, Ball D, Jett JR, Le Chevalier T, Lim E, Nicholson AG, et al. Non-small-cell lung cancer. Lancet Lond Engl. 2011;378(9804):1727–40.

4. Jarritt PH, Carson KJ, Hounsell AR, Visvikis D. The role of PET/CT scanning in radiotherapy planning. Br J Radiol sept 2006;79 Spec No 1:S27–S35.

5. Boellaard R, Delgado-Bolton R, Oyen WJG, Giammarile F, Tatsch K, Eschner W, et al. FDG PET/CT: EANM procedure guidelines for tumour imaging: version 2.0. Eur J Nucl Med Mol Imaging. 2015;42(2):328–54.

6. van Baardwijk A, Bosmans G, Boersma L, Buijsen J, Wanders S, Hochstenbag M, et al. PET-CT-based auto-contouring in non-small-cell lung cancer correlates with pathology and reduces interobserver variability in the delineation of the primary tumor and involved nodal volumes. Int J Radiat Oncol Biol Phys. 2007;68(3):771–8.

7. Schreurs LMA, Busz DM, Paardekooper GMRM, Beukema JC, Jager PL, Van der Jagt EJ, et al. Impact of 18-fluorodeoxyglucose positron emission tomography on computed tomography defined target volumes in radiation treatment planning of esophageal cancer: reduction in geographic misses with equal inter-observer variability: PET/CT improves esophageal target definition. Dis Esophagus Off J Int Soc Dis Esophagus ISDE. 2010;23(6):493–501.

8. Bradley JD, Paulus R, Komaki R, Masters G, Blumenschein G, Schild S, et al. Standard-dose versus high-dose conformal radiotherapy with concurrent and consolidation carboplatin plus paclitaxel with or without cetuximab for patients with stage IIIA or IIIB non-small-cell lung cancer (RTOG 0617): a randomised, two-by-two factorial phase 3 study. Lancet Oncol. 2015;16(2):187–99.

9. Aerts HJWL, van Baardwijk AAW, Petit SF, Offermann C, van LJ, Houben R, et al. Identification of residual metabolic-active areas within individual NSCLC tumours using a pre-radiotherapy (18) Fluorodeoxyglucose-PET-CT scan. Radiother Oncol J Eur Soc Ther Radiol Oncol. 2009;91(3):386–92.

10. Calais J, Thureau S, Dubray B, Modzelewski R, Thiberville L, Gardin I, et al. Areas of high 18F-FDG uptake on preradiotherapy PET/CT identify preferential sites of local relapse after chemoradiotherapy for non-small cell lung cancer. J Nucl Med Off Publ Soc Nucl Med. 2015;56(2):196–203.

11. Edet-Sanson A, Dubray B, Doyeux K, Back A, Hapdey S, Modzelewski R, et al. Serial assessment of FDG-PET FDG uptake and functional volume during radiotherapy (RT) in patients with non-small cell lung cancer (NSCLC). Radiother Oncol J Eur Soc Ther Radiol Oncol. 2012;102(2):251–7.

12. Vera P, Mezzani-Saillard S, Edet-Sanson A, Ménard J-F, Modzelewski R, Thureau S, et al. FDG PET during radiochemotherapy is predictive of outcome at 1 year in non-small-cell lung cancer patients: a prospective multicentre study (RTEP2). Eur J Nucl Med Mol Imaging. 2014;41(6):1057–65.

13. Kong FM, Ten Haken RK, Schipper M, Frey KA, Hayman J, Gross M, et al. Effect of Midtreatment PET/CT-adapted radiation therapy with concurrent chemotherapy in patients with locally advanced non-small-cell lung Cancer: a phase 2 clinical trial. JAMA Oncol. 2017;3(10):1358–65. https://doi.org/10.1001/jamaoncol.2017.0982.

14. Hatt M, Visvikis D. Defining radiotherapy target volumes using 18F-fluoro-deoxy-glucose positron emission tomography/computed tomography: still a Pandora's box?: in regard to Devic et al. (Int J Radiat Oncol Biol Phys 2010). Int J Radiat Oncol Biol Phys. 2010;78(5):1605.

15. Paulino AC, Johnstone PAS. FDG-PET in radiotherapy treatment planning: Pandora's box? Int J Radiat Oncol Biol Phys. 2004;59(1):4–5.

16. Nestle U, Schaefer-Schuler A, Kremp S, Groeschel A, Hellwig D, Rübe C, et al. Target volume definition for 18F-FDG PET-positive lymph nodes in radiotherapy of patients with non-small cell lung cancer. Eur J Nucl Med Mol Imaging. 2007;34(4):453–62.

17. Erdi YE, Mawlawi O, Larson SM, Imbriaco M, Yeung H, Finn R, et al. Segmentation of lung lesion volume by adaptive positron emission tomography image thresholding. Cancer. 1997;80(12 Suppl):2505–9.

18. Boellaard R, Krak NC, Hoekstra OS, Lammertsma AA. Effects of noise, image resolution, and ROI definition on the accuracy of standard uptake values: a simulation study. J Nucl med off Publ Soc. Nucl. Med. 2004;45(9):1519–27.

19. Krak NC, Boellaard R, Hoekstra OS, Twisk JWR, Hoekstra CJ, Lammertsma AA. Effects of ROI definition and reconstruction method on quantitative outcome and applicability in a response monitoring trial. Eur J Nucl Med Mol Imaging. 2005;32(3):294–301.

20. Doyeux K, Vauclin S, Hapdey S, Daouk J, Edet-Sanson A, Vera P, et al. Reproducibility of the adaptive thresholding calibration procedure for the delineation of 18F-FDG-PET-positive lesions. Nucl Med Commun may. 2013;34(5):432–8.

21. Schaefer A, Kremp S, Hellwig D, Rübe C, Kirsch C-M, Nestle U. A contrast-oriented algorithm for FDG-PET-based delineation of tumour volumes for the radiotherapy of lung cancer: derivation from phantom measurements and validation in patient data. Eur J Nucl Med Mol Imaging. 2008;35(11):1989–99.

22. Thureau S, Chaumet-Riffaud P, Modzelewski R, Fernandez P, Tessonnier L, Vervueren L, et al. Interobserver agreement of qualitative analysis and tumor delineation of 18F-fluoromisonidazole and 3′-deoxy-3′-18F-fluorothymidine PET images in lung cancer. J Nucl Med Off Publ Soc Nucl Med. 2013;54(9):1543–50.

23. Schaefer A, Vermandel M, Baillet C, Dewalle-Vignion AS, Modzelewski R, Vera P, et al. Impact of consensus contours from multiple PET segmentation methods on the accuracy of functional volume delineation. Eur J Nucl Med Mol Imaging. 2016;43(5):911–24.

24. Vauclin S, Doyeux K, Hapdey S, Edet-Sanson A, Vera P, Gardin I. Development of a generic thresholding algorithm for the delineation of 18FDG-PET-positive tissue: application to the comparison of three thresholding models. Phys med biol. 2009;54(22):6901.

25. Geets X, Lee JA, Bol A, Lonneux M, Grégoire V. A gradient-based method for segmenting FDG-PET images: methodology and validation. Eur J Nucl Med Mol Imaging. 2007;34(9):1427–38.

26. Onoma DP, Ruan S, Thureau S, Nkhali L, Modzelewski R, Monnehan GA, et al. Segmentation of heterogeneous or small FDG PET positive tissue based on a 3D-locally adaptive random walk algorithm. Comput Med Imaging Graph Off J Comput Med Imaging Soc dec. 2014;38(8):753–63.

27. Belhassen S, Zaidi H. A novel fuzzy C-means algorithm for unsupervised heterogeneous tumor quantification in PET. Med Phys mar. 2010;37(3):1309–24.

28. Dewalle-Vignion A-S, Betrouni N, Lopes R, Huglo D, Stute S, Vermandel M. A new method for volume segmentation of PET images, based on possibility theory. IEEE Trans Med Imaging. 2011;30(2):409–23.

29. Hatt M, Cheze le Rest C, Turzo A, Roux C, Visvikis D. A fuzzy locally adaptive Bayesian segmentation approach for volume determination in PET. IEEE Trans Med Imaging 2009;28(6):881–893.

30. Zaidi H, El Naqa I. PET-guided delineation of radiation therapy treatment volumes: a survey of image segmentation techniques. Eur J Nucl Med Mol Imaging. 2010;37(11):2165–87.

31. Vera P, Bohn P, Edet-Sanson A, Salles A, Hapdey S, Gardin I, et al. Simultaneous positron emission tomography (PET) assessment of metabolism with 18F-fluoro-2-deoxy-d-glucose (FDG), proliferation with 18F-fluoro-thymidine (FLT), and hypoxia with 18fluoro-misonidazole (F-miso) before and during radiotherapy in patients with non-small-cell lung cancer (NSCLC): a pilot study. Radiother Oncol jan. 2011;98(1):109–16.

32. Radiotherapy Dose Complement in the Treatment of Hypoxic Lesions Patients With Stage III Non-small-cell Lung Cancer - ClinicalTrials.gov. https://clinicaltrials.gov/ct2/show/NCT01576796?term=rtep&rank=6

33. Zar J. Biostatiscal analysis. 2nd ed. La Jolla: Prentice-Hall; 1984.

34. Aupérin A, Le Péchoux C, Rolland E, Curran WJ, Furuse K, Fournel P, et al. Meta-analysis of concomitant versus sequential radiochemotherapy in locally advanced non-small-cell lung cancer. J Clin Oncol Off J Am Soc Clin Oncol. 2010;28(13):2181–90.

35. Curran WJ, Paulus R, Langer CJ, Komaki R, Lee JS, Hauser S, et al. Sequential vs. concurrent chemoradiation for stage III non-small cell lung cancer: randomized phase III trial RTOG 9410. J Natl Cancer Inst. 2011;103(19):1452–60.

36. van Elmpt W, De Ruysscher D, van der Salm A, Lakeman A, van der Stoep J, Emans D, et al. The PET-boost randomised phase II dose-escalation trial in non-small cell lung cancer. Radiother Oncol J Eur Soc Ther Radiol Oncol. 2012;104(1):67–71.

37. Kelsey CR, Christensen JD, Chino JP, Adamson J, Ready NE, Perez BA. Adaptive planning using positron emission tomography for locally advanced lung cancer: a feasibility study. Pract Radiat Oncol. 2016;6(2):96–104.

38. Study of Positron Emission Tomography and Computed Tomography in Guiding Radiation Therapy in Patients With Stage III Non-small Cell Lung Cancer - ClinicalTrials.gov https://clinicaltrials.gov/ct2/show/NCT01507428?term=rtog+1106&rank=1.

39. Palie O, Michel P, Ménard J-F, Rousseau C, Rio E, Bridji B, et al. The predictive value of treatment response using FDG PET performed on day 21 of chemoradiotherapy in patients with oesophageal squamous cell carcinoma. A prospective, multicentre study (RTEP3). Eur J Nucl Med Mol Imaging. 2013;40(9):1345–55.

40. Study of Interest of Personalized Radiotherapy Dose Redistribution in Patients With Stage III NSCLC - ClinicalTrials.gov https://clinicaltrials.gov/ct2/show/NCT02473133?term=lung+rouen+pet&rank=6

24

Relation of baseline neutrophil-to-lymphocyte ratio to survival and toxicity in head and neck cancer patients treated with (chemo-) radiation

Beat Bojaxhiu[1,5]* [iD], Arnoud J. Templeton[2,5]*, Olgun Elicin[1], Mohamed Shelan[1], Kathrin Zaugg[4], Marc Walser[5], Roland Giger[3], Daniel M. Aebersold[1] and Alan Dal Pra[1]

Abstract

Background: A high neutrophil-to-lymphocyte ratio (NLR) is a marker of systemic inflammation and together with the platelet-to-lymphocyte ratio (PLR) is associated with worse outcomes in several solid tumors. We investigated the prognostic value of NLR and PLR in patients with head and neck squamous cell carcinoma (HNSCC) treated with primary or adjuvant (chemo)radiotherapy ((C)RT).

Methods: A retrospective chart review of consecutive patients with HNSCC was performed. Neutrophil-to-lymphocyte ratio and PLR were computed using complete blood counts (CBCs) performed within 10 days before treatment start. The prognostic role of NLR and PLR was evaluated with univariable and multivariable Cox regression analyses adjusting for disease-specific prognostic factors. NLR and PLR were assessed as log-transformed continuous variables (log NLR and log PLR). Endpoints of interest were overall survival (OS), locoregional recurrence-free survival (LRFS), distant recurrence-free survival (DRFS), and acute toxicity.

Results: We analyzed 186 patients treated from 2007 to 2010. Primary sites were oropharynx (45%), oral cavity (28%), hypopharynx (14%), and larynx (13%). Median follow-up was 49 months. Higher NLR was associated with OS (adjusted HR per 1 unit higher log NLR = 1.81 (1.16–2.81), $p = 0.012$), whereas no association could be shown with LRFS (HR = 1.49 (0,83-2,68), $p = 0.182$), DRFS (HR = 1.38 (0.65–3.22), $p = 0.4$), or acute toxicity grade ≥ 2. PLR was not associated with outcome, nor with toxicity.

Conclusion: Our data suggest that in HNSCC patients treated with primary or adjuvant (C)RT, NLR is an independent predictor of mortality, but not disease-specific outcomes or toxicity. Neutrophil-to-lymphocyte ratio is a readily available biomarker that could improve pre-treatment prognostication and may be used for risk-stratification.

Keywords: Head and neck, Squamous cell carcinoma, Inflammation, Neutrophil-to-lymphocyte ratio, Platelet-to-lymphocyte ratio, Toxicity

* Correspondence: beat.bojaxhiu@psi.ch; arnoud.templeton@claraspital.ch
[1]Department of Radiation Oncology, Inselspital, Bern University Hospital and University of Bern, Freiburgstrasse, 3010 Bern, Switzerland
[2]Department of Medical Oncology, St. Claraspital Basel and Faculty of Medicine, University of Basel, Basel, Switzerland
Full list of author information is available at the end of the article

Background

Risk stratification of patients diagnosed with head and neck squamous cell carcinoma (HNSCC) poses an important challenge [1]. Currently, some of the widely used factors are smoking and human papillomavirus (HPV) status, age, performance status, and tumor stage. Nomograms based on baseline characteristics can enhance prognostic prediction [2].

Inflammation is a hallmark of cancer [3], which is shown to play an important role in tumor development and progression [4–6]. An elevation of circulating neutrophil count is thought to be the result of tumor cells releasing cytokines, which stimulate the bone marrow to produce neutrophils [7–9]. Cytokines released by neutrophils also promote angiogenesis leading to tumor growth and metastasis [10–15]. There is an increasing interest in the use of hematological parameters as prognostic factors in malignancies. Neutrophil, lymphocyte, and platelet counts, either as individual values or in relation to each other, could be associated with the cancer prognosis [16, 17]. The neutrophil-to-lymphocyte ratio (NLR) is an emerging marker of host inflammation, which reflects the relation between circulating neutrophil and lymphocyte counts. It can be easily calculated from routine complete blood counts (CBCs) with differentiation. The independent prognostic value of NLR has been shown for a variety of solid malignancies [17–20]. In addition to NLR, the platelet-to-lymphocyte ratio (PLR) has also been shown to be a potential prognostic factor [2, 19]. Several studies involving HNSCC have shown an association between inflammation and worse prognosis [21–27]. However, information about the possible value of pretreatment NLR or PLR on toxicity is limited [18–29].

In this study, we retrospectively evaluated the prognostic impact of pretreatment NLR and PLR on oncological outcomes and toxicity in HNSCC patients treated with primary or adjuvant curative-intended (chemo-) radiotherapy ((C)RT). We hypothesized that elevated NLR and/or PLR are associated with detrimental survival; we also explored NRL and PLR associations with acute treatment-related toxicity since it has prognostic value in primary and adjuvant (C)RT for HNSCC [30, 31].

Methods

Patient selection

Medical records of HNSCC patients consecutively treated with primary or adjuvant curative-intent intensity-modulated radiation therapy with or without concomitant systemic therapy between January 2007 and December 2010 at the Department of Radiation Oncology, Inselspital, Bern University Hospital were retrospectively analyzed. Patients diagnosed with oral cavity (OCC), oropharynx (OC), hypopharynx (HC) and laryngeal cancers (LC) were included in the analysis. History of another malignancy within 5 years of diagnosis, prior radiation to the head and neck, non-squamous cell carcinoma histology, distant metastases, lack of differentiated CBC within 10 days before oncologic surgery or RT start, and early abortion of RT were defined as exclusion criteria. This study was approved by the local ethics committee (289/2014).

Treatment and follow-up

The standard treatment was based on institutional policies following the multidisciplinary tumor board decision as previously published [32, 33]. All cases were presented at the weekly institutional interdisciplinary head-and-neck tumor board. After completion of staging examinations and final TNM staging (AJCC), selection of treatment modalities and treatment sequencing were defined. The standard treatment in OCC was to perform surgery followed by adjuvant radiotherapy (RT) [30, 32], while in OC, HC and LC the joint recommendations of the multidisciplinary meeting was primary RT [31, 33]. Case-based decisions were made concerning the use of concomitant systemic therapy and up-front neck dissection. The delivery of radiotherapy, the definition of clinical target volume (CTV) and planned target volume (PTV) followed departmental guidelines [32, 33] based on international recommendations [34–36]. All treatment plans were contoured and calculated using Eclipse treatment planning system (Varian Medical Systems, Palo Alto, CA). The standard concomitant therapy consisted of cisplatin 100 mg/m2 day 1 in three-week intervals for all patients. In few cases of induction chemotherapy, cisplatin, docetaxel, and 5-fluorouracil were used. Patients not deemed medically fit for cisplatin chemotherapy because of pre-existing co-morbidities were evaluated for weekly treatment with monoclonal antibody cetuximab [37] or carboplatin three weekly. Pre-treatment CBC with differential values was used to calculate NLR and PLR.

Potential causes of changes in the CBC (e.g. infection, steroid use) were identified, and patients were excluded from the analysis. Patients were regularly followed, and toxicities were graded according to the National Cancer Institute (NCI) Common Terminology Criteria for Adverse Events (CTCAE) version 4.03 (https://evs.nci.nih.gov/ftp1/CTCAE/CTCAE_4.03/CTCAE_4.03_2010-06-14_QuickReference_5x7.pdf).

Statistical analysis

NLR was calculated by dividing absolute neutrophil count by absolute lymphocyte count measured in peripheral blood. PLR was calculated by dividing absolute thrombocyte count by absolute lymphocyte count. Due

Table 1 Patients' and disease characteristics

Age	
median (range), years	61 (41–88)
≤ 60, N (%)	86 (46)
> 60 to ≤70, N (%)	64 (34)
> 70 to ≤80, N (%)	27 (15)
> 80, N (%)	9 (5)
Gender, N (%)	
female	40 (22)
male	146 (79)
Smoking status	
never smoker	17 (6)
previous smoker	33 (31)
current smoker	58 (54)
missing	108
High risk alcohol consumption	
No	49 (46)
Yes	54 (51)
in the past	4 (4)
missing	79
Karnofsky Performance Status	
median (range)	90 (50–100)
> 70, N (%)	160 (86)
≤ 70, N (%)	26 (14)
Oncological resection of primary tumor	
yes	56 (30)
no	130 (70)
Induction chemotherapy	
yes	15 (8)
no	171 (92
Concomitant systemic therapy	
no	38 (20)
cisplatin or carboplatin	125 (67)
cetuximab	23 (12)
Site of primary tumor, N (%)	
oral cavity	52 (28)
oropharynx	83 (45)
hypopharynx	27 (15)
larynx	24 (13)
UICC stage, N (%)	
I	5 (3)
II	11 (6)
III	44 (24)
IV	126 (68)

Table 1 Patients' and disease characteristics *(Continued)*

Tumor grade, N (%)	
G1	1 (1)
G2	113 (61)
G3	72 (39)
Hemoglobin (g/dL)	
median (IQR)	13.3 (12.0–14.4)
missing	12
Neutrophil-to-lymphocyte ratio	
median (IQR)	3.28 (2.15–4.70)
missing	20
Platelet-to-lymphocyte ratio	
median (IQR)	189 (136–254)
missing	20

IQR inter-quartile range, *UICC* Union for International Cancer Control

to its non-normal distribution, NLR and PLR were $\log_e$-transformed to obtain symmetric distributions and then analyzed as continuous variables. Frequencies and percentages are reported for categorical variables, medians with range or interquartile range for continuous variables. The primary endpoint of the study was overall survival (OS), and the secondary endpoints were locoregional relapse-free survival (LRFS) and distant recurrence-free survival (DRFS). Time-to-event was calculated for OS, LRFS, and DRFS from the start of RT to death (OS), locoregional relapse (LRFS), and distant recurrence (DRFS), respectively, with censoring of patients without such events at last follow up. Median times to event were estimated using the Kaplan Meier method. The prognostic value of NLR and PLR, and other variables (i.e. age, gender, smoking status, Karnofsky Performance Status (KPS), UICC stage, tumor grade, hemoglobin level) were assessed by univariable Cox regression analysis. Subsequently, multivariable analysis with forward elimination was planned with inclusion of all variables with a p-value < 0.05 in the univariable analysis. The association of NLR and PLR with acute and late toxicities (i.e. pain, dermatitis, mucositis, dysphagia, xerostomia) was examined using logistic regression. Analyses were carried out using SPSS version 23 (IBM Corp., Chicago, IL). The threshold for statistical significance was set at $p < 0.05$, and no correction for multiple testing was performed.

Results

Patients

One hundred and eighty-six patients were included in the study. Patients' and disease characteristics are presented in Table 1. The majority of patients were male and in good performance status (KPS ≥ 70). The primary tumor was located in the oral cavity or oropharynx in approximately 75% of the cases, and more than half of all patients had UICC stage IVA or IVB disease. Median NLR and PLR were 3.28 and 189, respectively. There was a statistically significant correlation between NLR and PLR (Spearman's rho = 0.65, $p < 0.001$). Baseline NLR and PLR were not associated with gender, smoking status, site of the primary tumor, stage of disease or tumor grade.

Overall survival

At a median follow-up time of 40 months, 60 patients (32%) died; median OS was not reached. Higher NLR was associated with lower OS (Table 2). When dividing the population into two groups according to the median NLR, there was a significant OS difference between the groups (Fig. 1). For PLR there was a non-significant association between higher PLR and lower OS (Fig. 2). On univariable analysis $\log_e$ NLR was associated with OS. Also, older age, worse Karnofsky Performance Status (KPS ≤ 70), and UICC stage IV were associated with lower OS. Performance status, UICC stage IV and $\log_e$ NLR remained of prognostic value in multivariable analysis (Table 2).

Recurrence

Of the variables tested, only UICC stage IV was associated with increased loco-regional, distant, and any recurrence rate, whereas no association was found for all other variables tested (Table 3). Consequently, no multivariable analyses were conducted. In patients with high NLR, recurrences occurred earlier, but the correlation was not statistically significant (Fig. 3).

Toxicity

Rates and grades of the most common acute toxicities are summarized in Table 4. There was no correlation

between baseline NLR or PLR and the grade of toxicity (data not shown).

Discussion

NLR is the object of numerous previously published studies. Not only in oncology but also in other disciplines, blood counts reflecting the complexity of the immune system can be easily obtained at low costs, which may impact daily clinical practice. About 15–20% of all cancer deaths worldwide seem to be associated with underlying infections and inflammatory reactions [38]. Many triggers of chronic inflammation increase the risk of developing cancer. These triggers, for example, include microbial infections such as Helicobacter pylori (associated with stomach cancer), inflammatory bowel disease (associated with bowel cancer) and prostatitis (associated with prostate cancer) [38]. Despite conflicting studies, treatment with non-steroidal anti-inflammatory agents has been associated with reduced cancer incidence and mortality [38–41]. Increased NLR is associated with poorer outcomes in many solid tumors, be it early or advanced stage cancer [17]. An early decrease in NLR may be associated with more favorable outcomes and higher response rates [42], whereas an increase in NLR in the first weeks of treatment had the opposite effect [42].

In this study with a relatively large cohort of HNSCC patients treated with (C)RT with curative intention, an elevated NLR at baseline was associated with a shorter OS but not with disease recurrence or toxicities. Our findings of a negative prognostic role of NLR are in accordance with other studies [26, 43] that have investigated NLR in HNSCC. In contrast to our results, Rassouli et al. [44] have demonstrated a statistically significant impact of PLR on OS. Worth to note, such associations were observed at various cut-offs in different studies. They have also shown that an increased NLR was

Table 2 Univariable and multivariable Cox regression analysis of overall survival

		univariable analysis		multivariable analysis	
		HR (95% CI)	P	HR (95% CI)	P
Age	per 10 years older	1.32 (1.03–1.69)	0.026*		
Gender	male (vs. female)	1.17 (0.61–2.25)	0.639		
Smoking status	never smoker (vs. current/past)	0.66 (0.20–2.19)	0.492		
Karnofsky Performance Status	per 10 higher	0.76 (0.62–0.92)	0.005*	0.76 (0.62–0.98)	0.030*
UICC stage	IVA-B (vs. I-III)	1.87 (1.01–3.47)	0.045*		
Tumor grade	G3 (vs. G1-G2)	0.91 (0.54–1.54)	0.731		
Hemoglobin	per 1 g/dL higher	0.89 (0.77–1.04)	0.143		
log NLR	per 1 log NLR higher	1.81 (1.16–2.81)	0.009*	1.58 (1.01–2.47)	0.043*
log PLR	per 1 log PLR higher	1.62 (0.99–2.63)	0.054		

CI confidence interval, *G* tumor grade, *HR* hazard ratio, *log NLR* natural logarithm of neutrophil-to-lymphocyte ratio, *log PLR* natural logarithm of platelet-to-lymphocyte ratio, *UICC* Union for International Cancer Control; *statistically significant

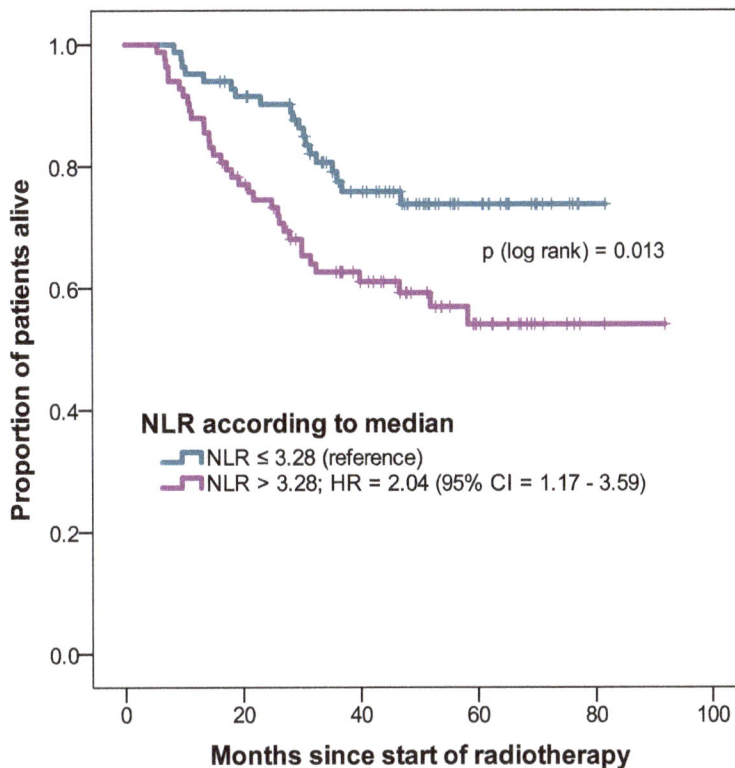

Fig. 1 Overall survival of NLR higher than median vs. equal or lower than median

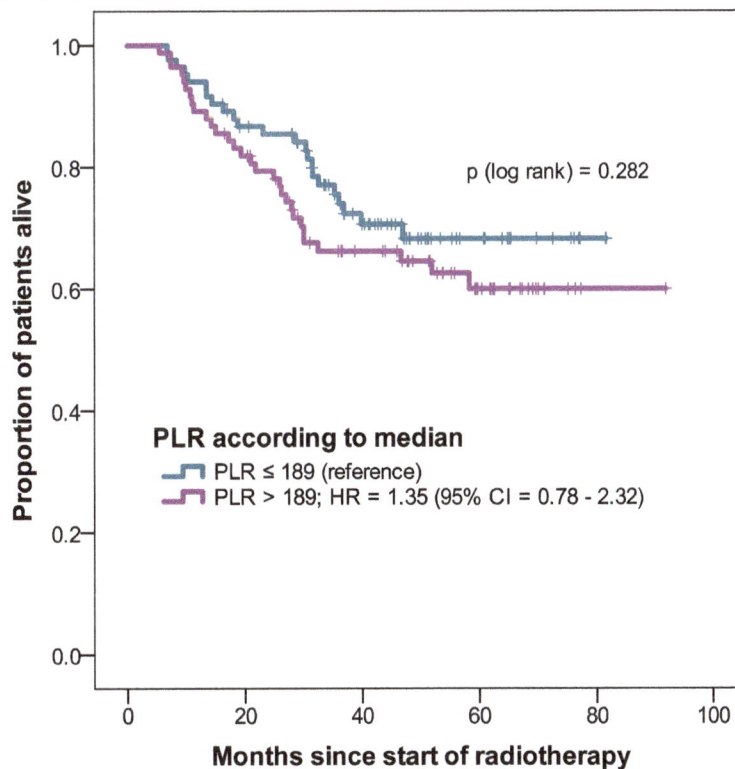

Fig. 2 Overall survival of PLR higher than median vs. equal or lower than median

Table 3 Univariable Cox regression analysis of recurrence

		Univariable analysis	
		HR (95% CI)	P
Loco-regional recurrence (38 events)			
Age	per 10 years older	1.08 (0.80–1.48)	0.607
Gender	male vs. female	1.21 (0.53–2.75)	0.648
Smoking status	never smoker (vs. current/past)	1.68 (0.34–8.31)	0.526
Karnofsky Performance Status	KPS over 70	0.55 (0.23–1.35)	0.191
UICC stage	IVA-B (vs. I-III)	3.43 (1.34–8.78)	0.010*
Tumor grade	G3 (vs. G1-G2)	0.78 (0.40–1.53)	0.477
Hemoglobin	per 1 g/dL higher	0.92 (0.76–1.13)	0.424
log NLR	per 1 log NLR higher	1.49 (0.83–2.68)	0.182
log PLR	per 1 log PLR higher	1.65 (0.88–3.10)	0.117
Distant recurrence (20 events)			
Age	per 10 years older	0.77 (0.49–1.22)	0.272
Gender	male	2.48 (0.57–10.7)	0.224
Smoking status	never smoker (vs. current/past)	0.04 (0.00–22.86)	0.314
Karnofsky Performance Status	KPS over 70	2.53 (0.34–18.94)	0.367
UICC stage	IV (vs. I-III)	9.91 (1.33–74.03)	0.025*
Tumor grade	G3 (vs. lower)	1.53 (0.64–3.68)	0.342
Hemoglobin	per 1 g/dL higher	1.11 (0.84–1.46)	0.472
log NLR	per 1 log NLR higher	1.38 (0.65–2.91)	0.400
log PLR	per 1 log PLR higher	1.44 (0.65–3.22)	0.371
Any recurrence (46 events)			
Age	per 10 years older	1.04 (0.78–1.28)	0.779
Gender	male	1.30 (0.61–2.79)	0.501
Smoking status	never smoker (vs. current/past)	0.60 (014–2.63)	0.501
Karnofsky Performance Status	KPS over 70	0.74 (0.33–1.65)	0.457
Localization	larynx or hypopharynx (vs. other)	1.24 (0.66–2.33)	0.497
UICC stage	IV (vs. I-III)	3.49 (1.48–8.24)	0.004*
Tumor grade	G3 (vs. G1-G2)	0.96 (0.53–1.74)	0.891
Hemoglobin	per 1 g/dL higher	0.95 (0.79–1.14)	0.948
log NLR	per 1 log NLR higher	1.49 (0.88–2.53)	0.134
log PLR	per 1 log PLR higher	1.55 (0.88–2.74)	0.128

CI confidence interval, *G* tumor grade, *HR* hazard ratio, *log NLR* natural logarithm of neutrophil-to-lymphocyte ratio, *log PLR* natural logarithm of platelet-to-lymphocyte ratio, *UICC* Union for International Cancer Control; *statistically significant*

not only associated with decreased OS but with higher recurrence rates too [44]; which was not shown in our cohort and another study from the United Kingdom [45].

Along with the increased NLR in malignant disease, a possible explanation for a lower OS could also be a cause of death not attributable to cancer, but other co-morbidities such as a cardiac cause where it could also be shown that an increased NLR is predictive for cardiac mortality [46]. It is also known that smokers have a "smoker's leukocytosis" [37, 38, 47, 48]. In our cohort, most patients are at least ex-smokers (80%), and at least one third continued smoking during and after

radiation. Therefore, it is possible that the patients with a smoker's leukocytosis have died earlier from smoking-related comorbidities [49].

Several limitations to our study should be considered. First, this was a retrospective analysis with possible selection bias and confounding variables. We included 16 patients (9%) with early-stage disease and 15 (8%) patients who had neoadjuvant chemotherapy, which may have introduced some heterogeneity to our cohort. Second, we were unable to capture data on HPV status systematically. Studies have shown an important interaction between HPV status, immunomodulation and

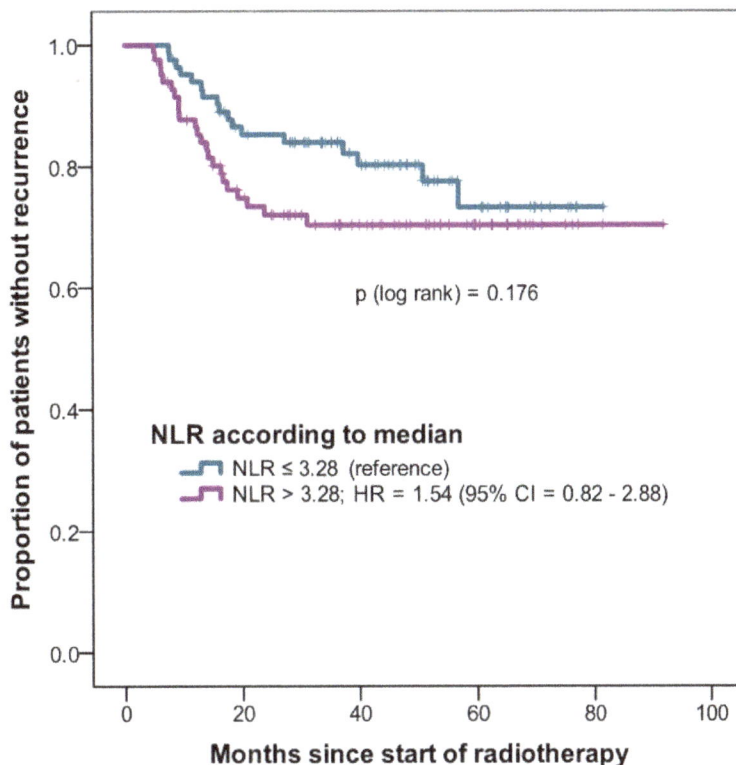

Fig. 3 Recurrence-free survival of NLR higher than median vs. equal or lower than median

clinical outcome [50]. Therefore, there might be different results in HPV-associated and unassociated tumors [51]. Since this is a retrospective study, there might be unknown causes of CBC changes that have not been identified. Beside patient and tumor-specific factors which may influence the complex cascades of the immune system, it must also be noted that despite clinical benefit, the dichotomization or grouping of continuous variables in statistical analysis is accompanied by a loss of the statistical power. To account for this, NLR and PLR were analyzed as (log-transformed) continuous variables. Lastly, an overestimation of statistical significance due to multiple testing is possible. Although these results should be validated in other cohorts, we reproduced some of the previously reported studies [26, 43] on the interface of systemic inflammatory pathways and OS. Therefore, we provide data on surrogate values for inflammation as predictors of clinical outcomes; however, a causal relationship and its impact on tumor aggressiveness or tumor microenvironment warrants further investigation.

Conclusion

Our data suggest that in HNSCC patients treated with primary or adjuvant (C)RT, NLR is an independent predictor of OS. NLR is a readily available biomarker that could improve pre-treatment risk stratification.

Table 4 Selected toxicities of 183 patients (toxicities of 3 patients missing)

	G1	G2	G3	G4
Symptoms prior to radiotherapy				
Pain	52 (28)	30 (16)	2 (1)	0
Dysphagia	52 (28)	32 (17)	11 (6)	0
Acute toxicities				
Pain	42 (23)	91 (49)	45 (24)	1 (1)
Dermatitis	44 (24)	117 (63)	22 (12)	0
Mucositis	31 (17)	110 (59)	40 (22)	0
Dysphagia	23 (12)	80 (43)	70 (38)	1 (1)
Xerostomia	63 (34)	8 (4)	0	0

Grades according to Common Terminology Criteria for Adverse Events (CTCAE) v4.03

Abbreviations

(C)RT: (Chemo)radiotherapy; CBCs: Complete blood counts; CI: Confidence interval; DRFS: Distant recurrence-free survival; G: Tumor grade; HC: Hypopharyngeal cancer; HNSCC: Head and neck squamous cell carcinoma; HR: Hazard ratio; IQR: Inter-quartile range; LC: Laryngeal cancer; log NLR: Natural logarithm of neutrophil-to-lymphocyte ratio; log PLR: Natural logarithm of platelet-to-lymphocyte ratio; LRFS: Locoregional recurrence-free survival; NLR: Neutrophil-to-lymphocyte ratio; OC: Oropharyngeal cancer; OCC: Oral cavity cancer; OS: Overall survival; PLR: Platelet-to-lymphocyte ratio; RT: Radiotherapy; UICC: Union for International Cancer Control

Acknowledgments

The authors thank Dr. Andreas Geretschläger and Dr. Michael Schmücking for their collaboration with the clinical data.

Funding

No funding was received.

Authors' contributions

Each author had participated sufficiently in the work to take public responsibility for appropriate portions of the content. AD, BB, and AT designed the study. AT performed the statistical analysis. BB collected the data and together with AT, KZ, OE, MW, MS, RG, and DMA interpreted the results. The manuscript was written by BB, AD and AT, and all other authors reviewed and finally approved the final manuscript.

Competing interests

No potential conflicts of interests are to declare.

Author details

[1]Department of Radiation Oncology, Inselspital, Bern University Hospital and University of Bern, Freiburgstrasse, 3010 Bern, Switzerland. [2]Department of Medical Oncology, St. Claraspital Basel and Faculty of Medicine, University of Basel, Basel, Switzerland. [3]Department of Otorhinolaryngology, Head and Neck Surgery, Inselspital, Bern University Hospital, Basel, Switzerland. [4]Department of Radiation Oncology, Stadtspital Triemli, Zürich, Switzerland. [5]Center for Proton Therapy, Paul Scherrer Institute, Villigen, Switzerland.

References

1. Curado MP, Boyle P. Epidemiology of head and neck squamous cell carcinoma not related to tobacco or alcohol. Curr Opin Oncol. 2013;25(3):229–34.
2. Templeton AJ, et al. Prognostic role of platelet to lymphocyte ratio in solid tumors: a systematic review and meta-analysis. Cancer Epidemiol Biomark Prev. 2014;23(7):1204–12.
3. Hanahan D, Weinberg RA. Hallmarks of cancer: the next generation. Cell. 2011;144(5):646–74.
4. Grivennikov SI, Greten FR, Karin M. Immunity, inflammation, and cancer. Cell. 2010;140(6):883–99.
5. O'Callaghan DS, et al. The role of inflammation in the pathogenesis of non-small cell lung cancer. J Thorac Oncol. 2010;5(12):2024–36.
6. Aggarwal BB, Vijayalekshmi RV, Sung B. Targeting inflammatory pathways for prevention and therapy of cancer: short-term friend, long-term foe. Clin Cancer Res. 2009;15(2):425–30.
7. Dumitru CA, Lang S, Brandau S. Modulation of neutrophil granulocytes in the tumor microenvironment: mechanisms and consequences for tumor progression. Semin Cancer Biol. 2013;23(3):141–8.
8. Tazzyman S, Niaz H, Murdoch C. Neutrophil-mediated tumour angiogenesis: subversion of immune responses to promote tumour growth. Semin Cancer Biol. 2013;23(3):149–58.
9. Ocana A, et al. Neutrophils in cancer: prognostic role and therapeutic strategies. Mol Cancer. 2017;16(1):137.
10. Bekes EM, et al. Tumor-recruited neutrophils and neutrophil TIMP-free MMP-9 regulate coordinately the levels of tumor angiogenesis and efficiency of malignant cell intravasation. Am J Pathol. 2011;179(3):1455–70.
11. Gregory AD, Houghton AM. Tumor-associated neutrophils: new targets for cancer therapy. Cancer Res. 2011;71(7):2411–6.
12. Demers M, Wagner DD. Neutrophil extracellular traps: a new link to cancer-associated thrombosis and potential implications for tumor progression. Oncoimmunology. 2013;2(2):e22946.
13. Cools-Lartigue J, et al. Neutrophil extracellular traps sequester circulating tumor cells and promote metastasis. J Clin Invest. 2013;123(8):3446–58.
14. Donskov F. Immunomonitoring and prognostic relevance of neutrophils in clinical trials. Semin Cancer Biol. 2013;23(3):200–7.
15. Tazzyman S, Lewis CE, Murdoch C. Neutrophils: key mediators of tumour angiogenesis. Int J Exp Pathol. 2009;90(3):222–31.
16. Takenaka Y, et al. Prognostic role of neutrophil-to-lymphocyte ratio in head and neck cancer: a meta-analysis. Head Neck. 2018;40(3):647-655.
17. Templeton AJ, et al. Prognostic role of neutrophil-to-lymphocyte ratio in solid tumors: a systematic review and meta-analysis. J Natl Cancer Inst. 2014;106(6):dju124.
18. Chowdhary M, et al. Post-treatment neutrophil-to-lymphocyte ratio predicts for overall survival in brain metastases treated with stereotactic radiosurgery. J Neuro-Oncol. 2018;139(3):689–97.
19. Proctor MJ, et al. A comparison of inflammation-based prognostic scores in patients with cancer. A Glasgow inflammation outcome study. Eur J Cancer. 2011;47(17):2633–41.
20. Guthrie GJ, et al. The systemic inflammation-based neutrophil-lymphocyte ratio: experience in patients with cancer. Crit Rev Oncol Hematol. 2013;88(1):218–30.
21. An X, et al. Elevated neutrophil to lymphocyte ratio predicts poor prognosis in nasopharyngeal carcinoma. Tumour Biol. 2011;32(2):317–24.
22. Fang HY, et al. Refining the role of preoperative C-reactive protein by neutrophil/lymphocyte ratio in oral cavity squamous cell carcinoma. Laryngoscope. 2013;123(11):2690–9.
23. He JR, et al. Pretreatment levels of peripheral neutrophils and lymphocytes as independent prognostic factors in patients with nasopharyngeal carcinoma. Head Neck. 2012;34(12):1769–76.
24. Khandavilli SD, et al. Serum C-reactive protein as a prognostic indicator in patients with oral squamous cell carcinoma. Oral Oncol. 2009;45(10):912–4.
25. Millrud CR, et al. The activation pattern of blood leukocytes in head and neck squamous cell carcinoma is correlated to survival. PLoS One. 2012;7(12):e51120.
26. Perisanidis C, et al. High neutrophil-to-lymphocyte ratio is an independent marker of poor disease-specific survival in patients with oral cancer. Med Oncol. 2013;30(1):334.
27. Grimm M, Lazariotou M. Clinical relevance of a new pre-treatment laboratory prognostic index in patients with oral squamous cell carcinoma. Med Oncol. 2012;29(3):1435–47.
28. Khoja L, et al. The full blood count as a biomarker of outcome and toxicity in ipilimumab-treated cutaneous metastatic melanoma. Cancer Med. 2016;5(10):2792–9.
29. Shaverdian N, et al. Pretreatment immune parameters predict for overall survival and toxicity in early-stage non-small-cell lung Cancer patients treated with stereotactic body radiation therapy. Clin Lung Cancer. 2016;17(1):39–46.
30. Wolff HA, et al. High-grade acute organ toxicity as positive prognostic factor in adjuvant radiation and chemotherapy for locally advanced head and neck cancer. Radiology. 2011;258(3):864–71.
31. Tehrany N, et al. High-grade acute organ toxicity and p16(INK4A) expression as positive prognostic factors in primary radio(chemo)therapy for patients with head and neck squamous cell carcinoma. Strahlenther Onkol. 2015;191(7):566–72.
32. Geretschläger A, et al. Outcome and patterns of failure after postoperative intensity modulated radiotherapy for locally advanced or high-risk oral cavity squamous cell carcinoma. Radiat Oncol. 2012;7:175.
33. Geretschläger A, et al. Definitive intensity modulated radiotherapy in locally advanced hypopharygeal and laryngeal squamous cell carcinoma: mature treatment results and patterns of locoregional failure. Radiat Oncol. 2015;10(1):20.
34. Gregoire V, et al. CT-based delineation of lymph node levels and related CTVs in the node-negative neck: DAHANCA, EORTC, GORTEC, NCIC, RTOG consensus guidelines. Radiother Oncol. 2003;69(3):227–36.
35. Eisbruch A, et al. Intensity-modulated radiation therapy for head and neck cancer: emphasis on the selection and delineation of the targets. Semin Radiat Oncol. 2002;12(3):238–49.
36. Eisbruch A, et al. Recurrences near base of skull after IMRT for head-and-neck cancer: implications for target delineation in high neck and for parotid gland sparing. Int J Radiat Oncol Biol Phys. 2004;59(1):28–42.
37. Bonner JA, et al. Radiotherapy plus cetuximab for squamous-cell carcinoma of the head and neck. N Engl J Med. 2006;354(6):567–78.
38. Mantovani A, et al. Cancer-related inflammation. Nature. 2008;454(7203):436–44.

39. Koehne CH, Dubois RN. COX-2 inhibition and colorectal cancer. Semin Oncol. 2004;31(2 7):12–21.

40. Flossmann E, et al. Effect of aspirin on long-term risk of colorectal cancer: consistent evidence from randomised and observational studies. Lancet. 2007;369(9573):1603–13.

41. Chan AT, Ogino S, Fuchs CS. Aspirin and the risk of colorectal cancer in relation to the expression of COX-2. N Engl J Med. 2007;356(21):2131–42.

42. Templeton AJ, et al. Change in neutrophil-to-lymphocyte ratio in response to targeted therapy for metastatic renal cell carcinoma as a prognosticator and biomarker of efficacy. Eur Urol. 2016;70(2):358–64.

43. Haddad CR, et al. Neutrophil-to-lymphocyte ratio in head and neck cancer. J Med Imaging Radiat Oncol. 2015;59(4):514–9.

44. Rassouli A, et al. Systemic inflammatory markers as independent prognosticators of head and neck squamous cell carcinoma. Head Neck. 2015;37(1):103–10.

45. Wong BY, et al. Prognostic value of the neutrophil-to-lymphocyte ratio in patients with laryngeal squamous cell carcinoma. Head Neck. 2016;38(1):E1903–8.

46. Kruk M, et al. Association of non-specific inflammatory activation with early mortality in patients with ST-elevation acute coronary syndrome treated with primary angioplasty. Circ J. 2008;72(2):205–11.

47. Kondo H, Kusaka Y, Morimoto K. Effects of lifestyle on hematologic parameters; I. analysis of hematologic data in association with smoking habit and age. Sangyo Igaku. 1993;35(2):98–104.

48. Kawada T. Smoking-induced leukocytosis can persist after cessation of smoking. Arch Med Res. 2004;35(3):246–50.

49. Friedman GD, Dales LG, Ury HK. Mortality in middle-aged smokers and nonsmokers. N Engl J Med. 1979;300(5):213–7.

50. Rachidi S, et al. Neutrophil-to-lymphocyte ratio and overall survival in all sites of head and neck squamous cell carcinoma. Head Neck. 2016;38 Suppl 1:E1068-74

51. Huang SH, et al. Prognostic value of pretreatment circulating neutrophils, monocytes, and lymphocytes in oropharyngeal cancer stratified by human papillomavirus status. Cancer. 2015;121(4):545–55.

25

A practical approach to estimating optic disc dose and macula dose without treatment planning in ocular brachytherapy using ^{125}I COMS plaques

Yongsook C. Lee, Shih-Chi Lin and Yongbok Kim[*]

Abstract

Background: It has been reported that proximity of the tumor to the optic disc and macula, and radiation dose to the critical structures are substantial risk factors for vision loss following plaque brachytherapy. However, there is little dosimetry data published on this. In this study, therefore, the relationship between distance from tumor margin and radiation dose to the optic disc and macula in ocular brachytherapy using ^{125}I Collaborative Ocular Melanoma Study (COMS) plaques was comprehensively investigated. From the information, this study aimed to allow for estimation of optic disc dose and macula dose without treatment planning.

Methods: An in-house brachytherapy dose calculation program utilizing the American Association of Physicists in Medicine Task Group-43 U1 formalism with a line source approximation in a homogenous water phantom was developed and validated against three commercial treatment planning systems (TPS). Then optic disc dose and macula dose were calculated as a function of distance from tumor margin for various tumor basal dimensions for seven COMS plaques (from 10 mm to 22 mm in 2 mm increments) loaded with commercially available ^{125}I seeds models (IAI-125A, 2301 and I25.S16). A prescribed dose of 85 Gy for an irradiation time of 168 h was normalized to a central-axis depth of 5 mm. Dose conversion factors for each seed model were obtained by taking ratios of total reference air kerma per seed at various prescription depths (from 1 mm to 10 mm in 1 mm intervals) to that at 5 mm.

Results: The in-house program demonstrated relatively similar accuracy to commercial TPS. Optic disc dose and macula dose decreased as distance from tumor margin and tumor basal dimension increased. Dose conversion factors increased with increasing prescription depth. There existed dose variations (<8%) among three ^{125}I seed models. Optic disc dose and macula dose for each COMS plaque and for each seed model are presented in a figure format. Dose conversion factors for each seed model are presented in a tabular format.

Conclusions: The data provided in this study would enable clinicians in any clinic using ^{125}I COMS plaques to estimate optic disc dose and macula dose without dose calculations.

Keywords: Ocular brachytherapy, ^{125}I, COMS plaques, Optic disc dose, Macula dose

* Correspondence: yongbokkim@email.arizona.edu
Department of Radiation Oncology, The University of Arizona, 3838 N.
Campbell Avenue, Building #2, Tucson, AZ 85719, USA

Background

Plaque brachytherapy is currently the most common treatment option for early stage or medium-sized intraocular tumors (≤10 mm in apical height and ≤ 16 mm in diameter for uveal melanomas) [1–3]. It offers equivalent tumor control and better quality of life such as eye preservation and vision retention in comparison to enucleation [3–5]. Various plaque designs were proposed and are clinically used in major institutions [6–8]. Nonetheless, Collaborative Ocular Melanoma Study (COMS) plaques have been widely used in most clinics since the COMS established standardized methods of plaque brachytherapy for medium-sized choroidal melanomas [3].

In plaque brachytherapy for intraocular tumors, major critical structures related to vision are lens, optic nerve (optic disc) and macula (fovea). A cataract, clouding of the lens, is the most common radiotherapy contraindication but a surgery can restore vision loss due to cataracts. On the other hand, radiation damage to the optic disc and macula can cause permanent vision loss which is usually not recoverable. Several studies reported outcomes for vision deterioration/loss following plaque brachytherapy [4, 5, 9–13]. Some of the studies revealed that proximity of the tumor to the optic disc and fovea, and radiation dose are substantial risk factors for vision loss [4, 5, 9]. However, there is a paucity of literature on the relationship between proximity of the tumor to the vision-related critical structures and radiation dose to them in plaque brachytherapy.

Therefore, this study has comprehensively examined the relationship between distance from tumor margin and radiation dose to the optic disc or macula in ocular brachytherapy using ^{125}I COMS plaques through a dosimetry study. By providing the dosimetry data, this study aims to enable clinicians (both ophthalmologist and radiation oncologist) in any clinic or institution using ^{125}I COMS plaques to predict optic disc dose and macula dose at the time of tumor size measurements without dose calculations in a treatment planning system (TPS).

The American Association of Physicists in Medicine (AAPM) Task Group (TG) 129 recommends that in dose calculations, heterogeneity corrections be accounted for non-tissue materials such as gold-alloy backing and silastic seed carrier insert in the plaque [3]. As of today, however, there is no commercially available TPS taking into account heterogeneity corrections. Furthermore, the hybrid method, homogeneous dose calculations multiplied by known heterogeneity correction factors, suggested by the AAPM TG 129, is limited to the obsolete ^{125}I seed model 6711 [3] and there is no correction factor provided for currently available ^{125}I seed models. Herein, in current clinical practice, the AAPM TG-43 dosimetry formalism with a line source approximation in a homogeneous water medium is widely used. In this study, dose calculations were performed based on the current clinical practice.

Methods

Determination of parameters required for treatment planning

Following COMS protocols [14], five parameters required for treatment planning were determined in an ophthalmologist's office. Tumor basal dimension at center in the direction from optic disc (BD, parameter #1) and distance from optic disc to tumor margin (DT, parameter #2) were measured in a fundus diagram. Tumor basal dimension at center in the direction from macula (BM, parameter #3) and distance from macula to tumor margin (MT, parameter #4) were also measured in the same fundus diagram. Tumor height (parameter #5), which determines a prescription depth, was measured using ultrasound. The fundus diagram in Fig. 1a illustrates BD, DT, BM and MT of the tumor and the cross section diagram of the eye in Fig. 1b shows apical height of the tumor. Adequate plaque size was determined by

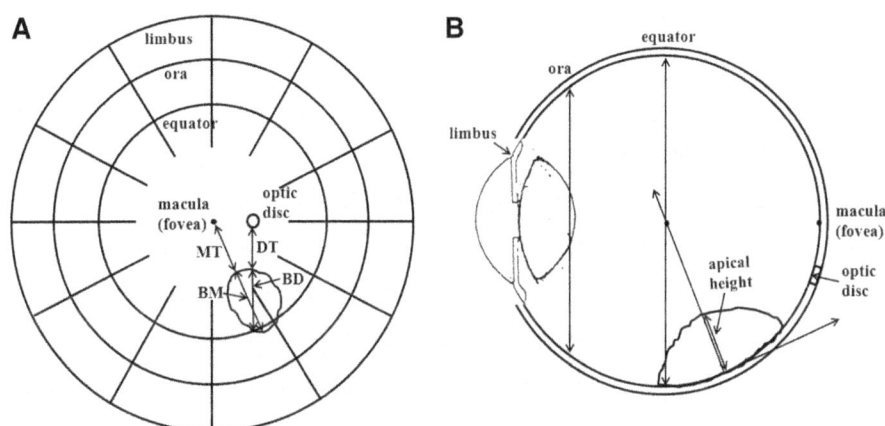

Fig. 1 a The fundus diagram illustrating BD, DT, BM and MT of the tumor and **b** the cross section diagram of the eye showing apical height of the tumor

adding a margin of 2–3 mm to the largest tumor dimension. Then this information was sent to the department of radiation oncology for treatment planning.

Validation of our in-house brachytherapy dose calculation program

For efficient calculations of optic disc dose and macula dose as a function of parameters mentioned above, an in-house brachytherapy dose calculation program was developed in MATLAB® software (vR2016a, MathWorks, Natick, MA) and validated against three commercial TPS for benchmark calculations in the literature [15]. The conventional AAPM TG-43 Update (TG-43 U1) dosimetry formalism with a line source approximation in a homogeneous water medium was incorporated into the in-house program. Parameters for the TG-43 U1 formalism including radial dose function (Table II in TG-43 U1) and anisotropy function (Table V in TG-43 U1) were taken from the TG-43 U1 [16]. The step size over distance "r" and polar angle "θ" for radial dose function and anisotropy function was coarser in the TG-43 U1 than that in Rivard et al. study. In our in-house program, linear interpolation was used to obtain radial dose function and anisotropy function values, while in Rivard et al., log-linear interpolation was used for radial dose function values and linear interpolation for anisotropy function values. Seed coordinates for COMS plaques taken from Table I in the AAPM TG 129 [3] were also incorporated into the program. In Rivard et al.'s benchmark test, doses at several points along the central-axis and at off-axis points for organs at risk (OARs) were calculated in commercial TPS for a 16 mm COMS plaque loaded with ^{125}I seeds (Amersham Oncoseed 6711). The TPS include P^3 (Pinnacle^3, v8.0dpl, Philips Medical Systems, Cleveland, OH), BV (BrachyVision™, v8.1, Varian Medical Systems, Inc., Palo Alto, CA) and PS (Plaque Simulator, v5.3.9, Eye Physics LLC, Los Alamitos, CA) which all use a line source approximation in homogeneous water phantoms [15]. In all three TPS, air-kerma strength (S_k) per seed (unit: $U = \mu Gym^2h^{-1}$) was kept the same (4.572 U) to deliver approximately 85 Gy to a central-axis depth of 5 mm for an irradiation time of 100 h. The central-axis depth is the distance along the plaque central-axis from the inner sclera. Central-axis and off-axis point doses for this benchmark test were calculated in our in-house program. Total reference air kerma (TRAK = S_k × irradiation time) per seed (unit: μGym^2) was kept the same (4.572 U × 100 h) as in the benchmark test. Then, for each point, our data were compared with those in Rivard et al.'s study by computing the modulus of a relative percent difference in dose using the following equation:

$$\left| D_{diff}^{Rel}(\%) \right| = \frac{|D_{in} - D_{ref}|}{D_{ref}} \times 100$$

where D_{in} is dose calculated in our in-house program and D_{ref} is reference dose from Rivard et al.'s study.

Calculations of optic disc dose and macula dose for standard COMS plaques loaded with ^{125}I seeds

Optic disc dose and macula dose for standard COMS plaques were calculated in the in-house program. Dose calculations were performed as a function of distance from tumor margin (DT or MT) up to 10 mm for various tumor basal dimensions (BD or BM) (<20 mm in 2 mm intervals). A prescribed dose of 85 Gy for an irradiation time of 168 h was normalized at a central-axis depth of 5 mm. The calculations were performed for all seven different-sized COMS plaques (from 10 mm to 22 mm in diameter in 2 mm increments) and for three currently, commercially available ^{125}I seeds models (IsoAid Advantage IAI-125A, Best Industries 2301 and Bebig I25.S16) of the seed models listed in the AAPM TG 129 [3]. Parameters in the dosimetry formalism for the three seed models were taken from the AAPM TG-43 U1 [16] and supplement to the AAPM TG-43 U1 [17].

Generation of dose conversion factors for different prescription depths

Since a prescription depth is determined based on the tumor apex (COMS protocols [14] or American Brachytherapy Society (ABS) guidelines [18]) and it is not always 5 mm, dose conversion factors for different prescription depths were generated in the in-house program. Optic disc dose and macula dose were calculated for prescription depths from 1 mm to 10 mm in 1 mm intervals. The prescribed dose (85 Gy) and irradiation time (168 h) were kept the same as for prescription depth of 5 mm. Then ratios of TRAK per seed to obtain 85 Gy to each prescription depth to that to 5 mm were taken as dose conversion factors. The calculations were performed for all seven COMS plaques and for the three seed models mentioned above.

Results

Validation of our in-house brachytherapy dose calculation program

Table 1 presents the comparison of central-axis dose values for a 16 mm COMS plaque loaded with ^{125}I seeds (model 6711) between our in-house program and three TPS used in Rivard et al.'s study [15]. Max| $D_{diff}^{Rel}(\%)$ | is the largest modulus of relative percent differences in dose between the two studies. Max| $D_{diff}^{Rel}(\%)$ | ranged from 0.32% to 2.35% and the largest

Table 1 The comparison of central-axis dose values (in Gy) for a 16 mm COMS plaque loaded with ^{125}I seeds (model 6711) calculated in our in-house program with those in three commercial treatment planning systems (TPS) in Rivard et al.'s study

d (mm)	CAX points	Current Study	Data from Table II in Rivard et al. [15]			Max$\|D_{diff}^{Rel}(\%)\|$
			P^3	BV	PS	
−1.0	Outer sclera	336.18	341	340	339	1.41
0.0	Inner sclera	258.79	261	261	260	0.85
1.0		202.10	203	203	202	0.44
2.0		160.48	161	161	160	0.32
3.0		128.68	129	129	128	0.53
4.0		103.91	104	104	103	0.88
5.0	Rx depth	84.52	84.4	84.5	83.9	0.74
6.0		69.26	69.2	69.2	68.8	0.67
7.0		57.27	57.2	57.2	56.9	0.65
8.0		47.73	47.7	47.7	47.4	0.70
9.0		40.12	40.0	40.0	39.8	0.81
10.0		34.00	33.9	33.9	33.7	0.89
11.3	Eye center	27.73	27.6	27.6	27.5	0.83
15.0		16.45	16.3	16.3	16.3	0.95
20.0		9.02	8.87	8.89	8.84	2.04
22.6	Opposite retina	6.83	6.70	6.70	6.67	2.35

P^3, BV and PS represent Pinnacle, BrachyVision and Plaque Simulator, respectively. Dose values were calculated for a prescribed dose of approximately 85 Gy to a central-axis depth of 5 mm ($S_k = 4.752$ U and irradiation time = 100 h) using a line source approximation of the AAPM TG-43 formalism and homogeneous water phantoms. Max$\|D_{diff}^{Rel}(\%)\|$ is the largest modulus of relative percent differences in dose between the two studies

difference (2.35%) occurred at the farthest dose point (22.6 mm, opposite retina).

Table 2 presents the comparison of doses at OAR points (fovea, optic disc center, lens center and lacrimal glad center) for four different plaque positions (#1-#4) between our study and Rivard et al.'s. From Fig. 3 in Rivard et al., the plaque positions #1, #2, #3 and #4 were centered on equator on temporal side (9 o'clock), on nasal side (3 o'clock), on superior side (12 o'clock) and on inferior side (6 o'clock), respectively [15]. Coordinates for the OARs were taken from Rivard et al. [15]. $\|D_{diff}^{Rel}(\%)\|$ was defined in the same way as for the central axis dose comparison except that D_{ref} was an average value of off-axis doses calculated from all TPS [15]. Off-axis dose differences between the two studies ranged from 0.40% to 1.52% except for the lacrimal gland point for plaque positions #1 (4.39%) and #3 (4.40%).

Optic disc dose and macula dose for standard COMS plaques loaded with ^{125}I seeds

Optic disc dose and macula dose for standard COMS plaques loaded with ^{125}I seeds (model IAI-125A) are shown in Figs. 2 and 3, respectively. Figure 2a-g presents optic disc dose as a function of DT up to 10 mm for various BDs in 2 mm intervals for seven COMS plaques when 85 Gy is prescribed at a central-axis depth of 5 mm for an irradiation time of 168 h. Optic disc dose

decreases with increasing DT and increasing BD. For the plaques ≥16 mm, however, there exist some regions where optic disc dose does not change much with DT (i.e., flat regions in Fig. 2d-g). This usually occurs within short distances (≤5 mm of DT) when BD is less than or equal to 5 mm. For example, for the 16 mm COMS plaque (Fig. 2d), the graph for BD = 1 mm does not vary a lot at <3 mm of DT and the graph for BD = 3 mm does not change much at <2 mm of DT, respectively. Plaque size also determines optic disc dose and the shape of dose curves. Macula dose is displayed in Fig. 3a-g as a function of MT for various BMs. Similar patterns to optic disc dose are observed. Optic disc dose and macula dose for the other two seed models (2301 and I25.S16) are presented as Additional file 1 (data not shown here).

There are variations of optic disc dose and macula dose among seed models. The maximum relative differences (%) in optic disc dose between IAI-125A and 2301, between IAI-125A and I25.S16, and between 2301 and I25.S16 are 7.74, 5.89 and 5.28%, respectively. Corresponding maximum relative differences (%) for macula dose are 7.39, 5.64 and 5.28%.

Dose conversion factors for different prescription depths

Dose conversion factors for different prescription depths from 1 mm to 10 mm in 1 mm intervals for standard COMS plaques loaded with ^{125}I seed (model IAI-125A) are tabulated in Table 3. Based on the COMS protocols

Table 2 The comparison of dose values (in Gy) at organs at risk points (fovea, optic disc center, lens center and lacrimal glad center) for four different plaque positions (#1-#4) [15] of the 16 mm COMS plaque loaded with ^{125}I seeds (model 6711) calculated in our in-house program with average off-axis dose values calculated from treatment planning systems used in Rivard et al.'s study

Plaque position	Off-axis location	Current Study	Data from Table III in Rivard et al. [15]	$|D_{diff}^{Rel}(\%)|$
#1	Fovea	16.50	16.3	1.25
	Optic disc	11.29	11.2	0.79
	Lens	21.59	21.5	0.40
	Lacrimal gland	40.92	39.2	4.39
#2	Fovea	16.50	16.3	1.25
	Optic disc	28.02	27.6	1.52
	Lens	21.59	21.5	0.40
	Lacrimal gland	7.19	7.1	1.22
#3	Fovea	16.50	16.3	1.25
	Optic disc	16.48	16.3	1.08
	Lens	21.59	21.5	0.40
	Lacrimal gland	40.92	39.2	4.40
#4	Fovea	16.50	16.3	1.25
	Optic disc	16.48	16.3	1.08
	Lens	21.59	21.5	0.40
	Lacrimal gland	7.19	7.1	1.22

Dose values were calculated for a prescribed dose of approximately 85 Gy to a central-axis depth of 5 mm ($S_k = 4.752$ U and irradiation time = 100 h) using a line source approximation of the AAPM TG-43 formalism and homogeneous water phantoms. $|D_{diff}^{Rel}(\%)|$ is a modulus of a relative percent difference in dose between the two studies

for tumors with apical height <5 mm [14], dose conversion factors were normalized to a depth of 5 mm. The factors increase with increasing prescription depth. The factors increase with increasing plaque size for a prescription depth <5 mm but the opposite is observed for a depth >5 mm. Table 3 is used for both optic disc dose and macula dose estimation when a prescription depth is not 5 mm. Dose conversion factors for the other two ^{125}I seed models (2301 and I25.S16) are provided as Additional file 2 (data not shown here). The differences of the factors among seed models increase with increasing prescription depth and decreasing plaque size. Maximum absolute differences between IAI-125A and 2301, between IAI-125A and I25.S16, and between 2301 and I25.S16 are 0.08, 0.1 and 0.02, respectively.

Estimation of optic disc dose without dose calculations: clinical application of this study

Optic disc dose (Fig. 2), macula dose (Fig. 3) and dose conversion factors (Table 3) presented in the current study can be conveniently used in clinic. As an example, there is a clinical case in which BD is 3 mm, DT is 3 mm and apical height is 4 mm. A clinician wants to prescribe 85 Gy to the tumor apex (i.e., 4 mm) using a 10 mm COMS plaque loaded with ^{125}I seeds (model IAI-125A). From the data obtained in this study, optic disc dose is about 145 Gy for the 10 mm COMS plaque and for a prescription depth of 5 mm (Fig. 2a). The dose

conversion factor for the 10 mm COMS plaque and for a prescription depth of 4 mm is 0.77 (Table 3). Thus, for this clinical case, expected optic disc dose is 112 Gy (=145 Gy × 0.77) which is lower than that when prescribed at 5 mm by 33 Gy. If tumor apex is higher (for instance, 6 mm) for the same tumor, optic disc dose for the same ^{125}I seed model is about 184 Gy (=145 Gy × 1.27) (Table 3).

Discussion

Our in-house brachytherapy dose calculation program demonstrated similar accuracy in brachytherapy dose calculations to commercial TPS. As presented in Tables 1 and 2, dose differences at central-axis and off-axis points between our in-house program and the three TPS used in Rivard et al.'s study were <2.4% except for the lacrimal gland point for plaque positions #1 and #3. Some seeds in plaque positions #1 and #3 have small polar angles (< 40 degrees) to the lacrimal gland point. At small polar angles, anisotropy function values vary more dramatically with polar angle than at large polar angles, leading to larger uncertainty in the interpolation of anisotropy function values. As mentioned in the Methods, Rivard et al.'s study used smaller step size over distance "r" and polar angle "θ" for anisotropy function than our in-house program (AAPM TG-43 U1), causing larger dose differences

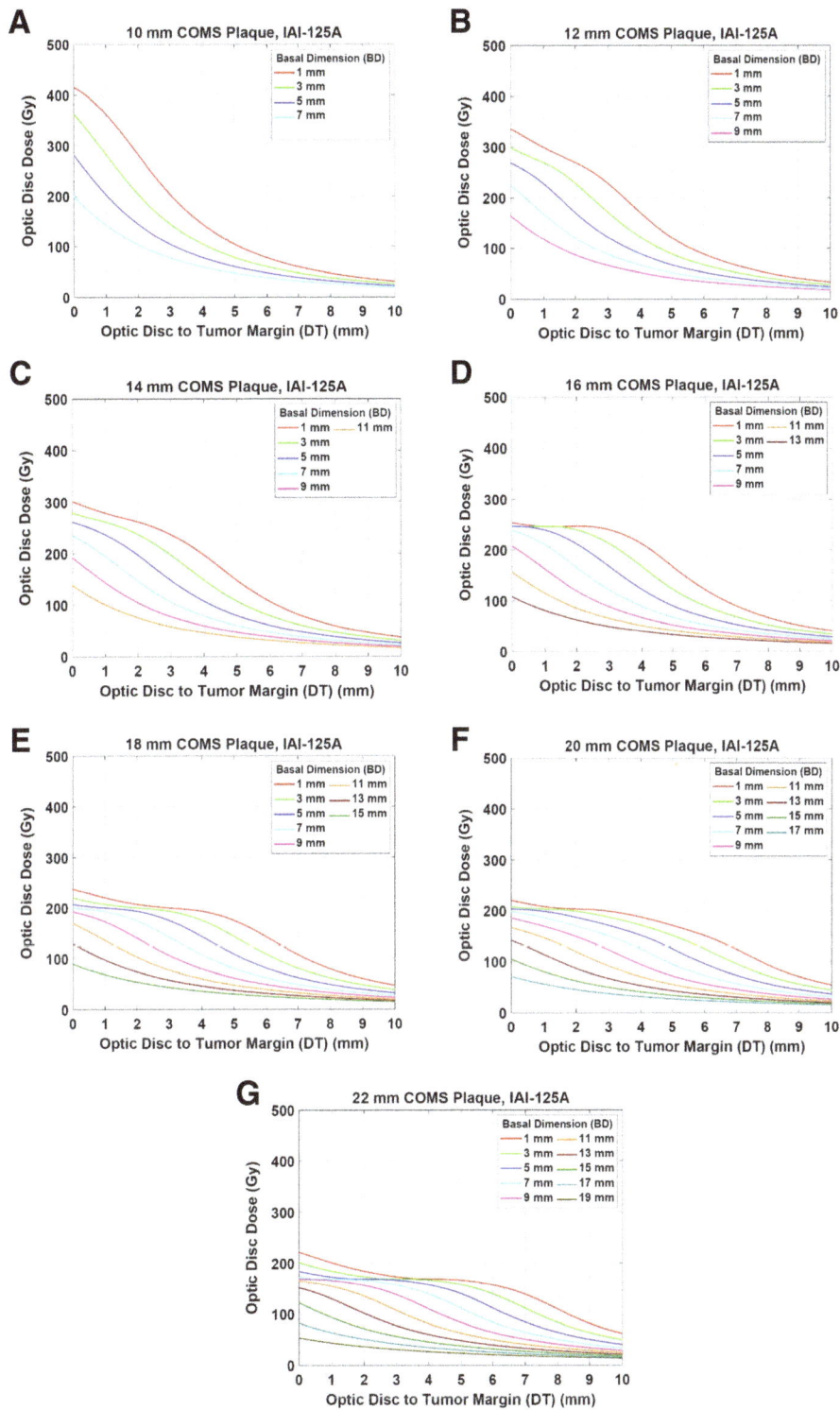

Fig. 2 a-g Optic disc dose as a function of optic disc-to-tumor margin distance (DT) for various tumor basal dimensions (BD) for seven COMS plaques loaded with ^{125}I seeds (model IAI-125A) when 85 Gy is prescribed to a central-axis depth of 5 mm

($\sim$ 4.4%) between the two studies at the lacrimal gland point for plaque positions #1 and #3 than at the other dose points.

This study showed that optic disc dose and macula dose strongly depend on distance from tumor margin (DT and MT) and tumor basal dimension (BD and BM).

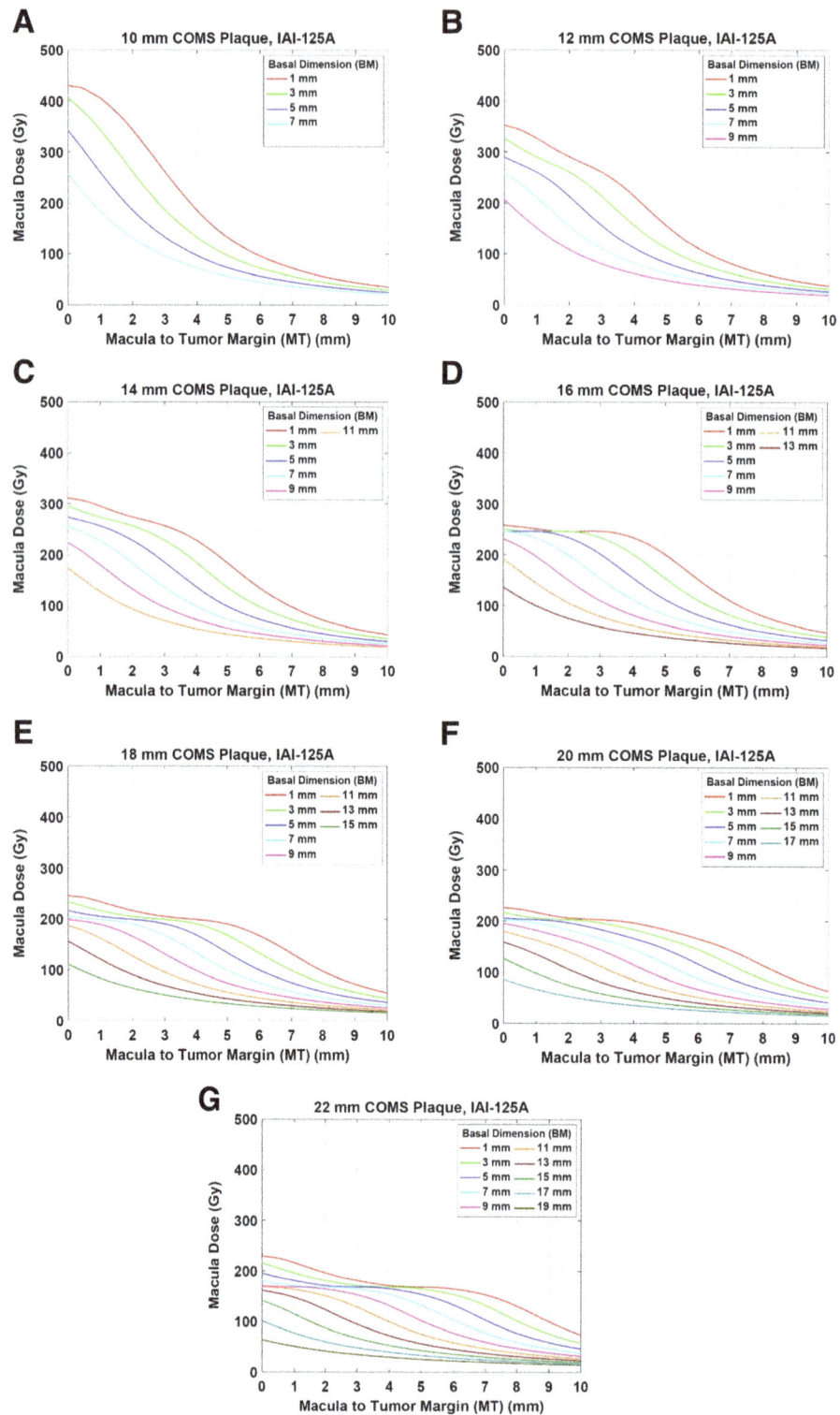

Fig. 3 a-g Macula dose as a function of macula-to-tumor margin distance (MT) for various tumor basal dimensions (BM) for seven COMS plaques loaded with ^{125}I seeds (model IAI-125A) when 85 Gy is prescribed to a central-axis depth of 5 mm

Table 3 Dose conversion factors (ratios of total reference air kerma per seed) for different prescription depths (1 mm – 10 mm in 1 mm intervals) for standard COMS plaques loaded with ^{125}I seeds (model IAI-125A). A reference depth for dose conversion factors is 5 mm

Prescription depth (mm)	Plaque size (mm) in diameter						
	10	12	14	16	18	20	22
1	0.29	0.33	0.37	0.42	0.44	0.47	0.47
2	0.41	0.45	0.48	0.52	0.55	0.58	0.59
3	0.57	0.60	0.63	0.66	0.68	0.70	0.71
4	0.77	0.78	0.80	0.81	0.83	0.84	0.85
5	1.00	1.00	1.00	1.00	1.00	1.00	1.00
6	1.27	1.25	1.23	1.22	1.20	1.18	1.18
7	1.59	1.54	1.50	1.47	1.43	1.40	1.38
8	1.95	1.88	1.82	1.76	1.69	1.64	1.61
9	2.37	2.27	2.18	2.10	2.00	1.92	1.87
10	2.84	2.71	2.59	2.48	2.34	2.24	2.17

In the COMS protocols, coordinates for the optic disc and macula are determined by the combination of these two parameters. Hence, the two parameters determine optic disc dose and macula dose. At close proximity (up to about 1 cm) of ^{125}I seeds (plaque), the inverse square law effect is severe. At farther distances, however, the radial dose function for ^{125}I seeds drastically decreases with distance because of its low photon energy (average energy: 28 keV) and consequently, rapid dose fall-off is observed. As a result, optic disc dose and macula dose decrease as DT and MT increase (Figs. 2 and 3), respectively. Optic disc dose and macula dose also decrease as BD and BM increase (Figs. 2 and 3), respectively because optic disc and macula become far away from the center of tumor as BD and BM increase, respectively. For plaques ≥16 mm, however, there are regions in which dose does not change much with distance (Figs. 2d-g and 3d-g). This occurs particularly for small basal dimensions at a tumor margin-to-critical structure distance ≤5 mm. As shown in Fig. 4a, for BD of 5 mm, as DT increases, an optic dose point becomes far away from seed #21 but simultaneously close to seeds #12 and #5. As a result, optic disc dose points between 2 mm and 4 mm of DT are in the same dose color map (three yellow dots in Fig. 4a) and optic disc dose is invariant within that region. On the other hand, for BD of 13 mm, an optic disc dose point becomes far away from seeds #12 and #5 with increasing DT. Therefore, each dose point between 2 mm and 4 mm is located in a different dose color map and optic disc dose decreases as DT increases (Fig. 4b). For the same reason, similar patterns are observed in macula dose (Fig. 3).

Optic disc dose and macula dose also have dependence on prescription depth and plaque size. The dependence can be explained with trends of dose conversion factors (Table 3) and TRAK values per seed (Table 4) as follows. First, for each plaque size, TRAK per seed to obtain a prescribed dose to a prescription depth increases with increasing prescription depth because a deeper prescription depth requires higher TRAK per seed. Hence, dose conversion factors increase with prescription depth. Second, for each prescription depth, TRAK per seed does not continuously decrease with increasing plaque size due to the number of seeds used in each COMS plaque (e.g., 24 seeds for 20 mm plaque and 21 seeds for 22 mm plaque). Thus, dose conversion factors do not always continuously increase (depth <5 mm) or decrease (depth >5 mm) with increasing plaque size. Third, TRAK per seed increases more rapidly with increasing prescription depth for smaller plaques than for larger plaques. The following example for seed model IAI-125A supports this trend. For the 10 mm plaque, TRAK per seed increases from 299.9 µGym^2 to 2923.5 µGym^2 (9.7-fold increase) when a prescription depth increases from 1 mm to 10 mm. On the other hand, for the 22 mm plaque, the increase of TRAK per seed by the depth increase from 1 mm to 10 mm is 4.6-fold (from 157.3 µGym^2 to 718.6 µGym^2). Thus, dose conversion factors increase more rapidly with increasing prescription depth for smaller plaques than for larger plaques, resulting in the increase in dose conversion factors with plaque size at a depth <5 mm but the decrease with plaque size at a depth >5 mm.

There exist dose differences among seed models. The differences are caused by differences of the parameters used in the AAPM TG-43 U1 dosimetry formalism which result from different seed geometry and internal construction among three seed models [16, 19]. As reported in the Results, the differences can be fairly significant (up to 7.7%) and similar results were reported by Thomson et al. [19]. Thomson et al. performed MC calculations for a 16 mm COMS plaque loaded with ^{125}I seeds under TG-43 assumptions (i.e., a homogeneous medium) and showed that doses differed by up to 11% for different seed models [19].

The results presented in this study will be beneficial to the clinic using ^{125}I COMS plaques and help improve current clinical practice as follows. First, this study would allow clinicians to estimate optic disc dose and macula dose without dose calculations. Figures 2 and 3 and Table 3 or the data in additional files can be easily looked up as in the example discussed in the Results. In this study, the calculations were based on a prescribed dose of 85 Gy. In clinical cases where a prescribed dose is different from 85 Gy (e.g., re-irradiation or treatment of benign lesions), a dose scaling factor (prescribed dose (Gy)/85 Gy) can be multiplied by optic disc dose or macula dose obtained in this study to estimate dose to the

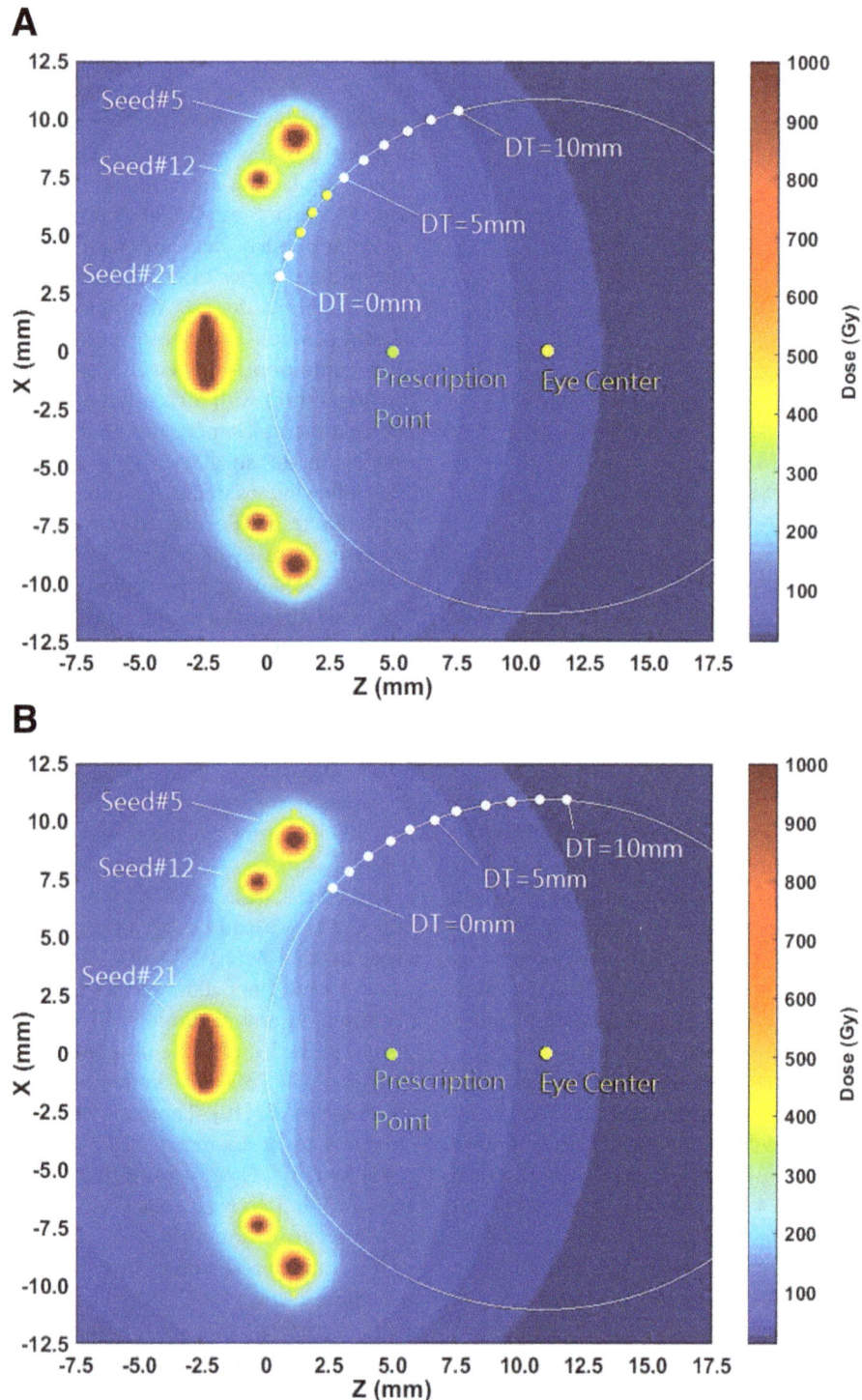

Fig. 4 Optic disc dose clouds for a 22 mm COMS plaque loaded with [125]I (model: IAI-125A) seeds for a tumor with **a** 5 mm basal dimension (BD) and **b** 13 mm basal dimension (BD). The positions in yellow (DT = 2 mm – 4 mm) in the **a** represent where dose does not change much

critical structures. Second, if an estimated dose to the OARs is high enough to be paid attention to, clinicians may take an action to reduce dose to the OARs by prescribing to a different depth or by the use of a notched

plaque [20]. As discussed in the example in the Results, prescribing 85 Gy to 4 mm (recent ABS guidelines [18]: prescribing at the tumor apex for all medium-sized choroidal melanomas) can give lower dose to the optic disc

Table 4 TRAK per seed (in μGym^2) for different prescription depths (1 mm – 10 mm in 1 mm intervals) for standard COMS plaques loaded with ^{125}I seeds (model IAI-125A)

Prescription depth (mm)	Plaque size (mm) in diameter						
	10	12	14	16	18	20	22
1	299.9	226.3	161.2	191.6	134.8	132.3	157.3
2	424.9	306.2	212.2	241.0	168.0	162.0	194.2
3	587.2	406.6	274.4	301.3	206.3	195.8	234.6
4	788.9	530.2	349.5	373.9	251.2	234.7	280.1
5	1030.6	677.1	438.1	459.8	303.2	279.4	331.2
6	1311.2	848.0	540.9	559.7	363.2	330.7	389.3
7	1634.7	1045.2	659.3	675.4	432.6	389.9	455.7
8	2008.7	1274.1	797.3	810.4	513.4	458.6	532.3
9	2438.7	1536.9	955.4	965.1	605.8	537.1	619.8
10	2923.5	1833.6	1133.9	1140.1	710.4	626.0	718.6

than prescribing 85 Gy to 5 mm (COMS protocols [14]: prescribing at 5 mm for the tumor apex <5 mm and to the apex for the tumor apex ≥5 mm [15]) (112 Gy vs. 145 Gy) due to lower TRAK per seed at a shallower depth. For the tumor apex ≥5 mm, prescribing dose to a shallower depth would reduce optic disc dose but tumor coverage can be compromised. Third, this study would enable clinicians to correlate clinical outcomes for vision with optic disc dose or macula dose. There have been no good published correlation data between clinical outcomes and radiation dose. If clinical outcomes for vision are available along with corresponding distance from tumor margin (DT and MT), tumor basal dimensions (BD and BM), plaque size, prescription depth, prescribed dose and seed model, one can correlate the outcomes with optic disc dose and macula dose which can be looked up from the results presented in this study. From the correlation data, clinicians can anticipate outcomes for vision for a given clinical situation and find a possible way to reduce dose to the critical structures before treatment. Furthermore, using the correlation data, tolerance dose to the optic disc or macula in ocular brachytherapy, which has not been known yet, can be investigated.

Conclusions

This study has comprehensively examined optic disc dose and macula dose as a function of distance from tumor margin in ocular brachytherapy using ^{125}I COMS plaques and has shown that dose to the critical structures has dependence on multiple parameters such as distance from tumor margin, tumor basal dimension, prescription depth, plaque size, and seed model. In any clinic or institution utilizing ^{125}I COMS plaques, the dosimetry data provided in this study can be looked up to estimate optic disc dose and macula dose without dose calculations in a TPS.

Abbreviations

AAPM: American Association of Physicists in Medicine; ABS: American Brachytherapy Society; BD: Tumor basal dimension at center in the direction from optic disc; BM: Tumor basal dimension at center in the direction from macula; COMS: Collaborative Ocular Melanoma Study; DT: Distance from optic disc to tumor margin; MT: Distance from macula to tumor margin; OARs: Organs at risk; S$_k$: Air-kerma strength; TG: Task group; TPS: Treatment planning system; TRAK: Total reference air kerma

Acknowledgements
None.

Funding
None.

Authors' contributions

YCL analyzed data and wrote a manuscript. SCL performed calculations and collected data. YK designed the study and analyzed data. All authors read and approved the final manuscript.

Competing interests

The authors declare that they have no competing interests.

References

1.　Fabian ID, Tomkins-Netzer O, Stoker I, Arora AK, Sagoo MS, Cohen VM. Secondary enucleations for uveal melanoma: a 7-year retrospective analysis. Am J Ophthalmol. 2015;160(6):1104–10 e1.

2.　Nag S, Quivey JM, Earle JD, Followill D, Fontanesi J, Finger PT, et al. The American brachytherapy society recommendations for brachytherapy of uveal melanomas. Int J Radiat Oncol Biol Phys. 2003;56(2):544–55.

3.　Chiu-Tsao ST, Astrahan MA, Finger PT, Followill DS, Meigooni AS, Melhus CS, et al. Dosimetry of (125)I and (103)Pd COMS eye plaques for intraocular tumors: report of task group 129 by the AAPM and ABS. Med Phys. 2012; 39(10):6161–84.

4.　Tseng V, Coleman A, Zhang Z, McCannel T. Complications from plaque versus proton beam therapy for choroidal melanoma: a qualitative systematic review. J Cancer Ther. 2016;7(3):169–85.

5.　Sagoo MS, Shields CL, Mashayekhi A, Freire J, Emrich J, Reiff J, et al. Plaque radiotherapy for juxtapapillary choroidal melanoma overhanging the optic disc in 141 consecutive patients. Arch Ophthalmol. 2008;126(11):1515–22.

6.　Finger PT. Finger's "slotted" eye plaque for radiation therapy: treatment of juxtapapillary and circumpapillary intraocular tumours. Br J Ophthalmol. 2007;91(7):891–4.

7.　Berry JL, Dandapani SV, Stevanovic M, Lee TC, Astrahan M, Murphree AL, et al. Outcomes of choroidal melanomas treated with eye physics: a 20-year review. JAMA Ophthalmol. 2013;131(11):1435–42.

8.　Karlsson M, Nilsson J, Lundell M, Carlsson TA. Monte Carlo dosimetry of the eye plaque design used at the St. Erik eye hospital for (125)I brachytherapy. Brachytherapy. 2014;13(6):651–6.

9.　Shields CL, Shields JA, Cater J, Gunduz K, Miyamoto C, Micaily B, et al. Plaque radiotherapy for uveal melanoma: long-term visual outcome in 1106 consecutive patients. Arch Ophthalmol. 2000;118(9):1219–28.

10.　Melia BM, Abramson DH, Albert DM, Boldt HC, Earle JD, Hanson WF, et al. Collaborative ocular melanoma study (COMS) randomized trial of I-125 brachytherapy for medium choroidal melanoma. I. Visual acuity after 3 years COMS report no. 16. Ophthalmology. 2001;108(2):348–66.

11.　Shields CL, Naseripour M, Cater J, Shields JA, Demirci H, Youseff A, et al. Plaque radiotherapy for large posterior uveal melanomas (> or =8-mm thick) in 354 consecutive patients. Ophthalmology. 2002;109(10):1838–49.

12.　Finger PT, Chin KJ, Duvall G. Palladium-103 for Choroidal Melanoma Study G. Palladium-103 ophthalmic plaque radiation therapy for choroidal melanoma: 400 treated patients. Ophthalmology. 2009;116(4):790–6 6 e1.

13.　Sagoo MS, Shields CL, Emrich J, Mashayekhi A, Komarnicky L, Shields JA. Plaque radiotherapy for juxtapapillary choroidal melanoma: treatment complications and visual outcomes in 650 consecutive cases. JAMA Ophthalmol. 2014;132(6):697–702.

14. COMS Manual of Procedures (Chapter 12. Radiation Therapy). http://pages. jh.edu/wctb/coms/manual/coms_chap12.pdf. Accessed 5 Nov 2018.

15. Rivard MJ, Chiu-Tsao ST, Finger PT, Meigooni AS, Melhus CS, Mourtada F, et al. Comparison of dose calculation methods for brachytherapy of intraocular tumors. Med Phys. 2011;38(1):306–16.

16. Rivard MJ, Coursey BM, DeWerd LA, Hanson WF, Huq MS, Ibbott GS, et al. Update of AAPM task group no. 43 report: a revised AAPM protocol for brachytherapy dose calculations. Med Phys. 2004;31(3):633–74.

17. Rivard MJ, Butler WM, DeWerd LA, Huq MS, Ibbott GS, Meigooni AS, et al. Supplement to the 2004 update of the AAPM task group no. 43 report. Med Phys. 2007;34(6):2187–205.

18. American Brachytherapy Society - Ophthalmic Oncology Task Force. Electronic address pec, Committee AO. The American brachytherapy society consensus guidelines for plaque brachytherapy of uveal melanoma and retinoblastoma. Brachytherapy. 2014;13(1):1–14.

19. Thomson RM, Rogers DW. Monte Carlo dosimetry for 125I and 103Pd eye plaque brachytherapy with various seed models. Med Phys. 2010;37(1):368–76.

20. Hegde JV, McCannel TA, McCannel CA, Lamb J, Wang P-C, Veruttipong D, et al. Juxtapapillary and circumpapillary choroidal melanoma: globe-sparing treatment outcomes with iodine-125 notched plaque brachytherapy. Graefes Arch Clin Exp Ophthalmol. 2017;255(9):1843–50.

Permissions

The contributors of this book come from diverse backgrounds, making this book a truly international effort. This book will bring forth new frontiers with its revolutionizing research information and detailed analysis of the nascent developments around the world.

We would like to thank all the contributing authors for lending their expertise to make the book truly unique. They have played a crucial role in the development of this book. Without their invaluable contributions this book wouldn't have been possible. They have made vital efforts to compile up to date information on the varied aspects of this subject to make this book a valuable addition to the collection of many professionals and students.

This book was conceptualized with the vision of imparting up-to-date information and advanced data in this field. To ensure the same, a matchless editorial board was set up. Every individual on the board went through rigorous rounds of assessment to prove their worth. After which they invested a large part of their time researching and compiling the most relevant data for our readers.

The editorial board has been involved in producing this book since its inception. They have spent rigorous hours researching and exploring the diverse topics which have resulted in the successful publishing of this book. They have passed on their knowledge of decades through this book. To expedite this challenging task, the publisher supported the team at every step. A small team of assistant editors was also appointed to further simplify the editing procedure and attain best results for the readers.

Apart from the editorial board, the designing team has also invested a significant amount of their time in understanding the subject and creating the most relevant covers. They scrutinized every image to scout for the most suitable representation of the subject and create an appropriate cover for the book.

The publishing team has been an ardent support to the editorial, designing and production team. Their endless efforts to recruit the best for this project, has resulted in the accomplishment of this book. They are a veteran in the field of academics and their pool of knowledge is as vast as their experience in printing. Their expertise and guidance has proved useful at every step. Their uncompromising quality standards have made this book an exceptional effort. Their encouragement from time to time has been an inspiration for everyone.

The publisher and the editorial board hope that this book will prove to be a valuable piece of knowledge for researchers, students, practitioners and scholars across the globe.

List of Contributors

Michela Buglione, Mauro Urpis, Liliana Baushi, Nadia Pasinetti, Paolo Borghetti, Sara Pedretti, Luca Triggiani, Diana Greco Stefano Maria Magrini and Stefano Ciccarelli1
Radiation Oncology Department, University and Spedali Civili Hospital – Brescia, P.le Spedali Civili 1 –, 25123 Brescia, Italy

Luigi Spiazzi, Rossella Avitabile, Alessia Polonini, Renzo Moretti, Federica Saiani and Alfredo Fiume
Medical Physics, Spedali Civili Hospital – Brescia, P.le Spedali Civili 1 –, 25123 Brescia, Italy

Yongjie Shui, Bicheng Zhang, Qiongge Hu and Li Shen
Department of Radiation Oncology, The Second Affiliated Hospital, Zhejiang University School of Medicine, Jiefang Road 88, Hangzhou 310009, People's Republic of China

Tao Ma, Xueli Bai and Tingbo Liang
Department of Hepatobiliary and Pancreatic Surgery, Zhejiang Provincial Key Laboratory of Pancreatic Disease, The Second Affiliated Hospital, Zhejiang University School of Medicine, Hangzhou 310009, People's Republic of China

Jianjun Wu and Qinghai Li
Department of Radiology, The Second Affiliated Hospital, Zhejiang University School of Medicine, Hangzhou 310009, People's Republic of China

Wei Yu, Xiaoqiu Ren, Yinglu Guo, Jing Xu and Qichun Wei
Department of Radiation Oncology, The Second Affiliated Hospital, Zhejiang University School of Medicine, Jiefang Road 88, Hangzhou 310009, People's Republic of China
Ministry of Education Key Laboratory of Cancer

Jae Pil Chung and Young Min Seong
Center for Ionizing Radiation, Division of Metrology for Quality of Life, Korea Research Institute of Standards and Science, 267 Gajeong-ro, Yuseong-gu, Daejon 34311, Korea

Tae Yeon Kim, Yona Choi and Kook Jin Chun
Department of Accelerator Science, Korea University Sejong Campus, 2511 Sejong-ro, Sejong 30019, Korea

Tae Hoon Kim
Department of Nuclear Engineering, Hanyang University College of Engineering, Seoul 04763, Korea

Hyun Joon Choi and Chul Hee Min
Department of Radiation Convergence Engineering, Yonsei University, 1 Yeonsedae-gil, Heungeop-myeon, Wonju 26493, Korea

Hamza Benmakhlouf
Department of Medical Radiation Physics and Nuclear Medicine, Karolinska University Hospital, SE-17176 Stockholm, Sweden

Hyun-Tai Chung
Department of Neurosurgery, Seoul National University College of Medicine, 101 Daehakro Jongno-gu, Seoul 03080, Korea

Pierfrancesco Franco, Francesca Arcadipane, Gabriella Furfaro, Elisabetta Trino, Stefania Martini, Giuseppe Carlo Iorio and Umberto Ricardi
Department of Oncology, Radiation Oncology, University of Turin, Via Genova 3, 10126 Turin, Italy

Berardino De Bari
Department of Radiation Oncology, Centre Hospitalier Régional Universitaire 'Jean Minjoz', Besançon, France

Alexis Lepinoy
Department of Radiation Oncology, Centre 'Paul Strauss', Strasbourg, France

Manuela Ceccarelli and Andrea Evangelista
Unit of Cancer Epidemiology and CPO Piedmont, AOU Citta' della Salute e della Scienza, Turin, Italy

Massimiliano Mistrangelo
Department of Surgical Sciences, University of Turin, Turin, Italy

Paola Cassoni
Department of Medical Sciences, Pathology Unit, University of Turin, Turin, Italy

Martina Valgiusti, Alessandro Passardi and Andrea Casadei Gardini
Department of Medical Oncology, Istituto Scientifico Romagnolo per lo Studio e la Cura dei Tumori (IRST) IRCCS, Meldola, Italy

Gilles Créhange
Department of Radiation Oncology, Centre 'Georges-François-Leclerc', Dijon, France

Ana Krivokuća, Milena Čavić, Siniša Radulović and Radmila Janković
Laboratory for Molecular Genetics, Institute of Oncology and Radiology of Serbia, Belgrade, Serbia

Jasmina Mladenović and Vesna Plesinac Karapandžić
Radiology and Radiotherapy Department, Institute of Oncology and Radiology of Serbia, Belgrade, Serbia

Stephan Beck
Medical Genomics, UCL Cancer Institute, University College London, London, UK

Snezana Susnjar
Medical Oncology Department, Institute of Oncology and Radiology of Serbia, Belgrade, Serbia

Miljana Tanić
Laboratory for Molecular Genetics, Institute of Oncology and Radiology of Serbia, Belgrade, Serbia
Medical Genomics, UCL Cancer Institute, University College London, London, UK

Sophie C. Huijskens, Irma W. E. M. van Dijk, Jorrit Visser, Brian V. Balgobind, D. te Lindert, Coen R. N. Rasch, Tanja Alderliesten and Arjan Bel
Amsterdam UMC, University of Amsterdam, Department of Radiation Oncology, Cancer Center Amsterdam, Meibergdreef 9, Amsterdam, The Netherlands

Christy Goldsmith
Guys and St Thomas' NHS Foundation Trust, London, UK

P. Nicholas Plowman
The London CyberKnife Centre, The Harley Street Clinic, 81 Harley Street, London W1G 8PP, UK
St. Bartholomew's Hospital, London, UK

Melanie M. Green and Roger G. Dale
Department of Surgery and Cancer, Imperial College London, London, UK

Patricia M. Price
The London CyberKnife Centre, The Harley Street Clinic, 81 Harley Street, London W1G 8PP, UK
Department of Surgery and Cancer, Imperial College London, London, UK

Yanzhu Lin, Kai Chen, Lei Zhao, Yalan Tao, Yi Ouyang and Xinping Cao
Department of Radiation Oncology, Sun Yat-sen University Cancer Center, State Key Laboratory of Oncology in South China, Collaborative Innovation Center for Cancer Medicine, 651 Dongfeng Road East, Guangzhou, Guangdong 510060, People's Republic of China

Zhiyuan Lu
Department of Oral and Maxillofacial Surgery, First Affiliated Hospital, Sun Yat-sen University, Guangzhou 510080, People's Republic of China

Wensha Yang
Department of Radiation Oncology, Cedars Sinai Medical Center, 8700 Beverly Blvd., Los Angeles, CA 90048, USA
Department of Biomedical Sciences, Biomedical Imaging Research Institute, Cedars Sinai Medical Center, Los Angeles, CA, USA

Zhaoyang Fan and Debiao Li
Department of Biomedical Sciences, Biomedical Imaging Research Institute, Cedars Sinai Medical Center, Los Angeles, CA, USA

Zixin Deng
Department of Biomedical Sciences, Biomedical Imaging Research Institute, Cedars Sinai Medical Center, Los Angeles, CA, USA
Department of Bioengineering, University of California, Los Angeles, Los Angeles, CA, USA

Jianing Pang and Xiaoming Bi
Siemens Healthineers, Los Angeles, USA

Benedick A Fraass, Howard Sandler and Richard Tuli
Department of Radiation Oncology, Cedars Sinai Medical Center, 8700 Beverly Blvd., Los Angeles, CA 90048, USA

M. Oertel, S. Scobioala, K. Kroeger, A. Baehr, U. Haverkamp and H.-T. Eich
Department of Radiation Oncology, Albert-Schweitzer Campus 1 A1, 48149 Muenster, Germany

L. Stegger and M. Schäfers
Department of Nuclear Medicine, Albert-Schweitzer Campus 1 A1, 48149 Muenster, Germany
Nicole Wiedenmann, Hatice Bunea, Andrei Bunea, Liette Majerus, Nils H. Nicolay and Anca L. Grosu

Department of Radiation Oncology, Medical Center University of Freiburg, Faculty of Medicine, University of Freiburg, Freiburg, Germany
German Cancer Consortium (DKTK), Partner Site Freiburg, Freiburg, German
German Cancer Research Center (DKFZ), Heidelberg, Germany

Hans C. Rischke
Department of Radiation Oncology, Medical Center University of Freiburg, Faculty of Medicine, University of Freiburg, Freiburg, Germany
Department of Nuclear Medicine, Medical Center University of Freiburg, Faculty of Medicine, University of Freiburg, Freiburg, Germany
German Cancer Consortium (DKTK), Partner Site Freiburg, Freiburg, German
German Cancer Research Center (DKFZ), Heidelberg, Germany

Lars Bielak, Alexey Protopopov, Ute Ludwig and Martin Büchert
Department of Radiology, Medical Physics, Medical Center University of Freiburg, Faculty of Medicine, University of Freiburg, Freiburg, Germany

Christian Stoykow, Michael Mix and Philipp T. Meyer
Department of Nuclear Medicine, Medical Center University of Freiburg, Faculty of Medicine, University of Freiburg, Freiburg, Germany
German Cancer Consortium (DKTK), Partner Site Freiburg, Freiburg, German
German Cancer Research Center (DKFZ), Heidelberg, Germany

Wolfgang A. Weber
Clinic for Nuclear Medicine, Technische Universität München, Munich, Germany

Jürgen Hennig and Michael Bock
Department of Radiology, Medical Physics, Medical Center University of Freiburg, Faculty of Medicine, University of Freiburg, Freiburg, Germany
German Cancer Consortium (DKTK), Partner Site Freiburg, Freiburg, Germany
German Cancer Research Center (DKFZ), Heidelberg, Germany

Wenzheng Sun
School of Information Science and Engineering, Shandong University, Qingdao, Shandong 266237, People's Republic of China
Department of Radiation Oncology, Duke University Cancer Center, Durham, NC 27710, USA

Mingyan Jiang
School of Information Science and Engineering, Shandong University, Qingdao, Shandong 266237, People's Republic of China

Jun Dang
Department of Oncology, The First Affiliate Hospital of Chongqing Medical University, Chongqing 400016, People's Republic of China

Panchun Chang
School of Electrical and Information Engineering, Qilu Institute of Technology, Jinan, Shandong 250200, People's Republic of China

Fang-Fang Yin
Department of Radiation Oncology, Duke University Cancer Center, Durham, NC 27710, USA

Liang Hong, Yun-xia Huang, Qing-yang Zhuang, Xue-qing Zhang, Li-rui Tang, Bu-hong Zheng, Jun-xin Wu and Jin-luan Li
Department of Radiation Oncology, Fujian Medical University Cancer Hospital, Fujian Cancer Hospital, Fuzhou 350014, China

Kai-xin Du and Xiao-yi Lin
Department of Radiation Oncology, Xiamen Humanity Hospital, Xiamen, China

Shao-li Cai
Biomedical Research Center of South China, Fujian Normal University, Fuzhou, China

Dennis J. Mohatt, Tianjun Ma, Naveed M. Islam and Harish K. Malhotra
Medical Physics Program, Jacobs School of Medicine and Biomedical Sciences, University at Buffalo, Buffalo, NY 14214-3005, USA
Department of Radiation Medicine, Roswell Park Cancer Institute, Buffalo, NY 14293, USA

Jorge Gomez and Anurag K. Singh
Department of Radiation Medicine, Roswell Park Cancer Institute, Buffalo, NY 14293, USA

David B. Wiant
Radiation Oncology, Cone Health Cancer Center, Greensboro, NC 27403, USA

Mark E Hwang, Paul J Black, Carl D Elliston, Brian A Wolthuis, Deborah R Smith, Cheng-Chia Wu and Israel Deutsch
Department of Radiation Oncology, Columbia University Medical Center, New York, New York 10032, USA

Sven Wenske
Department of Urology, Columbia University Medical Center, New York 10032, New York, USA

J. Krayenbuehl, M. Zamburlini, S. Tanadini-Lang and M. Guckenberger
Department of Radiation Oncology, University Hospital Zurich, Rämistrasse 100, CH-8091 Zurich, Switzerland

S. Ghandour and M. Pachoud
Department of Radiation Oncology, Hôpital Riviera-Chablais, Avenue de la Prairie 3, CH-1800 Vevey, Switzerland

J. Tol and W. F. A. R. Verbakel
Department of Radiotherapy, VU University Medical Center, De Boelelaan 1117, 1081, HV, Amsterdam, The Netherlands

Katharina Bell, Norbert Licht, Christian Rübe and Yvonne Dzierma
Department of Radiotherapy and Radiation Oncology, Saarland University Medical Centre, Kirrberger Str. Geb. 6.5/Saar, D-66421 Homburg, Germany

Halima Saadia Kidar and Hacene Azizi
Department of Physics, Ferhat Abbas Setif University, El Bez Compus, 19000 Setif, Algeria

Hanna Aula, Tanja Skyttä and Pirkko-Liisa Kellokumpu-Lehtinen
Faculty of Medicine and Life Sciences, University of Tampere, Tampere, Finland
Department of Oncology, Tampere University Hospital, Tampere, Finland

Suvi Tuohinen
Faculty of Medicine and Life Sciences, University of Tampere, Tampere, Finland
Heart Hospital, Tampere University Hospital, 33521 Tampere, Finland
Department of Cardiology, Heart and Lung Center, Helsinki University Hospital, Tampere 00029, Finland

Tiina Luukkaala
Research, Development and Innovation Center, Pirkanmaa Hospital District, Tampere, Finland
Health Sciences, Faculty of Social Sciences, University of Tampere, Tampere, Finland

Mari Hämäläinen and Eeva Moilanen
The Immunopharmacology Research Group, Faculty of Medicine and Life Sciences, University of Tampere and Tampere University Hospital, Tampere, Finland

Vesa Virtanen
Faculty of Medicine and Life Sciences, University of Tampere, 33014 Tampere, Finland
Heart Hospital, Tampere University Hospital, 33521 Tampere, Finland

Pekka Raatikainen
Department of Cardiology, Heart and Lung Center, Helsinki University Hospital, Tampere 00029, Finland

Julia Dreyer, Michael Bremer and Christoph Henkenberens
Department of Radiotherapy and Special Oncology, Medical School Hannover, Carl-Neuberg-Str. 1, 30625 Hannover, Germany

Tanja Sprave, Ingmar Schlampp, Rami Ateyah El Shafie, Jürgen Debus and Harald Rief
University Hospital of Heidelberg, Department of Radiation Oncology, Im Neuenheimer Feld 400, 69120 Heidelberg, Germany
Heidelberg Institute of Radiation Oncology (HIRO), Im Neuenheimer Feld 280, 69120 Heidelberg, Germany

Vivek Verma
Department of Radiation Oncology, Allegheny General Hospital, Pittsburgh, PA, USA

Robert Förster
University Hospital of Heidelberg, Department of Radiation Oncology, Im Neuenheimer Feld 400, 69120 Heidelberg, Germany
Heidelberg Institute of Radiation Oncology (HIRO), Im Neuenheimer Feld 280, 69120 Heidelberg, Germany
University Hospital Zurich, Department of Radiation Oncology, Raemistrasse 100, 8091 Zurich, Switzerland

Katharina Hees and Thomas Bruckner
Department of Radiation Oncology, Allegheny General Hospital, Pittsburgh, PA, USA
University Hospital of Heidelberg, Department of Medical Biometry, Im Neuenheimer Feld 305, 69120 Heidelberg, Germany

Tilman Bostel and Thomas Welzel
University Hospital of Heidelberg, Department of Radiation Oncology, Im Neuenheimer Feld 400, 69120 Heidelberg, Germany

Nils Henrik Nicolay
University Hospital of Heidelberg, Department of Radiation Oncology, Im Neuenheimer Feld 400, 69120 Heidelberg, Germany

Heidelberg Institute of Radiation Oncology (HIRO), Im Neuenheimer Feld 280, 69120 Heidelberg, Germany University Hospital of Freiburg, Department of Radiation Oncology, Robert-Koch-Strasse 3, 79106 Freiburg, Germany

Mélanie Guilhen, Christophe Hennequin, Idir Ouzaid, Ingrid Fumagalli, Valentine Martin, Sophie Guillerm, Pierre Mongiat-Artus, Vincent Ravery, François Desgrandchamps and Laurent Quéro
Radiation Oncology Department, Saint Louis Hospital, 1, avenue Claude Vellefaux, 75010 Paris, France

J. Ganem, R. Modzelewski, S. Hapdey and P. Vera
Nuclear Medicine Department, Henri Becquerel Cancer Centre and Rouen University Hospital, Rouen, France QuantIF-LITIS (EA [Equipe d'Accueil] 4108-FR CNRS [Fédération de Recherche-Centre National pour la Recherche Scientifique] 3638), Faculty of Medicine, University of Rouen, Rouen, France

S. Thureau and I. Gardin
Nuclear Medicine Department, Henri Becquerel Cancer Centre and Rouen University Hospital, Rouen, France QuantIF-LITIS (EA [Equipe d'Accueil] 4108-FR CNRS [Fédération de Recherche-Centre National pour la Recherche Scientifique] 3638), Faculty of Medicine, University of Rouen, Rouen, France Department of Radiotherapy and Medical Physics, Henri Becquerel Cancer Centre and Rouen University Hospital, Rouen, France

Beat Bojaxhiu
Department of Radiation Oncology, Inselspital, Bern University Hospital and University of Bern, Freiburgstrasse, 3010 Bern, Switzerland Center for Proton Therapy, Paul Scherrer Institute, Villigen, Switzerland

Arnoud J. Templeton
Department of Medical Oncology, St. Claraspital Basel and Faculty of Medicine, University of Basel, Basel, Switzerland Center for Proton Therapy, Paul Scherrer Institute, Villigen, Switzerland

Olgun Elicin, Mohamed Shelan, Daniel M. Aebersold and Alan Dal Pra
Department of Radiation Oncology, Inselspital, Bern University Hospital and University of Bern, Freiburgstrasse, 3010 Bern, Switzerland

Kathrin Zaugg
Department of Radiation Oncology, Stadtspital Triemli, Zürich, Switzerland

Roland Giger
Department of Otorhinolaryngology, Head and Neck Surgery, Inselspital, Bern University Hospital, Basel, Switzerland

Marc Walser
Center for Proton Therapy, Paul Scherrer Institute, Villigen, Switzerland

Yongsook C. Lee, Shih-Chi Lin and Yongbok Kim
Department of Radiation Oncology, The University of Arizona, 3838 N Campbell Avenue, Building #2, Tucson, AZ 85719, USA

Index